Andrew D.A. Maidment   Predrag R. Bakic
Sara Gavenonis (Eds.)

Breast Imaging

11th International Workshop, IWDM 2012
Philadelphia, PA, USA, July 8-11, 2012
Proceedings

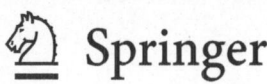 Springer

Volume Editors

Andrew D.A. Maidment
Predrag R. Bakic
Sara Gavenonis
University of Pennsylvania, Department of Radiology
3400 Spruce Street, 1 Silverstein Building, Philadelphia, PA 19014, USA
E-mail: {andrew.maidment, predrag.bakic, sara.gavenonis}@uphs.upenn.edu

ISSN 0302-9743   e-ISSN 1611-3349
ISBN 978-3-642-31270-0   e-ISBN 978-3-642-31271-7
DOI 10.1007/978-3-642-31271-7
Springer Heidelberg Dordrecht London New York

Library of Congress Control Number: 2012939850

CR Subject Classification (1998): I.4.3, I.4.6-7, I.4.9-10, I.4, J.3, I.6.3, I.5

LNCS Sublibrary: SL 6 – Image Processing, Computer Vision, Pattern Recognition,
and Graphics

Typesetting: Camera-ready by author, data conversion by Scientific Publishing Services, Chennai, India

Printed on acid-free paper

Springer is part of Springer Science+Business Media (www.springer.com)

Lecture Notes in Computer Science 7361

Commenced Publication in 1973
Founding and Former Series Editors:
Gerhard Goos, Juris Hartmanis, and Jan van Leeuwen

Preface

This volume of Springer's Lecture Notes in Computer Science presents the scientific proceedings of the 11th International Workshop on Breast Imaging (IWDM 2012), which was held July 8–11, 2012 in Philadelphia, Pennsylvania, USA. Formerly called the International Workshop on Digital Mammography, the new name recognizes the move in breast imaging towards more recent emerging technologies and multimodality imaging solutions. The IWDM meetings bring together a diverse group of researchers, clinicians and representatives of industry, who are jointly committed to developing technology for early detection and subsequent patient management of breast cancer. The conference series was initiated at a 1993 meeting of the SPIE in San Jose, with subsequent meetings hosted every two years by researchers around the world. Previous meetings have been held in York (1994), Chicago (1996), Nijmegen (1998), Toronto (2000), Bremen (2002), Durham (2004), Manchester (2006), Tucson (2008) and Girona (2010).

The IWDM 2012 was designed as a platform to present the latest technological developments and clinical experiences of novel breast imaging technologies, including digital mammography, tomosynthesis, CT, MR, ultrasound, optical and molecular imaging. Additional topics include multimodality imaging, image processing and visualization, and computer-aided imaging. A total of 120 papers were submitted to the conference from research groups in 24 countries. Each four-page extended abstract was reviewed in a fully-blinded process by at least two members of the Scientific Program Committee, which led to the final selection of 42 oral presentations and 58 poster presentations. The final 8-page papers were reviewed by the volume editors. Galley proofs were approved by the corresponding author(s) of each paper.

The proffered presentations were organized into 10 sequential oral sessions and 2 poster sessions during the two and a half day conference. The session titles give insight into the changes that have occurred in breast imaging in the 19 years since the first Digital Mammography conference in San Jose. Today digital mammography is the clinical standard of care. As a result, this year only one session was devoted to the technology of digital mammography, with a primary emphasis on image quality and radiation dose. Rather, one sees that digital mammography is the enabling technology for a number of new applications, including image-based breast cancer risk assessment. Thus, substantial work was presented on image-based measures of breast cancer risk, and other quantitative measures used in the detection, diagnosis, treatment and prevention of breast cancer.

A number of new and adjunctive technologies were also discussed in the workshop. In particular, digital breast tomosynthesis was heavily represented, both in papers covering system development and clinical application. Related topics in image processing, computer-aided diagnosis and quantitative imaging were also presented. Other new technologies including breast computed tomography and breast molecular imaging, and advances in adjunctive technologies including magnetic resonance imaging and ultrasound were well represented.

The invited speakers were chosen to illuminate the trends in breast imaging and stimulate future developments. In a trend spanning the last four IWDM meetings, tomosynthesis was again discussed in an invited lecture. This year, Emily F. Conant (University of Pennsylvania, USA) and Etta D. Pisano (Medical University of South Carolina, USA) presented "Tomosynthesis: Clinical Trials and Clinical Implementation". Thus, in a 6 year period, we have gone from papers covering the fundamentals of the technology and positing the role for tomosynthesis to papers discussing the successes of the technology.

John M. Lewin (Rose Breast Center, USA) presented a talk entitled "Contrast-enhanced Digital Mammography and Tomosynthesis – Review and Update". Contrast-enhanced breast radiography has the potential to combine the morphologic and functional signs of breast cancer. David A. Mankoff (University of Pennsylvania, USA) discussed "Molecular Imaging of the Breast: Clinical and Biological Considerations" in a complementary paper outlining numerous other applications of quantitative breast imaging. Katrina Armstrong (University of Pennsylvania, USA) provided a thought-provoking talk entitled "Moving to an Individualized Paradigm for Breast Cancer Screening and Prevention: Opportunities and Challenges". In this presentation, the role of imaging was reviewed in light of the larger clinical context of breast cancer. Finally, Martin J. Yaffe and Gina Clarke (University of Toronto, Canada) provided an overview of "Quantitative Imaging Techniques in Pathology for Management of Breast Cancer". In this presentation, they demonstrated how the role of imaging continues to expand and challenge researchers.

Finally, a meeting as large and successful as the IWDM 2012 is only possible through the tireless work of many people. The members of the Scientific Program Committee did an outstanding job in reviewing the papers and providing detailed critiques to the authors as part of the peer-review process. The local arrangements for the conference were skillfully handled by Lori Ehrich and Angela Scott, who are normally responsible for the continuing education program for the Department of Radiology at the University of Pennsylvania. Technical support of the meeting was provided by Joseph Chui of the Physics Section. Joe has worked hard to keep the various servers running and databases communicating together. Special thanks need to go to Roshan Karunamuni and Raymond Acciavatti who expended huge effort to put the 100 individual submissions into a single cohesive book. Finally, thanks go to Emily Conant and Mitch Schnall for helping to prepare the proposal for this meeting two years ago, and to Predrag Bakic and Sara Gavenonis for making this meeting a reality.

July 2012   Andrew D.A. Maidment

Organization

The 11th International Workshop on Breast Imaging (IWDM 2012) was organized by the Physics and Breast Imaging Sections of the Department of Radiology of the University of Pennsylvania. The organizers would like to acknowledge the following individuals for their assistance and hard work in making this workshop possible.

Scientific Program Committee

Susan M. Astley	University of Manchester, UK
Predrag R. Bakic	University of Pennsylvania, USA
Hiroshi Fujita	Gifu University, Japan
Sara Gavenonis	University of Pennsylvania, USA
Maryellen L. Giger	University of Chicago, USA
Nico Karssemeijer	University of Nijmegen, The Netherlands
Elizabeth A. Krupinski	University of Arizona, USA
Andrew D.A. Maidment	University of Pennsylvania, USA
Robert Marti	University of Girona, Spain
Joan Marti	University of Girona, Spain
Etta D. Pisano	Medical University of South Carolina, USA
Martin J. Yaffe	University of Toronto, Canada
Reyer Zwiggelaar	Aberystwyth University, UK

Local Organizing Committee

Raymond J. Acciavatti
Joseph H. Chui
Emily F. Conant
Lori Ehrich
Roshan Karunamuni
Mitchell Schnall
Angela Scott
Glenda Wortham

Table of Contents

Session 3: Tomosynthesis System Design

Poster Session 1

Session 4: Tomosynthesis - Image Quality and Dose

Session 5: Clinical Tomosynthesis

Session 6: Functional Breast Imaging

Session 7: Breast CT

Poster Session 2

Session 8: Computer-Aided Diagnosis and Image Processing

Session 9: Tomosynthesis Reconstruction

Session 10: Breast Density

Pre-clinical Evaluation of Tumour Angiogenesis with Contrast-Enhanced Breast Tomosynthesis

Melissa L. Hill[1,2], Kela Liu[1], James G. Mainprize[1], Ronald B. Levitin[1],
Rushin Shojaii[1,2], and Martin J. Yaffe[1,2]

[1] Sunnybrook Research Institute, Toronto, Canada
melissa.hill@sri.utoronto.ca
[2] Department of Medical Biophysics, University of Toronto, Toronto, Canada

Abstract. Contrast-enhanced digital breast tomosynthesis (CE DBT) has been proposed to image the effects of tumour angiogenesis. In this work we evaluate the relationship between CE DBT image signal and histopathology in an animal tumour model to provide evidence for the underlying basis for signal enhancement. A VX2 carcinoma was induced in the hind leg of 8 rabbits and grown for up to 3 weeks. Projection images from a 60 s contrast-enhanced CT acquisition were used to reconstruct CE DBT volumes. Fiducial markers implanted in the tumour provided a means for registration between images and stained whole-mount sections. The relationship between CE DBT image signal and angiogenesis marker expression was determined. A correlation was found between CE DBT image signal and dextran extravasation, which strengthened during washout, while no relationship was observed with CD31 staining. These results suggest that for clinical CE DBT, washout phase imaging will provide information on vascular permeability.

Keywords: Tomosynthesis, contrast-enhanced, angiogenesis, VX2, CD31, dextran.

1   Introduction

Formation of new blood vessels within tumours is essential for the growth and spread of cancer [1]. The combination of mammography and clinical iodinated contrast agents in contrast-enhanced digital mammography (CEDM) has been demonstrated to reveal vascular information similar to that provided by breast MRI, and recent approvals of a system for clinical use have been granted in the US, Canada and Europe. Clinical pilot studies of these systems have identified that the 2D nature of mammography may limit tumour detection sensitivity due to overlap of normal tissue signal that may mask small and/or weakly enhancing lesions in CEDM [2]. Contrast-enhanced digital breast tomosynthesis (CE DBT) offers the potential to overcome this limitation via 3D imaging. To date, CE DBT development has focused on image quality optimization, which is affected by a large parameter space including the acquisition geometry, imaging technique factors, the choice of reconstruction algorithm, and the subject breast characteristics [3–5]. As this modality moves toward the clinic it is

A.D.A. Maidment, P.R. Bakic, and S. Gavenonis (Eds.): IWDM 2012, LNCS 7361, pp. 1–8, 2012.

important to understand its diagnostic potential for appropriate medical application. As a first step towards an understanding of the pathology information potentially available from CE DBT images we aim to demonstrate the relationship between CE DBT image signal and histology markers for tumour angiogenesis. To our knowledge this is the first study of its kind for CE DBT. Similar work done in a CEDM clinical pilot study resulted in a poor correlation between imaging parameters and microvessel density [6]. The authors hypothesized that this finding could be attributed to the summation of tumour and normal tissue signals in CEDM, and that the signal is also related to functional parameters such as vessel permeability which were not captured in their study [6]. In this work we test both hypotheses with CE DBT in a rabbit tumour model.

2   Methods

2.1   Experimental Protocol

Under a protocol approved by the University Health Network Animal Care Committee, eight New Zealand White rabbits were inoculated with cell suspensions of VX2 carcinoma in the left hind leg. Although VX2 carcinoma does not strictly model the characteristics of breast cancers, this animal model allowed for tight control of experimental conditions and permitted registration between histopathology and *in vivo* images. This animal model was chosen because a vascularized tumour will grow to roughly the size of a small breast cancer (~1 cm) within 2 to 3 weeks and the leg can be easily immobilized to prevent motion artifact. To provide a range of tumour sizes and degrees of angiogenesis, four of the rabbits were imaged at 2 weeks and four at 3 weeks after inoculation. Immediately following imaging, the rabbits were sacrificed and tumours were excised for histology. A cone-beam CT system (eXplore Locus Ultra, GE Healthcare) with similar detector and geometry characteristics to DBT systems was used for imaging [7]. Full 3D datasets (416 projections) were acquired at 70 kVp, 50 mA with a W/Cu anode/filter combination at one second intervals for a one minute period in a perfusion protocol. Anesthetized tumour-bearing rabbits were injected intravenously with a single bolus of 1.5 ml/kg clinical iodinated contrast agent (Visipaque 270) at the onset of x-ray exposure. Post-sacrifice, 26 gauge catheters visible on both on x-ray and histology were implanted directly into the tumour as fiducial markers. The rabbit carcass with the tumour intact, and then the excised tumour embedded in agar were each imaged with CT to allow for registration between imaging and histology. About 20 minutes prior to sacrifice, 25 mg of 70 kDa biotinylated dextran (Invitrogen) was administered intravenously dissolved in 1 mL of saline solution for validation of vascular permeability. Immediately before sacrifice a second dose of contrast agent was administered for tumour visualization on post-sacrifice CT. Whole-mount sections of the tumour tissue and a control sample of the normal muscle from the contralateral leg were made for histopathological analysis. Serial sections were stained with haematoxylin and eosin (H&E) to identify tumour morphology, anti-CD31 (DAKO, clone JC70A) was used to detect vascular endothelium, and streptavidin-HRP (Vector Lab. Inc., Cat# SA-5004) was used to reveal biotinylated dextran extravasation.

2.2   Tomosynthesis Reconstruction

Projection images for DBT reconstruction with a SART algorithm were sampled post-acquisition as shown in Fig. 1. Fifteen projection images were sampled with regular spacing over a 42° angular extent such that the 0° projection aligned with the fiducial markers in the tumour, as determined using the post-sacrifice CT images (Fig. 1b).

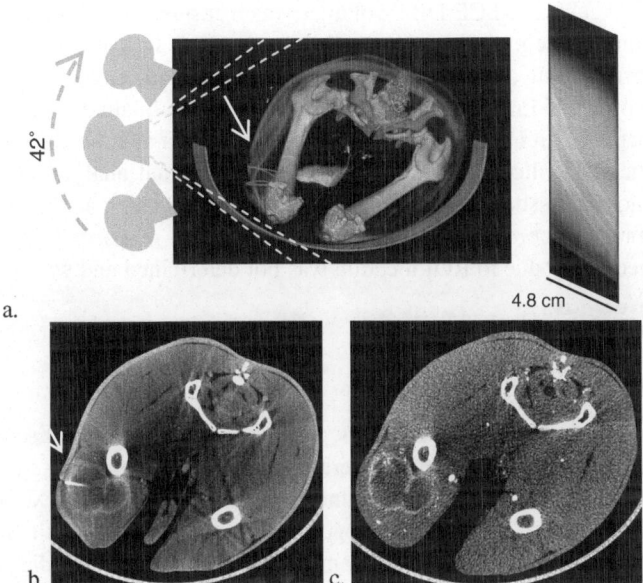

Fig. 1. Schematic of tomosynthesis image sampling from CT data. a) A surface rendering of post-sacrifice CT data illustrates the geometry of projection image sampling as determined from the fiducial marker (arrow) position; b) post-sacrifice CT axial slice; and c) perfusion CT axial slice. DBT reconstructions are generated from the perfusion scan data.

DBT volumes were reconstructed from the raw images acquired in the CT perfusion scans (Fig. 1c) with 0.2×0.2×1 mm voxels. To simulate radiation exposure at levels closer to a clinical DBT exam, for each projection angle, images acquired at the given angle from 7 individual time points were averaged together. For each perfusion scan, optically stimulated luminescent (OSL) chips (Landauer Inc.) were fixed to the inner thigh of the rabbit hind leg to monitor the dose to the animal. The OSL exposure readings were validated using measurements performed free in air and at the centre of a 10 cm diameter PMMA cylindrical phantom with an NRC calibrated farmer type ionization chamber (NE 2571) and electrometer (Fluke 35040). It was confirmed that the equivalent dose to water at the rabbit inner thigh was 0.058 ± 0.003 mGy/mAs, or 0.007 mGy per projection image. For one 15 projection image DBT dataset when averaging over 7 s is performed, the equivalent dose to water is about 0.73 mGy. In this study we evaluate a 5 time-point temporal subtraction CE DBT exam. The first post-contrast time point was chosen as 15 s, the time of peak arterial contrast-enhancement as determined from the signal in the left femoral artery in the perfusion CT dataset. Subsequent post-contrast volumes were reconstructed at 30, 45, and 55 s.

2.3   CE DBT Image Analysis

Analysis is performed on reconstructed DBT volumes subtracted between the first time point (4 s), where no contrast agent is present, and subsequent time points. The image signal in subtracted CE DBT volumes was measured as the mean voxel intensity within manually segmented regions of interest (ROI) in central slices through tumour and normal tissue. One ROI was placed in the tumour and another was selected within the corresponding muscle in the normal leg. A qualitative registration was performed between an H&E stained tumour tissue section and the CE DBT volume to determine the DBT slice number to use for tumour signal analysis. The DBT slice number for normal tissue ROI placement was determined using a constant offset from the right femur to approximate the location of excision of normal tissue. The measurement uncertainty due to ROI location was not determined and will be evaluated in future work.

2.4   Histological Analysis

Whole-mount specimen digitization was performed using a TISSUEscope^{TM} (Huron Technologies International), scanner operated in brightfield mode at 1 μm resolution. In this work serial sections were immunostained for CD31 and dextran with DAB (*3,3'*-diaminobenzidine) as the chromogen and counterstained with haemotoxylin. Tumour and normal tissue were each manually segmented from the digitized sections for quantification of DAB staining. To separate the stains, colour deconvolution [8] was applied to each segmented portion of the digitized slides using ImageJ software. The RGB values of haematoxylin and DAB for deconvolution were calibrated using single-stained slides, with a third colour vector defined as orthogonal to the other two. Each DAB-deconvolved section was transformed to grayscale and the staining was scored with an averaged threshold measure (ATM), which is a validated metric that quantifies the fractional area stained [9].

2.5   Statistical Analysis

To test for correlations between the CE DBT image signal and immunohistochemistry (IHC) staining the Pearson's correlation coefficient, r, was calculated. The relationship between the signal difference (SD) of tumour and normal tissue in CE DBT and the difference in ATM score in tumour and normal tissue was determined for each of CD31 and dextran immunostained tissue sections. Correlation between CD31 and dextran staining was also tested. Statistical significance was determined using the Student's t-test for a significance level of 0.05.

3 Results

All eight VX2 inoculations successfully resulted in a primary tumour in the hind leg. The average diameter as measured on H&E histology sections was 1.8 ± 0.4 cm after 2 weeks of growth and 2.8 ± 1.0 cm after 3 weeks growth. A representative VX2 tumour image dataset is presented in Fig. 2 in the DBT orientation (i.e. Fig. 1). A 0.2 mm thick CT slice is shown in Fig. 2a at the time of peak arterial contrast-enhancement. A 1 mm thick CE DBT slice from reconstructions subtracted between 15 s and 4 s time points is shown in Fig. 2b. The signal-vs-time curve in Fig. 2c plots mean CE DBT intensities in an ROI placed in the tumour and in the normal muscle. For comparison, the femoral artery CT signal is shown on the right y-axis to demonstrate the time-course of the intravascular contrast agent. In Fig. 2d, blue (haematoxylin) stain identifies nuclei and pink (eosin) dyes the cytoplasm. In Fig. 2e and 2f markers of angiogenesis, CD31 and 70 kDa dextran, are stained brown (DAB).

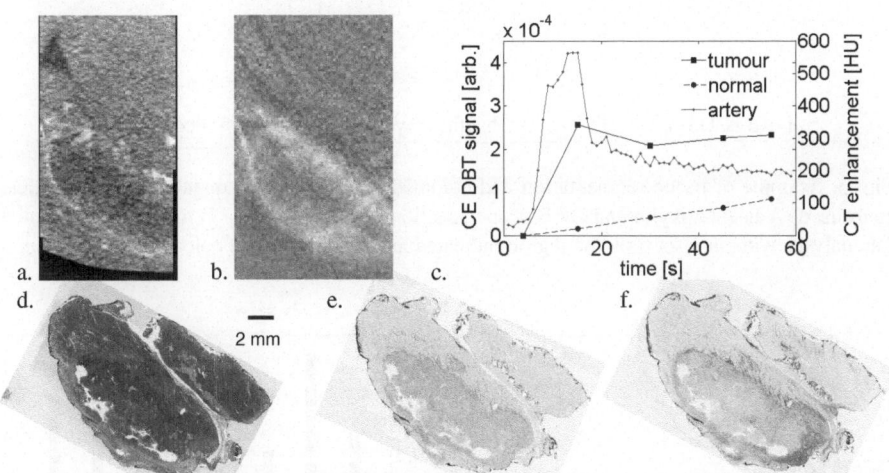

Fig. 2. Tumour at 3 weeks growth sliced perpendicular to the fiducials (Fig. 1), reconstructed in a) CT; and b) CE DBT. c) The CE DBT signal as a function of time in the tumour as compared to normal muscle and the CT signal in the femoral artery (right y-axis). Histology sections: d) H&E, e) CD31; and f) dextran each stained with DAB (brown).

Fig. 3 presents an example of colour deconvolution applied to a VX2 tumour. No pixels should be stained with the "third colour" because this indicates colour that is not included in DAB or haematoxylin. However, due to tissue processing and digitization artifacts and the fact that DAB is a light scatterer and not an absorber, some pixels are included in the third colour. In this example the fractional areas stained are 0.15, 0.15 and 0.03 for DAB, haematoxylin and the third colour respectively. This amount of the third colour is representative of the deconvolution performance observed for all sections evaluated in this study and is considered to be negligible.

The measurements of fractional area of DAB staining for CD31 and dextran in tumour and normal tissue are summarized in Fig. 4. The results are grouped so that rabbits numbered 1 to 4 have 2 weeks of tumour growth and rabbits 5 through 8 have 3 weeks of VX2 growth. Note that rabbit 4 did not receive a dextran injection.

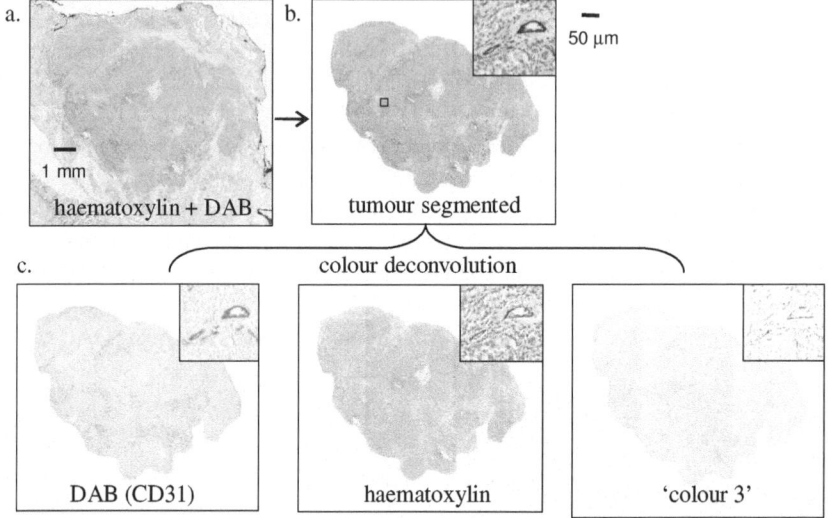

Fig. 3. Example of tissue segmentation and colour deconvolution for quantitative histological analysis. a) A haematoxylin and DAB stained section; b) tumour tissue is manually segmented for analysis, with an inset from the region indicated; and c) the result of colour deconvolution.

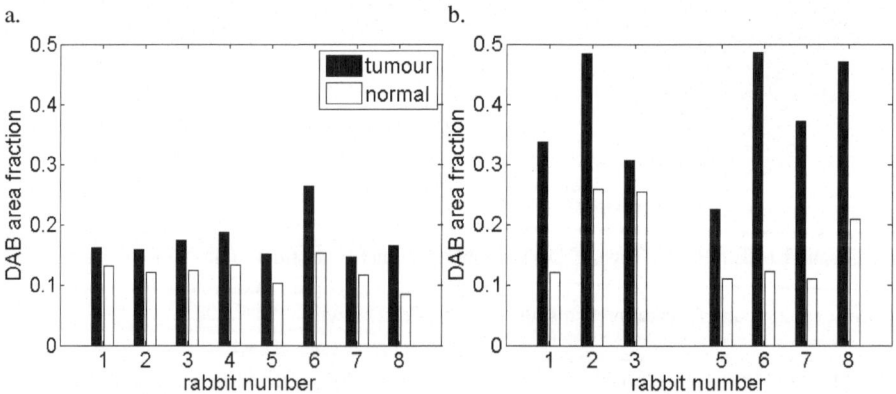

Fig. 4. Fractional area of DAB stained for a) CD31 and b) dextran in tumour and normal tissue

In Table 1 the results of correlation studies between the CE DBT signal difference at each reconstruction time point, and the fractional area (ATM score) stained with DAB in CD31 and dextran IHC sections. For each of the CE DBT and histology parameters, the difference between the tumour and normal tissue quantities are found, which largely eliminates the effect of any physiological differences between rabbits or changes in tissue processing conditions. The Pearson's correlation coefficient between CD31 and dextran area of staining was 0.39, with a p-value of 0.38.

Table 1. Pearson's Correlation coefficient, r, and corresponding p-value for the comparison of CE DBT signal difference (SD) and the difference in average threshold measurement (ATM) score in tumour and normal tissue for CD31 and dextran immunostained tissue sections

CE DBT SD $(S_{tumour} - S_{normal})$ at given time [s]	CD31 ATM score difference $(ATM_{tumour} - ATM_{normal})$		Dextran ATM score difference $(ATM_{tumour} - ATM_{normal})$	
	r	p	r	p
15	-.14	.74	.59	.16
30	.02	.96	.82	.02
45	.08	.85	.90	.006
55	.10	.81	.93	.003

4   Discussion

In this work we take the first step towards a validation of the source of the image signal in CE DBT. A VX2 tumour in rabbits provides a model for the study of the relationship between tumour angiogenesis and CE DBT image signal in a dynamic system. The use of a cone-beam CT permits rapid image acquisition to capture the contrast agent, while maintaining a similar geometry to existing DBT systems.

Angiogenesis was induced in all rabbits by the VX2 inoculation. Analysis of histology marker expression demonstrated reasonably consistent CD31 fractional area of staining across all rabbits. Neither CD31 expression, nor dextran extravasation had a clear association with the tumour size.

A statistically significant correlation between dextran staining area and the CE DBT signal difference was found from 30 s onwards, and the strength of the correlation increased with time. We know from the CT data, as shown in Fig 2c, that from 15 s onwards the arterial concentration of the contrast agent was decreasing, so the tumour tissue was in a washout phase when the dextran-CE DBT signal relationship became significant. Due to the size of dextran molecules chosen for use in this work, they are unlikely to extravasate from healthy endothelium, so the observation of dextran extravasation is a direct indication of increased vessel permeability. Thus, the results of this work show that the magnitude of CE DBT image signal in the washout phase is directly related to vascular permeability and interrogates the content of the extravascular extracellular space.

No relationship was observed between CE DBT signal and the fraction of CD31-stained area. Given that CE DBT has superior out-of-plane signal suppression compared with CEDM, it is unlikely that signal superposition is responsible for the lack of correlation in these parameters. Our finding that the CD31 and dextran fractional areas stained are not correlated suggests that there may be variability in vascular permeability and that some of the angiogenic microvessels may not be functional. Future work will include spatial correlation of dextran and CD31 staining to check for nonfunctional endothelium and immunostaining for vascular endothelial growth factor (VEGF), which is known to increase vascular permeability.

We believe this paper presents the first direct evidence of the relationship between vascular permeability at the cellular level and image signal in contrast-enhanced breast imaging. These results suggest that for clinical implementation of CE DBT, acquisition of one or more images during contrast agent washout could have diagnostic value since the image signal contains vessel permeability information in this phase.

Although the results of this work are very encouraging, the dependence of the CE DBT signal on blood flow and vascular volume is still not clear. Future work will include the evaluation of additional CE DBT image parameters such as enhancement and washout gradients and area under the curve, which may help tease out the relationship with other characteristics of angiogenesis. Furthermore, alternative IHC metrics should be evaluated, including microvessel density, especially for comparison with the literature, and an assessment of marker spatial distribution to quantify IHC-CE DBT correspondence such as between the dextran staining seen in Fig. 2f and the CE DBT rim enhancement in Fig. 2b. Finally, only a small tissue segment was evaluated in both histology and CE DBT. In future work, multiple sections of tissue will be evaluated on both histology and CE DBT to investigate tumour heterogeneity.

Acknowledgements. This project is funded by the Canadian Breast Cancer Foundation - Ontario Region and the Ontario Institute for Cancer Research. We thank Margarete Akens for her preparation of tumour cell suspensions and patient teaching, Sunmo Kim for his experimental support and Anguo Zhong for his vigilant animal care.

References

1. Folkman, J.: Incipient Angiogenesis. J. Natl. Cancer Inst. 92, 94–95 (2000)
2. Jong, R.A., Yaffe, M.J., Skarpathiotakis, M., Shumak, R.S., Danjoux, N.M., Gunesekara, A.: Contrast-enhanced digital mammography: initial clinical experience. Radiology 228, 842–850 (2003)
3. Carton, A.-K., Li, J., Chen, S., Conant, E., Maidment, A.D.A.: Optimization of Contrast-Enhanced Digital Breast Tomosynthesis. In: Astley, S.M., Brady, M., Rose, C., Zwiggelaar, R. (eds.) IWDM 2006. LNCS, vol. 4046, pp. 183–189. Springer, Heidelberg (2006)
4. Puong, S., Patoureaux, F., Iordache, R., Bouchevreau, X., Muller, S.: Dual-energy contrast enhanced digital breast tomosynthesis: concept, method, and evaluation on phantoms. In: Proc. SPIE, vol. 6510, p. 65100U (2007)
5. Samei, E., Saunders, R.S.: Dual-energy contrast-enhanced breast tomosynthesis: optimization of beam quality for dose and image quality. Phys. Med. Biol. 56, 6359–6378 (2011)
6. Dromain, C., Balleyguier, C., Muller, S., Mathieu, M.-C., Rochard, F., Opolon, F., Sigal, R.: Evaluation of tumor angiogenesis of breast carcinoma using contrast-enhanced digital mammography. Am. J. Roentgenol. 187, 528–537 (2006)
7. Du, L.Y., Lee, T.-Y., Holdsworth, D.W.: Image quality assessment of a pre-clinical flat-panel volumetric micro-CT scanner. In: Proc. SPIE, vol. 6142, p. 614216 (2006)
8. Ruifrok, A.C., Johnston, D.A.: Quantification of histochemical staining by color deconvolution. Anal. Quant. Cytol. Histol. 23, 291–299 (2001)
9. Choudhury, K.R., Yagle, K.J., Swanson, P.E., Krohn, K.A., Rajendran, J.G.: A Robust Automated Measure of Average Antibody Staining in Immunohistochemistry Images. J. Histochem. Cytochem. 58, 95–107 (2009)

The Effect of Amorphous Selenium Thickness on Imaging Performance of Contrast Enhanced Digital Breast Tomosynthesis

Yue-Houng Hu, David A. Scaduto, and Wei Zhao

Department of Radiology, State University of New York at Stony Brook,
L-4 120 Health Sciences Center, Stony Brook, New York, 11793-8460
yuehoung.hu@gmail.com, david.scaduto@stonybrook.edu,
wei.zhao@stonybrookmedicine.edu

Abstract. Digital breast tomosynthesis (DBT) and contrast enhancement (CE) for both DBT (CEDBT) and planar mammography (CEDM) are being investigated to increase conspicuity of malignant lesions. To image above the k-edge of iodine (33 keV), CEDBT requires x-ray energies higher than those of typical mammograms (~28 kVp). Increasing the thickness of the detector's amorphous selenium (a-Se) layer improves x-ray absorption and detective quantum efficiency (DQE), particularly at higher energies. For DBT, where systems are often designed with partially isocentric geometries, thicker a-Se layers may result in degradation of the modulation transfer function (MTF) for oblique views. We employed a cascaded linear system model to analyze the effect of oblique entry on MTF. Also, the model was experimentally validated using 200 and 300 μm a-Se flat panel imagers. Finally, we use an ideal-observer SNR model for projection and DBT imaging to optimize a-Se layer thickness for detectability of iodinated objects.

Keywords: digital breast tomosynthesis, contrast enhancement, amorphous selenium, cascaded linear system model, MTF, ideal observer signal to noise ratio.

1   Introduction

Detection of lesions in screening mammography suffers from the obscuring effect of projecting three-dimensional (3D) morphology onto a two-dimensional (2D) image. Digital breast tomosynthesis (DBT) has been the subject of much recent work and has been proposed as a method of removal of overlapping tissue through 3D tissue discrimination. DBT consists of the acquisition of a limited number of projection views over a limited angular range (<45°), from which a 3D image volume may be reconstructed and viewed as thin image slices (1 mm) parallel to the detector plane. Further, contrast enhancement (CE) for both planar mammography and 3D techniques (i.e. DBT and breast CT) has also been proposed as a method to increase lesion conspicuity by a) imaging the increased uptake of blood (through the use of contrast agents such as iodine) resulting from angiogenesis of malignant lesions; and by b) removal of background tissue through image subtraction using methods such as dual

A.D.A. Maidment, P.R. Bakic, and S. Gavenonis (Eds.): IWDM 2012, LNCS 7361, pp. 9–16, 2012.

energy (DE) subtraction and temporal subtraction (TS).[1-4] Both DE and TS involve imaging at tube energies well above the k-edge of iodine (33 keV) and above those of standard screening mammography (28 kVp) to increase the conspicuity of contrast uptake with respect to breast tissue. Increasing the thickness of the amorphous selenium (a-Se) layer will result in an increase in x-ray absorption, measured by the quantum detective efficiency (QDE), and detective quantum efficiency (DQE), particularly at higher energies. However, increasing a-Se thickness (d_{Se}) also leads to degradation of the modulation transfer function (MTF) for oblique views.[5] Using experimental methods, we determined the extent of the effect and use the results to validate theoretical predictions from a cascaded linear system model. The model was then used to determine the overall effects of a-Se layer thickness on object detectability in contrast enhanced digital mammography (CEDM) and contrast enhanced digital breast tomosynthesis (CEDBT).

2   Materials and Methods

Both CEDBT techniques (TS and DE subtraction) require the use of x-ray energies above the k-edge of iodine (33 keV), which is best achieved at the highest kVp (49 kVp) available in a mammography system.[6] Since this is much higher than those used in standard DBT (e.g. <32 kVp), a thicker x-ray detection layer, i.e. a-Se in direct conversion flat panel imagers (FPI), may be beneficial. Shown in Fig. 1(a) is a plot of the QDE as a function of d_{Se} for low energy (LE: 28 kVp W/Rh) and high energy (HE: 49 kVp W/Ti) views of a DE study. The benefit of increased a-Se layer thickness is clearly seen for HE imaging. However, it needs to be considered against other factors in DBT. Currently, most DBT systems employ a partially isocentric geometry, where the tube travels in an arc above a stationary detector. This geometry exacerbates image blur due to oblique entry of x-rays, particularly at higher angle projections. Fig. 1(b) is a schematic illustration of the lateral spread of energy absorption in the detector, which increases with angle of obliquity, x-ray energy, and d_{Se}.[5]

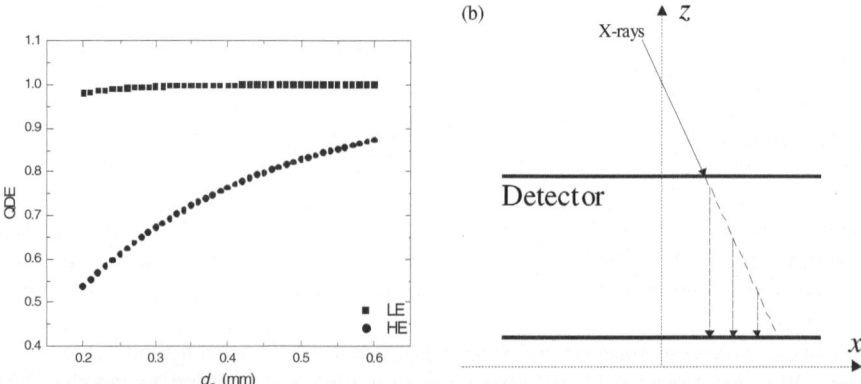

Fig. 1. A theoretical calculation of the improvement in QDE by increasing d_{Se} (a) as well as a schematic of the blurring effect of x-rays entering the detector at oblique angles (b)

2.1   Experimental Measurements of Detector Imaging Performance

A prototype Siemens Mammomat Inspiration unit[1], modified for CEDBT applications, was used for all experimental measurements. The system acquires 25 views over a nominal angular range of 45° with continuous tube motion with the most oblique view acquired at a tube angle of nominally 22°. The x-ray tube energy was enabled up to 49 kVp and three x-ray filters were employed including 0.050 mm rhodium (Rh) for LE acquisitions and 0.300 mm copper (Cu) or 1.000 mm titanium (Ti) for use on HE acquisitions. Measurements were acquired using either of two a-Se FPI, each with 85 μm pixel size. The FPI differed in d_{Se}, one with the standard d_{Se}= 200 μm and the other with d_{Se} increased to 300 μm.

LE and HE spectra were investigated employing gantry modes with stationary and moving x-ray tube (DBT). The MTF and noise power spectrum (NPS) were measured from the resulting projection images according to methods outlined previously.[7, 8] To calculate MTF, a 200 μm thick tungsten (W) edge was placed directly atop the detector cover (1.7 cm above the a-Se surface).

2.2   Cascaded Linear System Model

A cascaded linear system model for DBT was developed, validated, and modified for CE applications.[6, 9] Fig. 2 exhibits a simple flow chart for the model, which begins with a model of the projection domain imaging performance for a-Se detectors, which includes modulation transfer function (MTF) and noise power spectrum (NPS). The signal and NPS can be further modified with factors unique to DBT image acquisition, such as focal spot motion (FSM) and oblique entry of x-rays, which are followed by the logarithmic transformation. If image subtraction is implemented in the projection domain, then signal and NPS propagation for either DE subtraction or TS may be modeled.[6, 9-12] Additionally, a number of reconstruction filters may be applied including (1) ramp filter (H_{RA}); (2) spectral apodization filter (H_{SA}), which is in the form of a Hanning window applied in the tube-travel (x-) direction; and slice-thickness filter (H_{ST}), a Hanning window applied in the direction of gravity (z-).[13-15]

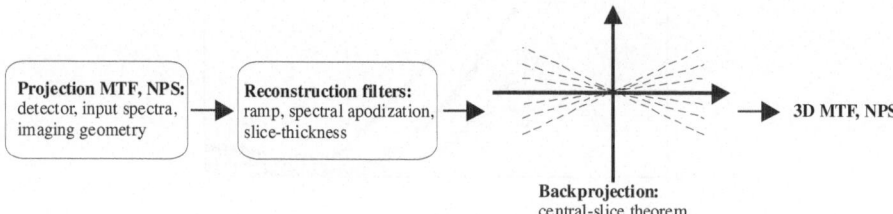

Fig. 2. Flow chart of the cascaded linear system model for CEDBT

---

[1] Caution: Investigations Device. Limited by US Federal law to investigational use.

The effects of d_{Se} on the MTF and NPS were incorporated into the projection image characteristics, as shown in Fig. 2. The effect of beam obliquity (which varies by projection angle) was determined, as outlined by Mainprize et al,[5], using:

$$T_\theta(f) = \frac{\left| \int_E E_{abs} \dfrac{1 - \exp(-\dfrac{\mu(E)d_{Se}}{\cos\theta} - i2\pi f d_{Se}\tan\theta)}{1 + i2\pi f \sin\theta / \mu(E)} \dfrac{d\varphi(E)}{dE} dE \right|}{\int_E E_{abs}\left[1 - \exp(-\dfrac{\mu(E)d_{Se}}{\cos\theta})\right]\dfrac{d\varphi(E)}{dE} dE} \tag{1}$$

where μ, φ, θ, and E_{abs} refer to the attenuation coefficient of a-Se, the x-ray spectrum, the x-ray incidence angle, and the absorbed energy, respectively.

The 2D projection image characteristics may be extended into 3D DBT following the central-slice theorem, as shown in Fig. 2. The projection MTF and NPS calculated at a specific angle is mapped along that same angle in 3D frequency space. The limited angular range of DBT results in incomplete coverage of the 3D frequency space. The resulting 3D MTF, $T(f_x, f_y, f_z)$, and NPS, $S(f_x, f_y, f_z)$, may be used to calculate the ideal observer signal-to-noise ratio (SNR), d', for an in-plane object according to:

$$d'^2_{in-plane} = \int\int \frac{\int K_c^2 \left[\left|O^2(f_x, f_y, f_z)\right| T^2(f_x, f_y, f_z) \right] df_z}{\int \left[S(f_x, f_y, f_z)\right] df_z} df_x df_y \tag{2}$$

where $O(f_x, f_y, f_z)$ and K_c describe the object's frequency components and contrast, respectively, for an ideal observer detection task.

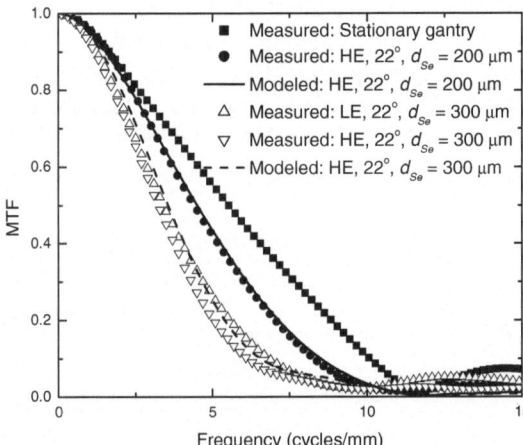

Fig. 3. Measured and MTF for an HE projection with stationary gantry ($d_{Se} = 200$, squares), and a 22° projection for HE ($d_{Se} = 200$, circles; $d_{Se} = 300$, downward triangles) and LE ($d_{Se} = 300$, upward triangles) views. The modeled data are included for HE projections with $d_{Se} = 200$ (solid line) and $d_{Se} = 300$ (dashed line).

3   Results and Discussion

3.1   Effect of Oblique X-ray Entry on Performance of Projection Views

The measured and modeled MTF from the two FPI are shown in Fig. 3. The results with a stationary gantry reflect the inherent MTF of the a-Se FPI, which has been investigated intensively.[16-19] The MTF is independent of the x-ray spectrum. Also plotted in Fig. 3 are the MTF for the 22° view of an HE DBT scan with d_{Se} = 200 and d_{Se} = 300, as well as the MTF for the 22° view of an LE DBT scan with d_{Se} = 300. Modeled data for both oblique HE views were included. In each of the DBT scans, additional blur is incurred due to the effect of FSM and oblique entry of x-rays. At 0° for the experimental DBT scan, the blur due to FSM was negligible. This is because the edge was placed at the surface of the detector housing, which essentially has no magnification. At the 22° view, the effect of oblique entry of x-rays is clearly visible. For the HE view with d_{Se} = 200, the MTF drops by approximately 30% at the Nyquist frequency (f_{NY}). With an FPI where d_{Se} = 300, the MTF drops by approximately 45% at f_{NY}. For the LE view, the effect of beam obliquity has a less pronounced effect on the MTF than in the HE case, where a significant drop between 5 and 10 cycles/mm is incurred at a 22° projection angle. In both oblique view HE cases, the modeled and measured data exhibit good agreement.

Although FSM and oblique entry of x-rays both introduce image blur as seen in the MTF measurements, they do not introduce noise correlation. As seen in Fig. 4, there is no change in the NPS with respect to projection angle for a single HE DBT scan using the 300 μm a-Se detector. As a result, the high frequency drop in DQE at oblique angles will be proportional to the square of the MTF..

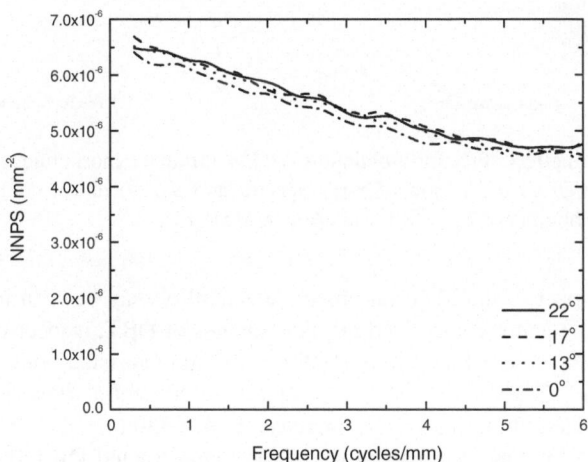

Fig. 4. Comparison of the NPS of a number of projection images of a HE DBT scan. Measurements were taken using an 300 μm a-Se FPI.

Our measurements showed that the DQE at zero cycles/mm improves by approximately 30% for the HE central view because of the thicker d_{Se}. However, due to oblique entry of x-rays, the DQE at f_{NY} decreases by a factor of 4 and 10 when comparing the $0°$ and $22°$ projection views for LE and HE imaging, respectively.

3.2   Effect of a-Se Thickness on DBT Detectability

Fig. 5(a) plots the modeled effect of the largest oblique x-ray entry angle $(34°)$ associated with the most oblique projection view $(22°)$ for the prototype CEDBT unit with different x-ray spectra and d_{Se}. Fig. 5(b) shows a comparison of the effects of reconstruction filter, x-ray obliquity $(22°)$, inherent detector MTF, and FSM . As seen in Fig. 5(a), increasing the d_{Se} has little effect on LE views. However, increasing the energy of the x-rays decreases the projection MTF due to increased blurring from the lateral spread of collection at oblique views. This effect is exacerbated when thicker detector is implemented. However, in spite of this effect, as seen in Fig. 5(b), the dominant blurring effect of oblique projection angles remains the effect of the reconstruction filters, particularly the slice-thickness filter.

a)   b)

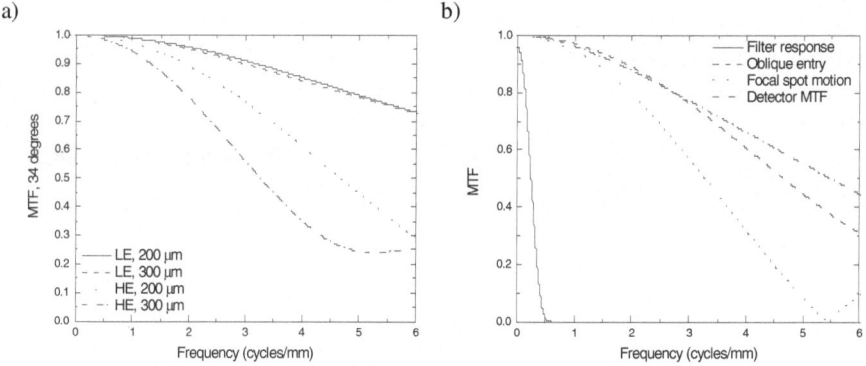

Fig. 5. Theoretical effect of the most oblique x-ray $(34°)$ from the most oblique tube angle $(22°)$ on projection MTF as a function of x-ray spectra and d_{Se} (a) and a comparison of filter response, x-ray obliquity of $22°$, FSM, and detector MTF (b)

The total impact of the MTF on object detectability may be seen in Fig. 6(a) and (b) for projection and reconstructed in-plane images of DBT, respectively. They both plots normalized d'^2 as a function of d_{Se} for a 300 μm Gaussian object in a DE DBT study. When the $22°$ projection view is compared to the central view, as shown in Fig. 6(a), there is a clear drop in d'^2 as d_{Se} increases above 350 μm. However, in Fig. 6(b), which plots the in-plane normalized d'^2 of the reconstructed DE DBT image of the object, there is no decrease in d'^2 as d_{Se} increases from 200 to 600 μm. This is because the effect of obliquity on MTF is negligible compared to the reconstruction filter. As a result, losses in d'^2 due to beam obliquity were found to be less than 0.4% in all cases.

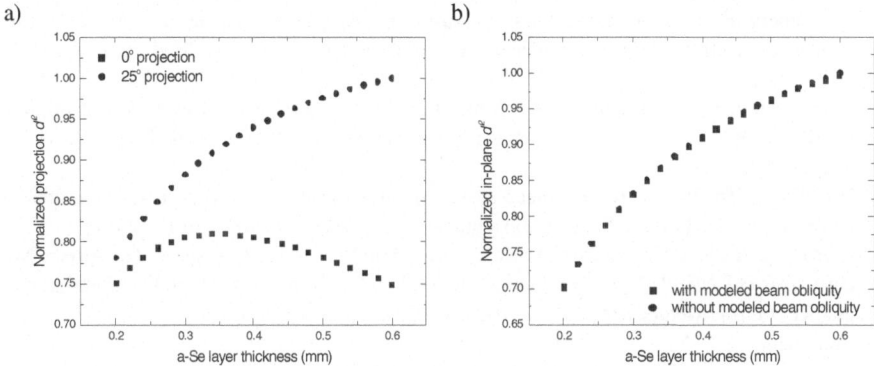

Fig. 6. Calculation of normalized d'^2 for a 300 μm object for projection views (a) and for reconstructed in-plane images (b) of a DE DBT scan (b) as a function of d_{Se} including the effect of oblique entry of x-rays (squares, i.e. central view for projection images) and not including oblique entry (circles)

4   Conclusion

Increasing the a-Se layer thickness may improve detector imaging performance for both CEDM and CEDBT by improving QDE at high energies. Due to the increased penetration and collection of HE photons, additional losses in MTF may be incurred at oblique views of a DBT scan. Since the noise remains uncorrelated, this MTF degradation directly translates to loss in DQE at high spatial frequencies. However, the losses in MTF at oblique views remain dominated by the effect of reconstruction filters and a net increase in detectability may be observed by increasing a-Se thickness for both CEDM and CEDBT applications.

Acknowledgments. We gratefully acknowledge the financial support from NIH (1 R01 CA148053 and 1 R01 EB002655), and Siemens Healthcare. We also acknowledge helpful discussions with Drs. Olivier Tousignant and Jonathan Greenspan, as well as Mr. Marc Hansrou from Anrad Corporation.

References

1. Carton, A.-K., Li, J., Albert, M., Chen, S., Maidment, A.D.A.: Quantification for contrast-enhanced digital breast tomosynthesis. In: Medical Imaging 2006: Physics of Medical Imaging, vol. 6142, pp. 61420D–61411D. SPIE, San Diego (2006)
2. Carton, A.-K., Lindman, K., Ullberg, C., Francke, T., Maidment, A.D.A.: Dual-energy subtraction for contrast-enhanced digital breast tomosynthesis. In: Medical Imaging 2007: Physics of Medical Imaging, vol. 6510, pp. 651007–651012. SPIE, San Diego (2007)
3. Carton, A.-K., Ullberg, C., Lindman, K., Francke, T., Maidment, A.: Optimization of a Dual-Energy Contrast-Enhanced Technique for a Photon Counting Digital Breast Tomosynthesis System. In: Krupinski, E.A. (ed.) IWDM 2008. LNCS, vol. 5116, pp. 116–123. Springer, Heidelberg (2008)

4. Fredenberg, E., Hemmendorff, M., Cederstrom, B., Aslund, M., Danielsson, M.: Contrast-enhanced spectral mammography with a photon-counting detector. Medical Physics 37, 2017–2029

5. Mainprize, J.G., Bloomquist, A.K., Kempston, M.P., Yaffe, M.J.: Resolution at oblique incidence angles of a flat panel imager for breast tomosynthesis. Med. Phys. 33, 3159–3164 (2006)

6. Hu, Y.-H., Zhao, W.: A 3D linear system model for the optimization of dual-energy contrast-enhanced digital breast tomosynthesis, pp. 79611C–79619C. SPIE (2011)

7. Carton, A.-K., Vandenbroucke, D., Struye, L., Maidment, A.D.A., Kao, Y.-H., Albert, M., Bosmans, H., Marchal, G.: Validation of MTF measurement for digital mammography quality control. Medical Physics 32, 1684–1695 (2005)

8. Maidment, A.D.A., Albert, M.: Conditioning data for calculation of the modulation transfer function. Medical Physics 30, 248–253 (2003)

9. Hu, Y.-H., Zhao, W.: Experimental quantification of lesion detectability in contrast enhanced dual energy digital breast tomosynthesis, pp. 83130A–83110A. SPIE (2012)

10. Richard, S., Siewerdsen, J.H.: Optimization of dual-energy imaging systems using generalized NEQ and imaging task. Medical Physics 34, 127–139 (2007)

11. Richard, S., Siewerdsen, J.H.: Cascaded systems analysis of noise reduction algorithms in dual-energy imaging. Medical Physics 35, 586–601 (2008)

12. Richard, S., Siewerdsen, J.H., Jaffray, D.A., Moseley, D.J., Bakhtiar, B.: Generalized DQE analysis of radiographic and dual-energy imaging using flat-panel detectors. Med. Phys. 32, 1397–1413 (2005)

13. Lauritsch, G., Haerer, W.H.: Theoretical framework for filtered back projection in tomosynthesis. In: Medical Imaging 1998: Image Processing, vol. 3338, pp. 1127–1137. SPIE, San Diego (1998)

14. Mertelmeier, T., Orman, J., Haerer, W., Dudam, M.K.: Optimizing filtered backprojection reconstruction for a breast tomosynthesis prototype device. In: Medical Imaging 2006: Physics of Medical Imaging, vol. 6142, pp. 61420F–61412F. SPIE, San Diego (2006)

15. Zhao, B., Zhao, W.: Three-dimensional linear system analysis for breast tomosynthesis. Medical Physics 35, 5219–5232 (2008)

16. Zhao, B., Zhao, W.: Imaging performance of an amorphous selenium digital mammography detector in a breast tomosynthesis system. Medical Physics 35, 1978–1987 (2008)

17. Zhao, W., Ji, W.G., Debrie, A., Rowland, J.A.: Imaging performance of amorphous selenium based flat-panel detectors for digital mammography: characterization of a small area prototype detector. Med. Phys. 30, 254–263 (2003)

18. Zhao, W., Ji, W.G., Rowlands, J.A., Debrie, A.: Investigation of imaging performance of amorphous selenium flat-panel detectors for digital mammography. In: Medical Imaging 2001: Physics of Medical Imaging, pp. 536–546. SPIE (2001)

19. Zhao, W., Rowlands, J.A.: Digital radiology using active matrix readout of amorphous selenium: Theoretical analysis of detective quantum efficiency. Medical Physics 24, 1819–1833 (1997)

Contrast Optimization in Clinical Contrast-Enhanced Digital Mammography Images

Juan-Pablo Cruz-Bastida[1], Iván Rosado-Méndez[1], Héctor Pérez-Ponce[1],
Yolanda Villaseñor[2], Héctor A. Galván[2], Flavio E. Trujillo-Zamudio[3],
Luis Benítez-Bribiesca[4], and María-Ester Brandan[1]

[1] Instituto de Física, Universidad Nacional Autónoma de México, 04511 DF, Mexico
{jpablocruz,brandan}@fisica.unam.mx
[2] Instituto Nacional de Cancerología, 14080 DF, Mexico
[3] Hospital Regional de Alta Especialidad de Oaxaca, 71256 Oaxaca, Mexico
[4] Hospital de Oncología, Centro Médico Nacional, IMSS, 06720 DF, Mexico

Abstract. CEDM is a radiological technique based on the use of digital mammography equipment and the injection of an iodinated contrast medium to enhance the visualization of tissues of interest. In previous works, our group has proposed a formalism for the use of dual-energy temporal CEDM, based on weighted subtraction of images, that has been applied with success to phantom data. This methodology requires the selection of ROIs by a radiologist, to determine the weight factors. In this work, we propose an alternative that improves the contrast in clinical images resulting from dual-energy temporal CEDM subtraction, while freeing the method from ambiguities due to the ROI selection by a radiologist. The new subtraction algorithm is based on the use of weight factors calculated pixel-by-pixel. The main result after evaluation of the methodology on images of 10 patients randomly chosen is a substantial improvement of the contrast (~5 times), reaching values that are similar to those obtained with single energy subtraction.

Keywords: Breast imaging, CEDM, contrast-enhanced digital mammography, contrast medium, angiogenesis, dual-energy, image subtraction.

1 Background

The increasingly common use of digital mammography worldwide, in addition to other well-known advantages over alternative breast imaging modalities, has profited from advanced applications that might improve early breast cancer detection [1]. One of these techniques is image subtraction under the administration of a contrast medium (CM) referred to as contrast-enhanced digital mammography (CEDM).

CEDM relies on the preferential CM uptake of aggressive cancers undergoing angiogenesis to enhance their visualization with respect to the structured breast background [2-3].

There are two modalities to perform CEDM, single energy temporal (SET) and dual-energy (DE) [2]. SET is based on the temporal differences between images

A.D.A. Maidment, P.R. Bakic, and S. Gavenonis (Eds.): IWDM 2012, LNCS 7361, pp. 17–23, 2012.

acquired prior and after the CM administration. DE focuses on the changes in the linear attenuation coefficient (μ) due to acquisition with different X-ray spectra. In all CEDM modalities the subtracted image is obtained as follows [4]

$$I_{sub} = \ln I\left(t_1, Q_1\right) - \alpha \ln I\left(t_2, Q_2\right) ,$$ (1)

where I is a mammographic image acquired at time t_i with an spectrum of quality Q_i. The weighting factor α compensates changes between the images due to acquisition with different beam qualities, so that the pixel values of the non-iodinated tissue becomes zero after the subtraction. Evidently, α has a value of 1 for SET.

2   The Dual-Energy-Temporal Formalism

2.1   Previous Proposal

Our group has proposed a formalism that combines both temporal and dual energy modalities (named dual-energy-temporal or DET subtraction) [5]. It is based on the acquisition of two *mask images* prior to the CM administration: one with a low energy X-ray spectrum (LE) and the other with a high energy one (HE). A series of *CM images* is acquired after the contrast medium administration, with the same radiological parameters as the HE mask.

First, all images are normalized by the mean pixel value (MPV) in a region of interest (ROI) identified by the radiologist as adipose tissue. Then, the LE mask is weight-subtracted from the CM images as indicated in Eq. (1). In this case (Eq. (2)), α is obtained as the ratio of MPVs in normal glandular tissue ROIs, also identified by the radiologist in the LE and HE masks I_{LE} and I_{HE}, respectively,

$$\alpha = \frac{\text{MPV}\left(\text{ROI}_{\text{glandular}}\left(I_{LE}\right)\right)}{\text{MPV}\left(\text{ROI}_{\text{glandular}}\left(I_{HE}\right)\right)} .$$ (2)

This proposal was successfully validated with phantom data [6], and the radiological parameters (detailed in section 3) were optimized [5] for SET and DET modalities in terms of mean glandular dose and contrast to noise ratio. SET and DET results reported here have followed this formalism.

A protocol for clinical application was approved by the ethics and research committees of the Mexico National Institute of Cancerology (INCan), and the preliminary analysis of clinical images has revealed the following limitations for DET:

- The definition of the glandular tissue ROI depends on the expertise of the radiologist to identify glandular regions on the breast. Thus, it can be subjective.
- After subtraction, the remaining structured noise –due to the spatial variations of breast glandularity– causes the contrast between lesion and normal glandular tissue to be relatively modest.

2.2   This Work Proposal

To compensate for spatial variations in glandular composition, and therefore increase the visualization of iodine, we have proposed two modifications to the original proposal that better fit it to the conditions in clinical images:

- To weight the images by a glandular density matrix G, obtained after Highnam [7], in order to emphasize the presence of glandular tissue in the image.
- To construct the factor α as a matrix whose elements $\hat{\alpha}_{ij}$ (Eq. (3)) are equal to the ratio between corresponding pixels in the LE and HE masks I_{LE} and I_{HE}, respectively,

$$\hat{\alpha}_{ij} = \frac{(I_{LE})_{ij}}{(I_{HE})_{ij}} \; . \tag{3}$$

The role of α as a matrix is the same as previously described for the weight factor.

Hence, in this proposed dual-energy-temporal formalism (referred to as DETm) the subtracted image I_{sub} is obtained as

$$I_{sub}(t) = \ln(G \circ I_{LE}) - \hat{\alpha} \circ \ln(G \circ I_{CM}(t)) \; , \tag{4}$$

where G is the glandular density matrix, I_{LE} is the LE mask, and I_{CM} is a contrast medium image acquired at time t.

3   Materials and Methods

Image Acquisition. Patients with suspicious lesions detected in routine mammography (BIRADS 4-5) were imaged with a Senographe DS system, following a CEDM optimized protocol that allows to perform DET and SET subtractions [5]. Two images were acquired prior to CM administration employing (anode/filter) Rh/Rh at 34 kV (LE mask), and 48 kV plus external 0.5cm Al (HE mask); four CM images were taken after CM administration, with same radiological parameters as HE mask. Iodine-based CM (Optiray® 300, 300 iodine mg per ml) was injected using an injection system, at a constant speed of 4 ml/s. The sequence of CM images allows the interpretation of iodine uptake in terms of dynamical absorption curves.

Imaging System Characterization. The implementation of DETm, particularly the calculation of G, requires the relationship between detector output signal and pixel value [7]. For this purpose, PMMA blocks of different thickness were imaged using the same radiological parameters as LE clinical images. The detector output signal was calculated following Lemacks formalism [8], and the MPVs in a 5×5 cm^2 ROI, centered at 6 cm from the edge of the detector, were calibrated. Lemacks formalism requires a knowledge of the X ray spectrum and the exposure during acquisition. In this case, X ray spectra were simulated based on Boone polynomial interpolation [9] and the correlation between X-ray tube charge (mAs) and air kerma at the entrance of the breast (mGy), was measured on the beam central axis, at 4.5 cm from the detector, with a mammography ionization chamber for a range of mAs values. Kerma values were then transformed to the appropriate distance according to the experimentally verified $1/r^2$ relation.

Image Processing. The raw (for processing) images of ten patients randomly chosen (among those who were part of the protocol) have been analyzed. Of each series, three images were considered for the evaluation of the subtraction formalisms: the two masks and the image taken 3 minutes after CM administration. Firstly, the images were aligned with respect to their LE mask with a moving least squares algorithm [10] and a median filter of radius 10 pixels was applied. Secondly, three subtraction formalisms were applied to the selected images: SET, DET and DETm, using a custom-made MATLAB® routine run in a personal computer with Windows® 7 and 1.80 GHz Intel® Core™ i7 processor.

Enhancement Evaluation. The resulting iodine enhancement in the subtracted image for each subtraction modality was evaluated in terms of contrast between the lesion and normal glandular tissue, according to Weber (Eq. (5)):

$$C = \frac{I_L - I_G}{I_G} , \tag{5}$$

where I_L is the MPV in the lesion and I_G is the MPV in a normal glandular tissue ROI. Lesion ROIs were selected by a radiologist in the LE mask, guided by subtracted images, while glandular ROIs were selected previous to any subtraction on the LE mask. To allow comparison, subtracted images were self-normalized and the resulting pixel values were mapped to an 8-bit gray scale.

4   Results

Figure 1 illustrates the image processing for a typical patient. Figs. 1A-C are "for presentation" LE and HE masks and CM image acquired at t=3 minutes, respectively. Fig. 1D is the SET subtraction of Figs. 1C minus 1B. The application of DET is shown in Fig. 1E. The background breast structure has been considerably reduced, the lesion is clearly visualized and the resulting contrast value (~0.3) depends strongly on the chosen ROIs for the adipose and normal glandular tissues. Fig. 1F is the processed image obtained with DETm. The breast structure has almost disappeared and the contrast value (~0.7) is greater than in DET (Fig. 1E).

These general features of the subtracted images are common to all the analyzed clinical cases (one of the patients did not show a significant iodine uptake and thus, contrast was always close to zero). Individual contrast values obviously differ from one patient to the other depending on the individual CM uptake, but values obtained with the proposed DETm formalism are consistently higher than with DET.

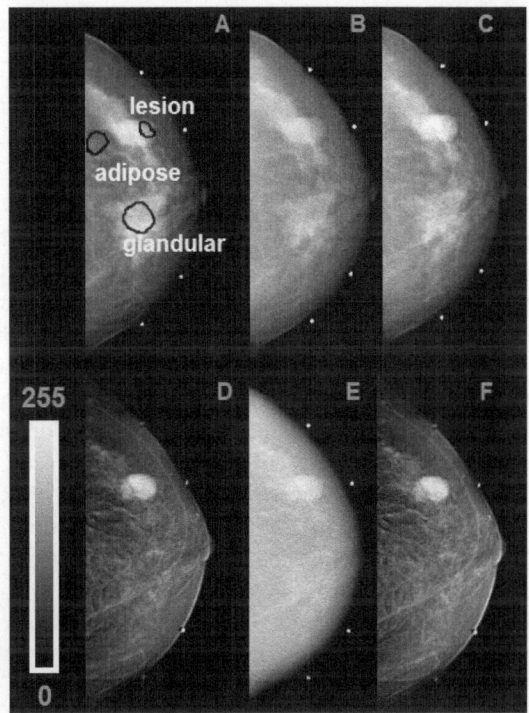

Fig. 1. Images for one patient. A and B are mask images acquired with LE and HE spectra, respectively. C is HE image 3 minutes after CM injection. D is subtracted image following SET formalism, E is DET result and F is DETm. Gray value bar represents pixel values after normalization of D, E and F. ROIs for adipose, glandular and lesion tissues are shown in A.

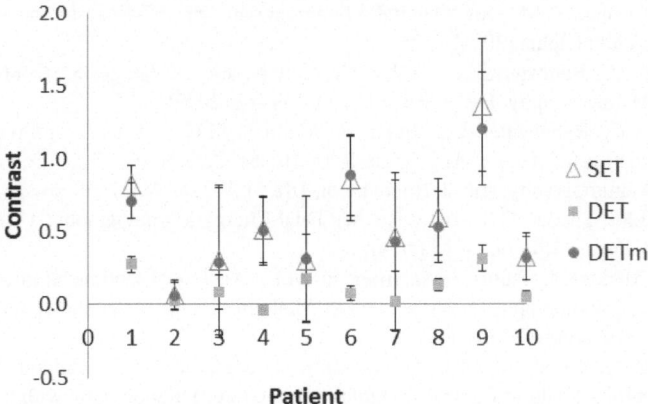

Fig. 2. Contrast between lesion and normal glandular tissue for SET, DET, and DETm modalities. Ten patients are reported

Figure 2 summarizes contrast values for all patients. Contrast derived from DETm is similar to that from SET, with differences (of about 10%) within the estimated uncertainties.

5   Discussion and Conclusions

These preliminary results suggest that the subtraction based on pixel-by-pixel weighting, compared with standard DET modality, improves the contrast in processed CEDM images while freeing the method from possible inconsistencies in the ROI determination (only the final evaluation of the contrast requires the definition of a region of interest.) Also, the image sharpness is apparently better, possibly due to the reduction of structural noise in DETm with respect to DET. Data from a sample of 10 patients leads to DETm contrast values similar to SET subtraction, suggesting that the energy- change compensation by the weight factor is done correctly. This feature was predicted by the DET formalism, as shown in Fig. 4(a) of Ref. 5. Computation time was considerably greater for DETm (~1 min per image subtraction) than for the other formalisms (~1 s) and this might be considered when evaluating the overall advantages of DETm. The pathological diagnosis and neoangiogenesis quantification are in process.

Acknowledgments. Authors acknowledge partial funding from DGAPA-UNAM grant PAPIIT 102610, and CONACyT Salud 2009-01-112374. JPCB acknowledges CONACyT scholarship for M. Sc. studies.

References

1. Yaffe, M.J.: Advanced Applications of Digital Mammography. In: Pisano, E.D., Yaffe, M.J., Kuzmiak, C.M. (eds.) Digital Mammography, pp. 67–76. Lippincott Williams & Wilkins, Philadelphia (2004)
2. Dromain, C., Balleyguier, C., Adler, G., Garbay, J.R., Delaloge, S.: Contrast-Enhanced Digital Mammography. Eur. J. Radiol. 69(1), 34–42 (2009)
3. Dromain, C., Balleyguier, C., Muller, S., Mathieu, M.C., Rochard, F., Opolon, P., Sigal, R.: Evaluation of Tumor Angiogenesis of Breast Carcinoma Using Contrast-Enhanced Digital Mammography. Am. J. Roentgenol. 187(5), W528–W537 (2006)
4. Boone, J.M., Shaber, G.S., Tecotzky, M.: Dual-Energy Mammography: a Detector Analysis. Med. Phys. 17(4), 665–675 (1990)
5. Rosado-Méndez, I., Palma, B.A., Brandan, M.E.: Analytical Optimization of Digital Subtraction Mammography with Contrast Medium Using a Commercial Unit. Med. Phys. 35(12), 5544–5557 (2008)
6. Palma, B.A., Rosado-Méndez, I., Villaseñor, Y., Brandan, M.E.: Phantom Study to Evaluate Contrast-Medium-Enhanced Digital Subtraction Mammography with a Full-Field Indirect-Detection System. Med. Phys. 37(2), 577–589 (2009)
7. Highnam, R., Brady, M., Shepstone, B.: A Representation for Mammographic Image Processing. Medical Image Analysis 1(1), 1–18 (1996)

8. Lemacks, M.R., Kappadath, S.C., Shaw, C.C., Liu, X., Whitman, G.J.: A Dual-Energy Subtraction Technique for Microcalcification Imaging in Digital Mammography–A Signal-to-Noise Analysis. Med. Phys. 29(8), 1739–1751 (2002)

9. Boone, J.M., Fewell, T.R., Jennings, R.J.: Molybdenum, Rhodium, and Tungsten Anode Spectral Models Using Interpolating Polynomials with Application to Mammography. Med. Phys. 24(12), 1863–1874 (1997)

10. Schaefer, S., McPhail, T., Warren, J.: Image Deformation Using Moving Least Squares. ACM Transactions on Graphics 25(3), 533–540 (2006)

Determination of System Geometrical Parameters and Consistency between Scans for Contrast-Enhanced Digital Breast Tomosynthesis

David A. Scaduto and Wei Zhao

Stony Brook University, Department of Radiology, Stony Brook, New York 11794
david.scaduto@stonybrook.edu, wei.zhao@stonybrookmedicine.edu

Abstract. Digital breast tomosynthesis (DBT) requires precise knowledge of acquisition geometry for accurate image reconstruction. Further, image subtraction techniques employed in dual-energy contrast-enhanced tomosynthesis require that scans be performed under nearly identical geometrical conditions. A geometrical calibration algorithm is developed to investigate system geometry and geometrical consistency of image acquisition between consecutive digital breast tomosynthesis scans, according to requirements for dual-energy contrast-enhanced tomosynthesis. Investigation of geometrical accuracy and consistency on a prototype DBT unit reveals accurate angular measurement, but potentially clinically significant differences in acquisition angles between scans. Further, a slight gantry wobble is observed, suggesting the need for incorporation of gantry wobble into image reconstruction, or improvements to system hardware.

Keywords: geometric calibration, tomosynthesis, dual-energy, contrast-enhanced tomosynthesis, flat-panel detector.

1 Introduction

Digital breast tomosynthesis (DBT) is a three-dimensional (3D) x-ray imaging modality that reduces the effect of anatomical clutter inherent to conventional screening mammography. In DBT, a number of x-ray projections are acquired over a limited angular range (e.g. ±25°), and reconstructed using a modified filtered back-projection algorithm into image slices parallel to the detector. In dual-energy contrast-enhanced DBT (CEDBT) an iodinated contrast agent is administered to the patient and consecutive tomosynthesis scans are acquired at energies above and below the K-edge of iodine. Using image subtraction techniques, an iodine-only image, virtually free of anatomical noise, can be obtained. [1] Previous studies in dual-energy computed tomography (CT) have shown that subtraction in the projection domain provides better performance than in the reconstruction domain. [2] In tomosynthesis, subtraction in the projection domain provides an additional advantage because it is not affected by reconstruction artifacts. However, implementing image subtraction in the projection domain requires that DBT datasets be acquired under nearly identical geometrical

A.D.A. Maidment, P.R. Bakic, and S. Gavenonis (Eds.): IWDM 2012, LNCS 7361, pp. 24–31, 2012.

conditions, with consistent angles of acquisition. Further, precise knowledge of acquisition geometry is critical for accurate image reconstruction. [3–5]

A number of calibration techniques have been developed for cone-beam CT and recently adapted for tomosynthesis, which utilize calibration phantoms with specific arrangements of embedded markers. Geometrical system parameters may be derived either through accurately known three-dimensional (3D) marker locations and their corresponding two-dimensional (2D) projections [6–9], or through specialized geometric arrangements of markers in the calibration phantom [5, 10].

In this paper we describe the phantom and calibration procedure developed for a prototype Siemens Inspiration DBT system to determine both its geometric parameters and reproducibility of the x-ray source trajectory, and discuss the impact of our findings in the implementation of CEDBT.

2   Materials and Methods

Our geometrical calibration procedure was developed for and tested on a Siemens Inspiration DBT system equipped with an amorphous selenium (a-Se) flat-panel detector with 85×85 μm pixel pitch. All image processing and calibration computations were performed in MATLAB (TheMathWorks, Natick, MA). We used a cylindrical acrylic phantom with 28 tungsten beads arranged in equi-angular separation of $24°$ and spiral pitch of 90 mm (Fig. 1), which is similar in concept to those widely used in geometric calibration of cone-beam CT. [8] The calibration procedure developed relates the 3D location of a marker to its 2D projection through a projection matrix, a description of the unique projective mapping of an object with respect to the x-ray source (Fig. 2). The calibration procedure is summarized as follows.

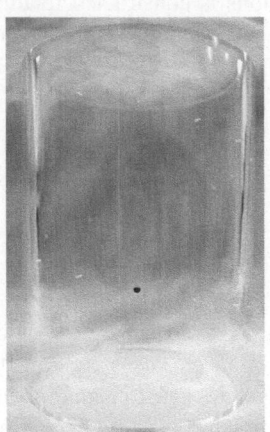 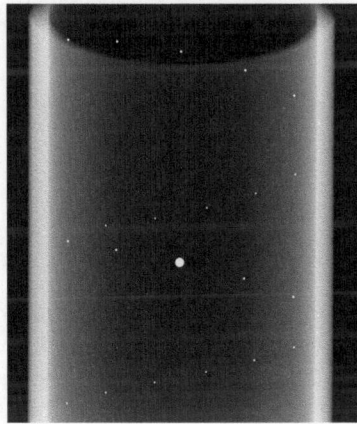

Fig. 1. Photograph (left) of the calibration phantom used in this study, and resulting x-ray projection image (right) of the phantom, with beads visible. The large central bead is used to define the origin of the phantom coordinate system, from which the nominal 3D coordinates of each bead on the spiral pattern could be determined.

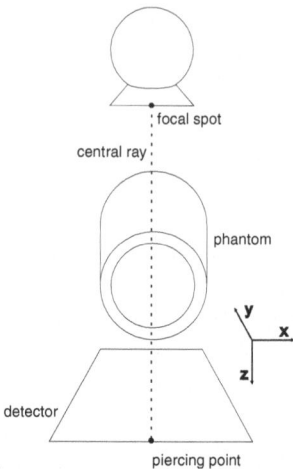

Fig. 2. Diagram of 3D phantom coordinate mapping to 2D detector plane

1. *Acquire phantom images:* The calibration phantom was compressed onto the detector cover to minimize relative phantom motion. Standard DBT scans were performed, with each scan containing 25 projection images (Fig. 1) acquired over a nominal angular range of ±25°.
2. *Determine bead coordinates in each projection image:* A bead detection algorithm evaluated bead shadows for size and eccentricity to determine the center coordinate of each projected bead.
3. *Make initial estimate of projection matrix*: An initial relationship between the 3D bead coordinates in the phantom and the 2D projected bead coordinates was determined algebraically. Briefly, a system of equations is constructed relating the 2D and 3D bead coordinates by elements of the 3×4 projection matrix P, such that

$$
\begin{bmatrix} u_i w \\ v_i w \\ w \end{bmatrix} = \begin{bmatrix} P_{11} & P_{12} & P_{13} & P_{14} \\ P_{21} & P_{22} & P_{23} & P_{24} \\ P_{31} & P_{32} & P_{33} & P_{34} \end{bmatrix} \begin{bmatrix} x_i \\ y_i \\ z_i \\ 1 \end{bmatrix} \tag{1}
$$

where $[u_i, v_i]$ represent the 2D bead coordinates in image space, and $[x_i, y_i, z_i]$ represent the 3D bead coordinates in phantom space. The weighting factor, w, maintains the homogeneity of the coordinates systems. Matrix multiplication, and elimination of the weighting factor, yields the following system of equations:

$$
\begin{bmatrix} P_{11}x_i + P_{12}y_i + P_{13}z_i + P_{14} - P_{31}x_iu_i - P_{32}y_iu_i - P_{33}z_i - P_{34} \\ P_{21}x_i + P_{22}y_i + P_{23}z_i + P_{24} - P_{31}x_iv_i - P_{32}y_iv_i - P_{33}z_i - P_{34} \end{bmatrix} = \begin{bmatrix} 0 \\ 0 \end{bmatrix} \tag{2}
$$

These expressions are used to construct a matrix, which includes the 3D bead coordinates and their corresponding 2D image coordinates. Singular value decomposition is employed to find a solution to the system of equations, representing a linear solution of the projection matrix.

4. *Minimize re-projection error:* The projection matrix is more accurately estimated by iteratively minimizing the square distance between measured bead coordinates and re-projected bead coordinates using the estimated P. We used the Levenberg-Marquardt nonlinear least-squares fit algorithm to minimize the objective function

$$E = \sum_i d\left([u_i, v_i]^T, P[x_i, y_i, z_i]^T\right)^2 .$$ (3)

Optimization is terminated when a minimum residual re-projection error is achieved.

5. *Decompose optimized projection matrix to derive source location*: The projection matrix may be factored into three component matrices, such that

$$P = K[R \,|\, t]$$ (4)

where the 3×3 rotation matrix R and the 3×1 translation vector t describe the orientation and location of the phantom with respect to the x-ray source, and the upper triangular intrinsic matrix K may be decomposed as

$$K = \begin{bmatrix} \alpha_x & s & u_0 \\ & \alpha_y & v_0 \\ & & 1 \end{bmatrix}$$ (5)

where α_x and α_y represent pixel-scaling factors, s represents a skew-parameter for non-square pixels, and u_0 and v_0 are coordinates of the piercing point where the central x-ray enters the x-ray detector.

Thus, these three matrices reveal detector orientation, source to detector distance and x-ray source location. For stationary detectors, the most important of these parameters is the x-ray source location with respect to the stationary detector.

3   Results

Using the method described above, projection matrices, P, were computed for each angle in a tomosynthesis scan, from which the x-ray source location (with respect to the detector plane) was derived. A plane of motion fitted to the source trajectory of each scan was found to be perpendicular to the detector, with a 0.85 degree rotation relative to the long axis of the detector plane (see Fig. 3). The deviation of the x-ray source from the fitted plane (wobble) was determined for a number of consecutive and non-consecutive scans to determine source orbit reproducibility between scans. The source trajectory appears reproducible; results for five consecutive scans are shown in Fig. 4.

A circular orbit was fit to the experimentally determined source locations; the origin of this circle represents the center of rotation. Gantry angles were computed for each acquisition location with respect to the source location at the stationary zero-angle position. These gantry angles were found to agree reasonably well with the nominal values recorded by the on-board inclinometer, differing by an average of 0.2 degrees, shown in Fig. 5.

Differences in the angles of acquisition between scans at each projection were registered both by the on-board inclinometer and the computed gantry angles. Several beads were tracked across projections for consecutive scans to study the effect of differences in acquisition angles between scans. The mean angular difference of 0.1 degrees resulted in a bead projection misalignment in the tube travel direction of 0.15 mm measured at the chest wall, and 0.22 mm measured 175 mm along the perpendicular to the chest wall, shown in Fig. 6. The misalignment in the direction perpendicular to tube travel was negligible, which suggests repeatable gantry trajectories, albeit with slight variations in projection angles between tomosynthesis scans.

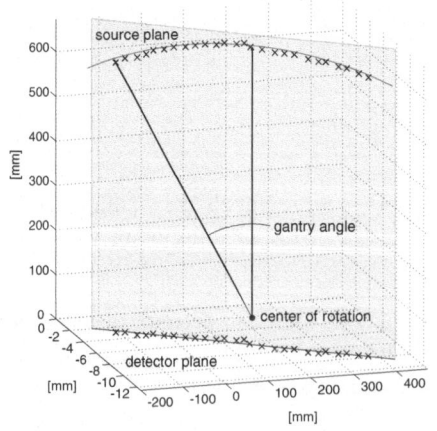
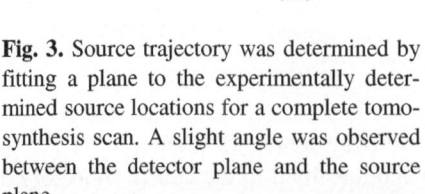
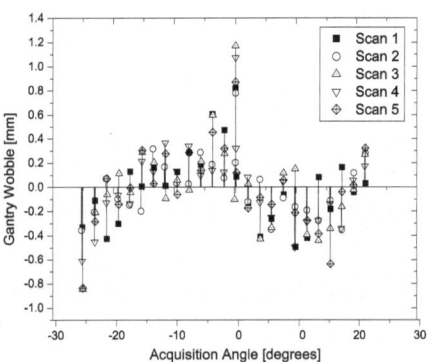

Fig. 3. Source trajectory was determined by fitting a plane to the experimentally determined source locations for a complete tomosynthesis scan. A slight angle was observed between the detector plane and the source plane.

Fig. 4. Deviation of the x-ray source from the fitted plane of motion (gantry wobble)

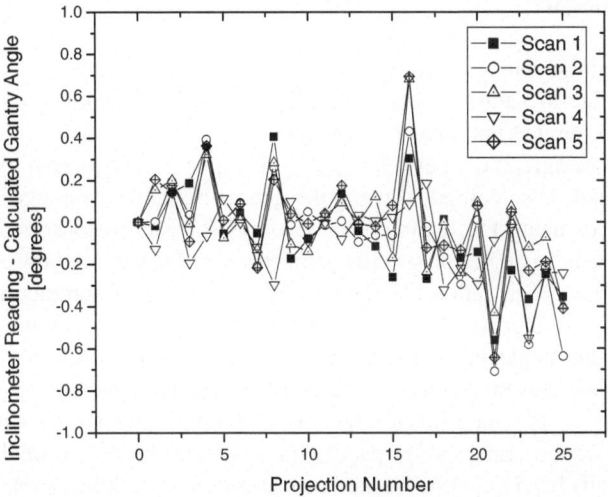

Fig. 5. Inclinometer accuracy was evaluated by comparing inclinometer readings with calculated gantry angles using calibration algorithm, and found to agree within ±0.7 degrees, with a mean difference of 0.2 degrees

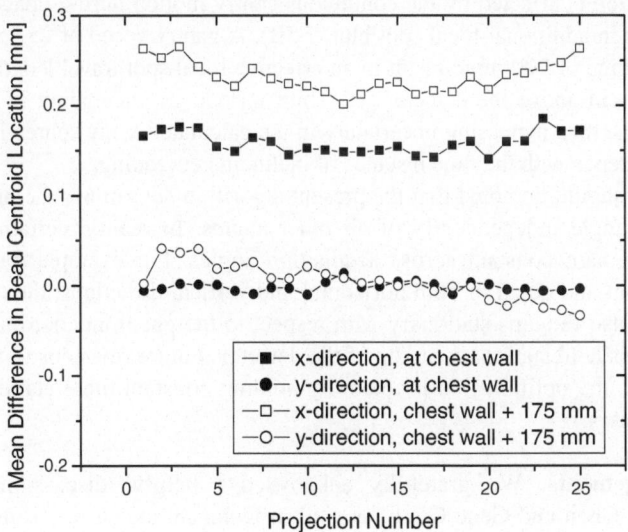

Fig. 6. Beads were tracked across projections for consecutive scans. A mean angular difference of 0.1 degrees between consecutives scans resulted in a mean bead projection misalignment of 0.15 mm at the chest wall, and 0.22 mm measured 175 mm from the chest wall.

4   Discussion

Our analysis of the source locations for complete scans indicates a deviation from the source plane due to gantry wobble, resulting in non-ideal acquisition geometry that should be incorporated into image reconstruction.

We find close agreement between angles of acquisition registered by the on-board inclinometer and those computed using the geometric calibration algorithm, assuring the reliability of using the inclinometer readings for each reconstruction. However, the exact acquisition angles at specific projections differ slightly between scans, suggesting that image registration may be needed if dual-energy subtraction is to be performed in projection space. It is important to note that the maximum misalignment due to projection angle inconsistency is ~2.5 pixels; patient motion is expected to further exacerbate this misalignment, necessitating image registration.

One strategy to facilitate image registration would be to place a small marker on the periphery of the compression paddle, i.e., outside the region of the breast. The projection of this bead could be tracked across consecutive scans, from which projection misalignments due to gantry angle inconsistency could be calculated, as described above.

Projection angle variations may ultimately be minimized by improving the synchronization between gantry motion and x-ray exposure.

It is important to note that the accuracy of source position determined during geometrical calibration is affected by the continuous gantry motion during image acquisition, which results in additional focal spot blur (FSB). A gantry speed of 25.45 mm/sec and an exposure time of 200 msec result in an effective focal spot travel length of 0.33 mm for objects 4 cm above the detector. This blur introduces uncertainty in the projected bead centroids, thus increasing uncertainty in the calculated x-ray source locations, and its correspondence with the time instance of inclinometer reading.

Finally, it should be noted that the present algorithm determines the projection matrix at each angle independently of all other angles. In reality, certain geometrical parameters remain constant across acquisition angles. For example, pixel pitch remains constant and equal in both horizontal and vertical directions; the orientation of the detector also remains stationary with respect to the phantom coordinate system if the phantom is held stationary on top of the detector. Future revisions to the algorithm will constrain the optimization problem by holding constant these stationary geometrical parameters.

Acknowledgements. We gratefully acknowledge helpful discussions with Drs. Guang-Hong Chen and Gene Gindi, as well as technical assistance from Mr. Yihuan Lu.

References

1. Carton, A.-K., Gavenonis, S.C., Currivan, J.A., Conant, E.F., Schnall, M.D., Maidment, A.D.A.: Dual-energy contrast-enhanced digital breast tomosynthesis—a feasibility study. The British Journal of Radiology 83, 344–350 (2010)

2. Yu, L., Liu, X., McCollough, C.H.: Pre-reconstruction three-material decomposition in dual-energy CT. In: Proceedings of SPIE, vol. 7258, pp. 72583V–72583V-8 (2009)
3. Li, X., Zhang, D., Liu, B.: Sensitivity analysis of a geometric calibration method using projection matrices for digital tomosynthesis systems. Medical Physics 38, 202–209 (2011)
4. Mainprize, J.G., Bloomquist, A., Wang, X., Yaffe, M.J.: Dependence of image quality on geometric factors in breast tomosynthesis. Medical Physics 38, 3090 (2011)
5. Cho, Y., Moseley, D.J., Siewerdsen, J.H., Jaffray, D.A.: Accurate technique for complete geometric calibration of cone-beam computed tomography systems. Medical Physics 32, 968 (2005)
6. Hartley, R., Zisserman, A.: Multiple view geometry in computer vision. Cambridge Univ. Press (2000)
7. Li, X., Zhang, D., Liu, B.: A generic geometric calibration method for tomographic imaging systems with flat-panel detectors—A detailed implementation guide. Medical Physics 37, 3844 (2010)
8. Strobel, N.K.: Improving 3D image quality of x-ray C-arm imaging systems by using properly designed pose determination systems for calibrating the projection geometry. In: Proceedings of SPIE, vol. 5030, pp. 943–954 (2003)
9. Chen, G.-H., Zambelli, J., Nett, B.E., Supanich, M., Riddell, C., Belanger, B., Mistretta, C.A.: Design and development of C-arm based cone-beam CT for image-guided interven-tions: initial results. In: Proceedings of SPIE, pp. 614210–614210-12. SPIE Press (2006)
10. Wang, X., Mainprize, J.G., Kempston, M.P., Mawdsley, G.E., Yaffe, M.J.: Digital breast tomosynthesis geometry calibration. In: Proceedings of SPIE, vol. 6510, pp. 65103B–65103B-11 (2007)

Initial Experience with Dual-Energy Contrast-Enhanced Digital Breast Tomosynthesis in the Characterization of Breast Cancer

Sara Gavenonis[1], Kristen Lau[1], Roshan Karunamuni[1], Yiheng Zhang[2], Baorui Ren[2], Chris Ruth[2], and Andrew D.A. Maidment[1]

[1] Department of Radiology, Hospital of the University of Pennsylvania,
Perelman School of Medicine at the University of Pennsylvania
{Sara.Gavenonis,Roshan.Karunamuni,Andrew.Maidment}@uphs.upenn.edu
[2] Hologic, Inc. Bedford, MA
{Yiheng.Zhang,Baurui.Ren,Chris.Ruth}@hologic.com

Abstract. An assessment is ongoing of the ability of dual energy contrast-enhanced digital breast tomosynthesis (CE-DBT) to depict the morphologic and vascular characteristics of breast cancer in comparison with breast MRI and digital mammography (DM). Eight patients with newly diagnosed breast cancer were imaged with an automated dual-energy CE-DBT system. High energy/low energy image pairs of the index breast were obtained at 1 pre- and 3 post-contrast timepoints. Post-contrast images were obtained after intravenous administration of Visipaque (1 mL/kg). Anatomic images were reconstructed using filtered backprojection, and contrast-enhanced images were generated using simple backprojection followed by temporal or dual-energy subtraction. Dual-energy CE-DBT was able to demonstrate the index malignant lesion in 7 of 8 patients (9 of 10 lesions). Morphologic characteristics including margin detail and associated microcalcifications were qualitatively concordant with DM. Vascular characteristics were identifiable qualitatively on post-processed images in some cases, and judged to be qualitative concordant with breast MRI.

1   Introduction

On imaging, malignant breast lesions are characterized by both structural and functional features[1-4]. Currently, multimodality imaging provides complementary information that is useful in the assessment and staging of breast cancer. However, while MRI can provide vascular information about breast lesions [5-6], it has lower spatial resolution than digital mammography and microcalcifications are not directly visible on MRI. Conversely, projection digital mammography can demonstrate morphology with high spatial resolution, but is susceptible to artifacts from superimposed tissues and does not provide functional information about breast lesions.

CE-DBT can potentially integrate into one breast imaging tool many of the strengths of existing multimodality imaging while also avoiding some limitations of existing modalities. The unique combination into a single imaging modality of the ability to

A.D.A. Maidment, P.R. Bakic, and S. Gavenonis (Eds.): IWDM 2012, LNCS 7361, pp. 32–39, 2012.

acquire functional characteristics of breast lesions together with high spatial resolution similar to digital mammography results in a potentially powerful breast imaging tool. An additional strength of CE-DBT lies in the underlying technology of digital breast tomosynthesis (DBT), which circumvents the limitations of two-dimensional projection mammography. DBT is an emerging x-ray based breast imaging technique in which high resolution tomographic images of the breast are obtained at a dose comparable to projection mammography [11, 12]. In clinical trials, DBT provides improved sensitivity and specificity relative to projection mammography[12].

Thus, the purpose of this study was to assess the ability of dual-energy CE-DBT to demonstrate morphologic and vascular characteristics of breast cancer in comparison with breast MRI and digital mammography. Our hypothesis is that these features of breast cancers will be demonstrable on CE-DBT images.

2   Methods

2.1   Acquisition Protocol

This prospective research study received IRB approval and is HIPAA compliant. After informed consent was obtained, 8 patients (age range 48 – 68 years) with newly diagnosed breast cancer were imaged with an automated dual-energy CE-DBT system (Hologic, Bedford MA). High energy/Low energy image pairs of the index breast were obtained at 1 pre and 3 post-contrast timepoints. Dynamic post-contrast images were obtained after intravenous administration of Visipaque (1 mL/kg) using a power injector (2-3 ml/sec). Images were reconstructed using backprojection (Figure 1). Subtraction images were generated and reviewed (dual energy and temporal). In this preliminary study, no motion correction processing was applied. Qualitative comparison with breast MRI and DM in each case was performed.

DM: DM was obtained as part of the standard clinical workup, prior to diagnosis.

MRI: The breast MRI was performed either before or after the CE-DBT exam (6 on the same day, 1 the day after MRI, and one 12 days after MRI.) MRI was performed with the patient prone in a 1.5-T scanner (Siemens) with a dedicated surface breast coil array. For contrast imaging, a rapid bolus injection of 0.1 mmol/kg gadobenate dimeglumine (MulitHance, Bracco Diagnostics Inc, Princeton, NJ) followed by a saline flush was administered (via peripheral intravenous access). The clinical breast MRI protocol includes the following series: pre-contrast T1-weighted, pre-contrast T2-weighted fat suppressed, pre-contrast T1-weighted fat suppressed, dynamic post-contrast T1-weighted fat suppressed (3 timepoints, 90 second intervals), delayed axial T1-weighted fat suppressed. Sagittal subtraction images are generated.

CE-DBT: Each patient underwent unilateral CE-DBT using the Hologic Selenia Dimensions CE-DBT prototype system (Table 1). Patients were seated for the duration of the exam. Initial pre-contrast DBT high and low energy pair in the MLO projection (or optimal projection for visualization of the index lesion) was obtained (7 MLO, 1 XCCL). The low energy series was used as an unenhanced anatomic baseline for tomographic assessment of microcalcifications and margin analysis. The high energy series was used as the tomographic mask for temporal subtraction. The breast remained in this compression for the remainder of the study. Then, a contrast injection of 1ml/kg iodixanol (Visipaque-320,GE Healthcare Inc., Princeton, NJ) was made(via peripheral intravenous access) using a power injector followed by a saline flush. Three post-contrast high energy/low energy (HE/LE) image sets were obtained (20 seconds, 1 minute 25 seconds, and 3 minutes 25 seconds after injection commencement.) The timing of the post-injection CE-DBT images is based on prior work for breast MRI with multiple post-contrast time points [10]. The breast with the index lesion was then decompressed. Our current technique results in a mean glandular dose of approximately 3.0 mGy per HE/LE image set for a 4.5 cm breast. Current total procedure time is less than 8 minutes.

Table 1. Hologic Prototype CE-DBT system

Target	W
kVp	49 (HE) / 32 (LE)
Filter	Cu (HE) / Al (LE)
SID	70 cm
Detector	3 fps, 2x2 binning
Angular Range	15°
Scan Time	7.3 seconds
Projections	22, 11(HE), 11(LE) interleaved

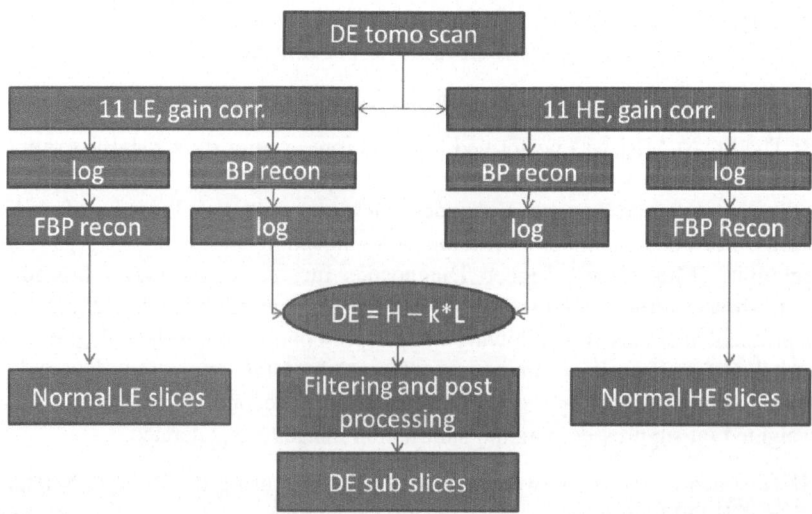

Fig. 1. Dual Energy Processing. FBP = Filtered Back Projection, BP = Back Projection. Source DE tomosynthesis images were post processed per this schematic to create the images for clinical interpretation.

2.2   Image Interpretation

Images were reviewed by a fellowship-trained breast imager. The size of the index lesion (at least the greatest linear dimension) was measured. Findings regarding the margins of the index lesion were recorded using descriptors in the ACR BIRADS lexicon. Vascular enhancement kinetics were assessed and characterized as Persistent, Plateau, or Washout for the index lesion (as per the BI-RADS lexicon[1]).

Ratings on a 10-point scale (10 = best, equivalent to DM) of the conspicuity of margins on CE-DBT relative to DM and on MRI relative to DM were recorded. Similarly, the visibility of any associated microcalcifications on CE-DBT and MRI were separately evaluated relative to DM and recorded.

3   Results

Dual-energy CE-DBT was able to demonstrate the index malignant lesion in 7 of 8 patients (9 of 10 lesions). The one lesion in one patient that was not demonstrated was secondary to a far posterior location of the tumor, which was not an area that could be imaged mammographically (the finding had been detected on physical exam and evaluated with ultrasound).

Morphologic characteristics including margin detail were visualized on CE-DBT. Presence of associated microcalcifications were visualized on CE-DBT processed images in 4/4 lesions with associated microcalcifications. Benign microcalcifications away from the index lesion were visualized and characterized as benign on tomosynthesis images in 1 case. Qualitative concordance with digital mammography was judged to be achieved. Vascular characteristics were identifiable qualitatively on post-processed dual energy subtraction images in 4 cases. Qualitative concordance with breast MRI was judged to be achieved in those cases. (Table 2) (Figures 2 and 3)

4   Discussion

CE-DBT can potentially integrate into one breast imaging tool many of the strengths of existing multimodality imaging while also avoiding some limitations of existing modalities. The unique combination into a single imaging modality of the ability to acquire functional characteristics of breast lesions together with high spatial resolution similar to digital mammography results in a potentially powerful breast imaging tool. An additional strength of CE-DBT lies in the underlying technology of digital breast tomosynthesis (DBT), which circumvents the limitations of two-dimensional projection mammography. DBT is an emerging x-ray based breast imaging technique in which high resolution tomographic images of the breast are obtained at a dose comparable to projection mammography [11, 12]. In clinical trials, DBT provides improved sensitivity and specificity relative to projection mammography[12].

Table 2. Case Summary. For numerical scales, 10 = best, equivalent to DM

Case	Le-sion	Size (mm) ML, SI, AP if available		Margins		Enhancement Kinetics (if available)		Margin conspicuity relative to DM		Microcalcification conspicuity relative to DM	
		CE-DBT	MRI	CE-DBT	MRI	CE-DBT	MRI	CEDBT	MRI	CE-DBT	MRI
1		9 x 5 x 6	14 (AP)	Indistinct, irregular	Irregular	Persistent	Persistent	7	6	-	-
2		24 (SI) x 59 (AP)	50 (AP)	Segmental non-mass like	Segmental non-mass like	Persistent	Persistent	-	-	9	1
3		15 (SI) x 13 (AP)		Spiculated	Spiculated	Not seen	Present, No descriptor reported	10	8	9 (benign)	1
4		Not seen, too far posterior	13 (SI) x 15 (AP)	-	Irregular	Not seen	Present, No descriptor reported	-	7	-	-
5	1	6 x 12	9	Linear	Linear	Not seen	Present, No descriptor reported	-	-	8	1
	2	6 x 13	10	Indistinct, irregular	Irregular, associated non-mass like	Not seen	Avid	10	10	8	1
6	2	24 x 21	25 AP (index)	Spiculated	Spiculated, associated non-mass like	Rapid, persistent	Rapid, persistent	10	8	-	-
7	1	8 x 27	88 x 38 both findings	Calcifications	N/A	Not seen	Present, No descriptor reported	-	-	10	1
	2	9 x 14		Irregular	-	Not seen	Present, No descriptor reported	10	8	-	-
8		20 x 31	23 x 25	Spiculated	Irregular	Rapid washout	Rapid	10	7	-	-

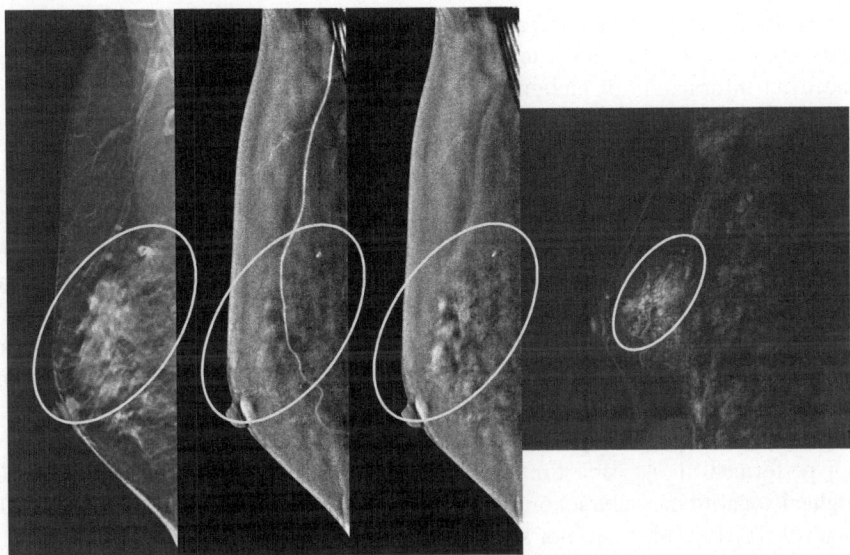

Fig. 2. DCIS. Segmental clumped enhancement in the upper breast. From left to right: Pre-contrast low energy DBT, Post-contrast DE subtraction at 20 s, Post-contrast DE subtraction at 3 m 25 s, and subtraction image from breast MRI at 3 min. Clip at site of prior biopsy.

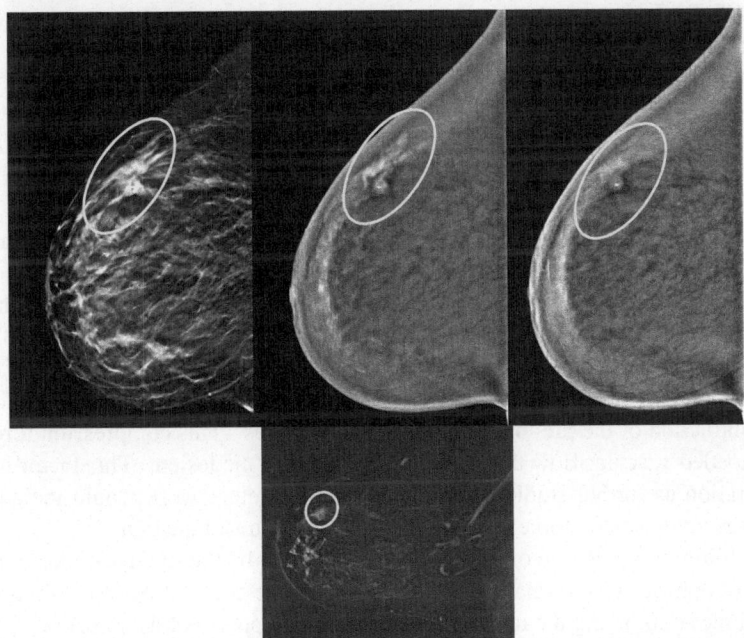

Fig. 3. Invasive ductal carcinoma. Irregular enhancing mass in the upper breast, with washout kinetics. From left to right: Pre-contrast low energy DBT, Post-contrast DE subtraction at 20 s, Post-contrast DE subtraction at 3 m 25 s, and (bottom) subtraction MRI at 3 min.

Early preliminary studies[7] have demonstrated that CE-DBT using an iodinated vascular contrast agent has the potential to demonstrate morphology and vascular enhancement information of malignant breast lesions concordant with that of MRI. A temporal subtraction CE-DBT technique was performed in 13 patients, where one pre- and one or more post-contrast tomosynthesis time-points are acquired using a spectrum beyond the K-edge of iodine (32.3 keV). Logarithmic subtraction yields iodine-enhanced images. In this early pilot group, 11 of 13 patients had malignancy [6 invasive ductal carcinoma; 4 DCIS; and 1 invasive lobular carcinoma]. Suspicious enhancing lesions were demonstrated in 10 of 11 cases of pathology proven breast cancer using this temporal subtraction CE-DBT technique. Also, when present, spiculated margins were more conspicuous on CE-DBT than on breast MRI. Furthermore, one case of breast cancer was initially detected by CE-DBT, and was only demonstrated on MRI on repeat imaging.

Additional early investigations into a dual-energy technique for CE-DBT have been performed[8]. At each time point, iodine-enhanced images are calculated by weighted logarithmic subtraction of the low-energy and high-energy (LE and HE) images[9, 10, 13, 14]. In a pilot study of one patient[8] with a known malignancy, a combined temporal and dual-energy CEDBT technique was performed with a total mean glandular radiation dose within prescribed limits for x-ray breast imaging (6.48mSv for this patient with a breast thickness of 5 cm in compression). In addition to providing morphologic and vascular information about the malignant lesion, dual energy CE-DBT also appeared more resilient to motion artifacts when compared with temporal subtraction CE-DBT in this one case.

Thus, the purpose of the current study was to assess more fully the ability of dual-energy CE-DBT to demonstrate morphologic and vascular characteristics of breast cancer in comparison with breast MRI and digital mammography. Our hypothesis that these features of breast cancers will be demonstrable on CE-DBT images is supported by the qualitative results obtained to date.

One of the technical factors that may have led to nonvisualization of the index lesion is the location of the finding. In one case, the finding was far posterior and could not be visualized on mammographic techniques, as the region could not be included in the image. This is not a limitation that is unique to tomosynthesis or CE-DBT.

Another factor that may have influenced contrast agent uptake is that in this current series, the breast remained in compression for the injection in order to allow for temporal subtraction of the pre image from the post images. This compression force may have impeded vascular flow through the breast and to the lesion. This factor is under consideration as further studies are planned. Thus, future work would include optimizing the compression force used (if any) during contrast injection.

In addition, visualization of uptake may be affected by the timing of image acquisition post-contrast. Either imaging too early or too late could affect this. Future work also includes optimizing the image acquisition timing post contrast injection.

If there were associated microcalcifications, these findings were very well demonstrated on the CE-DBT study. In future work, if vascular enhancement visualization can be optimized, then this would facilitate correlation of any visualized enhancement with the calcifications.

5   Significance and Future Directions

The results from this pilot study support the hypothesis that CE-DBT can demonstrate both high-resolution morphologic features of breast cancers (including microcalcifications) and vascular characteristics that are qualitatively concordant with DM and breast MRI. Additional reader studies are planned. Furthermore, CE-DBT may also theoretically offer quantitative evaluation of contrast uptake and perfusion given the linear relationship between attenuation and contrast-agent concentration. Additional work in this exciting direction is also planned.

This work is supported in part by Grant IRG-78-002-31 from the American Cancer Society, and Grant UL1RR024134 from the National Center For Research Resources.

References

1. American College of Radiology (ACR) BI-RADS® - Mammography. In: ACR BreastImaging Reporting and Data System, Breast Imaging Atlas, 4th edn. American College of Radiology, Reston (2003)
2. Schnall, M., Orel, S.: Breast MR imaging in the diagnostic setting. Magn. Reson Imaging Clin N Am. 14(3), 329–337 (2006)
3. Kaiser, W.A., Zeitler, E.: MR imaging of the breast: fast imaging sequences with and without Gd-DTPA.Preliminary observations. Radiology 170, 681–686 (1989)
4. Morris, E.A.: Breast cancer imaging with MRI. Radiol. Clin North Am. 40(3), 443–466 (2002)
5. Kuhl, C.: The current status of breast MR imaging. Part I. Choice of technique, image interpretation, diagnostic accuracy, and transfer to clinical practice. Radiology 244(2), 356–378 (2007)
6. Kuhl, C.K.: Current status of breast MR imaging. Part 2. Clinical applications. Radiology 244(3), 672–691 (2007)
7. Chen, S.C., Carton, A.K., Albert, M., Conant, E.F., Schnall, M.D., Maidment, A.D.: Initial clinical experience with contrast-enhanced digital breast tomosynthesis. Acad. Radiol. 14(2), 229–238 (2007)
8. Carton, A.K., Gavenonis, S.C., Currivan, J.A., Conant, E.F., Schnall, M.D., Maidment, A.D.: Dual-energy contrastenhanceddigital breast tomosynthesis–a feasibility study. Br. J. Radiol. 83(988), 344–350 (2010)
9. Lewin, J.M., Isaacs, P.K., Vance, V., Larke, F.J.: Dual-energy contrast-enhanced digital subtractionmammography: Feasibility. Radiology 264, 261–268 (2003)
10. Diekmann, F., Freyer, M., Diekmann, S., et al.: Evaluation of contrast-enhanced digital mammography. Eur. J. Radiol. (November 18, 2009)
11. Niklason, L.T., Christian, B.T., Niklason, L.E., et al.: Digital tomosynthesis in breast imaging. Radiology 205(2), 399–406 (1997)
12. Poplack, S.P., Tosteson, T.D., Kogel, C.A., Nagy, H.M.: Digital breast tomosynthesis: initial experience in 98women with abnormal digital screening mammography. AJR Am. J. Roentgenol. 189(3), 616–623 (2007)
13. Diekmann, F., Diekmann, S., Taupitz, M., et al.: Use of iodine-based contrast media in digital full-fieldmammography–initial experience. ROFO-Fortschritte auf dem Gebiet der Rontgenstrahlen und derBildgebenden V 175(3), 342–345 (2003)
14. Dromain, C., Thibault, F., Muller, S., et al.: Dual-energy contrast-enhanced digital mammography: initialclinical results. EurRadiol. Electronic publication September 14 (2010)

Mammographic Segmentation and Risk Classification Using a Novel Binary Model Based Bayes Classifier

Wenda He[1], Erika R.E. Denton[2], and Reyer Zwiggelaar[1]

[1] Department of Computer Science,
Aberystwyth University, Aberystwyth, SY23 3DB, UK
{weh,rrz}@aber.ac.uk
[2] Department of Radiology,
Norfolk & Norwich University Hospital, Norwich NR4 7UY, UK
erika.denton@nnuh.nhs.uk

Abstract. Clinical research has shown that the sensitivity of mammography is significantly reduced by increased breast density, which can mask some tumours due to dense fibroglandular tissue. In addition, there is a clear correlation between the overall breast density and mammographic risk. We present an automatic mammographic density segmentation approach using a novel binary model based Bayes classifier. The Mammographic Image Analysis Society (MIAS) database was used in a quantitative and qualitative evaluation. Visual assessment on the segmentation results indicated a good and consistent extraction of mammographic density. With respect to mammographic risk classification, substantial agreements were found between the classification results and ground truth provided by expert screening radiologists. Classification accuracies were 85% and 78% in Tabár and Breast Imaging Reporting and Data System (Birads) categories, respectively; whilst in the corresponding low and high categories, the classification accuracies were 93% and 88% for Tabár and Birads, respectively.

1 Introduction

Breast cancer is the most common cancer in the UK and across Europe [1]. It has been considered a major health problem, and it is estimated that between one in eight and one in twelve women will develop breast cancer during their lifetime [2]. An evident rise in breast cancer and the lack of understanding of the disease development makes early breast cancer detection crucial. Clinical evidence has indicated a strong correlation between mammographic density and the likelihood of a woman developing breast caner; and the sensitivity of mammography is significantly reduced by increased breast density, which can mask some tumours due to dense fibroglandular tissue. Due to radiologist subjective appraisal of mammograms, automatic mammographic risk assessment is expected to play a significant role in the development of breast screening programs and computer

A.D.A. Maidment, P.R. Bakic, and S. Gavenonis (Eds.): IWDM 2012, LNCS 7361, pp. 40–47, 2012.
© Springer-Verlag Berlin Heidelberg 2012

aided mammography, in order to reduce inter and intra observer variability in risk classification.

Using mammographic parenchymal patterns, Tabár *et al.* have proposed a mammographic modelling scheme based on mixtures of four building blocks composing the normal breast anatomy (i.e. nodular, linear, homogeneous and radiolucent). Nodular densities mainly corresponds to Terminal Ductal Lobular Units (TDLU); linear densities correspond to either ducts, fibrous or blood vessels; homogeneous densities correspond to fibrous tissue which appears as bright areas in mammographic images, hides the underlying normal TDLU, ducts and their alterations; radiolucent areas are related to adipose fatty tissue which appears as dark areas in mammographic images [3]. Wolfe [4] used different mammographic parenchymal patterns to divide mammograms into four risk classes. Strongly influenced by such a modelling approach, Boyd *et al.* [5] developed a method to measure percentage mammographic densities using a computer-aided technique, and divided mammograms into six categories.

In mammographic risk assessment, inter and intra observer variability are introduced due to radiologist's subjective appraisal of mammograms. To standardise mammography reporting, and to reduce confusion in breast imaging interpretations, the American College of Radiology's Breast Imaging Reporting and Data System (Birads) [6] was developed as a quality assurance tool, covers the significant relationship between increased breast density and decreased mammographic sensitivity in detecting cancer [7]. Mammographic breast composition is categorised into four patterns: 1) Birads I, the breast is almost entirely fat ($< 25\%$ glandular); 2) Birads II, the breast has scattered fibroglandular densities ($25\% - 50\%$); 3) Birads III, the breast consists of heterogeneously dense breast tissue ($51\% - 75\%$); and 4) Birads IV, the breast is extremely dense ($> 75\%$ glandular). Such a quantitative measure suggests the use of an accurate and repeatable mammographic density segmentation technique, to perform automatic mammographic risk assessment, and allows quantification of change in the relative proportion of dense breast tissue [3]. Fig. 1 shows example mammographic images.

Various methods have been investigated to perform mammographic density segmentation. Early research [8,9,10] focused on estimating parameters for statistical models, which were subsequently used to segment the fibroglandular tissue. Such approaches led to more sophisticated model parameter estimation, based on detailed knowledge of the mammographic system and the imaging parameters, which is refereed to as the Standard Mammogram Form (SMF) [11]. Grey-level histogram information [12,13], and texture features [14,15] are commonly used for mammographic segmentation and risk classification. A statistical based texton technique [16] was employed to model the whole mammogram; and the statistical distributions over a texton dictionary (histogram information) was used as basis for mammographic risk classification. Texture features were directly extracted from mammographic images in [17], and the ratio of segmented fatty and dense breast tissue were used for automatic classification of breast density.

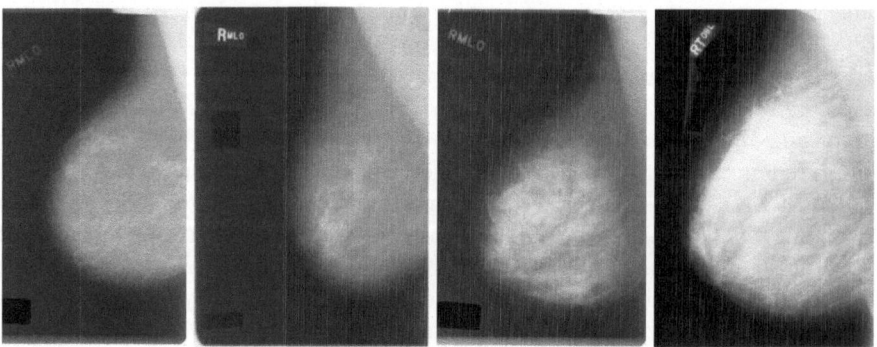

Fig. 1. Mammographic images with respect to Birads risk classification. From left to right showing Birads I-IV, corresponding from low to high mammographic risk.

This paper investigates mammographic density segmentation using texture features derived from grey-level histograms, and a novel binary model matching pattern based Bayes classifier. The extracted texture features contain not only periodic aspect but also spatial and geometric information; which are expected to be rich and discriminative for glandular tissue with distinct characteristics. The developed method was quantitatively evaluated, and the Mammographic Image Analysis Society (MIAS) database [18] was used to facilitate the experiment.

2   Data and Method

The MIAS database contains 321 available images (file mdb295ll is excluded for historical reasons). A total of 643 mammographic patches (199 nodular, 253 linear, 70 homogeneous and 121 radiolucent) were subsampled from randomly selected mammograms by an expert mammographic screening radiologist. The collection of the patches consists of representative Tabár's mammographic building block samples, covering various sizes of anatomical structures, densities and risk categories. In addition, for 136 mammographic patches, tissue specific regions were annotated in detail.

The proposed method can be broken down into the following stages: 1) breast tissue feature extraction, 2) mammographic building block model generation, 3) building a binary model based Bayes classifier, 4) mammographic segmentation, and 5) mammographic risk classification.

To extract texture features of various mammographic building blocks, four sets (i.e. nodular, linear, homogeneous and radiolucent) of mammographic patches containing tissue specific samples were used, regardless of the associated risk class for the original mammograms. As a multi-resolution approach, a set of square windows (i.e. 41, 31 and 21 pixels) were used to compute local texture features. The window sizes were determined using local patches, based on a range of breast anatomical structures (*e.g.* from large to small structures) and Fourier analysis. For each pixel, three grey-level histograms are constructed; the number of bins were empirically defined as 250, 150 and 50, respectively. For each histogram, 11 histogram features are computed to encode various texture features: contrast C, energy E_1, skewness S, kurtosis K, entropy E_2, homogeneity H, standard deviation SD, and moments up to the fourth order $M_{1,2,3,4}$. Therefore, with respect to a histogram bin configuration, a feature vector of 33 dimensions (11 features × 3 resolutions) is generated. The feature extraction resulted in a total of 12 sets of feature vectors (4 tissue types × 3 histogram bin configurations). Note that for each type of tissues, about 5,000,000 pixels were randomly sampled.

The resultant feature vectors were fed into K-means clustering to group similar texture features as a means of establishing mammographic building block models. This clustering processing is performed over the feature vectors generated for one mammographic building block and one of the three histogram bin configurations, at a time. Empirical testing on the detail annotated mammographic patch segmentation and visual assessment on the correctness of the segmentation, indicated that the optimal number of cluster centres for nodular, linear, homogeneous and radiolucent tissue types were 3, 5, 2, and 7, respectively. This resulted in a total of 9, 15, 6, and 21 models for the four mammographic building blocks, respectively.

At the stage of building the binary model based Bayes classifier, the mammographic building blocks were separated into three groups based on the density characteristics, where linear and radiolucent tissue are considered non-dense tissue, and nodular and homogeneous tissue are considered semi-dense and dense tissue, respectively. To build the classifier, four sets of mammographic patches with detail annotations were used. The same feature extraction was applied to each pixel of a specific mammographic building block; the resultant feature vector is compared with the learnt tissue models, using the nearest neighbour methodology. The similarity comparison was performed with the tissue models associated with one histogram bin configuration at a time. The closest match mammographic building block is labelled as a binary value 1, or otherwise 0. This process generates a binary pattern (see Fig. 2 for example). The three binary codes are converted to the corresponding decimal numbers to facilitate building the classifier. In particular, the counts of these decimal values are allocated into three look up tables (LUTs) for dense, semi-dense and non-dense tissue, respectively. The size of such a look up table is defined as 9 (possible decimal values for three digits binary

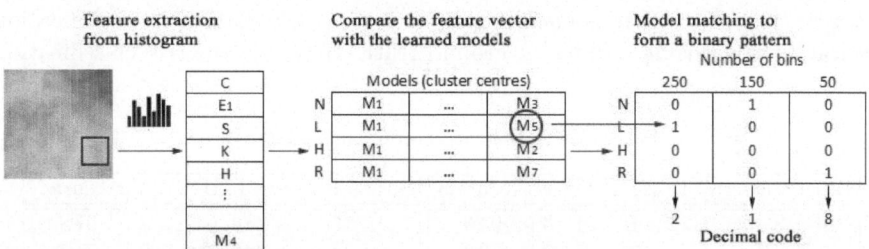

Fig. 2. Example binary model pattern. N, L, H and R denote nodular, linear, homogeneous and radiolucent, respectively.

code) $\times$ 9 $\times$ 9 bins. The dense (i.e. homogeneous), semi-dense (i.e. nodular) and non-dense (i.e. linear and radiolucent) tissue prior probabilities are calculated as: $nPixels = nPixels(tissue) + nPixels(\neg tissue)$, $priorProbability(tissue) = \frac{nPixels(tissue)}{nPixels}$, $priorProbability(\neg tissue) = \frac{nPixels(\neg tissue)}{nPixels}$; where '$nPixels$' indicates number of total pixels of a specific (*e.g.* homogeneous) and other types of tissue (*e.g.* nodular, linear and radiolucent). The probabilities for a particular tissue belonging to a specific tissue and non-tissue classes are calculated as: $probability(D_{1,2,3}|tissue) = \frac{nPixels(tissue)[D_{1,2,3}]}{nPixels(tissue)}$, $probability(D_{1,2,3}|\neg tissue) = \frac{nPixels(\neg tissue)[D_{1,2,3}]}{nPixels(\neg tissue)}$; where $D_{1,2,3}$ indicate the converted decimal values. The mammographic segmentation process is straightforward, where tissue class of an unseen pixel is determined by calculating the probability of it being one of the four mammographic building blocks; it is labelled to the observed tissue class where the probability is the highest. The tissue probability is calculated as: $A = LUTs(tissue)[D_1][D_2][D_3] \times priorProbability(tissue)$, $B = LUTs(\neg tissue)[D_1][D_2][D_3] \times priorProbability(\neg tissue)$, $tissueProbablity = \frac{A}{A+B}$. The relative proportions of dense, semi-dense and non-dense tissue were calculated from the resultant mammographic segmentation; and mammographic risk classification was performed using the derived tissue proportions and leave-one (woman)-out methodology.

3   Results

All the available images in the MIAS database were used in the evaluation. Example mammographic segmentation is shown in Fig. 3. Tab. 1 (left) shows classification accuracies for discriminating between Tabár's categories. Total accuracy was 85%, whilst the accuracy for the corresponding low (Tabár I and II/III) and high (Tabár IV and VI) category was 93%. To avoid bias and determine the robustness of the classifier, we also performed classification based on Birads categories. Classification results as seen in Tab. 1 (right), were in 78% and 88% accuracies for Birads four categories, and the corresponding low and high category, respectively. Note that the ground truth used is based on the majority risk classification rated by three expert radiologists; when using an alternative ground truth based on an expert screen radiologist, the accuracies achieved in 74% and 87% for Birads four categories, and the corresponding low and high category, respectively. It is encouraging to see small variances in classification accuracies when using a different ground truth. However, the risk classification

Table 1. Classification confusion matrices

Tabár Pattern	I	II/III	IV	V	Accuracy	Birads Pattern	I	II	III	IV	Accuracy
I	112	0	4	3	94%	I	84	0	1	2	97%
II/III	14	74	5	0	80%	II	13	73	17	0	71%
IV	7	1	70	3	80%	III	0	17	73	4	78%
V	1	0	9	18	64%	IV	0	2	12	23	62%

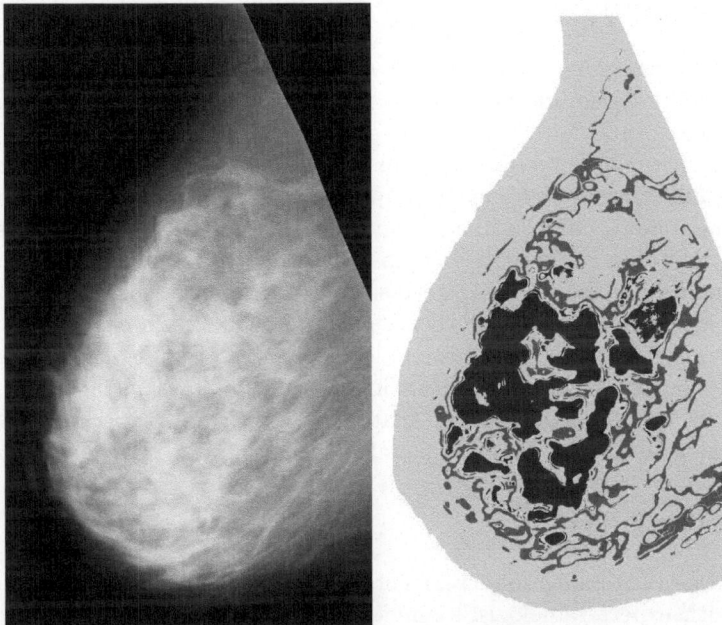

Fig. 3. Example segmentation (mdb108rl); non-dense, semi-dense and dense tissue are colour coded yellow, red and blue, respectively

performance seems to be better when using the ground truth based on Tabár's risk scheme. This may due to the training mammographic pathes containing tissue specific structures (i.e. mammographic building blocks) were subsampled based on Tabár's scheme. Visual assessment indicated that radiolucent tissue models may be over trained. The number of models for homogeneous type of tissue is relatively less than other types of mammographic building blocks, which may reflect that homogeneous tissue is less represented in the segmentation. Note that the numbers of Tabár V and Birads IV are relatively low.

4   Discussion

The prior knowledge of probabilities to be a tissue and non-tissue pixel can be constructed to serve as our best estimation, provided the number of sampling pixels is large enough. In our case the number of pixel sampled for each type of tissue was about 1,000,000, which seems to be sufficient to build a statistically meaningful classifier. At the same time, an unbalanced number of training samples can lead to under or over training, which should be avoided.

All the patches were normalised to zero mean and unit variance during the training stage to reduce intensity distribution variance (*e.g.* contrast and brightness). This process can potentially alter inter and intra class variation, which makes it difficult to draw decision lines in the feature space; a poorly separated decision space can lead to unsatisfactory segmentation results when using a model driven segmentation. The use of binary model as basis of the classifier is a probability based approach, which seems to be robust in dealing with inter and intra class variation.

The number of annotated regions for nodular is relatively small, and may not cover the full range of anatomical samples; therefore it may not be adequate to be a strong training dataset. In addition, visual inspection indicated that some of the annotated data is less precise which may be related to hand tremor and other limitations during the manual process; as a consequence the annotation data contains artifacts and noise which are not beneficial for the feature extraction and the subsequent model generation, leading to incorrect segmentation.

Future work will focus on algorithm improvement (*e.g.* using balanced training data across various densities and anatomical structures, experimenting other feature extraction technique) and possible evaluation in a clinical environment.

5   Conclusions

The developed mammographic segmentation has shown anatomically consistent results with expert radiologist's annotations. All the available images in the MIAS database were used in the evaluation based on both Tabár and Birads risk categories. Strong correlations were found between the classification results. The total classification accuracies were 93% and 85% in Tabár's categories and the corresponding low and high category, respectively; 88% and 78% accuracies in Birads categories and the corresponding low and high category, respectively. The novelty aspect and primary finding of this study are: 1) using a novel binary model matching pattern as basis to train a Bayes classifier and 2) the developed probability based classifier is robust in dealing with inter and intra class variation. The initial segmentation results are promising; the developed method can be found useful in quantification of change of relative proportion of dense tissue, as means of aiding radiologists' estimation in mammographic risk assessment.

References

1. Office for National Statistics. Cancer statistics registrations: Registrations of cancer diagnosed in 2007, england. MB1(38) (2010)
2. Bray, F., McCarron, P., Parkin, D.M.: The changing global patterns of female breast cancer incidence and mortality. Breast Cancer Research 6(6), 229–239 (2004)
3. Tabár, L., Tot, T., Dean, P.B.: Breast Cancer: The Art And Science Of Early Detection With Mamography: Perception, Interpretation, Histopatholigic Correlation, 1st edn., December 16. Georg Thieme Verlag (2004)
4. Wolfe, J.N.: Risk for breast cancer development determind by mammographic parenchymal pattern. Cancer 37(5), 2486–2492 (1976)
5. Boyd, N.F., Byng, J.W., Jong, R.A., Fishell, E.K., Little, L.E., Miller, A.B., Lockwood, G.A., Tritchler, D.L., Yaffe, M.J.: Quantitative classification of mammographic densities and breast cancer risk: results from the canadian national breast screening study. Journal of the National Cancer Institute 87, 670–675 (1995)

6. American College of Radiology. Breast Imaging Reporting and Data System BI-RADS, 4th edn. American College of Radiology, Reston (2004)
7. Sickles, E.A.: Wolfe mammographic parenchymal patterns and breast cancer risk. American Journal of Roentgenology 188(2), 301–303 (2007)
8. Aylward, S.R., Hemminger, B.M., Pisano, E.D.: Mixture modeling for digital mammogram display and analysis. In: The 4th International Workshop on Digital Mammography, pp. 305–312. Kulwer Academic Publishers (1998)
9. Ferrari, R.J., Rangayyan, R.M., Borges, R.A., Frère, A.F.: Segmentation of the fibro-glandular disc in mammograms using gaussian mixture modelling. Medical & Biological Engineering & Computing 42(3), 378–387 (2004)
10. Selvan, S.E., Xavier, C.C., Karssemeijer, N., Sequeira, J., Cherian, R.A., Dhala, B.Y.: Parameter estimation in stochastic mammogram model by heuristic optimization techniques. IEEE Transactions on Information Technology in Biomedicine, 685–695 (2006)
11. Highnam, R., Brady, M.: Mammographic Image Analysis. Kluwer Academic Publishers, London (1999)
12. Oliver, A., Freixenet, J., Zwiggelaar, R.: Automatic classification of breast density. In: Proceedings of the 2005 International Conference on Image Processing, vol. 2, pp. 1258–1261 (2005)
13. Zwiggelaar, R., Denton, E.R.E.: Mammographic risk assessment and local greylevel appearance histograms. In: 10th International Conference on Information Technology and Applications in Biomedicine, p. 1 (2010)
14. Marias, K., Petroudi, S., English, R., Adams, R., Brady, M.: Subjective and computer-based characterisation ofmammographic patterns. In: The 6th International Workshop on Digital Mammography, pp. 552–556 (2002)
15. Petroudi, S., Marias, K., English, R., Brady, M.: Classification of mammogram patterns using area measurements and the standard mammogram form (smf). In: Medical Image Analysis and Understanding, pp. 197–200 (2002)
16. Petroudi, S., Kadir, T., Brady, M.: Automatic classification of mammographic parenchymal patterns: A statistical approach. In: Engineering in Medicine and Biology Society, vol. 1, pp. 798–801 (2003)
17. Oliver, A., Freixenet, J., Marti, R., Pont, J., Perez, E., Denton, E.R.E., Zwiggelaar, R.: A novel breast tissue density classification framework. Information Technology in BioMedicine 12, 55–65 (2008)
18. Suckling, J., Parker, J., Dance, D., Astley, S., Hutt, I., Boggis, C., Ricketts, I., Stamatakis, E., Cerneaz, N., Kok, S., Taylor, P., Betal, D., Savage, J.: The mammographic images analysis society digital mammogram database. In: Dance, Gale, Astley, Gairns (eds.) Excerpta Medica. International Congress Series, vol. 1069, pp. 375–378. Elsevier (1994)

Intensity-Based MRI to X-ray Mammography Registration with an Integrated Fast Biomechanical Transformation

Thomy Mertzanidou[1], John H. Hipwell[1], Lianghao Han[1], Zeike Taylor[2],
Henkjan Huisman[3], Ulrich Bick[4], Nico Karssemeijer[3], and David J. Hawkes[1]

[1] Centre for Medical Image Computing, University College London,
Gower Street, WC1E 6BT London, UK
[2] Department of Mechanical Engineering, The University of Sheffield,
Mappin Street, S1 3JD Sheffield, UK
[3] Diagnostic Image Analysis Group, Radboud University Nijmegen Medical Centre,
P.O. Box 9102, 6500 HC Nijmegen, The Netherlands
[4] Department of Radiology, Charite Universitätsmedizin Berlin,
10117 Berlin, Germany
t.mertzanidou@cs.ucl.ac.uk

Abstract. Determining MRI to X-ray mammography correspondence is a clinically useful task that is challenging for radiologists due to the large deformation that the breast undergoes. In this work we propose an intensity-based registration framework with a new integrated transformation module that uses a biomechanical model of the breast in order to simulate the mammographic compression. The breast model is patient-specific and is extracted from the MRI of the patient. The transformation model has seven degrees of freedom and uses a fast explicit Finite Element (FE) solver that runs on the graphics card, enabling it to be fully integrated into the optimisation scheme. The iteratively updated parameters include both parameters of the biomechanical model simulation, and also rigid transformation parameters of the breast geometry model. The framework was tested on five clinical cases. The mean registration error was $7.6 \pm 2.4mm$ for the CC and $10.2 \pm 2.3mm$ for the MLO view registrations, indicating that this could be a useful clinical tool.

Keywords: multimodal registration, 2D/3D registration, FEM-based transformation model.

1 Introduction

MRI is often used as a complementary modality to X-ray mammography to investigate symptomatic patients and women with dense breasts. However, identifying corresponding regions can be problematic, due to the differences in image appearance and the large breast deformation between the two modalities. Women are lying prone in the MR scanner with their breasts pendulous, while during X-ray mammography acquisition women are standing with their breast compressed

A.D.A. Maidment, P.R. Bakic, and S. Gavenonis (Eds.): IWDM 2012, LNCS 7361, pp. 48–55, 2012.
© Springer-Verlag Berlin Heidelberg 2012

between two plates. There are typically two images acquired, one Cradio-Caudal (CC) and one Medio-Lateral Oblique (MLO) view. An automated MRI to X-ray registration algorithm would be a valuable tool that could help radiologists in the diagnosis and management of breast cancer.

Previously, authors have used feature-based techniques for this task ([1], [2]). However these cannot be easily integrated into clinical practice, as the robust selection of corresponding, distinctive features from both breast MR and X-ray images remains unresolved. In addition the possibility of mismatched features can lead to the need for impractical, manual interaction.

A patient-specific FE modelling approach that simulates mammographic compression was proposed by Ruiter et al. [3]. This implementation used the breast outline for alignment and applied displacements on the breast surface in two stages: once in the direction of the projection to match the chest wall to nipple distance and once in the perpendicular direction to account for the anisotropic behaviour of the breast and match the breast outline. More recently, a FEM-based approach with a contact model was proposed [4]. This employed an iterative intensity-based registration framework. However, the updated parameters were limited to the degree of compression and the 2D rotation of the simulated mammogram.

We have previously investigated the performance of an intensity-based framework using simpler transformation models, such as an affine transformation [5] and a statistical deformation model learnt from biomechanical simulations [6]. In this work, we are using the same iterative optimisation framework with a new patient-specific FEM-based transformation model.

The original contribution of our technique, compared to other approaches that used biomechanical modelling for the same application, is the use of an intensity-based registration framework with an iterative update of both the model parameters and the rigid transformation parameters. This is enabled by the use of an integrated transformation module that runs on the Graphics Processing Unit (GPU) [7], providing shorter execution times than commercial packages.

2 Methodology

In our method, patient-specific biomechanical models are built from the pre-contrast MRI of the subject. Initially, we segment the breast volume from the background using a simple region-growing algorithm and then apply Gaussian smoothing and downsample the extracted binary mask to an isotropic volume of $10mm$ resolution, to produce smooth meshes and reduce the computational cost of the FE solver. The surface mesh is extracted using a VTK implementation of the marching cubes algorithm and the tetrahedral elements are extracted using the opensource software package TetGen[1]. A typical breast model of the five used in this study consists of around $2,500$ elements and 800 nodes.

We are using a nearly incompressible and hyperelastic neo-Hookean model for modelling [8]. This is transversely isotropic, to account for the reinforcement of

---

[1] http://tetgen.berlios.de/

biomechanical properties from fiber-like connective tissues in a preferred direction that was previously observed [9]. We simulate the plate compression using a frictionless contact model and we approximate the position of the pectoral muscle nodes to lie on a plane, constraining their movement to be planar.

The transformation model consists of seven parameters which are iteratively updated during registration. Four of these account for the positioning of the breast before compression. More specifically these are:

- Two translations within the plane perpendicular to the direction of the projection
- Two rotations, one for the rotation of the breast about the anterior-posterior axis (rolling) and one about the superior-inferior axis (in-plane rotation).

The remaining three transformation parameters control the material properties and the compression simulation of the FEM deformation. These are:

- Amount of compression - constrained between: no compression (0%) and 90% of the maximum distance between the nodes in the direction of the projection
- Ratio of tissue enhancement coefficient - constrained between $[0-512]$ (range taken from the literature [9])
- Poisson's ratio - constrained between 0.45 and 0.499

The compression is simulated using the same amount of displacement for both compression plates. The optimised parameter is the distance between the two plates. We assume that the breast tissue is homogeneous with Young's modulus $4kPa$.

Before registration, the MRI intensities are transformed to X-ray attenuation using the methodology described in [5]. This new volume and the real X-ray mammogram are the inputs to the registration pipeline. The breast volume is positioned above the detector and the distance between the X-ray source and the detector is fixed and extracted from the DICOM file of the mammogram ($f = 660mm$). The initial translation parameters are set such that the centre of mass of the volume is projected onto the centre of mass of the real mammogram. This provides a good initial position for registration, which is important for the optimisation scheme in order to converge to a global minimum. The rotation parameters are initialised to 0°for the CC view mammogram registrations, while for the MLO view the roll is set to 45°, to account for the different direction of the projection, and the in-plane rotation is set to 30°, as the breast in MLO view mammograms appears to have an in-plane rotation.

To avoid resampling the 3D volume into the transformed position and then ray-casting using this new volume grid, the transformation is performed as the ray transverses the 3D grid of the undeformed, moving volume. More specifically, during the registration process we use ray-casting from the 2D target space through the 3D grid of the moving image and integrate the intensities of each transformed intersection of the ray with the 3D grid. For a point x_i, which is the intersection of the ray with the volume grid of the moving image, the transformation is given by the equation:

$$T(x_i) = T_{2rigid}(T_{non-rigid}(T_{1rigid}(x_i)))$$ (1)

where $T_{1rigid}(x_i) = T_{translation}(R_{in-plane}(x_i))$ and $T_{2rigid}(x_i) = R_{rolling}(x_i)$. The non-rigid transformation $T_{non-rigid}$ is the interpolated displacement at the current position x_i and is computed by the FE solver at the current parameter position.

The geometry of the model is stored in an *xml* file, which is used as an additional input into the registration pipeline. The optimised parameters are part of a transformation module that is integrated in the Insight Toolkit [10], without requiring the geometry model to be reloaded at each iteration of the algorithm. This implementation also provides the flexibility to use different similarity measures and optimisation techniques.

At each iteration the model is transformed using a rigid transformation and an FE compression simulation and it is projected into 2D using a perspective ray-casting projection. The similarity measure used is normalised cross correlation and the optimisation scheme is hill climbing. The value of each parameter p at iteration i is given by:

$$p^i = p^{i-1} \pm \frac{step}{w(p)}$$ (2)

where $w(p)$ is a scalar weight factor that controls the relative magnitude of the step size *step* for each parameter. At each iteration one parameter is updated, that which results in the largest increase of the similarity measure, at the current relative step size. The parameter p_i is updated only if the similarity increases and the *step* is decreased if the similarity does not improve using the current parameters.

In our current implementation the algorithm requires approximately 2 hours for each registration, on a single core, 64-bit machine, with a 2.8GHz processor. A typical registration task converges usually within 30 iterations (approximately 450 simulations). The performance can be further optimised to include a GPU implementation of the ray-casting algorithm.

3   Experiments

For validation, we used clinical data from five patients. The MR images of two cases had a voxel size of $[0.7 \times 0.7 \times 1.3]mm^3$, two had $[0.7 \times 0.7 \times 2]mm^3$ and one had $[0.9 \times 0.9 \times 1]mm^3$. The X-ray mammograms of three patients had pixel size $[0.1 \times 0.1]mm^2$, one had $[0.07 \times 0.07]mm^2$ and one $[0.08 \times 0.08]mm^2$. All mammograms were resampled by a factor of 10 for registration, to reduce the computational cost of the ray-casting and more closely match the MRI resolution.

Three of the above patients had lesions visible in both the MRIs and in the CC and MLO view mammograms. The annotations of these lesions were used as ground truth correspondences between the modalities. The other two patients had an MRI and X-ray compatible clip that was used as a known corresponding point.

For each registration, the error was calculated as the 2D Euclidean distance between the centre of mass of the annotation/clip position in the X-ray mammogram and the centre of mass of the MRI annotation/clip position projected into 2D at the final registration position. We consider this metric more appropriate than an overlap measure for our application, as the size of the annotations can vary significantly both between different patient pathologies and between the two modalities, since they measure different physical properties of the tissue.

The registration results for all cases are shown in Table 1, where our approach is compared against an affine transformation [5]. For the CC view the FEM transformation performs better with a mean error of $7.6 \pm 2.4mm$, compared to $13 \pm 7.1mm$ of the affine, while for the MLO view the mean error ($10.2 \pm 2.3mm$) is comparable to the affine transformation ($11 \pm 4.7mm$). We can also see that the variance of the registration error is smaller for our FEM-based transformation model than the affine, showing that the performance of this technique is more consistent. Example registration results are shown for two patients with annotations in Figure 1 and the two patients with clips in Figure 2.

Table 1. Registration error (in mm) of our FEM transformation method and comparison with an affine transformation [5]. The clip cases are patients p4 and p5.

	p1	p2	p3	p4	p5	mean	std
FEM CC	8.0	6.8	7.2	4.8	11.4	7.6	2.4
Affine CC	14.6	13.5	3.7	9.9	23.4	13.0	7.1
FEM MLO	12.2	11.5	10.3	11.1	6.2	10.2	2.3
Affine MLO	11.9	7.2	9.4	7.7	18.9	11.0	4.7

4   Discussion

In Figure 1 it is clear that the two modalities can give different estimates of the lesion size. In general, the projections of the MRI annotations appear larger than the ones on the X-ray images. This difference can be partially explained by the fact that the two modalities measure different physical properties of the tissue and also by the effect of the manual annotations, which are generally harder to perform accurately for 3D structures. Moreover, when the lesions are deformed during registration, their radius can be reduced in the direction of the projection and consequently increased in the perpendicular plane. This is expected since we are using a homogeneous material for the FEM simulations and therefore the lesions are not modelled as rigid structures.

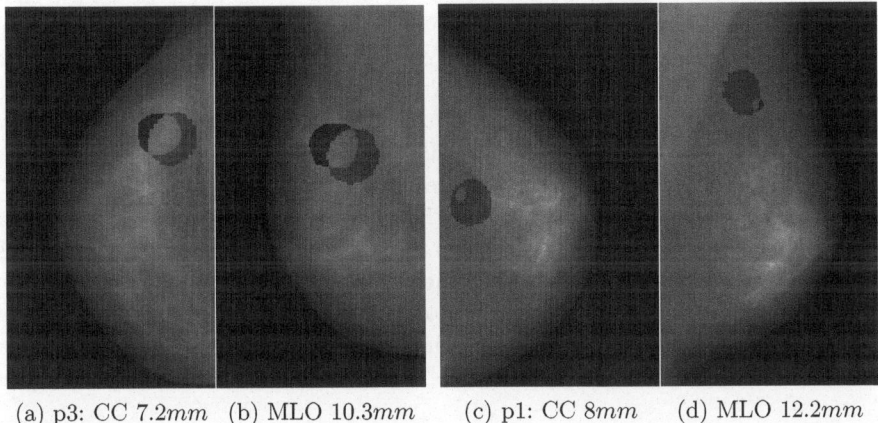

(a) p3: CC 7.2*mm*   (b) MLO 10.3*mm*   (c) p1: CC 8*mm*   (d) MLO 12.2*mm*

Fig. 1. Registration results for two patients, p1 and p3. The X-ray annotation is shown in red and the projection of the MR annotation in green; their overlap is yellow. Inevitably each modality can give different estimates of lesion size, but all cases show overlap.

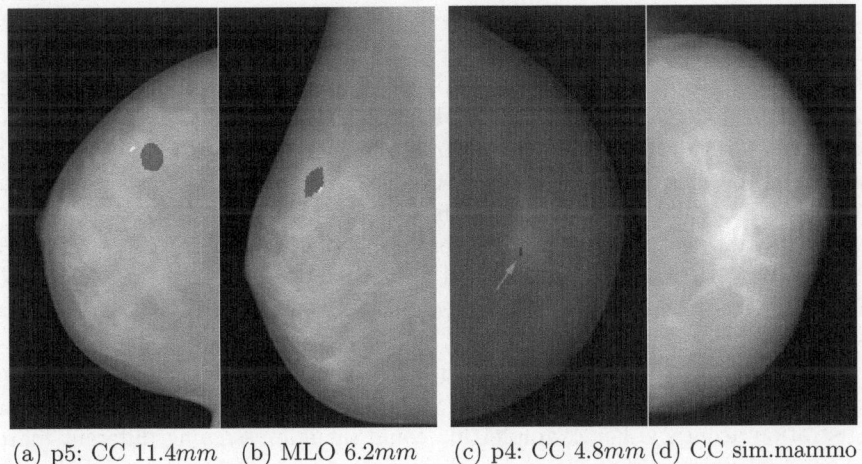

(a) p5: CC 11.4*mm*   (b) MLO 6.2*mm*   (c) p4: CC 4.8*mm* (d) CC sim.mammo

Fig. 2. Registration results for the two patients with MR and X-ray compatible clips, p4 and p5. The clip location on the X-ray mammogram is visible as the high intensity region (and a red arrow for p4). The MR annotation is shown in green. For the patient p4 we also show the simulated CC X-ray mammogram (d).

Table 1 shows that our proposed FEM-based transformation model is less accurate for the MLO than the CC view registrations. One factor that might have contributed to this difference is our modelling of the pectoral muscle that is currently approximated with a plane. As the effect of the pectoral muscle is larger for the MLO view, we expect our approximation to be less accurate for these registrations than for the ones of the CC view mammograms. Also the muscle is excluded from the simulation but is visible in the mammogram. Further validation tests on a larger data set will show whether there is a significant difference in the algorithm's performance between the two views.

Compared to other patient-specific FEM-based methods used for this task, quantitative results on clinical cases showed a mean error of 4.3mm on 6 cases [3], and in a more recent semi-automated implementation of the same approach 11.8±6.5mm on CC view mammograms of 11 patients [11]. However, meaningful comparison is not possible unless an algorithm could be tested on the same data sets. We would welcome the opportunity to do this on a common data set.

5   Conclusion

We have presented a framework for an intensity-based MRI to X-ray mammography registration using a novel iteratively updated FEM breast compression simulation. The results on five clinical data sets indicate that this could be a useful tool and potential aid to breast cancer detection and diagnosis.

We believe that the proposed method, in which we simultaneously optimise both the pose, via four degrees of freedom, and the biomechanical model parameters, via a further three degrees of freedom, provides the most physically realistic transformation model to date, for this application. In addition, incorporating this transformation model into an intensity-based registration framework, maximises the amount of information used by the optimisation, increasing the likelihood of the correct transformation being obtained.

The only interactive step of the current implementation is the pectoral muscle segmentation. However automated methods exist [12], which could be incorporated into our method, to create a fully-automated pipeline suitable for clinical use.

Finally, future work includes further validation on a larger data set and investigation of the effect that a more accurate modelling of the breast has on the registration accuracy. For example this could include assigning different material properties to the fibro-glandular, the adipose tissue, the tumour and the skin and also precise modelling of the boundary between the pectoral muscle and the breast.

Acknowledgements. This work was funded by the European 7th Framework Program, HAMAM, ICT-2007.5.3. The authors would like to thank the Radboud University Nijmegen Medical Centre for the MRI and X-ray mammography data with annotations and the Charite Universitätsmedizin Berlin for the clip cases used in this study.

References

1. Behrenbruch, C., Marias, K., Armitage, P., Moore, N., English, R., Clarke, J., Brady, M.: Fusion of contrast-enhanced breast MR and mammographic imaging data. Medical Image Analysis 7, 311–340 (2003)
2. Marti, R., Zwiggelaar, R., Rubin, C., Denton, E.: 2D-3D correspondence in mammography. Cybernetics and Systems 35, 85–105 (2004)
3. Ruiter, N., Stotzka, R., Muller, T., Gemmeke, H., Reichenbach, J., Kaiser, W.: Model-Based registration of X-ray Mammograms and MR images of the female breast. IEEE Transactions on Nuclear Science 53, 204–211 (2006)
4. Lee, A., Rajagopal, V., Reynolds, H., Doyle, A., Nielsen, P., Nash, M.: Breast X-ray and MR image fusion using Finite Element Modeling. In: MICCAI Workshop on Breast Image Analysis, pp. 129–136 (2011)
5. Mertzanidou, T., Hipwell, J., Cardoso, M., Zhang, X., Tanner, C., Ourselin, S., Bick, U., Huisman, H., Karssemeijer, N., Hawkes, D.: MRI to X-ray mammography registration using a volume-preserving affine transformation. Medical Image Analysis (in press, 2012)
6. Mertzanidou, T., Hipwell, J., Han, L., Huisman, H., Karssemeijer, N., Hawkes, D.: MRI to X-ray mammography registration using an ellipsoidal breast model and biomechanically simulated compressions. In: MICCAI Workshop on Breast Image Analysis, pp. 161–168 (2011)
7. Taylor, Z., Comas, O., Cheng, M., Passenger, J., Hawkes, D., Atkinson, D., Ourselin, S.: On modelling of anisotropic viscoelasticity for soft tissue simulation: Numerical solution and GPU execution. Medical Image Analysis 13, 234–244 (2009)
8. Han, L., Hipwell, J., Tanner, C., Taylor, Z., Mertzanidou, T., Ourselin, S., Hawkes, D.: Development of patient-specifc biomechanical models for predicting large breast deformation. Physics in Medicine and Biology 57, 455–472 (2012)
9. Tanner, C., White, M., Guarino, S., Hall-Craggs, M., Douek, M., Hawkes, D.: Large breast compressions – Observations and evaluation of simulations. Medical Physics 38, 682–690 (2011)
10. The Insight Segmentation and Registration Toolkit (ITK), http://www.itk.org
11. Hopp, T., Baltzer, P., Dietzel, M., Kaiser, W., Ruiter, N.: 2D/3D image fusion of X-ray mammograms with breast MRI: visualizing dynamic contrast enhancement in mammograms. Int. Journal of Computer Assisted Radiology and Surgery (2011) (in press)
12. Gubern-Merida, A., Kallenberg, M., Marti, R., Karssemeijer, N.: Fully automatic fibroglandular tissue segmentation in breast MRI: atlas-based approach. In: MICCAI Workshop on Breast Image Analysis, pp. 73–80 (2011)

Comparison of Experimental, MANTIS, and hybridMANTIS X-ray Response for a Breast Imaging CsI Detector

Diksha Sharma* and Aldo Badano

Division of Imaging and Applied Mathematics,
Center for Devices and Radiological Health, Food and Drug Administration,
10903 New Hampshire Ave, Silver Spring, MD 20993 USA
{diksha.sharma,aldo.badano}@fda.hhs.gov

Abstract. Simulations have become a very important tool in studying the details of the physical processes underlying imaging systems. With the current generation of many-core computer architectures, it has become possible to have realistic simulations in reasonable computing times. In this work, we briefly describe hybridMANTIS, a fast Monte Carlo tool for simulating indirect x-ray detectors that uses a hybrid approach to maximize the utilization of CPUs and GPUs in a workstation. hybridMANTIS is based on the MANTIS code with an improved geometrical model. Moreover, hybridMANTIS can run on GPUs for maximum computational efficiency. We compare hybridMANTIS results on point response and modulation transfer function for a CsI scintillator screen against experimental and MANTIS results. For quantitative analysis, we calculate the root mean square (RMS) difference and Swank factors for simulated and experimental data. We find that hybridMANTIS matches the experimental results as good as or better than MANTIS, especially in the high spatial frequency range. The RMS values were lower (0.025, 0.028 for 40 and 70 kVp input spectra respectively) for hybridMANTIS than for MANTIS (0.049, 0.075 respectively) when compared to experimental data. The comparison of Swank factors suggests that hybridMANTIS and MANTIS are both consistent with the experimental data. Our models of detector response are useful tools for the design and optimization of breast imaging systems and for improved description of the forward problem in reconstruction algorithms.

Keywords: Monte Carlo, scintillator detector, MANTIS, Graphics Processing Units (GPU).

1 Introduction

The detailed analysis of imaging systems requires thorough understanding of the underlying physical processes through theory, experiments and simulations.

---

* Corresponding author.

A.D.A. Maidment, P.R. Bakic, and S. Gavenonis (Eds.): IWDM 2012, LNCS 7361, pp. 56–63, 2012.

With the advent of parallel computer architectures, it is now possible to perform realistic simulations, especially an advantage in medical imaging, where large number of images are required to obtain low uncertainities in performance estimates. Some examples of computationally intensive simulation tools include PENELOPE [1] and MANTIS [2] for performing x-ray, electron and optical photon transport. Graphics Processing Units (GPU) are suitable for problems like optical photon transport involving independent photon histories. To overcome this problem, we describe and perform initial validation studies for a novel hybrid Monte Carlo approach using CPUs and GPUs in parallel. We refer to it as hybridMANTIS. It is a fast Monte Carlo package for modeling indirect x-ray imagers.

2   Methods

In this section we summarize the hybrid concept, present key features of hybridMANTIS, and explain the methods used for validation of hybridMANTIS with MANTIS and experimental data.

2.1   Hybrid Concept

The hybrid approach can be applied to any problem consisting of two processes. The first process runs in a CPU and the other can be run independently in a GPU. This approach can provide a balanced utilization of the CPUs and GPUs in a single or multiple workstations. For this work, we consider the x-ray and electron transport as process 1, which runs in a CPU and the optical transport as process 2 (runs in a GPU). Process 1 outputs the energy and locations of energy deposition events in the scintillator and buffers them. This buffer is sent to process 2 which calculates the number of optical photons to be simulated and transports them. By the time the GPU transports these optical photons, the CPU simulates more x-ray transport and re-fills the buffer. Thus both process 1 and 2 are run in parallel [3].

2.2   hybridMANTIS

PENELOPE 2006 was used for the x-ray and electron transport. The modeled x-ray source was a 30 μm diameter circular parallel beam with two energy spectra at 40 and 70 kVp. Cesium Iodide (CsI) was used as detector material. The optical photons were transported using fastDETECT2, a rewrite of the optical transport code DETECT2 used in MANTIS. It offers improved features as compared to DETECT2 in terms of columnar geometry description and computational efficiency. PENELOPE generates the locations and deposited energy of the interaction events which are used by fastDETECT2 to sample optical photons following a Poisson distribution. An optical photon can either be absorbed (at the top surface or in the bulk) or lost (exits the detector boundary) or detected (at non-ideal sensor plane located at the bottom of the detector) during its transport. In addition,

Table 1. Simulation parameters for hybridMANTIS

Detector lateral dimensions	50 x 50 mm^2
Detector thickness	170 μm
Column radius	5.1 μm
Refractive index of columns	1.8 (Cesium Iodide)
Refractive index inter-col. space	1.0 (Air)
Top surface absorption fraction	0.1
Bulk absorption coefficient	0.0001 μm^{-1}
Surface roughness coefficient	0.2
Minimum dist. to next column	1 μm
Maximum dist. to next column	280 μm
Non-ideal sensor reflectivity	0.25
Input X-ray spectra	40 and 70 kVp
Light yield	55 optical photons per keV

to accurately model the roughness of surface walls we implemented the roughness model used in MANTIS. The simulation parameters are given in Table 1 (see Ref. [3] for details).

hybridMANTIS addresses some of the limitations of MANTIS. For instance MANTIS stores all columnar array details in memory, making it difficult to model large area detectors. In hybridMANTIS, we solve this issue by modeling columns on the fly, which means that the columnar array details are computed dynamically. Once a photon travels out of a column, we sample a distance uniformly between a minimum and maximum value to locate the new column. The photon is then transported to the surface of this new column. Another limitation of MANTIS is that due to its regular columnar arrangement, it does not match the randomness of real columnar structure. To compensate for this, a uniform CsI layer is added at the bottom of the detector to allow photons to travel laterally at different angles, thus matching the experimental response. In hybridMANTIS, as the columns are modeled on the fly, they can be described with randomness in terms of shape, size, tilt angle and material properties. We have implemented an algorithm (referred to as columnar crosstalk) to allow photons to cross over to the adjacent column without undergoing reflection or refraction. This simulates regions where columns are physically connected as seen in the scanning electron microscope (SEM) image of the screen in Fig. 1 (left). For this work, we implemented a linear model of crosstalk with depth (see right image of Fig. 1).

hybridMANTIS simulations were performed using one core of an Intel® Core i7 920 CPU and an NVIDIA® GeForce GTX 580 GPU[1]. C language was used for programming on the CPU and CUDA (version 4.0) for the GPU. MANTIS

---

[1] The mention of commercial products herein is not to be construed as either an actual or implied endorsement of such products by the Department of Health and Human Services. This is a contribution of the Food and Drug Administration and is not subject to copyright.

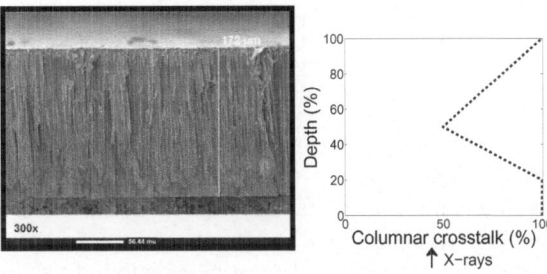

Fig. 1. (Left) SEM image of the screen (courtesy Radiation Monitoring Devices Inc., Watertown MA) used for comparison of hybridMANTIS with the experimental results in this work. (Right) Columnar crosstalk model as a function of depth. Here depth is defined in the direction of x-rays entrance. In the first 20% of the detector, all the photons can crossover to adjacent columns. This crossover decreases linearly to half at 50% depth, and then increases linearly back to 100% crossover at the sensor plane of the detector.

simulations were performed using one core of Intel® Xeon® E5410 CPU. hybridMANTIS source codes are available for free download at http://code.google.com/p/hybridmantis.

2.3 Experimental and MANTIS Data

Freed *et al.* [4] validated MANTIS simulation results against four CsI scintillator screens with different properties. For the experiments, they measured the point response functions (PRF) for all the screens for 40 and 70 kVp spectra and at four incidence angles (0°, 15°, 30° and 45°). A 30-μm pinhole was used in front of the x-ray beam. MANTIS simulations incorporated the details of the geometrical structure for each specific screen and were produced with 500,000 x-ray histories. For comparison in this work, we have used their experimental and MANTIS data for only one screen, shown in Fig. 1 (left) at 0° incidence angle. Its manufacturer specifications can be found in Table 1, and MANTIS simulation parameters in Table 2 of Reference [4].

2.4 Simulation Output and Data Analysis

All PRFs were obtained for an area of 909×909 μm^2 around the center of the sensor plane using a 9 μm pixel pitch and have been normalized by their maximum value. Line spread functions (LSF) were calculated by integrating each column or row of the PRF and the modulation transfer functions (MTF) were calculated as the discrete Fourier transform of the LSF. Pulse-height spectra (PHS) were generated for all hybridMANTIS simulations.

We compare the data quantitatively based on the root mean square difference between the experimental and simulated MTF data averaged over the range (0.1,10) mm^{-1}.

$$RMS = \sqrt{\frac{1}{N} \sum_{i=1}^{N} (e_i - s_i)^2} \tag{1}$$

where N is the number of spatial frequency bins in the range $(0.1,10)$ mm^{-1}, e_i is the experimental and s_i is the simulated MTF data. In addition, we also calculate the Swank or information factor (A_s) for comparison with MANTIS. A_s characterizes the noise associated with converting x-ray to optical (light) energy and can be obtained from the PHS. A_s can be calculated using the zeroth (m_0), first (m_1) and second moments (m_2) of the PHS [5],

$$A_s = \frac{m_1^2}{m_0 m_2}. \tag{2}$$

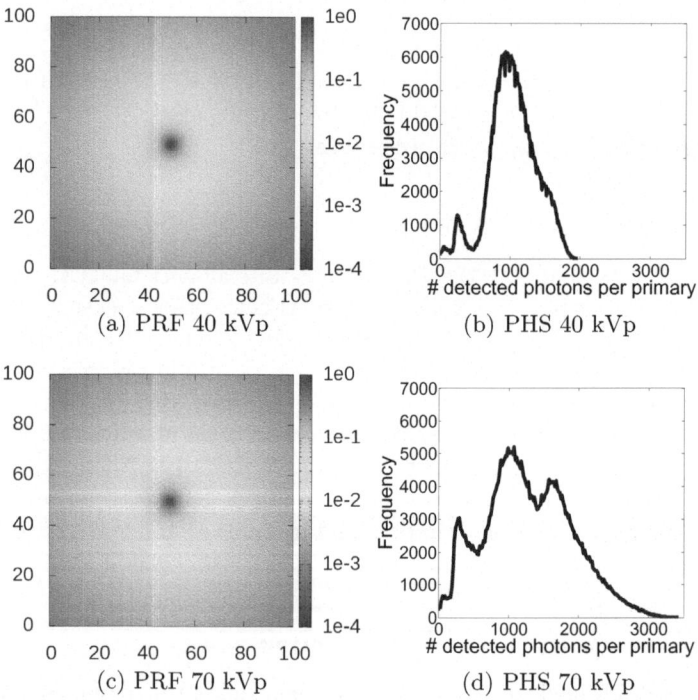

Fig. 2. PRF and PHS for 40 and 70 kVp spectra using hybridMANTIS

3   Results and Discussion

We compare our hybridMANTIS results against MANTIS and experimental data for the two input spectra (40 kVp and 70 kVp). All the hybridMANTIS results shown in this work are for simulating 1 million x-ray histories. Table 1 lists the

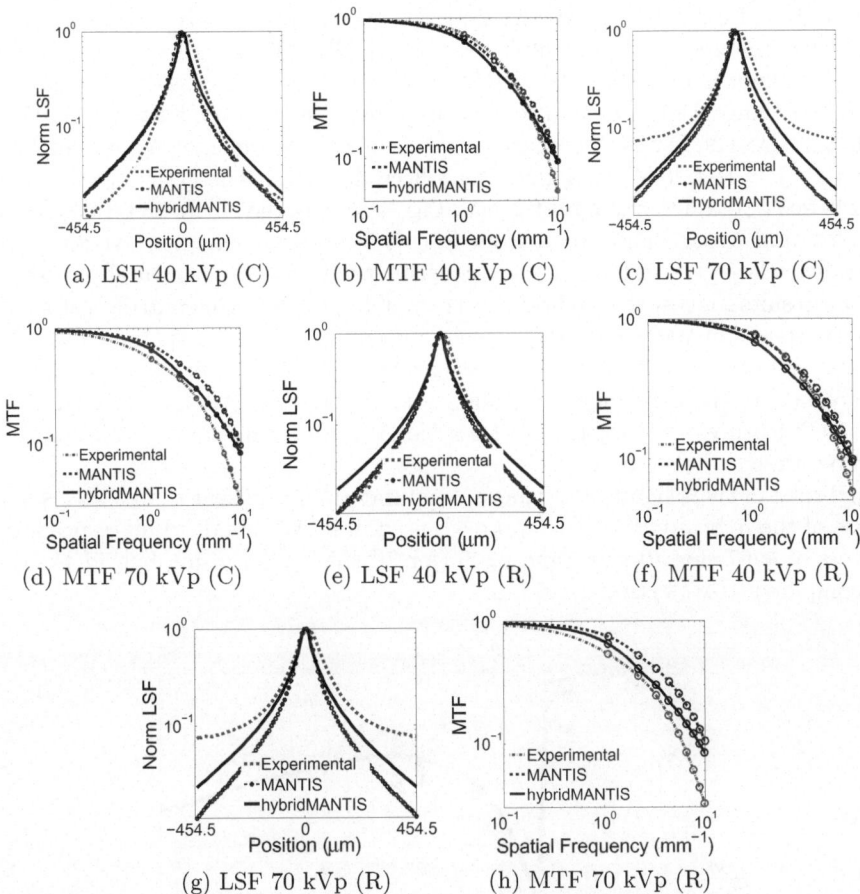

Fig. 3. LSF and MTF comparison of experimental, MANTIS and hybridMANTIS data for the two spectra. LSFs (a-d) are obtained by integrating each column of the PRF (marked with C) while (e-h) are obtained by integrating the PRF row-wise (marked with R). MTFs are the discrete fourier transform of the LSF.

simulation parameters used for hybridMANTIS. Fig. 2 shows the PRF and corresponding PHS for hybridMANTIS simulations. We observe that the PHS changes significantly between the two spectra due to the difference in the relative photoelectric fraction. Fig. 3 provide the LSF and MTF comparisons between the simulation and experimental results. Figs. 3 (a) to (d) show the LSF by integrating each column of the PRF while plots (e) to (h) integrate each row. We do not observe any significant difference between the two types of LSF calculations. From Fig. 3 we observe that hybridMANTIS matches the experimental better than MANTIS especially at higher spatial frequencies and for 70 kVp spectra.

We calculated the RMS values for comparing hybridMANTIS and MANTIS simulations with the experimental data. RMS was calculated using MTFs from Fig. 3 (b, d). When comparing hybridMANTIS with the experimental data, RMS values are 0.025 and 0.028 for the 40 and 70 kVp spectra respectively. For comparing MANTIS with experimental results, we obtain RMS of 0.049 (40 kVp) and 0.075 (70 kVp). hybridMANTIS has lower RMS values and thus matches the experimental better than MANTIS. In addition, we used the A_s as a metric for the validation of hybridMANTIS. For this comparison we used the experimental A_s obtained by Zhao *et al.* in Ref. [6,5]. This data was collected for monoenergetic input from 2 to 140 keV, obtained in steps of 2 keV. Fig. 4 depicts the A_s for hybridMANTIS, MANTIS and experimental data from Ref. [6,5] at these energies. We see that both hybridMANTIS and MANTIS are consistent with the experimental results.

Our results suggest that hybridMANTIS matches the experimental data as good as or better than MANTIS for this screen, especially in the high spatial frequency range. We postulate that this is because hybridMANTIS more closely follows the realism of the columnar array due to its on-the-fly geometry and columnar crosstalk features as compared to MANTIS. A more comprehensive comparison will be presented elsewhere.

hybridMANTIS is significantly more computationally efficient than MANTIS because of the hybrid CPU-GPU approach used in it. We obtained high speed-up factors of 4967 (for 40 kVp) and 4209 (for 70 kVp) when using hybridMANTIS as compared to MANTIS.

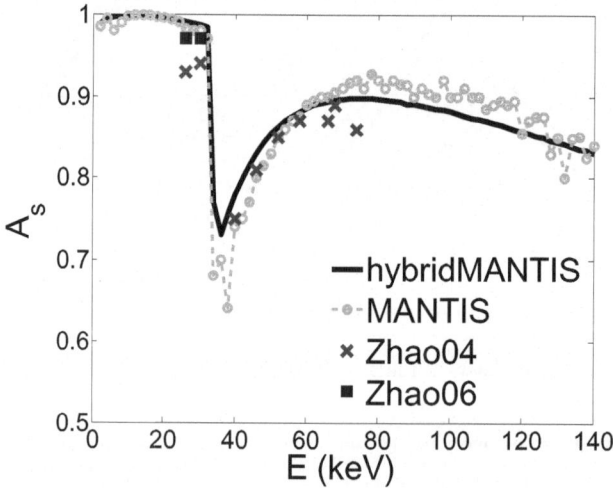

Fig. 4. Swank factor (A_s) comparison of hybridMANTIS with MANTIS and experimental data (from Ref. [6,5])

4   Conclusion

We described hybridMANTIS and highlighted its key features in comparison with MANTIS. The hybridMANTIS point response and modulation transfer function results were compared against experimental and MANTIS results obtained from

Reference [4]. We calculated root mean square and Swank factor and demonstrated that hybridMANTIS matches the experimental results as good as or better than MANTIS for the screen considered in this work, especially in the high spatial frequency range. Our hybridMANTIS package is computationally more efficient than MANTIS achieving speed-ups of up to 4967 over MANTIS. This package can facilitate the design and optimization of breast imaging systems and modeling for reconstruction algorithms.

Acknowledgement. The authors thank M. Freed for sharing the experimental data she obtained and reported on in Ref. [4].

References

1. Salvat, F., Fernández-Varea, J., Sempau, J.: *PENELOPE-2006: A code system for Monte Carlo simulation of electron and photon transport*. Nuclear Energy Agency / OECD (2006), www.oecd-nea.org/science/pubs/2006/nea6222-penelope.pdf
2. Badano, A., Sempau, J.: MANTIS: combined x-ray, electron and optical Monte Carlo simulations of indirect radiation imaging systems. Physics in Medicine and Biology 51(6), 1545–1561 (2006)
3. Sharma, D., Badal, A., Badano, A.: hybridMANTIS: a CPU-GPU Monte Carlo method for modeling indirect x-ray detectors with columnar scintillators. Physics in Medicine and Biology 57(8), 2357–2372 (2012)
4. Freed, M., Miller, S., Tang, K., Badano, A.: Experimental validation of Monte Carlo (MANTIS) simulated x-ray response of columnar CsI scintillator screens. Medical Physics 36(11), 4944–4956 (2009)
5. Zhao, W., Ristic, G., Rowlands, J.A.: X-ray imaging performance of structured cesium iodide scintillators. Medical Physics 31(9), 2594–2605 (2004)
6. Lubinsky, A.R., Zhao, W., Ristic, G., Rowlands, J.A.: Screen optics effects on detective quantum efficiency in digital radiography: Zero-frequency effects. Medical Physics 33(5), 1499–1509 (2006)

Breast Mass Classification Using Orthogonal Moments

Fabián Narváez and Eduardo Romero

CIM&LAB
Faculty of Medicine
Universidad Nacional de Colombia
Bogotá, Colombia
{frnarvaeze,edromero}@unal.edu.co

Abstract. Automatic classification of breast masses in mammograms has been considered a major challenge. Mass shape, margin and density define the malignancy level according to a standardized description, the BI-RADS lexicon. Unlike other approaches, we do not segment masses but instead, we attempt to describe entire regions. In this paper, continuos (Zernike) and discrete (Krawtchouk) orthogonal moments were used to characterize breast masses and their discriminant power to classify benign and malign masses, was assessed. Firstly, Regions of Interest selected by an expert are projected onto two sets of orthogonal polynomials functions, continuous and discrete, thereby drawing shape global information onto a feature space. Using a simple euclidean metric between vectors, the projected images are automatically classified as benign or malign by a k-nearest neighbor strategy. The parameter space is characterized using a set of 150 benign and 150 malign images. The whole method was assessed in a set of 100 masses with different shape and margins and the classification results were compared against a ground truth, already provided by the database. These results showed that discrete Krawtchouk outperformed Zernike moments, reaching an accuracy rate of $90,2\%$ (compared to 81% for Zernike moments), while the area under the curve in a ROC evaluation yielded $Az = 0.93$ and $Az = 0.85$ for the Krawtchouk and Zernike strategies, respectively.

Keywords: Breast mass, Zernike moments, krawtchouk moments, Orthogonal moments.

1 Introduction

Breast cancer is the most frequently diagnosed cancer in women and is considered as the largest public health problem in women population worldwide [1]. This disease is fully curable when an early diagnosis is achieved and mammography is the more efficient method for visualizing abnormalities in these stages [2]. However, mammographic interpretation is a really difficult task, especially when a mass is present, due to its high inter and intra observer variability. Previous studies have

A.D.A. Maidment, P.R. Bakic, and S. Gavenonis (Eds.): IWDM 2012, LNCS 7361, pp. 64–71, 2012.

reported that between 10% and 25% of breast cancer are not detected in mammography, a finding that has been associated to the variability introduced by the observer. The American College of Radiology has therefore designed a protocol, currently known as the *Breast and Imaging Report and Database System* (BI-RADS) that has permitted to standardize the radiological work flow and to improve the radiological reading reproducibility [3]. This agreement established that radiologic semiology signs are shape, margin and mass density. Ultimately, development of Computer Assisted Diagnosis Systems (CAD) for mammography has decreased this observer variability since the radiologists can support their diagnosis using the evidence stored in a particular database, becoming a well accepted clinical practice to assist radiologists [4]. However, for mass detection and/or classification, these systems have reported poor accuracy. In breast mass analysis, the feature extraction process plays the most important role because its effectiveness directly determines the system performance. A main problem is then that those extracted features have to be discriminative enough to represent different kinds of pathological characteristics.

In the context of image analysis, shape analysis based on moments theory have been used to distinguish between different objects, characters, aircrafts, chromosomes, and industrial parts [5]. Since Hu [6] introduced moments invariants, moments and functions of moments have been widely used because of their ability to represent global features of an image [7]. However, these moments are not orthogonal in general, whereby this representation is redundant and can be hardly used for reconstruction. However, Teague [8] suggested the use of Legendre and Zernike polynomials by an appropriate approximation of the integrals [9], allowing minimal information redundancy, low noise and high image reconstruction capability. Previous works have reported that Zernike moments perform better than others continuous orthogonal moments [10], but their geometric and numerical error have limited their use. Orthogonal polynomials were firstly introduced by Mukundan et al. [7], who proposed a set of discrete orthogonal moment functions, based on the discrete Tchebichef polynomials. Another new set of discrete orthogonal moment functions, based on the discrete Krawtchouk polynomials, was presented by Yap et al. [11]. It was shown therein that discrete orthogonal moments perform better than conventional continuous orthogonal moments in terms of image representation. These investigations suggest the Krawtchouk moments are better suited for shape analysis. Furthermore the Krawtchouk moments can be used to extract local features of an image, unlike other orthogonal moments, which generally capture the global features.

In previous works, many approaches based on moments analysis have been proposed for classification of masses in mammography [12,13,14]. Most of them are higher dependent of previous segmentation, in which morphology is described using Zernike moments [14].

In this paper we proposed a breast mass characterization strategy based on a set of discrete orthogonal functions, known as krawtchouk polynomials. This set of bases has permitted to define a new type of discrete orthogonal moments, which are herein formulated, implemented and evaluated on a breast mass classification problem. We evaluate the performance of both continuous (Zernike) and discrete (Krawtchouk) orthogonal moments. Firstly, these regions are projected onto a set of orthogonal polynomials functions, continuous and discrete, respectively. Once these basic features are computed, a further dimensionality reduction is achieved using a standard Principal Component Analysis (PCA), reducing the Krawtchouk initial descriptor from 820 to 30 and the Zernike descriptors, from 961 to 40 dimensions. Finally, these features are classified using a K-nearest-neighbor strategy under a Euclidean metric. The strategy was assessed by classifying a set of 100 masses with different shapes and margins, using as the ground truth the radiologist's annotation, already provided by the data base. Results showed that discrete Krawtchouk moments obtained an accuracy of $90, 2\%$ for the classification task, in contrast with 81% obtained with Zernike moments, while the area under the curve in a ROC evaluation yielded $Az = 0.93$ and $Az = 0.85$ for the Krawtchouk and Zernike strategies, respectively. The rest of this article is organized as follows: next section presents the methodology, results are shown in section 3 and the last section discusses future works and conclusions.

2   Methodology

After the radiologist selects a mass, the corresponding Region of Interest ROI is pre-processed to enhance the mass shape. Unlike other approaches, we do not segment masses but instead, we attempt to describe entire region. Afterward, this ROI is transformed to any of the spaces defined by any of the selected bases, either Zernike or Krawtchouk. The number of selected moments is set by determining a polynomial order that achieves a good reconstruction error for both types of representations, in this case, an order of 50 was found to produce a low reconstruction error(0.23 and 0.196 Zernike or Krawtchouk moments respectively). This polynomial order generates a number of basic features, 961 for the Zernike moments and 820 for the Krawtchouk moments. Once these basic features are computed, a further reduction of dimensionality is achieved using a standard Principal Component Analysis (PCA), setting a Zernike descriptor of 40 and Krawtchouk of 30 dimensions, which preserve a 85% of variability in the data for both descriptor, respectively. Finally, regions are classified with a K-nearest-neighbor strategy using Euclidean distance.

2.1   RoI Pre-processing

Breast mass analysis is very likely one of the most difficult radiological examinations since these images capture a very complicated anatomical object with a limited spatial resolution. Every image was herein size reduced using 16-8 bit conversion technique [15] , stretched to the maximum and minimum gray level values ([0, 255]) followed by a bin reduction from 256 to 12 bins, adaptively equalizing the histogram so that structural details were preserved. This step aims to conserve exclusively what is relevant for the classification task. Resultant images were smoothed out by a median filter to remove the remaining noise. Figure 1 shows an example of the resultant preprocessed images (benign and malign masses).

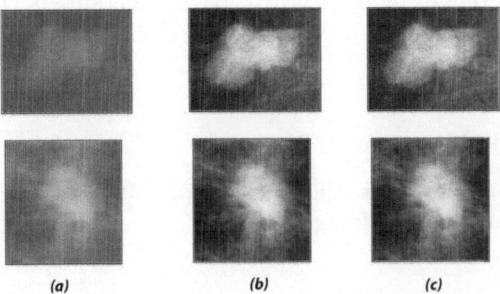

(a) (b) (c)

Fig. 1. RoI pre-processing: RoIs of columns (a) original images, (b) stretched images, (c) images with bin reduction

2.2 Zernike Moments

According to BI-RADS, the two more important properties for diagnosis are shape and texture [3,16,17]. Teague [8] suggested that the use of orthogonal bases in terms of the Legendre and Zernike polynomials are good shape descriptor but also rotation-invariant, robust to noise and constitute multiresolution shape representations [18]. Zernike polynomials based representation turns out to be more robust to noise [9], allowing reconstruction with minimal losses. The Zernike polynomials are a set of complex polynomials which form an orthogonal complete set $V_{pq}(x,y)$ within the unitary circle [8] and are defined as:

$$V_{pq}(x, y) = R_{pq}(r)e^{jq\theta}, r \in [-1, 1] \tag{1}$$

where $r = \sqrt{x^2 + y^2}$ is the vector magnitude and $\theta = tan^{-1}\left(\frac{y}{x}\right)$ its angle.

In general, the Zernike Moments are defined as:

$$Z_{pq} = \frac{p+1}{\pi} \int_{-\pi}^{\pi} \int_{0}^{1} [V_{pq}(r,\theta)]^* f(r,\theta)rdrd\theta \tag{2}$$

where $f(r, \theta)$ is the image in polar coordinates. With a numerical approximation, the complex Zernike moments are derived from the real-valued radial polynomials, given by:

$$R_{pq}(r) = \sum_{s=0}^{(p-|q|)/2} (-1)^s \frac{(p-s)!}{s!(\frac{p+|q|}{2} - s)!(\frac{p-|q|}{2} - s)!} r^{p-2s} \tag{3}$$

where p and q are subjected to $p - |q|$ is even, $0 \leqslant |q| \leqslant p$, and $p \geqslant 0$. Then the complex Zernike moments of order p, with q repetitions for an image intensity function $f(x, y)$ are given by:

$$Z_{pq} = \frac{p+1}{\pi} \sum_{x} \sum_{y} V_{pq}^*(x, y) f(x, y) \tag{4}$$

where $*$ stands for the conjugated complex of $V_{pq}(x, y)$.

Since that the domain of the Zernike basis functions is the unitary circle, images are mapped to the unitary circle and their centers must coincide with the unitary circle center [19,9] .

2.3 Krawtchouk Moments

The basis functions of Krawtchouk moments are the discrete orthogonal Krawtchouk polynomials satisfying

$$\sum_{x=0}^{N} j(x)k_n(x)k_n(x) = \rho(N,n,p)\delta_{pq}, 0 \leqslant m, n \leqslant N \tag{5}$$

where $\rho(N,n,p) = \binom{N}{n} p^n(1-p)^n$, and $q = (1-p)$. The explicit hypergeometric (F) representation of the Krawtchouk polynomial is given by [11] as

$$K_n(x) = q^n \binom{x}{n} F\left(-n, x - N; x - n; -\frac{p}{q}\right) \tag{6}$$

and the weight function $j(x) = \binom{N}{x} p^x q^{N-x}$.

Krawtchouk moments [11], unlike Zernike and Legendre moments, belong to the class of discrete orthogonal moments. Therefore, implementation of these moments does not involve any numerical approximation. Moreover, Krawtchouk polynomials do not require coordinate space transformations. Krawtchouk moments with order $m + n$ are defined as

$$K_{nm}(x) = [\rho(N,n,p)\rho(N,m,p)]^{-1} \sum_{x=0}^{N-1} \sum_{y=0}^{N-1} j(x)k_n(x)j(y)k_m(y)f(x,y) \tag{7}$$

for $m, n = 0, 1, 2, ...N$ where $k_n(x)$ and $k_m(y)$, given by (6) are used as the basis set. The inverse moment transform is used to reconstruct the image and is defined by

$$f(x,y) = \sum_{m=0}^{N} \sum_{n=0}^{N} K_{nm}k_n(x)k_m(y) \tag{8}$$

2.4 Reconstruction Error

The normalized (RMS) root-mean-square error (ε) is used for measuring the accuracy of the moments in reconstructing the image and is determined as

$$\varepsilon = \sqrt{\frac{\sum_i \sum_j [f(i,j) - F(i,j)]^2}{\sum_i \sum_j [f(i,j)]^2}} \tag{9}$$

where $f(i,j)$ and $F(i,j)$ are the original and reconstructed images, respectively.

A minimum image reconstruction error calculating the root-mean-square (RMS), shown in Table 1 for both Krawtchouk and Zernike moments, allowed to choose the optimum order of moments to be used in the classification task.

Table 1. Minimum Reconstruction Error (RMS)

Max. Order	Krawtchouk	Zernike
10	0.796	1.032
20	0.624	0.742
30	0.323	0.532
40	0.281	0.319
50	**0.196**	**0.230**
60	0.179	0.779
70	0.176	1.299
80	0.172	1.298

An order of 50 was chosen since it generates a low reconstruction error for both Zernike and Krawtchouk moments.

3   Experimental Results

The strategy was evaluated on a total of 100 RoIs, including pathological masses previously annotated as benign and malign by a group of radiologists, extracted from the *Digital Database for Screening Mammography (DDSM)* [20]. This dataset was split into training (300) and test (100), (50 benign-50 malign) subsets. Classification performance was evaluated by K-NN strategy using the euclidean distance as the space metrics since this classifier has been successfully used as a baseline in image annotation tasks [21]. The optimal number of used RoIs was estimated by a 10-fold cross validation assessment (k=7). The Zernike strategy, set to 40 dimensions by the PCA method, reported an accuracy of 81%. The obtained confusion matrix reads as: $accuracy = \frac{TP+TN}{TP+FP+FN+TN}$, where TP is the number of True Positives, TN true negatives, FP false positives, FN false negatives, respectively.

The performance of classification was evaluated by the area under the ROC curve, which reported a $Az = 0.85$ as illustrated in Figure 2. The ROC curve was generated using a threshold value to make a classification decision, which were proportional to each K-nearest distance [22].

On the other hand, Krawtchouk strategy with 50 order moments was evaluated. For this, a vector feature was reduced to a set of 30 features by PCA analysis. Results reported an accuracy of 90.2%, while the area under the curve in a ROC evaluation yielded $Az = 0.93$. Figure 2 present the classification performance for Krawtchouk and Zernike moments, respectively.

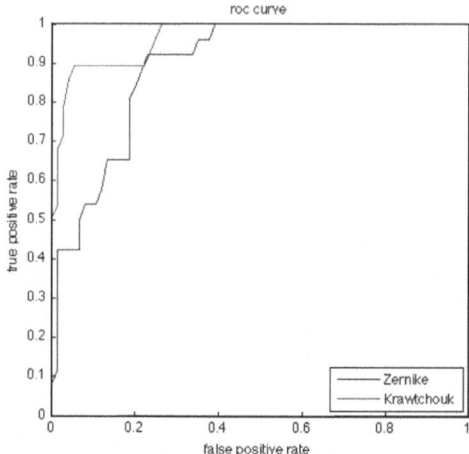

Fig. 2. Classification results : ROC curves for Zernike and Krawtchouk moments

4   Conclusions and Future Works

The use of Krawtchouk moments for describing shape of mammography masses was evaluated in this paper. The performance by using this descriptor in a bening-malign classification task was evaluated using images obtained from a well known public database. Classification was performed using a single K-NN classifier. Results were compared with description performed by the state of the art shape descriptor, named Zernike moments, which have been used previously for breast mass representation. Experimental results indicate that the shape descriptor based on the Krawtchouk moments improve they obtained by the use of the Zernike moments. Future works include the fusion of this descriptor with other visual features such as texture that allows to improve the classification performance in the most challenging tasks.

Acknowledgment. This work was partially funded by the Ecuadorian government through Secretaría Nacional de Educación Superior, Ciencia y Tecnología (SENESCYT), Grant: 20110958 "CONVOCATORIA ABIERTA 2011" and by the project: Anotación Automática y Recuperación por Contenido de Imágenes Radiológicas usando Semántica Latente" Grant: 110152128803, "CONVOCATORIA COLCIENCIAS 521 de 2010".

References

1. Society, A.C.: Cancer facts & figures 2008. Technical report, ACS (2008)
2. Buseman, S., Mouchawar, J., Calonge, N., Byers, T.: Mammography screening matters for young women with breast carcinoma. Cancer 97, 352–358 (2003)

3. ACR: Illustrated Breast Imaging Reporting and Data System (BI-RADS), 3rd edn. American College of Radiology, Reston (1998)
4. Nishikawa, R.M.: Current status and future directions of computer-aided diagnosis in mammography. Computerized Medical Imaging and Graphics 31, 224–235 (2007)
5. Mukundan, R., Ramakrishnan, K.R.: Moment Functions in Image Analysis: Theory and Applications. World Scientific, Singapore (1998)
6. Hu, M.K.: Visual pattern recognition by moment invariants. IRE Transactions on Information Theory 8(2), 179–187 (1962)
7. Mukundan, R., Ong, S.H., Lee, P.A.: Image analysis by tchebichef moments. IEEE Trans. Image Process 10(9), 1357–1364 (2001)
8. Teague, M.R.: Image analysis via the general theory of moments. J. Optical Soc. Am. 70, 920–930 (1980)
9. Wee, C.Y., Paramesran, R.: On the computational aspects of zernike moments. Image and Vision Computing 25, 967–980 (2007)
10. Yin, J., Pierro, A., Wei, M.: Analysis for the reconstruction of a noisy signal based on orthogonal moments. Appl. Math. Comput. 132(2), 249–263 (2002)
11. Yap, P., Paramesran, R., Ong, S.: Image analysis by krawtchouk moments. IEEE Trans. Image Process. 12(11), 1367–1377 (2003)
12. Tahmasbi, A., Saki, F., Shokouhi, S.B.: Classification of benign and malignant masses based on zernike moments. Computers in Biology and Medicine 41, 726–735 (2011)
13. Oliver, A., Torrent, A., Llado, X., Marti, J.: Automatic diagnosis of masses by using level set segmentation and shape description. In: International Conference on Pattern Recognition, pp. 2528–2531 (2010)
14. Wei, C.H., Chen, S.Y., Liu, X.: Mammogram retrieval on similar mass lesions. Computer Methods and Programs in Biomedicine 3, 1–15 (2010)
15. AbuBaker, A.A., Qahwaji, R.S., Aqel, M.J., Saleh, M.H.: Mammogram image size reduction using 16-8 bit conversion technique. International Journal of Biological and Medical Sciences 2, 103–110 (2006)
16. Homer, M.J.: Mammographic Interpretation: A Practical Approach, 2nd edn., New York (1997)
17. Maggio, C.D.: State of the art of current modalities for the diagnosis of breast lesions. Eur. J. Nucl. Med. Mol. Imaging 31(suppl.1), S56–S69 (2004)
18. Kim, H., Kim, J.: Region-based shape descriptor invariant to rotation, scale and translation. Signal Proc.: Image Communication 16, 87–93 (2000)
19. Narváez, F., Díaz, G., Romero, E.: Automatic BI-RADS Description of Mammographic Masses. In: Martí, J., Oliver, A., Freixenet, J., Martí, R. (eds.) IWDM 2010. LNCS, vol. 6136, pp. 673–681. Springer, Heidelberg (2010)
20. Heath, M., Bowyer, K., Kopans, D., Moore, R., Kegelmeyer, W.P.: The digital database for screening mammography. In: Yaffe, M.J. (ed.) Proceedings of the Fifth International Workshop on Digital Mammography, pp. 212–218. Medical Physics Publishing (2001)
21. Makadia, A., Pavlovic, V., Kumar, S.: A New Baseline for Image Annotation. In: Forsyth, D., Torr, P., Zisserman, A. (eds.) ECCV 2008, Part III. LNCS, vol. 5304, pp. 316–329. Springer, Heidelberg (2008)
22. Fawcett, T.: An introduction to roc analysis. Pattern Recognition Letters 27, 861–874 (2006)

A Task-Specific Argument for Variable-Exposure Breast Tomosynthesis

Stefano Young[1,*], Andreu Badal[2], Kyle J. Myers[2], and Subok Park[2]

[1] University of Arizona, College of Optical Sciences, Tucson, Arizona, USA
[2] FDA Center for Devices and Radiological Health,
Division of Imaging and Applied Mathematics, Silver Spring, Maryland, USA
`syoung@optics.arizona.edu`

Abstract. Digital breast tomosynthesis (DBT) is a young technology, and the current imaging protocols are not yet fully optimized. Numerous recent studies have focused on optimizing DBT scan geometries, but the optimal DBT scan geometry is inextricably linked to the exposure delivery scheme. It is possible that alternative, variable-exposure delivery schemes could change our understanding of the optimal DBT scan. There is a need for strategies to evaluate and optimize DBT exposure delivery on a task- and patient-specific basis. To this end, we developed a simulation framework that uses fast, GPU-enabled Monte Carlo simulations and linear observer models to evaluate variable-exposure DBT systems. We tested three different exposure schemes: Equal, Central, and Oblique exposure. Preliminary results indicate that for the specific task of detecting a small signal in low density breast phantoms (15%), the alternative Central and Oblique exposure schemes may increase detectability.

Keywords: tomosynthesis, breast, variable-exposure, task-specific, image quality.

1 Introduction

Digital breast tomosynthesis (DBT) is a young technology, and researchers in the field generally agree that the current imaging protocols are not fully optimized. Numerous recent studies have focused on optimizing DBT scan geometries in a task-specific manner. However, the optimal DBT scan geometry for a particular task is inextricably linked to the exposure delivery scheme. Thus, it is important to study how to optimize exposure delivery alongside optimizing the scan geometry. It is possible that alternative, variable-exposure delivery schemes could change our understanding of the optimal DBT scan. There is a need for strategies to evaluate and optimize DBT exposure delivery on a task- and patient-specific basis. Due to the many variables in this optimization problem, there is an additional need for fast, accurate software tools for virtual DBT system evaluation.

---

* Corresponding author.

A.D.A. Maidment, P.R. Bakic, and S. Gavenonis (Eds.): IWDM 2012, LNCS 7361, pp. 72–79, 2012.

2 Methods

We are developing a virtual trial engine for DBT system evaluation. The virtual DBT trial engine involves six computational steps:

1. Generate an ensemble of breast phantoms.
2. Frame the image quality problem with a specific, clinically-relevant task.
3. Simulate DBT projection data with scatter.
4. Model detector noise.
5. Postprocess the data for analysis of raw or reconstructed images.
6. Perform model observer (linear discriminant) analysis.
   Adjust parameters of interest in steps #1-6 and repeat.

With this approach, it is possible to evaluate various DBT systems by appropriately modifying interesting parameters at each step in the virtual trial. In the following subsections, we provide more detail on each of the steps.

2.1 Generate an Ensemble of Breast Phantoms

We used the UPENN breast phantom model[1] to generate ensembles of 400 voxelized phantoms for each of three different percent density classes: 15%, 25%, and 40% (Fig. 1). Each phantom contained randomly-varying compartments of adipose (gray) and fibroglandular (white) tissue.

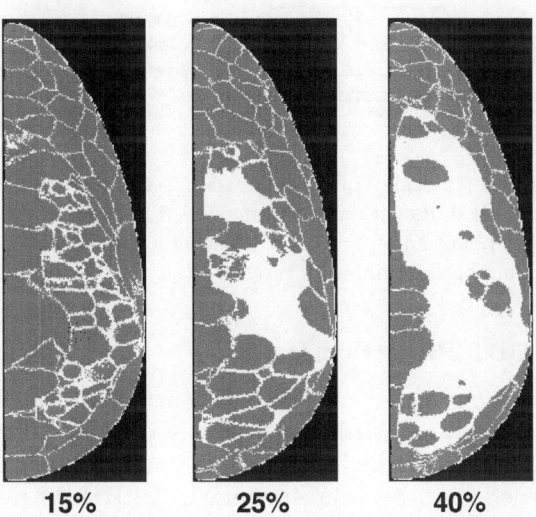

Fig. 1. Example compressed breast phantoms (ML slices) from three different density classes

2.2   Frame the Image Quality Problem

We simulated a detection task by embedding identical spherical masses into half
of the breast phantoms at the center-of-rotation of the x-ray source arc (Fig.
2). We repeated the task for two signal sizes – small (3 mm) and large (8 mm).
Each mass was inserted into a phantom by changing the density coefficients of
the voxels at the signal location from the existing background density to 1.044
g/cm^3. The fibroglandular and adipose tissue densities were set to 1.035 and
0.928 g/cm^3 based on previously published values[2]. The voxel size was 500
microns, so the small signal occupied a volume of 112 voxels and the large signal
occupied a volume of 2096 voxels.

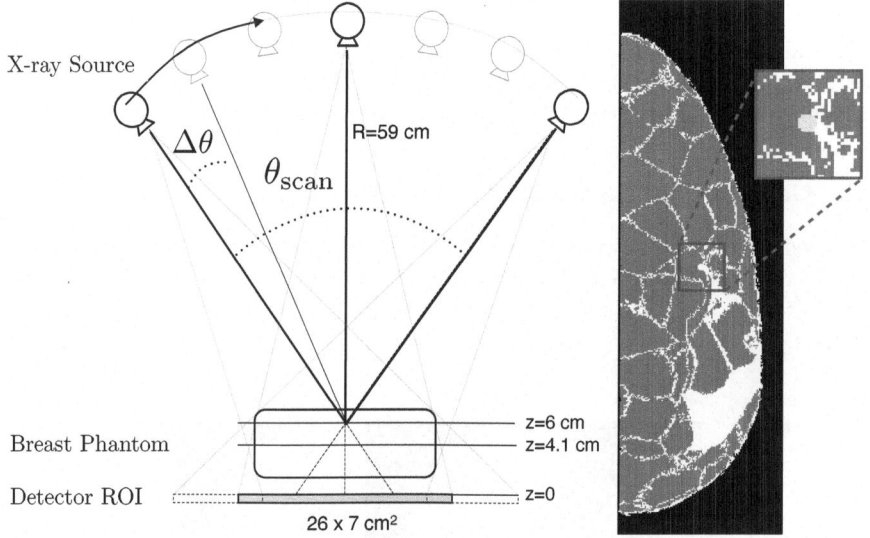

Fig. 2. Schematic (not to scale) of the simulated partial-isocentric DBT geometry
(left). The detector ROI shifts with projection angle. The right image is a slice through
a 25% density breast phantom at z = 6 cm, showing a small signal (in yellow) as well
as random overlapping background structures.

2.3   Simulate DBT Projection Data

To generate projection images, we used the open source MC-GPU[3] Monte
Carlo code appropriately modified for partially-isocentric DBT geometries. MC-
GPU takes advantage of the highly-parallelized architecture of current GPUs.
To model a polyenergetic x-ray source, we used CDRH/FDA measured spectral
data[4] in conjunction with the parameters in Table 1. For a single phantom, MC-
GPU can easily handle 10^{11} or 10^{12} photon histories on recent GPU hardware.
For ensembles of hundreds of phantoms, however, we chose to evaluate two lower
exposure levels – 1.5×10^9 and 10^{10} photons per phantom – to reduce the time
required for the virtual trials.

Table 1. X-ray source parameters for generating MC-GPU input spectrum

Target/Filter	Tungsten/Al (0.9 mm)
kVp	28 kVp, 13° anode angle
HVL	0.537 mm Al
Mean x-ray energy	20.04 keV

We considered a simple 3-projection DBT acquistion $(0°, \pm 48°)$ with three different exposure-delivery schemes. In the first scheme – Equal exposure – each projection received 1/3 of the total photons. The next two schemes were chosen based on the fact that the thickness of tissue increases roughly with the cosine of the projection angle. In the "Central exposure" scheme, the oblique projections received 1/3 of the total times the cosine of the projection angle. In other words, the 48° projection consumed $\frac{N_0}{3} \cos 48°$ photons. The 0° projection received the remaining photons, or $N_0(1 - \frac{2}{3} \cos 48°)$. In the "Oblique exposure" scheme, the 0° projection consumed $\frac{N_0}{3} \cos 48°$ photons while the oblique projections each received $\frac{N_0}{6}(3 - \cos 48°)$ photons. These three exposure-delivery methods are summarized in Table 2.

Table 2. Exposure fractions (fraction of the total photons) at each of the 3 projection angles for three different exposure-delivery schemes:

	$-48°$	$0°$	$48°$
Equal exposure	1/3	1/3	1/3
Central exposure	$\frac{1}{3} \cos 48°$	$1 - \frac{2}{3} \cos 48°$	$\frac{1}{3} \cos 48°$
Oblique exposure	$(3 - \cos 48°)/6$	$\frac{1}{3} \cos 48°$	$(3 - \cos 48°)/6$

2.4   Model Detector Noise

In MC-GPU, a 26 x 7 cm^2 perfectly-absorbing detector was used with 100 micron pixels (2600 x 700 total pixels). Thus, the data in this study only suffered from object/anatomical noise due to the randomly-varying phantom backgrounds and quantum noise due to the finite sampling of x-ray photons. We neglected other sources of detector noise (e.g. scatter in the scintillator, electronic noise) to study the variable-exposure effects in relative isolation.

2.5   Postprocess for Analyzing Raw or Reconstructed Images

If we are interested in hardware evaluation only – i.e. finding the upper limits of signal detectability before reconstruction – we can apply model observers directly to the raw projection data. The dimensions of the projection data are large, however, which presents difficulties for model observers. Park et. al. have shown that Laguerre-Gauss (LG) channels are fairly robust for capturing statistical information from various signals in non-Gaussian randomly-varying backgrounds[6]. To reduce the dimensionality problem, we applied 5 LG channels to each of the projections (Fig. 3) and concatenated the resulting channel outputs. The channel width parameter σ approximately matched the signal diameter in the central projection ($\sigma = 25$ for 3 mm signals, $\sigma = 75$ for 8 mm signals).

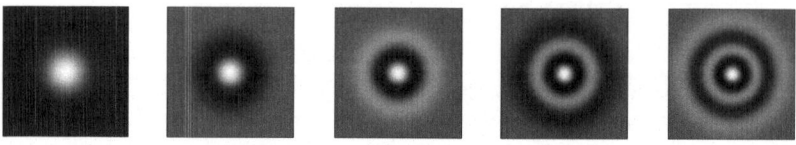

Fig. 3. The 5 Laguerre-Gauss channels used for dimensionality reduction

There is scant literature on how to design optimal data-reducing channels for 3D breast imaging modalities like DBT. In model observer design, the goal is typically to "tune" the channel parameters (i.e. LG width and number of channels) to the task for maximum signal detectability with as few channels as possible. This reduces the risk of unstable observer models due to finite sample size effects[5]. In previous studies using noisefree raytracing images with a Poisson model for high-exposure noise and a 3 mm signal, we plotted AUC at the 0° projection angle as a function of the number of channels for three representative widths $\sigma = 10, 25,$ and 50 called "Skinny", "Medium", and "Broad" channels (Fig. 4). In this study, the percent density was 25% and condition number regularization was used to stabilize the data covariance. Fig. 4 indicates that the Medium ($\sigma = 25$) channel profile was best tuned to the task, reaching an asymptotic AUC limit after approximately 5 channels.

2.6   Perform Model Observer/Linear Discriminant Analysis

To evaluate signal detectability, we used a linear discriminant classifier applied to the concatenated channel outputs from three projection angles. We have used this approach previously[8], and it has since been called a 3Dp channelized Hotelling observer (CHO)[7]. We used functions provided in Matlab's Statistical Toolbox (v7.6) to estimate the linear classifiers and perform ROC analysis on the channel outputs. For each set of 400 DBT scans, we divided the channel outputs into 200 for training the discriminant and 200 for testing/computing ROC curves and AUCs. In each subset of 200 phantoms, half contained signals.

3   Results

For a total exposure of 1.5×10^9 photons, we computed AUC values for each exposure delivery scheme, and repeated the process for 3 different ensembles of breast phantoms having percent densities 15%, 25%, and 40%. The results for 15% and 25% densities are shown in Figs. 5 and 6. At 40% density, the task was too difficult and the mean AUCs were ≈ 0.5 for all three exposure schemes.

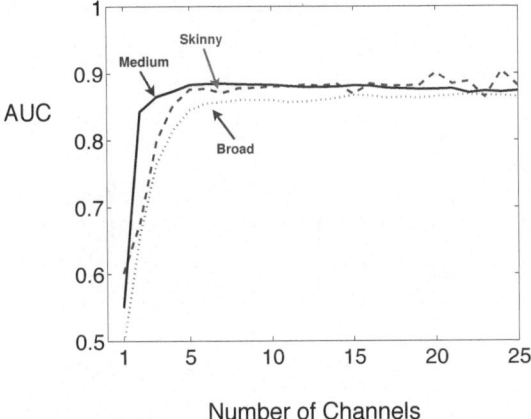

Fig. 4. AUC versus the number of channels at the $0°$ projection angle for three different channel sizes: $\sigma = 10$ (Skinny), 25 (Medium), and 50 (Broad). The medium ($\sigma = 25$) channel width appears to be best suited for the 3 mm signal detection task and reaches an asymptote after 5 channels

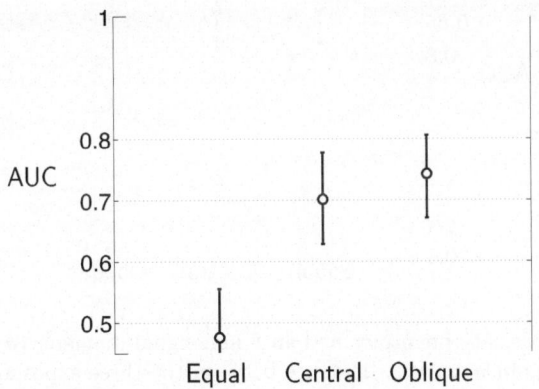

Fig. 5. For 15% density phantoms and a 3 mm signal diameter, we found a significant increase in AUC with alternative exposure schemes. Error bars are 95% confidence intervals computed from 1000 bootstrap samples.

In the Equal exposure scheme, the 3 mm signal was undetectable in 15% density phantoms (AUC ≈ 0.5). With Central and Oblique exposure schemes, however, we found a statistically significant increase in AUC (Fig. 5). Similarly, for the 25% density phantoms, Central and Oblique exposure schemes gave higher mean AUCs, though the 95% bootstrap confidence intervals overlapped slightly in this case (Fig. 6).

For comparison with the challenging task of detecting a 3 mm signal, we evaluated the same exposure schemes with a larger 8 mm signal embedded into

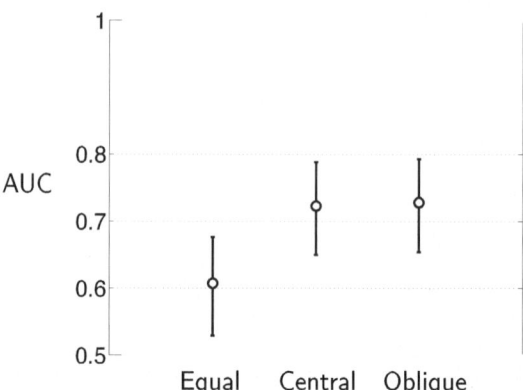

Fig. 6. For 25% density phantoms and a 3 mm signal diameter, Central and Oblique exposure schemes gave higher mean AUCs, though the error bars overlapped slightly. Error bars are 95% confidence intervals computed from 1000 bootstrap samples.

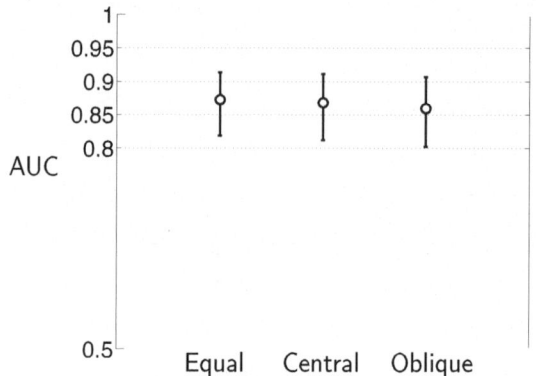

Fig. 7. For 25% density phantoms and an 8 mm signal diameter ($\sigma = 75$), there was no statistically significant AUC difference between the three exposure methods. Error bars are 95% confidence intervals computed from 1000 bootstrap samples.

the 25% density phantoms (Fig. 7). We also increased the total exposure from 1.5×10^9 to 10^{10} photons. Fig. 7 shows that there was no significant difference between the AUCs in the large signal case.

4   Conclusions and Future Work

The preliminary results in this work suggest that for the specific task of detecting a small (3 mm) signal at the center-of-rotation in an ultra-low-dose DBT scan, alternative exposure schemes may improve detectability. Comparing Figures 6 and 7 for the same density class, we expect that any AUC improvements will be task-depdendent. Central or Oblique exposure schemes may increase the detectability of small spherical signals in low-exposure scans, but this does not necessarily apply to other types of signals. At high total exposure levels, this effect could disappear completely. The results of this preliminary study should not be construed as a rule – rather, they provide evidence that variable-exposure schemes may offer image quality advantages in some specific scenarios.

Future challenges are to increase the realism of the DBT simulations, improve the observer model, and broaden the scope of the experiments to perform optimization over a range of clinically-relevant tasks and exposure schemes. To incorporate the correlation information between the angular projections, we applied 2D LG channels to each projection and concatenated the output vectors; but there are other variants such as 3D LG channels that could offer theoretical or practical advantages in detectability experiments[7]. In this study, we were plagued by large error bars in all of the AUC calculations. This is likely caused by using a small sample set of 400 phantoms for training and testing the model observer. We should investigate the effects of sample size on our AUC results. While MC-GPU has made it possible to simulate hundreds of low-dose DBT scans in less than a day, we are still far from the thousands of scans needed to reduce the statistical uncertainty in our AUC estimates. In future work, we plan to investigate hybrid analytical/Monte Carlo approaches that allow us to scale up to a larger optimization space while still taking advantage of MC-GPU's state-of-the-art scatter modeling capabilities.

References

1. Bakic, P.R., Zhang, C., Maidment, A.D.A.: Development and Characterization of an Anthropomorphic Breast Software Phantom Based upon Region-Growing Algorithm. Med. Phys. 38(6), 3165–3176 (2011)
2. Johns, P.C., Yaffe, M.J.: X-ray characterisation of normal and neoplastic breast tissues. Phys. Med. Biol. 32(6), 675–695 (1987)
3. Badal, A., Badano, A.: Accelerating Monte Carlo simulations of photon transport in a voxelized geometry using a massively parallel graphics processing unit. Med. Phys. 36(11), 4878–4880 (2009)
4. Jennings, R.J., Quinn, P.W., Fewell, T.R.: Measured x-ray spectra for mammography. In: 43rd Annual Meeting of the AAPM, 7129 (2001)
5. Fukunaga, K., Hayes, R.R.: Effects of Sample Size in Classifier Design. IEEE Trans. Patter Anal. Mach. Intell. 11(8), 873–885 (1989)
6. Witten, J.M., Park, S., Myers, K.J.: Partial Least Squares: A Method to Estimate Efficient Channels for the Ideal Observers. IEEE Trans. Med. Imaging. 29(4), 1050–1058 (2010)
7. Platisa, L., Goosens, B., Vansteenkiste, E., Park, S., Gallas, B.D., Badano, A., Philips, W.: Channelized Hotelling observers for the assessment of volumetric imaging data sets. J. Opt. Soc. Am. A. 28(6), 1145–1163 (2011)
8. Young, S., Park, S., Anderson, S.K., Badano, A., Myers, K.J., Bakic, P.: Estimating breast tomosynthesis performance in detection tasks with variable-background phantoms. In: Proc. SPIE, vol. 7258, p. 1 (2009)

Detective Quantum Efficiency of a CsI-CMOS X-ray Detector for Breast Tomosynthesis Operating in High Dynamic Range and High Sensitivity Modes

Tushita Patel[1], Kelly Klanian[2], Zongyi Gong[1], and Mark B. Williams[1,2]

[1] Department of Physics
[2] Department of Biomedical Engineering,
University of Virginia, Charlottesville, Virginia, USA
mbwilliams@virginia.edu

Abstract. The spatial frequency dependent detective quantum efficiency (DQE) of a CsI-CMOS x-ray detector was measured in two operating modes: a high dynamic range (HDR) mode and a high sensitivity (HS) mode. DQE calculations were performed using the IEC-62220-1-2 Standard. For detector entrance air kerma values between ~7 µGy and 60 µGy the DQE is similar in either HDR mode or HS mode, with a value of ~0.7 at low frequency and ~ 0.15 – 0.20 at the Nyquist frequency $f_N = 6.7$ mm^{-1}. In HDR mode the DQE remains virtually constant for operation with K_a values between ~7 µGy and 119 µGy but decreases for K_a levels below ~ 7 µGy. In HS mode the DQE is approximately constant over the full range of entrance air kerma tested between 1.7 µGy and 60 µGy but kerma values above ~75 µGy produce hard saturation. Quantum limited operation in HS mode for entrance kerma as small as 1.7 µGy makes it possible to use a large number of low dose views to improve angular sampling and decrease acquisition time.

Keywords: detective quantum efficiency, breast tomosynthesis, CMOS, sensitivity, hybrid imaging.

1 Introduction

X-ray tomosynthesis of the breast promises to improve upon planar mammography in terms of visualization of small lesions, especially among women with radiodense breast tissue. However, the requirements associated with the acquisition of a series of rapid, low exposure projection images place greater demands on x-ray detectors used in tomosynthesis compared to those in planar FFDM. In particular, high quality, low dose tomosynthesis requires detectors with high x-ray absorption efficiency, high frame rates with low read noise, and low dark noise.

We are developing a dual modality tomosynthesis (DMT) breast scanner that merges x-ray tomosynthesis and molecular imaging tomosynthesis modalities within a single system to provide co-registered three-dimensional (3D) anatomic images and radiotracer maps [1]. When acquiring x-ray tomosynthesis images, the x-ray tube and detector simultaneously rotate about the stationary, mildly compressed breast. Because of our use of the step-and-shoot method, tomosynthesis image acquisition time

A.D.A. Maidment, P.R. Bakic, and S. Gavenonis (Eds.): IWDM 2012, LNCS 7361, pp. 80–87, 2012.

is longer than desirable (nearly 2 minutes), significantly increasing the possibility of motion artifacts. With the goal of decreasing overall acquisition time, we would like to replace the acquisition method with continuous gantry motion with the help of the 2923MAM CMOS detector from Dexela, a PerkinElmer company (London). The 2923MAM has 75 micron detector elements in a 3888x3072 matrix, for an overall sensitive area of approximately 29 cm x 23 cm. With no pixel binning the maximum frame rate is 17 fps, rising to up to 78 fps for 4x4 binning. The 2923MAM tested here includes a columnar CsI converter. All measurements described here were performed without pixel binning.

The spatial dependent detective quantum efficiency (DQE(u)) is the most generally used indicator of how efficiently the detector can process the input x-ray signal. For this reason, the widely accepted IEC-62220-1-2 Standard was followed to test the Dexela 2923MAM CMOS x-ray detector [2]. There are two possible operating modes for the Dexela detector: a high dynamic range (HDR) mode and a high-sensitivity (HS) mode. A comparison was made between the DQE for HDR mode operation and HS mode operation over a range of entrance exposures that were less than or comparable to a single projection view in a typical tomosynthesis acquisition.

2   Methods and Materials

The IEC Protocol 62220-1-2 was followed in calculating the DQE for the Dexela 2923MAM CMOS detector, though minor modifications were made as described in the following sections. As given in the IEC protocol, the equation for the frequency dependent DQE is:

$$DQE(u) = T^2(u) \cdot (NPS_{in}(u)/ NPS_{out}(u)) \tag{1}$$

$T(u)$ is the modulation transfer function (MTF), $NPS_{in}(u)$ is the noise power spectrum at the input of the detector, and $NPS_{out}(u)$ is the noise power spectrum of the output images. The posterior-to-anterior direction (23cm dimension of the detector) is parallel to the rows in the image and is designated as x in position space or u in frequency space. The direction parallel to the image columns in the 29 cm dimension of the detector will be denoted as y in position space or v in frequency space. NPS_{in} is determined by Eq (2):

$$NPS_{in} = K_a \cdot SNR_{in}^2 \tag{2}$$

where K_a is air kerma in units of $1/(mm^2 \cdot \mu Gy)$ and SNR_{in}^2 is the squared signal-to-noise ratio of the input signal per unit air kerma, which is a constant provided in Table 2 of IEC-62210-1-2 for a given target/filter combination.

2.1   Geometry and Radiation Quality

The distance between the focal spot and the closest point on the detector surface is 81cm. The x-ray tube contains a tungsten target, exit window filtration of 0.76 mm of beryllium, and an external filter of 0.050 mm of rhodium. Addition external filtration of 1.4 mm of Al was added to match the half value layer (HVL) of 0.75mm of Al specified in the IEC Protocol for W/Rh target/filter systems operated at 28 kVp. As per protocol requirements, all images and measurements were taken at a tube voltage of 28 kVp. From this setup, we were able to use 5975 $(mm2 \cdot \mu Gy)^{-1}$ as the SNR_{in}^2 value for a tungsten target, 50μm rhodium filter at 28 kVp.

2.2   Detector Response and Determination of Conversion Function

The conversion function is the relationship between the large area detector output (i.e. average pixel value) in a corrected image and the input x-ray fluence. Prior to the determination of the average pixel value in all of the images used, corrections were made to the raw images (replacement of bad pixels, dark image subtraction, and flat-fielding) as permitted by the standard. The conversion function was then used to convert pixel values into units of fluence. For many digital x-ray detectors, this relationship is linear to a high degree in which case the conversion function reduces to a proportionality constant and a pixel value offset.

The detector response was measured for each mode by recording the average pixel value over a range of input kerma values in the uncorrected images. A Radcal Accu-Pro ion chamber was used for determining the air kerma, and inverse square law corrections were made to calculate the exposure at the detector surface

2.3   MTF and NPS$_{out}$

The MTF was measured using a straight-edged piece of tungsten rather than the aluminum test device suggested by the IEC Standard. The presampling MTF was calculated using a program based upon the method described by Fujita et al [3]. It was written by our lab in the Interactive Data Language programming environment (IDL; Research Systems, Boulder, Colorado).

The protocol was followed in determining NPS$_{out}$ for each exposure. An ROI chosen within the image for the NPS calculation had dimensions of 17.85cm x 27.48cm corresponding to an area of 8720320 pixels^2. The final 2D NPS$_{out}$ was found by averaging over noise power spectra from 459 overlapping 256x256 pixel sub-regions within the ROI. The 1-D NPS$_{out}$(u) was obtained by averaging over 7 rows above and 7 rows below the $v = 0$ mm^{-1} frequency axis. The same was done for NPS$_{out}$(v) about the $u = 0$ mm^{-1} frequency axis. Additionally, per the IEC standard an optional 2D second-order polynomial fit was subtracted from each ROI to remove low frequency noise prior to NPS estimation.

3   Results

3.1   Detector Response and Conversion Function

Figure 1 is a plot of the mean pixel value, within a region of interest (ROI) drawn at the focal spot projection in uncorrected images, versus exposure. The portion of each curve in Figure 1 that is linear has been fit with a linear equation and projected forward to show the detector's deviation from a linear response at higher input fluences.

The highest tested air kerma levels chosen for each mode are just below the point at which the detector stops behaving linearly with increasing fluence. The air kerma levels tested here are 1.69 µGy, 3.57 µGy, 7.34 µGy, 15.1 µGy, 30.0 µGy, and 60.1 µGy for HS mode. The same levels were tested in HDR mode with two additional levels at 89.9 µGy and 119 µGy.

The conversion function for both modes is shown in Figure 4. In HDR mode, the conversion function slope is 0.008388 ADU·mm2/photon and in HS mode it is 0.02750 ADU·mm2/photon. The zero fluence values shown in Fig. 4 are due primarily to DC offset values digitally added to each pixel value during the dark subtraction and uniformity correction procedures.

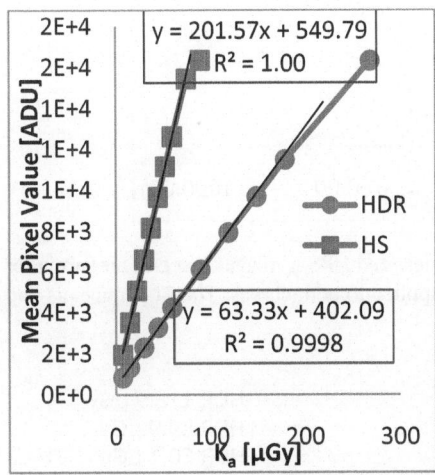

Fig. 1. Mean pixel value versus air kerma. Pixel values come from uncorrected images taken with nothing in the x-ray beam except for the internal and external filters. Least squares fits are shown to the portion of each curve exhibiting linear behavior.

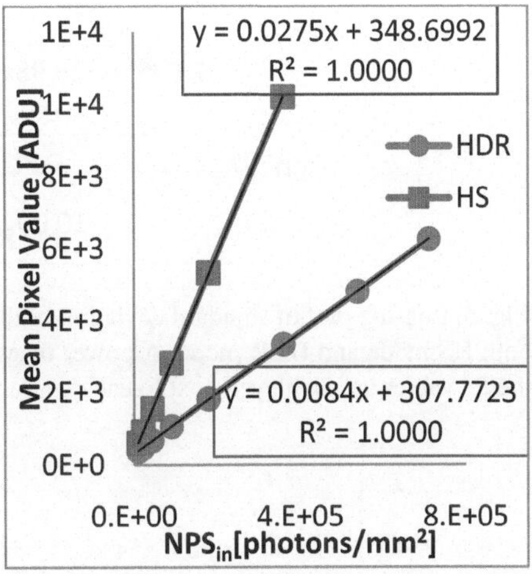

Fig. 2. Conversion function in both HDR mode and HS mode. A linear fit was applied to each curve and the fit equation and R-squared values are shown next to each curve.

3.2   NPS$_{out}$

As an additional quantification of image noise, a log-log plot of the standard deviation σ in the NPS$_{out}$ images versus K_a is shown in Fig. 3 for both HS mode and HDR mode. In all cases it was verified that the integral of the 2-D NPS between ±Nyquist frequencies was equal to σ^2. As a measure of quantum limited behavior a power fit was applied to both curves. The fit equation and the R^2 value are shown next to each curve.

3.3   DQE

Figs. 4 and 5 are plots of DQE(u) and DQE(v), respectively for HDR mode. Figs. 6 and 7 are plots of DQE(u) and DQE(v), respectively for HS mode. A subset of all exposures tested is shown in each figure. Data are plotted within a frequency range of 0 mm^{-1} to the Nyquist frequency of 6.67 mm^{-1}. The 0 mm^{-1} frequency points were omitted since it does not correspond to an achievable physical quantity.

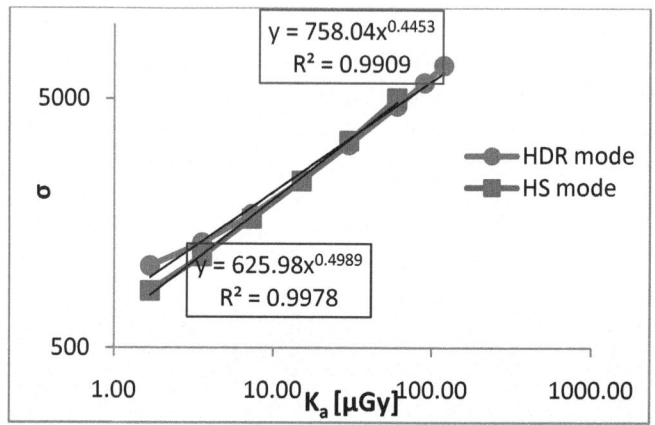

Fig. 3. Log-log plot of standard deviation of the linearized NPS$_{out}$ images σ versus air kerma for both HS mode and HDR mode. A power fit was applied to both curves. The fit parameters and the R^2 values are displayed next to each curve.

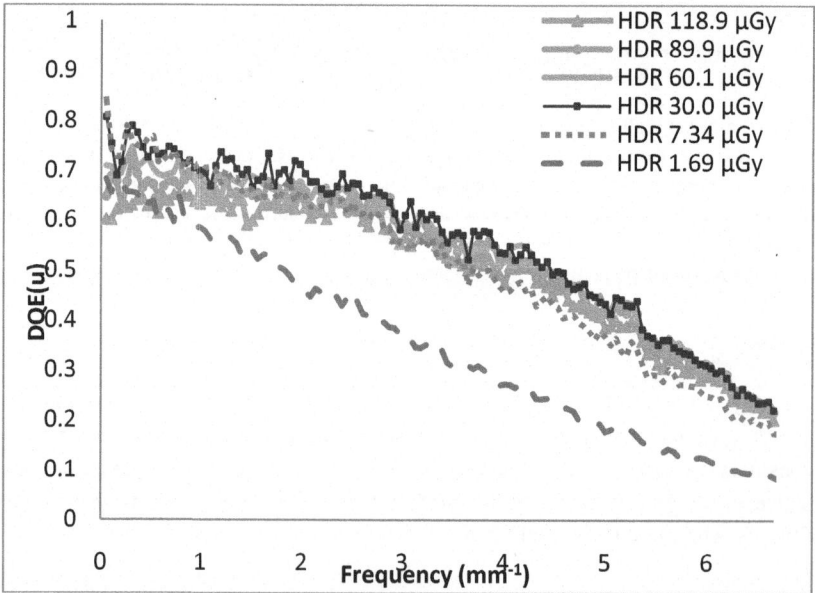

Fig. 4. DQE along detector rows at the tested exposure levels of 1.69 μGy, 7.34 μGy, 30.0 μGy, 60.1 μGy, 89.9 μGy and 118.9 μGy in HDR mode

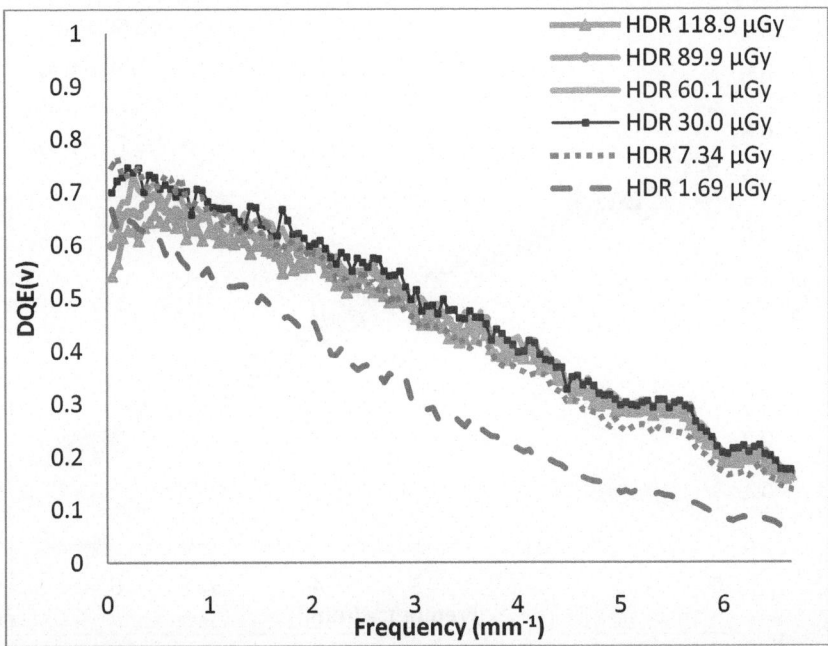

Fig. 5. DQE along detector columns at the tested exposure levels of 1.69 μGy, 7.34 μGy, 30.0 μGy, 60.1 μGy, 89.9 μGy and 118.9 μGy in HDR mode

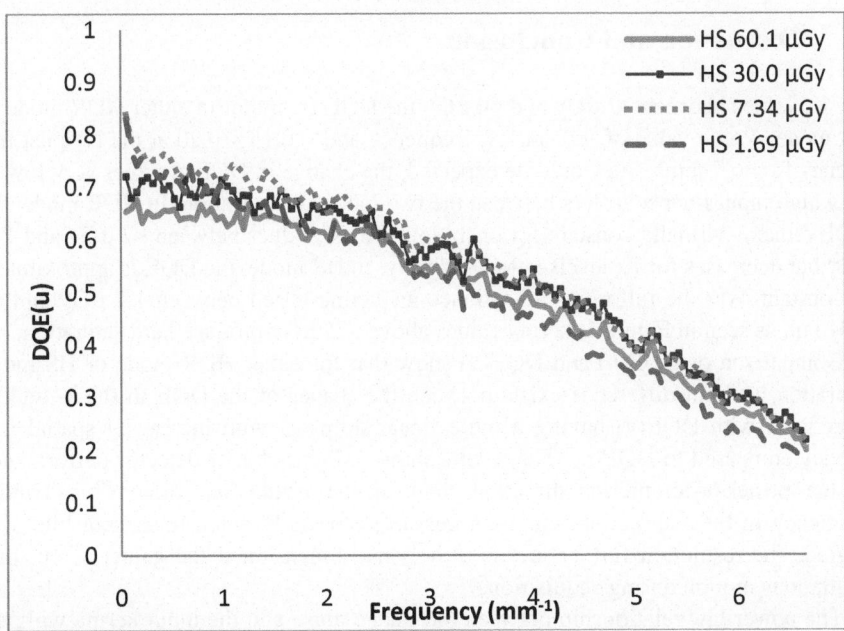

Fig. 6. DQE along detector rows at the tested exposure levels of 1.69 μGy, 7.34 μGy, 30.0 μGy, and 60.1 μGy in HS mode

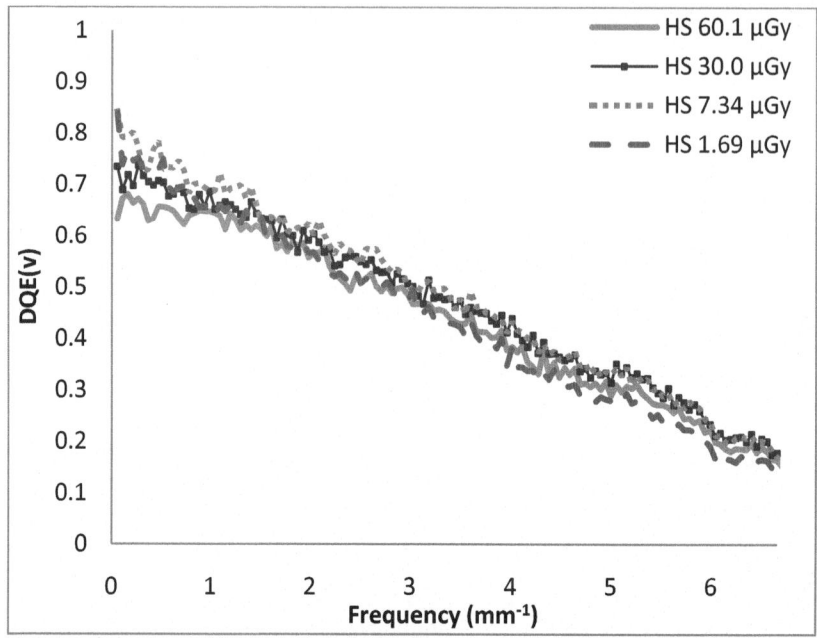

Fig. 7. DQE along detector columns at the tested exposure levels of 1.69 μGy, 7.34 μGy, 30.0 μGy, and 60.1 μGy in HS mode.

4   Discussion and Conclusion

For K_a values between ~7 μGy and 60 μGy the DQE is similar in either HDR mode or HS mode, with a value of ~0.7 at low frequency and ~ 0.15 – 0.20 at the Nyquist frequency $f_N = 6.7$ mm^{-1}. As would be expected, the change in DQE at either very low or very high input fluence differs between the two modes of operation. In HDR mode, the DQE remains virtually constant for operation with K_a values between ~7 μGy and 119 μGy but decreases for K_a levels below ~ 7 μGy. In HS mode, the DQE is approximately constant over the full range of entrance air kerma tested between 1.7 μGy and 60 μGy but, as seen in Figure 1, kerma values above ~75 μGy produce hard saturation.

Comparison of DQE(u) and DQE(v) show that for either HDR mode or HS mode operation, a slight difference exists between the shapes of the DQE in the x- and y-directions, with DQE(v) having a more linear drop off with increasing spatial frequency compared to DQE(u). The results show a slightly better detector performance in the posterior-to-anterior direction than in the orthogonal dimension. Higher efficiency in the x-direction will be necessary, especially when focal spot blur will degrade the resolution further in this orthogonal dimension if the gantry is put into continuous motion during acquisition.

The power law relationship between the image noise and the input kerma with exponent of ~0.5 (Figure 3) shows that the image variance increases approximately linearly with increasing input fluence as would be expected for quantum limited operation. However, in addition to the deviation from quantum limited operation at low exposure in HDR mode operation, there is a slight deviation at high exposure in either mode most prominently in HDR mode.

The fact that quantum limited operation is available in HS mode for entrance kerma as small as 1.7 μGy makes it possible to use a very large number of very low dose views in order to improve angular sampling and decrease artifacts since there would be minimal penalty in terms of the effects of system noise. However the choice of number of views must also take into account the maximum acceptable tomosynthesis scan time, maximum available detector frame rate, and the optimal x-ray tube settings for a given subject. For example, a tomosynthesis scan of a 5 cm thick acrylic phantom using a Hologic Dimensions scanner in Autofilter mode results in a full scan detector entrance kerma of 340 μGy, corresponding to 200 1.7 μGy views. Operated at its maximum full resolution frame rate of 17 fps, this would correspond to an 11.8 second scan time for the 2923MAM. A more practical choice might be 85 views in 5 seconds with a detector entrance kerma of 4 μGy per view. Of course, for a given breast type the desirable full scan kerma is dependent on the detector, beam quality, and reconstruction algorithm used. Using the maximum possible number of views may not necessarily maximize image quality, so these are example possibilities only. System-specific image optimization studies are required to determine the best acquisition parameters.

In summary, the two operating modes of the 2923MAM together provide high DQE over a large exposure range. The combined abilities of very low dose operation and rapid readout make dense angular sampling tomosynthesis feasible with acceptably short overall scan time and without image degradation from system noise.

Acknowledgements. This work was supported by the National Institutes of Health (R01 CA149130) and Susan G. Komen for the Cure (KG100479).

References

1. Williams, M.B., Judy, P.G., Gunn, S., Majewski, S.: Radiology 255, 191 (2010)
2. International Electrotechnical Commission. Medical electrical equipment—Characteristics of digital X-ray imaging devices—Parts 1-2: Determination of the detective quantum efficiency - Detectors used in mammography. IEC 62220-1-2, Geneva: IEC (2007)
3. Fujita, H., Tsai, D.Y., Itoh, T., Doi, K., Morishita, J., Ueda, K., Ohtsuka, A.: IEEE Trans. Med. Imag. 11, 34 (1992)

Multimodal Classification of Breast Masses in Mammography and MRI Using Unimodal Feature Selection and Decision Fusion

Jan M. Lesniak[1], Guido van Schie[2], Christine Tanner[1], Bram Platel[2], Henkjan Huisman[2], Nico Karssemeijer[2], and Gabor Székely[1]

[1] Computer Vision Laboratory, Sternwartstrasse 7, Eidgenössische Technische Hochschule Zürich, 8092 Zürich, Switzerland
jlesniak@vision.ee.ethz.ch
[2] Radboud University Nijmegen Medical Centre, Department of Radiology, Geert Grooteplein Zuid 18, 6525 GA Nijmegen, The Netherlands

Abstract. In this work, a classifier combination approach for computer aided diagnosis (CADx) of breast mass lesions in mammography (MG) and magnetic resonance imaging (MRI) is investigated, using a database with 278 and 243 findings in MG resp. MRI including 98 multimodal (MM) lesion annotations. For each modality, feature selection was performed separately with linear Support Vector Machines (SVM). Using nonlinear SVMs, calibrated unimodal malignancy estimates were obtained and fused to a multimodal (MM) estimate by averaging. Evaluating the area under the receiver operating characteristic curve (AUC), feature selection raised AUC from 0.68, 0.69 and 0.72 for MG, MRI and MM to 0.76, 0.73 and 0.81 with a significant improvement for MM (P=0.018). Multimodal classification offered increased performance compared to MG and MRI (P=0.181 and P=0.087). In conclusion, unimodal feature selection significantly increased multimodal classification performance and can provide a useful tool for generating joint CADx scores in the multimodal setting.

1 Introduction

Multimodal breast imaging is becoming of increasing clinical interest, enabling the exploitation of complementary diagnostic characteristics of the individual imaging modalities. One example is combined mammography (MG) and dynamic contrast enhanced-magnetic resonance imaging (DCE-MRI), which is being investigated e.g. for screening of high-risk patients [1]. In parallel, multimodal decision support systems for computer aided diagnosis (CADx) are researched with the focus of providing decision support based on a combination of modalities [2] [3].

In multimodal CADx systems, different information fusion strategies can be pursued, including pooling of image features or joining classifier decisions [4]. Pooling features from MG-MRI CADx allows to exploit complementary effects of multimodality directly in feature space as one classifier is trained on the joint

A.D.A. Maidment, P.R. Bakic, and S. Gavenonis (Eds.): IWDM 2012, LNCS 7361, pp. 88–95, 2012.
© Springer-Verlag Berlin Heidelberg 2012

feature set [3]. Conversely, a decision fusion scheme joins the final output scores of multiple classifiers, which may be particularly useful if classifiers were trained on different feature sets [5].

Often multimodal breast imaging databases comprise more unimodal than multimodal imaging data [6]. In this situation, a decision fusion approach allows to exploit the entire breadth of unimodal imaging and generate multimodal scores at the same time. Particularly if the multimodal subset is relatively small, the approach of unimodal decision fusion may contribute to stability of feature selection and classification, as a smaller feature space and more training data can be considered.

In this work, the fusion of two independent CADx systems (MG and MRI) to generate a multimodal malignancy estimate was investigated. In total, a database of 278 findings in MG and 243 findings in MRI was available, whereas 98 of these findings comprised joint MG-MRI multimodal imaging. 53 features were extracted from each MG view and 46 from MRI. Unimodal CADx employed linear Support Vector Machines (SVM) for feature selection in a first stage to filter less relevant features which may impair SVM classification performance [7] [8]. Finally, nonlinear SVMs were used for lesion classification [9]. Unimodal malignancy estimates were fused by averaging, which has shown to be an effective and robust classifier combination method [5]. The performance of the generated malignancy estimates was evaluated using receiver operating characteristic (ROC) analysis.

2   Materials and Methods

2.1   Image Database

The database consisted of full field digital MG images from 179 patients including craniocaudal (CC) and mediolateral oblique (MLO) views, comprising 243 findings (115 benign, 128 malignant) which manifested as masses, architectural distortions or asymmetries. Analogously, MRI data from 209 patients were available with 278 annotated findings (122 benign, 156 malignant). Lesion outlines were provided by radiologists including links of lesions across views or modalities. A subset of 90 patients had joint MG-MRI image sessions with 98 (31 benign, 67 malignant) multimodal (MM) lesions visible in both modalities. The ground truth for classification was obtained by biopsy for all malignant lesions. Benign lesions were either proven by biopsy or their benign characteristics were confirmed in follow-up imaging.

2.2   Features

For each annotated region in MG, 53 image features including neural network based malignancy likelihoods, context, spiculation, gradient, linear texture, morphology, location and density descriptors were extracted for each view [10]. The features from CC and MLO were pooled so that each MG feature vector consisted of 106 features. In case a finding was only visible in one view, the features vectors have been completed by duplication of features from the other view. In DCE-MRI, 46 descriptors were available per annotated lesion including kinetic, pharmacokinetic and morphological features. High spatial resolution images were used to derive kinetic curve and morphology characteristics such as baseline, initial enhancement and washout characteristics resp. lesion size, compactness, elongation and others [11]. Based on a series of low resolution images at a higher repetition frequency, voxel-based pharmacokinetic parameters such as extracellular volume V_e, volume transfer coefficient K_{Trans} and rate constant K_{ep} of the kinetic model were obtained [12].

2.3   SVM-Based Feature Selection and Classification

Support Vector Machines (SVM) were used for feature selection and classification. For labeled training data of the form $(x_i, y_i), i \in \{1, \ldots, l\}$, where x_i represents the feature vector and $y_i \in \{-1, 1\}$ the label of finding i, a decision function

$$f(x) = w^T \phi(x) + b \qquad (1)$$

is fitted with weight vector w and bias value b representing a separating hyperplane. Nonlinear decision boundaries in the input data space can be obtained by projecting the data using a mapping $\phi(x)$. SVMs find the separating hyperplane by maximizing distances to its closest data points thus embedding it in a large margin between the classes. This can be expressed via the optimization problem:

$$\min_{w,b} p(w) + C \sum_{i=1}^{l} max(1 - y_i f(x_i), 0), \qquad (2)$$

where C serves as a user-defined regularization parameter for elements inside the margin and $p(w)$ acts as a penalty term on the coefficients of the weight vector w. Choosing an L1 penalty term $p(w) := \|w\|_1 = \sum_{i=1}^{l} |w_i|$ leads to sparse solutions. In linear classification with $\phi(x) := x$ this approach can be used for feature selection as "uninformative" features are assigned zero weight, with C controlling the sparsity of the solution [13].

Lesion malignancy scores were computed based on an L2 penalty ($p(w) := \|w^2\|_2 = \sum_{i=1}^{l} w_i^2$) and nonlinear classification using a Gaussian kernel $K(x, x') = \phi(x)^T \phi(x') = exp(-\gamma \| x - x' \|^2)$, leaving the regularization weight C and the kernel width γ as a free parameters. The decision scores of the nonlinear SVM were translated into probability estimates in the interval $[0, 1]$ using Platt's probabilities, i.e. by fitting a sigmoid curve to pooled decision scores from training data which were generated by leave-one-out cross validation [14]. For lesions visible in MG and MRI the unimodal malignancy estimates were joined into a multimodal (MM) score by averaging the calibrated SVM output scores [5].

2.4   Evaluation

The quality of the malignancy estimations was characterized using ROC analysis and computing the area under the curve (AUC). Differences between AUC (including 95% confidence intervals (CI) and two-tailed p-values) were assessed using the bootstrapping method with 5000 times resampling as described in [15]. Differences in AUC were considered statistically significant at the $\alpha = 0.05$ level.

3 Experiments and Results

3.1 Feature Selection

First the free parameter C_{fs} for feature selection using L1-penalized linear SVM (L1P-SVM) was determined. For this purpose, two unimodal validation data sets consisting of 108 findings in MG (63 benign, 45 malignant) resp. 157 findings in MRI (59 benign, 75 malignant) were selected from patients in the database with only unimodal data and therefore were not part of the multimodal data set. Each data set was split using 10-fold cross validation (CV) and the optimal penalty parameter C_{fs} was determined by grid search over $C_{fs} \in \{10^i | i = -3, -2, -1, 0, 1, 2, 3\}$. In each fold the data were standardized by subtracting the mean and dividing by the standard deviation computed on training data. For MG and MRI, $C_{fs}^{opt} = 0.1$ resp. $C_{fs}^{opt} = 10$ maximized AUC with $AUC_{MG} = 0.73$ and $AUC_{MR} = 0.77$. Finally, the L1P-SVM was fit to the entire standardized validation data set using C_{fs}^{opt}, yielding 15 features for MG and 18 features for MRI.

For MG, the selected set comprised 5 CC and 10 MLO view features (4 likelihood, 5 (iso-)density, two spiculation and single features measuring gradient, contrast, morphology and distance to the nipple). In MR, the selected feature set comprised 3 baseline, 3 relative enhancement, two washout characteristic, 5 morphology features and 5 pharmacokinetic parameters (two for K_{Trans}, one for K_{ep} and two for V_e).

3.2 Lesion Classification

Nonlinear Gaussian SVM classification with Platt's score calibration was used to generate malignancy estimates. For each of the multimodal lesions two unimodal classification scores - MG and MRI - and a multimodal score were generated as follows.

The set of multimodal lesions was split according to a leave-one-patient-out cross validation scheme (LOPO-CV), resulting in 90 folds (see Section 2.1). For each fold, the unimodal feature spaces were separately processed. For MG, the multimodal training data were joined with the independent MG data which were not part of the multimodal data set and a dedicated MG classifier was trained using the MG features. For MRI, the procedure was carried out analogously. The data were standardized using the mean and the standard deviation computed on the training data. The parameters for the Gaussian SVM were found by grid search over 10-fold CV inside the training data. The kernel width γ was estimated as the median of all pairwise distances in the training data and C^{opt} was selected using grid search over $C \in \{10^i | i = -3, -2, -1, 0, 1, 2, 3\}$ maximizing AUC on the training set. For lesions which appeared in MG and MRI, a multimodal (MM) malignancy estimate was computed by averaging the MG and MRI scores.

The procedure was carried out using the complete feature sets for MG resp. MRI and the reduced feature sets obtained from feature selection.

Table 1. AUC comparison of the MG, MRI and MM scores obtained when using all 106 available features for MG resp. 46 for MRI in SVM classification and a reduced number of features for MG and MRI with 15 and 18 features, respectively

	All features		Selected features		
Score Type	AUC	95% CI	AUC	95% CI	P-Value
MG	0.68	[0.56,0.79]	0.76	[0.66,0.86]	0.056
MRI	0.69	[0.57,0.79]	0.73	[0.63,0.83]	0.071
MM	0.72	[0.59,0.83]	**0.81**	[0.71,0.89]	**0.018**

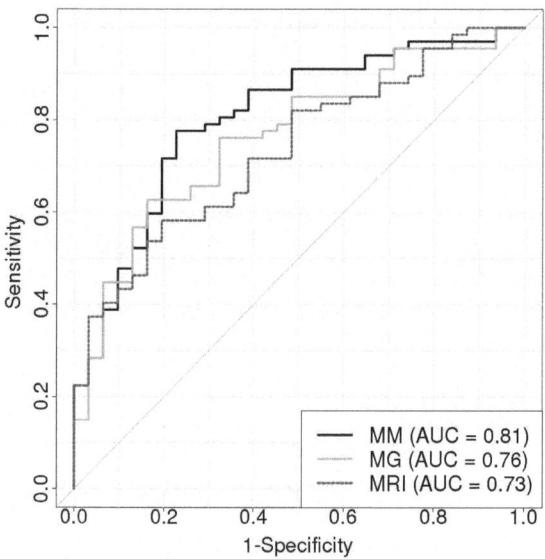

Fig. 1. ROC curves for mammography (MG), MRI and multimodal (MM) CADx using 15 features for MG and 18 features for MRI lesion classification

Using all features, parameter estimation for MG chose an average $\bar{C}_{MG}^{opt} = 4.6$ with standard deviation $sd = 10.88$ during LOPO-CV. Using the reduced feature set $\bar{C}_{MG}^{opt} = 1$ with $sd = 0$ was found during CV. For MRI, using all features resulted in $\bar{C}_{MR}^{opt} = 2.6$ with $sd = 3.44$ respectively $\bar{C}_{MR}^{opt} = 1$ with $sd = 0$ for the reduced feature set, indicating less varying models learned for MG and MR when less features were used. The corresponding AUC for MG, MRI and MM is reported in Table 1. Using the complete feature sets available, the performance of MG and MR was approximately similar. Averaging their scores resulted in a mild performance increase compared to sole unimodal scoring. By using the reduced feature sets, AUC generally increased, whereas MG offered mildly better classification than MRI. In addition, the joint MM score showed a significant improvement in AUC (P = 0.018) and exhibited the best performance obtained in this study. Comparison of the MG, MRI and MM score (see Figure 1) showed that no statistically significant performance difference was obtained between MM and MG (P=0.181) as well as MM and MR (P=0.087). The difference between MR and MM score was more pronounced than between MG and MM.

4   Discussion and Conclusion

In this work, a multimodal breast lesion classification system was proposed relying on fusion of two independent, unimodal CADx systems. Each unimodal CADx system employed L1-penalized SVM feature selection on independent unimodal data and a nonlinear SVM for classification, whereas the final multimodal malignancy estimates were averaged in order to generate a single multimodal decision score.

The dimensionality of the unimodal feature spaces was reduced by filtering features prior to classification. Using L1-penalized SVM classification allowed for a straightforward feature selection scheme which required little effort in terms of parametrization. Relevant feature sets were successfully identified comprising 14 % (MG) and 39% (MRI) of the original feature sets. Particularly in the case of MG, a relatively large feature set was available which resulted from pooling features from CC and MLO view. For both unimodal classifiers, feature selection reduced the variance of the learned models and thus contributed to better generalization. Both unimodal CADx systems benefited from feature selection, while leading to a statistically significant performance improvement in multimodal classification despite only using unimodal feature selection.

The available database reflected an often encountered situation where more unimodal than multimodal data is available. Consequently, the adopted training scheme was tailored to utilize the entire available breadth of unimodal data. The actual decision fusion was carried out by averaging calibrated unimodal SVM malignancy estimates, which caused an improvement over unimodal classification yielding the best AUC observed in this study. A similar observation was reported by Yuan et al. [3], who found a significant increase in AUC from 0.74 (MG) resp. 0.78 (MRI) to 0.87 for multimodal CADx, adopting a feature selection and classification scheme in multimodal feature space. Although in our study the improvement by multimodal CADx was not statistically significant, the joining of unimodal scores by averaging appears as a feasible solution to merge a single multimodal malignancy estimate that can be presented to an observer in MG-MRI CADx in addition to or in lieu of unimodal scores.

In summary, this work described a decision fusion-based system for multimodal classification of breast mass lesions in MG and MRI using L1-penalized SVM feature selection and subsequent nonlinear SVM classification. It could be demonstrated that unimodal feature selection caused a significant increase in multimodal classification performance. Calculating a multimodal malignancy estimate by averaging of unimodal decision scores allowed for a noteworthy increase in performance over unimodal CADx alone and can provide a useful tool for generation of a single joint CADx score in the multimodal setting.

Directions for future work include the evaluation of additional training schemes for multimodal classification as well as the investigation of automated strategies for multimodal lesion linking, such as learning of multimodal feature correspondences.

Acknowledgements. This work was funded by the European 7th Framework Program, HAMAM, ICT-2007.5.3.

References

1. Kuhl, C.K., Kuhn, W., Schild, H.: Management of women at high risk for breast cancer: new imaging beyond mammography. The Breast 14(6), 480–486 (2005)
2. Horsch, K., Giger, M.L., Vyborny, C.J., Lan, L., Mendelson, E.B., Hendrick, R.E.: Classification of breast lesions with multimodality computer-aided diagnosis: observer study results on an independent clinical data set. Radiology 240(2), 357 (2006)
3. Yuan, Y., Giger, M.L., Li, H., Bhooshan, N., Sennett, C.A.: Multimodality Computer-Aided Breast Cancer Diagnosis with FFDM and DCE-MRI. Academic Radiology 17(9), 1158–1167 (2010)
4. Constantinos, S.P., Pattichis, M.S., Micheli-Tzanakou, E.: Medical imaging fusion applications: An overview. In: Conference Record of the Thirty-Fifth Asilomar Conference on Signals, Systems and Computers 2001, vol. 2, pp. 1263–1267. IEEE (2001)
5. Kittler, J., Hatef, M., Duin, R.P.W., Matas, J.: On combining classifiers. IEEE Transactions on Pattern Analysis and Machine Intelligence 20(3), 226–239 (1998)
6. Bhooshan, N., Giger, M.L., Drukker, K., Yuan, Y., Li, H., McCann, S., Newstead, G., Sennett, C.: Performance of Triple-Modality CADx on Breast Cancer Diagnostic Classification. In: Martí, J., Oliver, A., Freixenet, J., Martí, R. (eds.) IWDM 2010. LNCS, vol. 6136, pp. 9–14. Springer, Heidelberg (2010)
7. Ng, A.Y.: Feature selection, l 1 vs. l 2 regularization, and rotational invariance. In: Proceedings of the Twenty-First International Conference on Machine Learning, p. 78. ACM (2004)
8. Weston, J., Mukherjee, S., Chapelle, O., Pontil, M., Poggio, T., Vapnik, V.: Feature selection for svms. Advances in Neural Information Processing Systems, 668–674 (2001)
9. Chen, Y.-W., Lin, C.-J.: Combining svms with various feature selection strategies. In: Guyon, I., Nikravesh, M., Gunn, S., Zadeh, L. (eds.) Feature Extraction. Studies in Fuzziness and Soft Computing, vol. 207, pp. 315–324. Springer, Heidelberg (2006)
10. Hupse, R., Karssemeijer, N.: Use of Normal Tissue Context in Computer-Aided Detection of Masses in Mammograms. IEEE Transactions on Medical Imaging 28(12), 2033–2041 (2009)

11. Platel, B., Huisman, H., Laue, H., Mus, R., Mann, R., Hahn, H., Karssemeijer, N.: Computerized characterization of breast lesions using dual-temporal resolution dynamic contrast-enhanced mr images. In: Workshop on Breast Image Analysi in conjunction with the 14th International Conference on Medical Image Computing and Computer Assisted Intervention, MICCAI 2011 (2011)
12. Veltman, J., Stoutjesdijk, M., Mann, R., Huisman, H.J., Barentsz, J.O., Blickman, J.G., Boetes, C.: Contrast-enhanced magnetic resonance imaging of the breast: the value of pharmacokinetic parameters derived from fast dynamic imaging during initial enhancement in classifying lesions. European Radiology 18(6), 1123–1133 (2008)
13. Fan, R.E., Chang, K.W., Hsieh, C.J., Wang, X.R., Lin, C.J.: Liblinear: A library for large linear classification. The Journal of Machine Learning Research 9, 1871–1874 (2008)
14. Chang, C.C., Lin, C.J.: Libsvm: a library for support vector machines. ACM Transactions on Intelligent Systems and Technology (TIST) 2(3), 27 (2011)
15. Robin, X., Turck, N., Hainard, A., Tiberti, N., Lisacek, F., Sanchez, J.C., Muller, M.: Proc: an open-source package for r and s+ to analyze and compare roc curves. BMC Bioinformatics 12(1), 77 (2011)

Comparison of Lesion Size Using Area and Volume in Full Field Digital Mammograms

Jelena Bozek[1], Michiel Kallenberg[2], Mislav Grgic[1], and Nico Karssemeijer[2]

[1] University of Zagreb, Faculty of Electrical Engineering and Computing,
Unska 3, HR-10000 Zagreb, Croatia
[2] Radboud University Nijmegen Medical Centre, Department of Radiology,
Geert Grooteplein Zuid 18, 6525 GA Nijmegen, The Netherlands
jelena.bozek@fer.hr

Abstract. The size of a lesion is a feature often used in computer-aided detection systems for classification between benign and malignant lesions. However, size of a lesion presented by its area might not be as reliable as volume of a lesion. Volume is more independent of the view (CC or MLO) since it represents three dimensional information, whereas area refers only to the projection of a lesion on a two dimensional plane. Furthermore, volume might be better than area for comparing lesion size in two consecutive exams and for evaluating temporal change to distinguish benign and malignant lesions. We have used volumetric breast density estimation in digital mammograms to obtain thickness of dense tissue in regions of interest in order to compute volume of lesions. The dataset consisted of 382 mammogram pairs in CC and MLO views and 120 mammogram pairs for temporal analysis. The obtained correlation coefficients between the lesion size in the CC and MLO views were 0.70 (0.64-0.76) and 0.83 (0.79-0.86) for area and volume, respectively. Two-tailed z-test showed a significant difference between two correlation coefficients (p=0.0001). The usage of area and volume in temporal analysis of mammograms has been evaluated using ROC analysis. The obtained values of the area under the curve (AUC) were 0.73 and 0.75 for area and volume, respectively. Although a higher AUC value for volume was found, this difference was not significant (p=0.16).

Keywords: digital mammography, temporal change, lesion classification, CAD, breast density.

1 Introduction

In developed computer-aided detection (CAD) systems one of the features that has been used for the classification between benign and malignant lesions is the size computed as the area of a lesion [1]. However, since the mammogram is a two dimensional projection of a three dimensional breast, the area of a lesion visible in two mammographic views, namely craniocaudal (CC) and mediolateral oblique (MLO), might differ. To overcome this issue one could calculate volume of a lesion, as the volume might be a more reliable feature that should remain

A.D.A. Maidment, P.R. Bakic, and S. Gavenonis (Eds.): IWDM 2012, LNCS 7361, pp. 96–103, 2012.
© Springer-Verlag Berlin Heidelberg 2012

the same in both views and might be better for use in CAD systems than the area of a lesion. In addition, volume might give reliable information about the lesion seen in two consecutive exams, i.e. for evaluating temporal change in the size of a lesion. Since benign lesions have tendency to stay the same over time and malignant lesions tend to grow, volume might be a useful feature for distinguishing between benign and malignant lesions in temporal comparison of digital mammograms.

Volume of dense tissue in digital mammograms can be computed using the method developed by van Engeland et al. [2]. In this study we investigated the use of volume as a measure of lesion size compared to area. We were interested in the area and volume of a lesion in CC and MLO views. We hypothesized that the effective radius of a lesion obtained from volume is more similar in the two views than the one obtained from area. Additionally, we analysed the effective radius obtained from area and volume in the temporal mammogram pairs. In particular, we explored the possibility of volume as a feature to distinguish benign and malignant lesions in temporal comparison of mammograms.

2   Method

2.1   Dataset

Digital mammograms for this study were collected from the screening-institution Preventicon, Utrecht, the Netherlands, where they were acquired with a Hologic Selenia FFDM system. All mammograms used in the study have a visible lesion that has been biopsy proven as benign or malignant. In this study under the term lesion we consider masses, architectural distortion and bilateral asymmetry. We have included only lesions that are projected within the breast area, i.e. not overlapping with the pectoral muscle.

The dataset for the analysis of area and volume performance for CC and MLO views consisted of 382 digital mammogram pairs with lesion visible in both views, of which 164 were benign and 218 malignant lesions. For the temporal analysis the dataset comprised 120 mammogram pairs, of which 74 benign and 46 malignant lesions that were visible in both prior and current mammogram. All FFDM mammograms were downsampled to a resolution of 200 microns using bilinear interpolation.

2.2   Area and Volume Computation

The center location of each region that contained a lesion was annotated by a radiologist and was used as a seed point for automated segmentation. The segmentation method is based on the region boundary information and grey level distribution of a region of interest around the lesion. The best contour is selected using an optimisation technique known as dynamic programming. The method is explained in detail in [3].

For each pixel in the segmented region we have determined the thickness of dense tissue based on a physical model of image acquisition. The model proposed by van Engeland et al. [2] assumes that the breast is composed of two types of tissue, dense glandular tissue and fatty tissue. The attenuation of a mixture of dense and fatty tissue at a given location is given by

$$\frac{I}{I_0} = \int_{E=0}^{\infty} p(E)e^{-\mu_f(E)h_f - \mu_d(E)h_d}dE \tag{1}$$

where I is the X-ray exposure, $p(E)$ is the normalized photon energy spectrum, μ_d and μ_f are linear attenuation coefficients for dense and fatty tissue, respectively, and h_d and h_f are thicknesses of dense and fatty tissue, respectively.

Since in an unprocessed full field digital mammograms pixel values are proportional to the total exposure $I(\mathbf{r})$, the image model is obtained from (1) by replacing exposure value (I) with pixel value (g)

$$\frac{g(\mathbf{r})}{g_0} = \int_{E=0}^{\infty} p(E)e^{-\mu_f(E)h_f(\mathbf{r}) - \mu_d(E)h_d(\mathbf{r})}dE$$

$$= \int_{E=0}^{\infty} p(E)e^{-\mu_f(E)h(\mathbf{r}) - (\mu_d(E) - \mu_f(E))h_d(\mathbf{r})}dE. \tag{2}$$

In this equation the normalized photon energy spectrum $p(E)$ and the attenuation coefficients $\mu_f(E)$ and $\mu_d(E)$ are known from the empirical data. Computation of the dense breast tissue thickness $h_d(\mathbf{r})$ would be straightforward if it would be possible to determine breast thickness $h(\mathbf{r})$ and the pixel value associated with the incident X-ray beam g_0. Unfortunately, it is not easy to accurately obtain estimates of these parameters in practice.

Hence, van Engeland et al. [2] applied thickness correction transform on the mammogram in which a layer of adipose tissue with attenuation coefficients $\mu_f(E)$ and thickness $H - h(\mathbf{r})$ was added to the breast. In the obtained image the following relation holds

$$\frac{\bar{g}(\mathbf{r})}{g_0} = \int_{E=0}^{\infty} p(E)e^{-\mu_f(E)H - (\mu_d(E) - \mu_f(E))h_d(\mathbf{r})}dE \tag{3}$$

In this image pixel values only vary with dense tissue thickness. By setting $h_d(\mathbf{r})=0$ in (3) image model for purely fatty tissue is obtained as

$$\frac{\bar{g}_f}{g_0} = \int_{E=0}^{\infty} p(E)e^{-\mu_f(E)H}dE. \tag{4}$$

By substituting the pixel value of fatty tissue $\bar{g}_f$ in (3) we obtain

$$\frac{\bar{g}(\mathbf{r})}{\bar{g}_f} = \frac{\int_{E=0}^{\infty} p(E)e^{-\mu_f(E)H - (\mu_d(E) - \mu_f(E))h_d(\mathbf{r})}dE}{\int_{E=0}^{\infty} p(E)e^{-\mu_f(E)H}dE} \tag{5}$$

In principle, $h_d(\mathbf{r})$ can be solved from this equation if H is known. However, due to the internal calibration with a fatty tissue pixel value, the value of H is not critical anymore.

To simplify the computations, van Engeland et al. [2] computed effective attenuation coefficients for fatty and dense tissue. The effective attenuation coefficients depend on acquisition parameters and are computed as a function of the anode and filter material, tube voltage and breast thickness H. For typical spectra used in mammographic imaging this attenuation can very well be approximated by an exponential function. As such, we obtain the logarithm of attenuation written as

$$\ln \frac{I}{I_0} \approx -\mu_{f,\text{eff}} h_f - \mu_{d,\text{eff}} h_d$$
$$= -\mu_{f,\text{eff}}(H - h_d) - \mu_{d,\text{eff}} h_d \tag{6}$$

where H is breast thickness, and $\mu_{f,\text{eff}}$ and $\mu_{d,\text{eff}}$ are effective attenuation coefficients for fatty and dense tissue, respectively. By applying the exponential approximation (6) and rewriting (5) with the effective attenuation coefficients $\mu_{f,\text{eff}}$ and $\mu_{d,\text{eff}}$ the explicit dependency of H dissapears. The thickness of dense tissue at a location $\mathbf{r}$ is obtained by the following relation

$$h_d(\mathbf{r}) = -\frac{1}{\mu_{d,\text{eff}} - \mu_{f,\text{eff}}} \ln \frac{\bar{g}(\mathbf{r})}{\bar{g}_f}. \tag{7}$$

From the obtained thickness and area of the lesion we have computed its volume. For the comparative analysis of the performance of area and volume as a measure of lesion size we have computed effective radiuses as follows:

$$r_{\text{eff,area}} = \sqrt{\frac{A}{\pi}} \tag{8}$$

$$r_{\text{eff,volume}} = \sqrt[3]{\frac{3V}{4\pi}} \tag{9}$$

where A is area and V volume of the segmented region.

3   Results

The comparison of area and volume was performed for the corresponding lesions in the CC and MLO views as well as in the temporal mammogram pairs using the effective radiuses. In order to evaluate volume compared to area in CC and MLO views we computed Pearson's correlation coefficient. The correlation plots for all data, i.e. both benign and malignant lesions, are presented in Fig. 1. The correlation coefficient between CC and MLO views for the area of a lesion is 0.70, with 95% confidence interval 0.64-0.76. The correlation coefficient between CC view and MLO view for the volume of a lesion is 0.82, with 95% confidence interval 0.79-0.86. The significance of the difference between two correlation

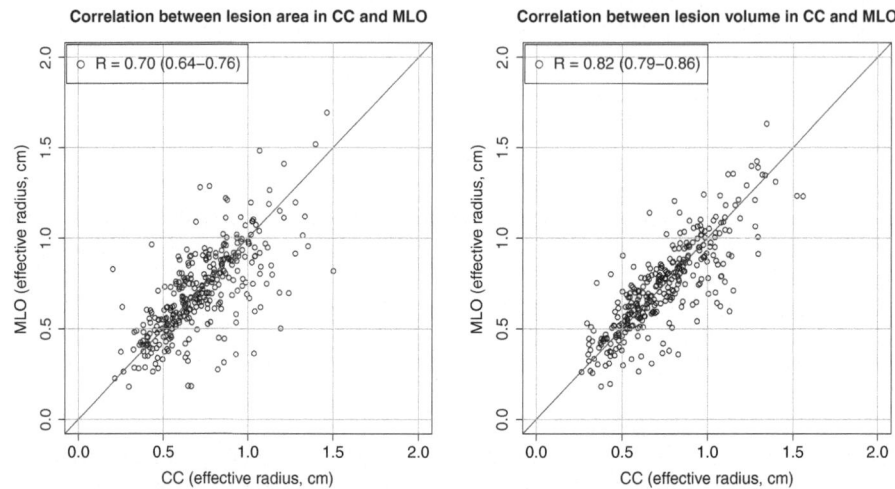

Fig. 1. Correlation for effective radiuses of lesion area and lesion volume between CC and MLO views

coefficients was assessed with a two-tailed z-test. The obtained z-score was 4.03 which corresponds to the p-value of 0.0001 and shows that the difference is significant.

For the analysis of temporal mammogram pairs we used Pearson's correlation coefficient between current and prior mammogram for lesion area and volume. Correlation plots for temporal change in area and volume in subsequent screening intervals for benign and malignant lesions are presented in Fig. 2. The correlation coefficient for the area of a lesion is 0.79, with 95% confidence interval 0.68-0.86, for benign lesions and 0.63, with 95% confidence interval 0.38-0.79, for malignant lesions. The correlation coefficient for the volume of a lesion is 0.86, with 95% confidence interval 0.79-0.91, for benign lesions, and 0.69, with 95% confidence interval 0.47-0.83, for malignant lesions.

Assuming that benign lesions are stable and malignant lesions grow, we used change of lesion size as an indicator of malignancy and computed the receiver operating characteristic (ROC) curve using change in lesion size as a single feature. The feature was computed in two ways, using size of a lesion in the current view and in the prior view obtained by

$$A_{\text{diff}} = A_{\text{current}} - A_{\text{prior}} \tag{10}$$

$$V_{\text{diff}} = V_{\text{current}} - V_{\text{prior}} \tag{11}$$

where A_{current} and A_{prior} are areas of a lesion in the current and prior view, and V_{current} and V_{prior} are volumes of a lesion in the current and prior view.

ROC curves for area and volume change were plotted using the ROCR package [4] and are shown in Fig. 3. The obtained values of the area under the curve (AUC) were 0.73, with 95% confidence interval 0.62-0.82, and 0.75, with 95% confidence interval 0.66-0.85, for area and volume, respectively. However, use of volume compared to area did not show significant improvement in distinguishing between benign and malignant lesions as assessed by bootstrapping (p=0.16) using the pROC package [5].

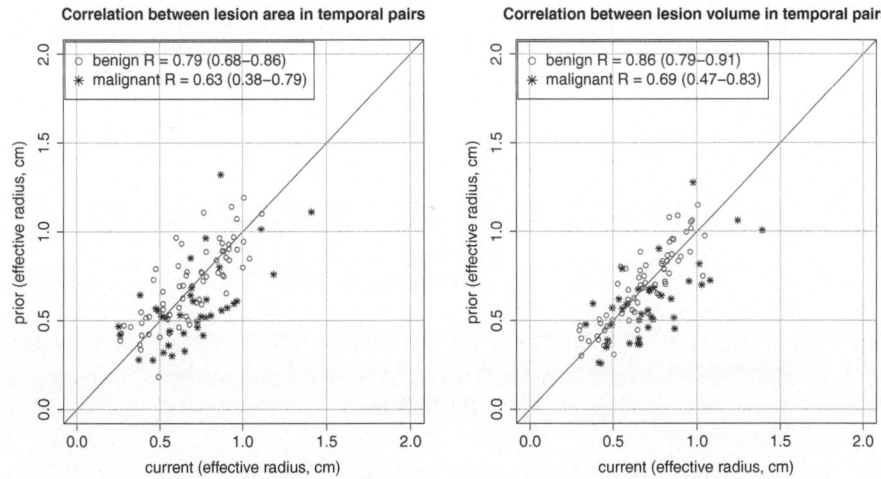

Fig. 2. Correlation for effective radiuses of lesion area and lesion volume between current and prior mammogram

4   Discussion

To the best of our knowledge this is the first paper that validates lesion volume size both in CC and MLO digital mammograms and in temporal mammogram pairs. Results showed that when comparing area and volume of a lesion in the CC and MLO views, area is less consistent between the views than volume, which suggests that volume is a more accurate feature for assessing the size of a lesion. These results suggest that volume might be a better feature in CAD systems for measuring size of a lesion than area.

Although in the temporal analysis volume did not significantly outperform area in its performance of distinguishing between benign and malignant lesions, results indicate that it might be a better feature for representing size of a lesion.

Obviously, results depend on the lesion segmentation method that was employed. It is remarked that when lesions are embedded in fatty tissue it will not affect the volume estimates if lesions are oversegmented, as the area outside

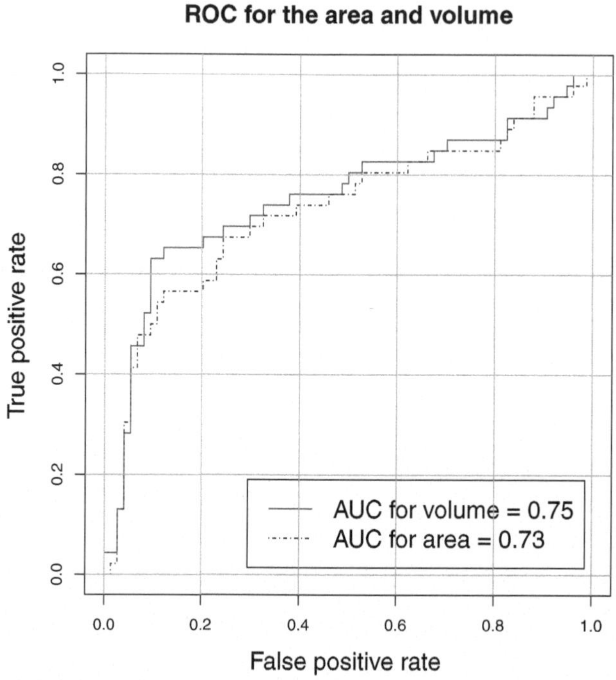

ROC for the area and volume

Fig. 3. ROC curves for the area and volume of a lesion

the lesion will not contribute to its volume due to the fact that in this area dense tissue thickness will be zero. This makes volume a more robust feature.

Acknowledgements. The work in this paper was conducted under the research project "Intelligent Image Features Extraction in Knowledge Discovery Systems" (036-0982560-1643), supported by the Ministry of Science, Education and Sports of the Republic of Croatia. These materials are based on work financed by the Croatian Science Foundation. The financial support for presenting this paper was provided by the Foundation of the Croatian Academy of Sciences and Arts, which is gratefully acknowledged.

References

1. Hupse, R., Karssemeijer, N.: Use of normal tissue context in computer-aided detection of masses in mammograms. IEEE Transactions on Medical Imaging 28, 2033–2041 (2009)
2. van Engeland, S., Snoeren, P.R., Huisman, H., Boetes, C., Karssemeijer, N.: Volumetric breast density estimation from full-field digital mammograms. IEEE Transactions on Medical Imaging 25, 273–282 (2006)

3. Timp, S., Karssemeijer, N.: A new 2D segmentation method based on dynamic programming applied to computer aided detection in mammography. Medical Physics 31, 958–971 (2004)
4. Sing, T., Sander, O., Beerenwinkel, N., Lengauer, T.: ROCR: visualizing classifier performance in R. Bioinformatics 21, 3940–3941 (2005)
5. Robin, X., Turck, N., Hainard, A., Tiberti, N., Lisacek, F., Sanchez, J.C., Mueller, M.: pROC: an open-source package for R and S+ to analyze and compare ROC curves. BMC Bioinformatics 12, 77 (2011)

Very High Contrast and Very High Spatial Resolution 2-D, 2.5-D and 3-D Breast Tissue Visualization under X-ray Dark Field Imaging

Masami Ando[1,*], Qingkai Huo[1], Shu Ichihara[2], Tokiko Endo[2], Tetsuya Yuasa[3], Naoki Sunaguchi[4], and Kensaku Mori[5]

[1] RIST, Tokyo University of Science, Noda, 278-8510 Japan
msm-ando@rs.noda.tus.ac.jp, ddllhqk76@gmail.com
[2] Department of Advanced Diagnosis, NMC, Nagoya, 460-0001 Japan
shu-kkr@umin.ac.jp, endot@nnh.hosp.go.jp
[3] Faculty of Engineering, Yamagata University, Yonezawa, 992-8510 Japan
yuasa@yz.yamagata-u.ac.jp
[4] Photon Factory, KEK, Oho 1-1, Tsukuba, Ibaraki 305-0801 Japan
kuroiinazuma@gmail.com
[5] Graduate School of IS, Nagoya University, Nagoya, 464-8603 Japan
kensakum@gmail.com

Abstract. A parallel x-ray beam that is made by an asymmetric-cut Bragg monochromator-collimator (MC) is incident on breast tissue so that the beam containing information from the breast tissue is incident upon a Laue-case angle analyzer (LAA). This beam is subsequently split into a forward diffracted beam and a separate diffracted beam. We acquire two beams simultaneously each of which contains relating angular information on specimen so that one can deduce simultaneously angular information at each pixel. In this paper, we propose an imaging system using dark-field imaging (XDFI) for 2D image, CT measurement and 2.5D image (tomosynthesis) based on a tandem system of Bragg- and Laue-case crystals with two CCD cameras, along with a data-processing method to extract information on refraction from the measured entangled intensities by use of rocking curve fitting with polynomial functions. Reconstructed images of soft tissues are presented and described.

Keywords: X-ray dark-field imaging, synchrotron radiation, refraction contrast, 2D image, 2.5D (tomosynthesis) image, 3D image, breast tissue, breast cancer.

1   Introduction

Imaging based on the phase-contrast term δ produces much greater contrast in the case of medical soft tissues consisting of low Z-elements than imaging based on the absorption term β, where $n = 1 - \delta - i\beta$ is the complex refractive index. Up to now, a variety of imaging methods have been proposed [1-3]. Currently, the diffraction

---

* Corresponding author.

A.D.A. Maidment, P.R. Bakic, and S. Gavenonis (Eds.): IWDM 2012, LNCS 7361, pp. 104–110, 2012.

enhanced imaging (DEI) method [4] by means of a Bragg-case analyzer which detects the incident beam angular deviation due to refraction is the most widespread method utilized in medical applications. This is due to the imaging geometry having an affinity to tomographic imaging [5-8]. DEI-CT (computed tomography) has been developed into an excellent method to delineate biological soft tissues, with further potential to develop other medical science applications [9,10].

The deflection angle, $\Delta (x,y: k)$ associated with a refraction contrast which is the basic component of dark-field imaging can be described as follows:

$$\Delta (x,y: k) \propto - \int_{z0}^{z1} \partial \, \delta(x,y,z: k) / \partial x \, dz, \qquad (1)$$

where $\delta(x,y,z: k)$ is related to the refractive index, $n = 1 - \delta(x,y,z: k)$, z is the direction of the x-ray beam, z_0 and z_1 mean the coordinates where the x-rays come into and out from a sample, respectively, and let refraction take place along the x axis so that (z,x) should be the incidence plane and y is vertical to the plane (z,x).

In our imaging system the x-ray optics named XDFI (x-ray dark-field imaging) was proposed [11], where the Laue geometry of diffraction in a (+ , -) parallel achromatic arrangement is essential so that image contains no effect of the wavelength spread, that may otherwise blur the contrast. Two beams, one I_o toward the direction of the forward diffraction and the other I_G corresponding to the diffracted direction from an analyzer crystal plate, can be expressed if the x rays undergo no absorption, as follows:

$$Io = sin^2(t\pi/\sqrt{1+W^2} / \Lambda)/(1 + W^2), \qquad (2)$$

$$I_G = ((cos^2 (t\pi/\sqrt{1+W^2} / \Lambda) + W^2)/(1 + W^2), \qquad (3)$$

$$Io + I_G = 1, \qquad (4)$$

, where t, W, Λ are the crystal thickness, the deviation of the angle from the Bragg condition, expressed as $W = 2\Lambda \, sin\theta_B \, v/c (\theta - \theta_B - \Delta\theta_0)$, and the extinction distance, expressed as $\Lambda = v/c \, cos\theta_B / P/\chi_G/$ where v relates to the x-ray photon energy hv, θ_B the Bragg angle, P the polarization factor and χ_G is the polarizability, expressed as $\chi_G = \beta v\eta - r_e (v/c)^2 F_G /\pi V_C$, where r_e is the classical radius of electron, F_G the crystal structure from factor and V_C is the volume of unit cell. $\Delta\theta_0 = 2(1-n)/sin^2\theta_B$. Equations (2) and (3) can be simplified as

$$Io|_{W=0} = sin^2 (t\pi/\Lambda) \qquad (5)$$

and

$$I_G|_{W=0} = cos^2 (t\pi/\Lambda) \qquad (6)$$

at $W=0$ so that these Io and I_G oscillate between 0% and 100% reflection at every thickness change of the analyzer, $\Delta t = p\Lambda/2$, where p is an integer, while keeping the relation between them, $Io + I_G = 1$. Δt corresponds to 62.5 μm in case of 4,4,0 reflection at 35 keV. Its corresponding x-ray photon energy ΔE should be approximately 3.05 keV. If one can achieve these conditions, that can give $Io = 0\%$, one can obtain dark-field imaging. In this paper is described application of XDFI to medical imaging.

2   Experimental: Optic of X-ray Dark-Field Imaging

An explanation is given as follows: first prepare an extremely straight forward beam by MC (monochromator-collimator) as shown in Fig .1 using asymmetric diffraction [12]. In Figure 1 is shown a sketch of a typical XDFI optics where diffracting planes of both MC and LAA (Laue angle analyzer) are in a parallel arrangement. FD (forward diffraction) corresponds to Io and D (diffraction) to I_G. Object is located between MC and LAA. FD corresponds to dark-field imaging Io and D bright-field one I_G.

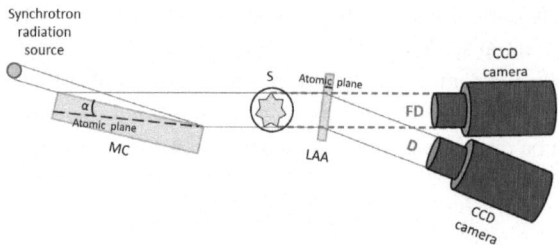

Fig. 1. The XDFI system where the thickness of LAA (Laue angle analyzer) was chosen so that the x-ray intensity of the forward diffraction FD becomes zero at $w=0$. Since one can obtain two beams one FD and the other D can save.

We have chosen the asymmetric factor $b = \sin(\Theta_B - \alpha)/\sin(\Theta_B + \alpha)$, where Θ_B is 10.6° for 440 diffraction and 35keV and α is 10.2°, to be 0.05, that can provide a divergence of the beam incident onto the object of 0.28 μrad. We would like to emphasize that our system can thus provide complete dark- and bright- imaging simultaneously by a single shot. Further, the dark-field imaging consists of mapping of the refraction in an object without background. All of the previous work should belong to the category between bright-field imaging and dark-field imaging, including that by Ingal and Beliaevskaya [2] in the Laue geometry. Although the background of their imaging could be reduced to some extent, it was not hundred percent by tuning the angular position of an analyzer so that the Bragg angle would be $|W|>>0$.

An experiment was performed at beamline BL14C [13] using a radiation source from a 5 Tesla vertical wiggler at the 2.5 GeV Photon Factory so that the polarization of the radiation is vertical. This means that the plane of incidence that comprises the incident x-rays and the diffracted x-rays is horizontal. That the plane of incidence gives us a big advantage over the vertical plane of incidence because one can set up the whole imaging system on the same horizontal plane that is usually a steel plate.

X-ray images were picked up by CCD cameras (Photonic Science, pixel number: 4008×2670, pixel size: 12.5×12.5 μm^2, FOV: 49 mm horizontal and 33 mm vertical size). An object placed upon a rotational stage is inserted between MC and LAA, and the rotational axis of the object is parallel to that of rotation axis of MC and LAA. The angular positions of the MC and LAA are fixed after being adjusted before measurement data is collected whereupon the object axis is rotated for CT data acquisition. The monochromatic vertical size is 33 mm at the station BL14C and the incident horizontal beam size is 8 mm before MC and is expanded to a square parallel beam by an asymmetrical Bragg-case MC to cover the full object width. The beam impinges on the object and is refracted and absorbed by the object. The beam containing internal information of the object impinging LAA is split into the FD and the D beam as shown in Fig. 1. The LAA is adjusted at half up the peak, and at half down the valley of the rocking curves for the D and FD beams, respectively. The Bragg-case MC plays not only the role of collimating and expanding the beam, but also that of smoothing the rocking curves which have many ripples of the LAA. Since the LAA with size of $\Phi 80$ mm $\times 0.29$ mm^T requests no deformation of the diffracting planes, by that means the radius of curvature should be greater than 2 km. The LAA was vertically set and attached onto a surface of a 2 mm thick mirror polished Be plate with size of 100 mm $\times$ 100 mm.

The nearly plane-wave x-rays from MC that enter object S may receive a very small refraction effect, either left or right or both directions, against the incident beam direction. Let's introduce a simplified model of object. The x rays which exit from the object S may possess information. An angle analyzer crystal LAA which takes place diffraction corresponding to Io, such as $Io = 0\ \%$ at $|W| \leq 1$. Mathematically convolution of Io or I_G and S may result in two diffraction profiles. Io corresponding to FD shows high reflectivity for almost all angular ranges, except for the central position $|W| \leq 1$. What happens to the beam from the object because of effect due to this angular filter which apparently has no central part. This can be called dark-field imaging. This means that almost all refraction information the object has can remain in a visual image with no background.

Since the theory described in (5) thickness of LAA to fulfill the condition of dark-field imaging has to be fixed with the precision of μm; if final t shows a different value than theory still one can find out a way to adjust the condition of (5) such as tilting the LAA so that one can change an apparent x-ray path length in LAA to adjust t. Furthermore tuning the x-ray photon energy in keV is equivalent too.

3   Result of 2D Image

Fig. 2 shows two kinds of views of nodular adenosis, one pathological picture stained with hematoxyline and eosin and the other x-ray photo taken with XDFI. The arrow indicates lobular.

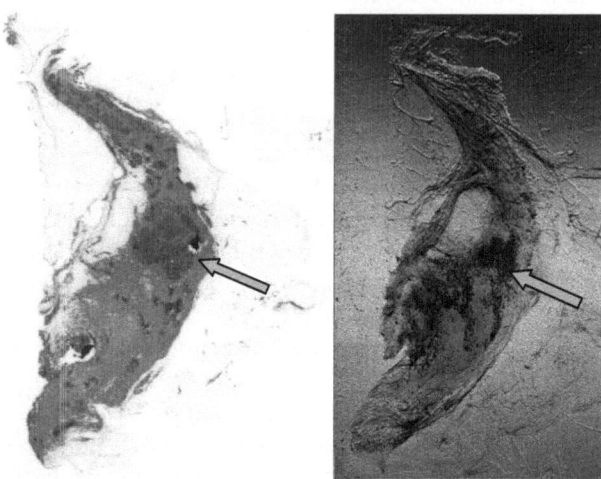

Fig. 2. Pathological view (left) and the XDFI (right) of nodular adenosis. An arrow in the XDFI corresponds to the arrow shown in the pathological view so that the XDFI can reveal lobular as well by x-ray refraction contrast.

A variety of approaches to deduce refraction component have been proposed [14-20]. Chapman *et al.* has made a pioneering work of first extracting information on refraction from the both D intensity and the FD in the LAA system using an algorithm based on linear approximation [14]. Later, Maksimenko used the tail of the Bragg reflection curve to reflect nonlinear relations between the intensity gray scale and the angular deviation due to refraction [15]. Yuasa et al proposed a wave theory [16] to visualize soft tissue with refraction-based contrast. Also Bushuev et al proposed another approach based on wave theory [17]. As an approach to acquire purely refracted component Kitchen et al [18] introduced a concept to obtain ratio between the beam. The incidence angle was used to find the closest match to the intensity ratio using a linear fit between a look-up table prepared from ratio of the two rocking curves. They showed a beautiful 2-D image of a rabbit pup thorax. On the other hand, it is necessary extract more precisely refraction angles toward reconstruction of tomography. Sunaguchi et al improved the precision of extraction of refraction angle without absorption using the polynomial fitting of rocking curves [19], which is used in the present paper.

4   Result of 3D Image

In order to reconstruct a CT image, a set of projections are collected by repeating the measurement procedure while rotating the object. Then, the reconstruction algorithm for refraction-contrast CT [20] is applied to projections of refraction-angle estimated with the proposed method above. We refer to the imaging scheme as DFI-CT following DEI-CT. The condition of XDFI [10] has been selected so that it has the deepest FD profile and the highest D profile, respectively so that one can obtain the largest black and white range of grey scale of x-ray intensity that can be converted to angular information.

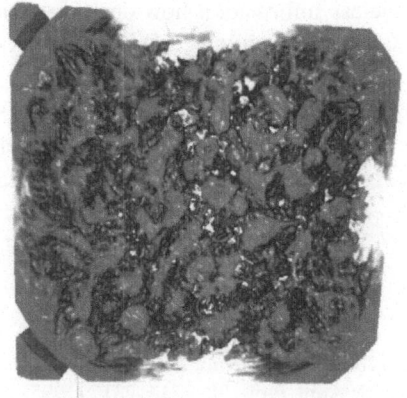

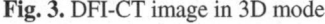

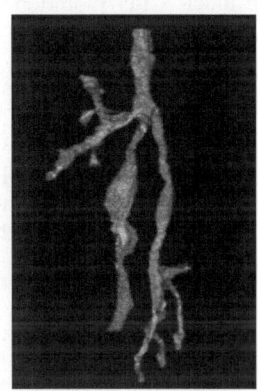

Fig. 3. DFI-CT image in 3D mode   **Fig. 4.** Milk duct of DCIS

We imaged a soft tissue sample of ductal carcinoma in situ (DCIS) that was removed surgically from a breast-cancer patient[19]. The sample size was $2.5 \times 2.1 \times 4.5$ cm^3, and put in an acrylic cylinder filled with alcohol. The number of projections acquired corresponded to 900. Fig. 3 shows the reconstruction in 3D mode. Fig. 4 shows a 3D image of a milk duct consisting of 5 branches that has a relation to the structure of Fig. 3. The overall configuration of fibrous and adipose tissue has shown well correlation in between refraction and pathological views. In conventional absorption based X-ray CT, the DCIS itself, except for calcification which sometimes occurs in secretory or necrotic material, has hardly been depicted. Clear 3D view of lobular carcinoma with the spatial resolution of 7 μm has also been successfully visualized [21].

5   Result of 2.5D (Tomosynthesis) Image

Furthermore attempt was made to reconstruct a tomosynthesis (TS) image [22]. From the point of view of bringing the refraction-based X-ray contrast into clinical issue the authors do not think 3D image is appropriate because patient might has to be exposed to

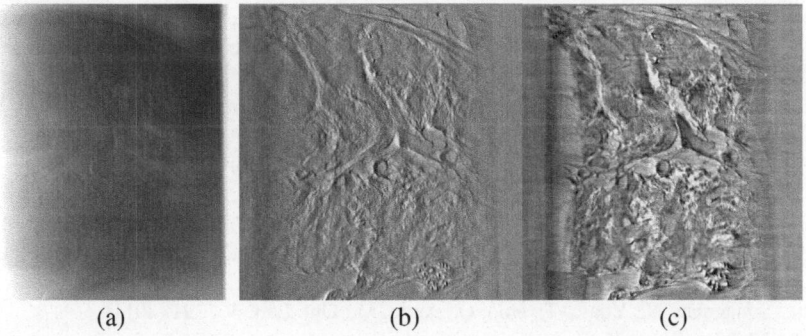

(a)   (b)   (c)

Fig. 5. Three ways of reconstruction of a DCIS specimen. A classical shift-and-add TS, novel sgn+shepp filter back projection TS image and sgn+shepp filter back projection CT image.

too much x-ray radiation dose. Nevertheless information how deep one critical part locates in breast is always of use so that trial of obtaining 2.5D image if not complete 3D information is under way.

Acknowledgement. This work is supported in part by a Grant-in-Aid for Scientific Research (No. 22591353) from the Ministry of Education, Culture, Sports, Science and Technology (MEXT) in Japan, and in part by a Grant-in-Aid for Clinical Research from the National Hospital Organization. The experiment was performed under the approval of the PAB at KEK under No. 2008S2-002, 2011G-672 for use of the Photon Factory.

References

1. Fitzgerald, R.: Physics Today 63(7), 23 (2000)
2. Ingal, V.N., Beliaevskaya, E.A.: J. Phys. D: Appl. Phys. 28, 2314–2317 (1995)
3. Davis, T.J., Gao, D., Gureyev, T.E., Stevenson, A.W., Wilkins, S.W.: Nature 373, 595–598 (1995)
4. Chapman, D., Thomlinson, W., Johnston, R.E., Washburn, D., Pisano, E., Gmür, N., Zhong, Z., Menk, R., Arfelli, F., Sayers, D.: Phys. Med. Biol. 42, 2015 (1997)
5. Dilmanian, F.A., Zhong, Z., Ren, B., Wu, X.Y., Chapman, D., Orion, I., Thomlinson, W.C.: Phys. Med. Biol. 45, 933 (2000)
6. Maksimenko, A., Ando, M., Sugiyama, H., Yuasa, T.: Appl. Phys. Lett. 86, 124105 (2005)
7. Huang, Z., Kang, K., Li, Z., Zhu, P., Yuan, Q., Huang, W., Wang, J., Zhang, D., Yu, A.: Appl. Phys. Lett. 89, 041124 (2006)
8. Yuasa, T., Maksimenko, A., Hashimoto, E., Sugiyama, H., Hyodo, K., Akatsuka, T., Ando, M.: Optics Letters 31(12), 1818 (2006)
9. Ichihara, S., Ando, M., Maksimenko, A., Yuasa, T., Sugiyama, H., Hashimoto, E., Yamasaki, K., Mori, K., Arai, Y., Endo, T.: Virchows Arch. 452, 41 (2008)
10. Ando, M., Bando, H., Endo, T., Ichihara, S., Hashimoto, E., Hyodo, H., Kunisada, T., Gang, L., Maksimenko, A., Mori, K., Shimao, D., Sugiyama, H., Yuasa, T., Ueno, E.: European Journal of Radiology 68, S32 (2008)
11. Ando, M., Maksimenko, A., Sugiyama, H., Pattanasiriwisawa, W., Hyodo, K., Uyama, C.: Jpn. J. Appl. Phys. 41, L1016 (2002)
12. Kohra, K.: J. Phys. Soc. Jpn. 17, 589 (1962)
13. Ando, M., Satow, Y., Kawata, H., Ishikawa, T., Spieker, P., Suzuki, S.: Nucl. Instr. & Meth. A264-1, 144–148 (1986)
14. Chapman, D., Thomlinson, W., Arfelli, F., Gmuer, N., Zhong, Z., Menk, R., Johnson, R.E., Washburn, D., Pisano, E., Sayers, D.: Rev. Sci. Instrum. 67(1) (1996)
15. Maksimenko, A.: Appl. Phys. Lett. 90, 154106 (2006)
16. Yuasa, T., Sugiyama, H., Zhong, Z., Maksimenko, A., Dilmanian, F.A., Akatsuka, T., Ando, M.: JOSA 22, 2622 (2005)
17. Bushuev, V.A., Guskova, M.A.: Bull. Russ. Acad. Sci. Phys. 69, 253 (2005)
18. Kitchen, M.J., Pavlov, K.M., Hooper, S.B., Vine, D.J.K., Siu, K.W., Wallace, M.J., Siew, M.L.L., Yagi, N., Uesugi, K., Lewis, R.A.: Eur. J. Radiol. 68, S49 (2008)
19. Sunaguchi, N., Yuasa, T., Huo, Q., Ichihara, S., Ando, M.: Appl. Phys. Letters 97, 153701-1-153701-3 (2010)
20. Sunaguchi, N., Yuasa, T., Huo, Q., Ando, M.: Opt. Lett. 36, 391 (2011)
21. Ichihara, S., et al.: (in preparation)
22. Sunaguchi, N., Yuasa, T., Huo, Q., Ichihara, S., Ando, M.: Appl. Phys. Letters 99, 103704-103704-3 (2011)

Detecting Clusters of Microcalcifications with a Cascade-Based Approach

Alessandro Bria, Claudio Marrocco,
Mario Molinara, and Francesco Tortorella

DIEI, Università degli Studi di Cassino e del Lazio Meridionale
Cassino (FR), Italy
{a.bria,c.marrocco,m.molinara,tortorella}@unicas.it

Abstract. In this paper we present a cascade-based framework to detect clusters of microcalcifications on mammograms. The algorithm is based on a sliding window technique where a detector is structured as a "cascade" of simple boosting classifiers with increasing complexity. Such a method couples the effectiveness of the cascade approach with the RankBoost algorithm that is aimed at maximizing the area under the ROC curve and represents a good choice when dealing with unbalanced data sets.

Keywords: Computer aided detection, mammography, clusters of microcalcifications, cascade of classifiers, RankBoost.

1 Introduction

When grouped in cluster, microcalcifications (μCs) can be an important indicator of breast cancer, since they appear in 30%-50% of cases diagnosed by mammographic screenings [1] . To help radiologists in the diagnostic decision, various Computer Aided Detection (CAD) systems have been recently proposed, especially based on machine learning techniques such as Support Vector Machines [2,3,4,5] or ensemble classifiers [6,7,8] . These methods rely on a sliding subwindow which scans the entire image and on a dichotomizer (i.e., a two-class classifier) classifying each subwindow as positive (containing μCs) or negative (no μCs). However, these approaches present a high computational burden due to the huge number of subwindows to be analyzed and the complexity of the classifier. An useful solution to these problems is to employ an ensemble of classifiers structured as a "cascade" of dichotomizers with increasing complexity. As highlighted in [9], where such a method has been applied for the detection of human faces, a cascade-based approach exhibits both a low computational complexity and good performance.

In this paper we propose a cascade of classifiers built for the detection of μCs clusters. Accordingly, we have devised a huge set of features suitable for the shape of the μCs, among which the learning algorithm selects the most discriminating ones. The proposed learning procedure employs RankBoost [10] as dichotomizer since it has been proved [11] to maximize the area under the ROC curve (AUC). This makes it a good choice when dealing with strongly

A.D.A. Maidment, P.R. Bakic, and S. Gavenonis (Eds.): IWDM 2012, LNCS 7361, pp. 111–118, 2012.

unbalanced data sets, as is the case with the detection of μC on mammograms. The cascade detector not only locates the candidate regions, but it also provides a confidence degree for each of them which estimates the probability of the presence of a μC. The detector's outputs are finally conveyed to a clustering algorithm which uses both the spatial and probabilistic data to detect clusters. Experiments accomplished on a full-field digital mammographic database show that the cascade approach obtains good results in comparison with a monolithic detector based on RankBoost.

2   Method

The proposed approach for the detection of clusters of μCs is based on a three steps process which is composed as follows. Firstly, we employ a supervised learning framework for the detection of μCs based on a cascade of classifiers trained to classify mammographic subwindows as likely-μCs or background. A confidence degree which conveys the probability of the presence of a μC is also associated to each likely-μCs subwindow by the cascade. Secondly, a post-processing step translates and merges likely-μCs subwindows into likely-μCs regions which roughly identify the segmented μCs. Finally, these regions go through a clustering step which uses both the spatial and probabilistic information to detect clusters. In the following subsections we detail each of these steps.

2.1   Microcalcifications Detection

The underlying idea is to employ a sequence of node classifiers with increasing complexity. A given subwindow passes to the next node if the current node classifies it as containing a μC, otherwise it is rejected. The majority of subwindows containing easily detectable background are discarded by the early nodes, while the most likely-μC subwindows go through the entire cascade. As a result, the detection rate D and false positive rate F of a cascade composed by n nodes is given by

$$D = \prod_{i=1}^{n}(d_i) \quad F = \prod_{i=1}^{n}(f_i) \tag{1}$$

where d_i and f_i are the detection rate and false positive rate of the ith node respectively. Such approach, which showed to be effective also in other fields [9], allows us to face the learning task in a more effective way. In fact, while it is hard for a monolithic classifier to ensure both a good sensitivity and a good specificity, the cascade provides a high constant sensitivity and a growing specificity through the stages obtained by connecting more simpler classifiers with high sensitivity and sufficient specificity. As an example, to build a detector having $D = 0.990$ and $F = 0.001$ it would be sufficient to build 6 node classifiers, each with $t_i = 0.999$ and $f_i = 0.3$. In this way, the first stages of the cascade have to face a simpler task (rejecting the most distinguishable background regions), while the last stages are specialized to discriminate between actual μC's and the most confusing background configurations. This should reduce the number of false positives produced by the detector and concentrate the computational complexity of the system on the last classifiers of the cascade.

To describe the region to be classified, some groups of Haar-like features are used. For the first group the value of each feature is calculated as the difference between the sum of pixels belonging to adjacent rectangular regions, aimed at capturing edge and elongated patterns (see Fig. 1a). For the second group, the value is calculated in a similar way, but the support regions are two concentric rectangles, so being more suitable for the granule-like shape of μCs (see Fig. 1b). The third group is constituted by the 45 degrees-rotated version of the features of the first two groups (see Fig. 1c). The features of the first two groups are evaluated very quickly thanks to the *integral image* [9], while for the rotated features a particular representation of the image is introduced, similar to the *integral image*, but suited for the calculation of tilted rectangle areas. All features are stretched and shifted across all possibile combinations on the subwindow, leading to tens of thousands of features. As a consequence it stands out the need of a feature selection mechanism embedded in each node classifier during the training phase.

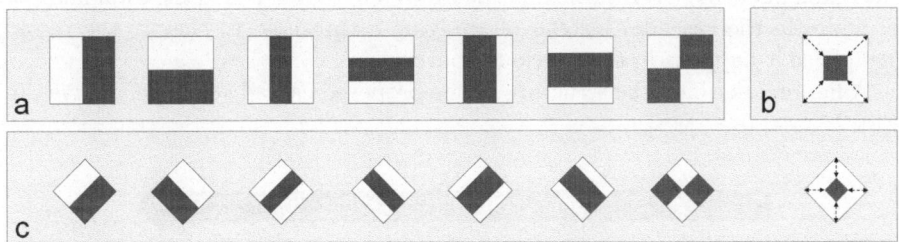

Fig. 1. The Haar-like feature groups used by the proposed cascade of classifiers. (a) Some examples of the first group. (b) An example of the second group. (c) Some examples of the third group.

Each node classifier is actually an ensemble classifier which builds a "strong classifier" $H_i(\mathbf{x})$ as a linear combination of "weak classifiers", added in subsequent rounds. At each round, a weak classifier is built by picking up the feature which provides the best weighted *bipartite ranking* on positive and negative samples. In other words, if we consider all the pairs made by a positive sample and a negative sample (*crucial pair*) and consider how the two samples are ordered according to a particular feature, the feature chosen is the one that minimizes the weighted number of misranked crucial-pairs. After that, the samples forming misranked crucial-pairs are given a weight so that they are more influential in the following rounds. Such approach was inspired by *RankBoost* [10], a boosting machine learning algorithm not based on a cascade mechanism. It allows us to build node classifiers aimed at maximizing the area under the ROC curve (AUC). In our application, this is a quality index for the classifier certainly more appropriate than accuracy which is used in other boosting algorithm such as *AdaBoost*. Moreover, AUC is independent of the a priori probabilities of the two classes and this makes it a good choice when dealing with unbalanced data sets.

As we said before, a consequence of the arrangement in a cascade is that different nodes face different problems. This is considered during the learning phase, when each node is trained with the training set used by the previous node reduced by extracting the negative samples correctly classified by the previous node. In this way, the training set for each node describes faithfully the problem to be faced. It is worth noting that the learning phase require, for each node, a *validation set* different from the training set and necessary to tune the classifier in order to provide the required d_i and f_i. Also the validation set is updated in the same way as the training set. The described learning mechanism obviously causes that a high number of negative samples is removed from both the training and the validation sets, thus significantly altering the original balancing between positive and negative samples. For this reason, a huge *pool* of negative samples is set apart for refilling and re-balancing the sets after a node is trained.

A particular strategy is adopted for the last node of the cascade that does not reject negative subwindows, but it merely associates to each subwindow arriving to it a confidence degree about the presence of a μC. This is achieved by using the real number $H_n(\mathbf{x})$ returned by the last node classifier (n is the total number of nodes in the cascade) instead of applying a threshold to classify the tested sample as it happens in the previous nodes.

A figure describing the structure of the proposed cascade classifier is given in Fig. 2.

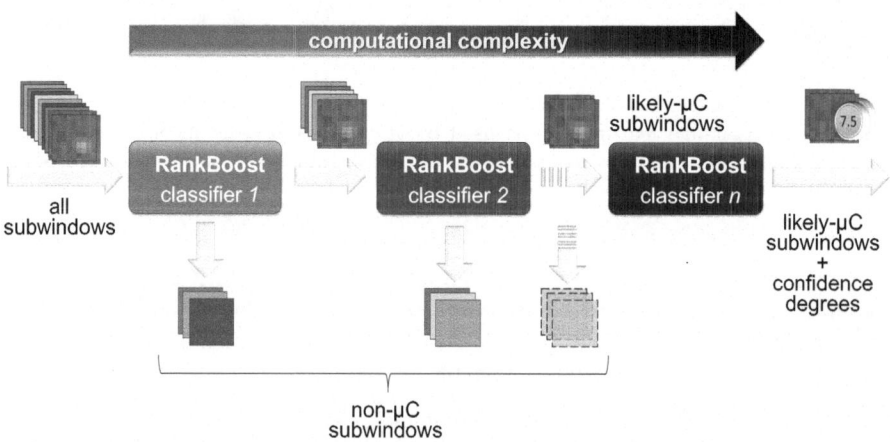

Fig. 2. The proposed cascade-based μC-classifier

2.2   Post-Processing Step

Since sliding subwindows can overlap each other, multiple likely-μC subwindows are usually detected around the same μC region. A post-processing step which translates the overlapping subwindows into regions is therefore needed. Accordingly, we employ an *accumulation matrix*, whos values are computed as follows. Firstly the matrix is initialized with the same dimensions of the tested image and with zero values. Secondly, for each likely-μC subwindow detected, the values inside the square of side k centered on that subwindow are incremented by 1. Finally, the connected regions of the accumulation matrix are found and a confidence degree is associated to each of them by computing the mean of the confidence degrees of the subwindows belonging to that region. Such regions represent a rough segmentation of the μCs, so that their centroid can be used as the associated spatial coordinate.

2.3   The Clustering Algorithm

Since the number of clusters in the image is unknown, clustering algorithms relying on this information (e.g. k-means) cannot be used. Therefore we employ a sequential clustering algorithm described in [12] that constructs the cluster according to the sequence of μC-regions submitted to the algorithm. The sequence is ordered according to the confidence degree since regions that have a higher confidence degree can more probably represent microcalcifications. In this way, the first points that the algorithm will consider are those with the highest probability of being microcalcifications. During the aggregation, each cluster C_i is represented by its the centroid c_i, assumed as the center of mass of the μC-regions belonging to the cluster, each weighted by its confidence degree. A new μC-region is added to C_i if the distance between its centroid and c_i is less than a given threshold R. In this case the centroid c_i is recalculated, otherwise a new cluster C_{i+1} containing the μC-region will be created. In this way, the centroid of the cluster moves towards the direction where the regions are more dense and with higher confidence degrees.

3   Results

The experimental results were performed using 198 full-field digital mammograms extracted from a non-public database. All the images were labeled by experts, who accurately segmented the μCs and marked the clusters of μCs by a poligonal line. In order to estabilish the size of subwindows, we firstly made a statistical evaluation of the typical size of a μC. We found that a subwindow of 12×12 pixels, corresponding to 1.2 mm$\times$1.2 mm, can contain the 99% of the μCs. Next, we extracted the training data from 90 of the 198 images using non-overlapped subwindows of 12 x 12 pixels, so obtaining more than 2.000 positive and about 400.000 negative samples. In order to have a sufficiently wide pool suited for the cascade approach, the set of negative samples was oversampled by adding a huge number of subwindows partially overlapped with those already present in the set, for a total number of about 12.000.000 negative samples. We used 20.000 and 60.000 of such negative samples for the training and the validation set respectively, while the remaining have been used for the pool.

The positive samples were equally distributed between the training set and the validation set.

The cascade detector has been built with $d_i = 0.99$ and $f_i = 0.3$. The training stage produced 13 nodes employing respectively 22, 26, 33, 43, 44, 28, 38, 29, 28, 32, 28, 30, 26 features automatically selected from the 11.879 possible ones. The overall detection and false positive rate obtained by the cascade on the validation set were 0.87 and 8.83×10^{-3} respectively.

We fixed the parameter k of the post processing to $k = 4$ since this configuration has been found to provide the best results. The threshold R of the clustering algorithm was fixed to $R = 8$ mm as suggested by the experts. Only clusters with at least three μCs were considered.

To have a comparison with a non-cascade boosting approach, a monolithic RankBoost detector has been implemented and trained with the same training data and feature set of the cascade detector. We have built several models (with different sizes for the set of negative samples and different numbers of boosting rounds) and picked the best one in order to have a fair comparison. The best results were obtained with a training set of 400.000 negative samples and 100 boosting rounds.

The cascade detector and the monolithic one were evaluated on the remaining 108 images of the initial set of 198 mammograms. 100 of such images contained one ore more clusters of μCs, while the remaining 8 ones did not contain any cluster. The evaluation has been performed in terms of Free-response Receiver Operating Characteristics (FROC) curve, that plots the True Positive Rate, i.e., the number of clusters correctly detected in the test set, versus the False Positive per image, i.e., the number of detected non-clusters per image. The criterion used to evaluate a cluster detection as true or false is based on the area of intersection between the automatically detected clusters and the labeled clusters and it is detailed as follows. Given the area $\mathcal{A}(L)$ of a labeled cluster L, the area $\mathcal{A}(C)$ of cluster C detected by the classifier, the total number of labeled clusters l and automatic detected clusters c, we have:

- a *true positive* if $\mathcal{A}(L \cap \bigcup_{i=1}^{c}(\mathcal{A}(C_i)) \geq \mathsf{CF}_{lab} \cdot \mathcal{A}(L)$ where CF_{lab} is the groundtruth coverage factor;
- a *false negative* if $\mathcal{A}(L \cap \bigcup_{i=1}^{c}(\mathcal{A}(C_i)) < \mathsf{CF}_{lab} \cdot \mathcal{A}(L)$;
- a *false positive* if $\mathcal{A}(C \cap \bigcup_{i=1}^{l}(\mathcal{A}(L_i)) < \mathsf{CF}_{auto} \cdot \mathcal{A}(C)$ where CF_{auto} is the detected clusters coverage factor.

We have experimentally fixed the coverage factors as $\mathsf{CF}_{lab} = 0.3$ and $\mathsf{CF}_{auto} = 0.1$ by visual inspection of the obtained results with the help of an expert.

The curves which show the result of the comparison are reported in Fig. 3 and were obtained by varying the threshold on the confidence degree associated to likely-μC regions. The comparison shows that the cascade approach significatively outpeforms the monolithic RankBoost. In particular, at 1.0 false positive per image the detection rate of the cascade classifier is 0.95, while the RankBoost's one is 0.71, with a gain of about 25%. It is also worth noting that the cascade approach reduced the elaboration time of 55% with respect to the RankBoost approach.

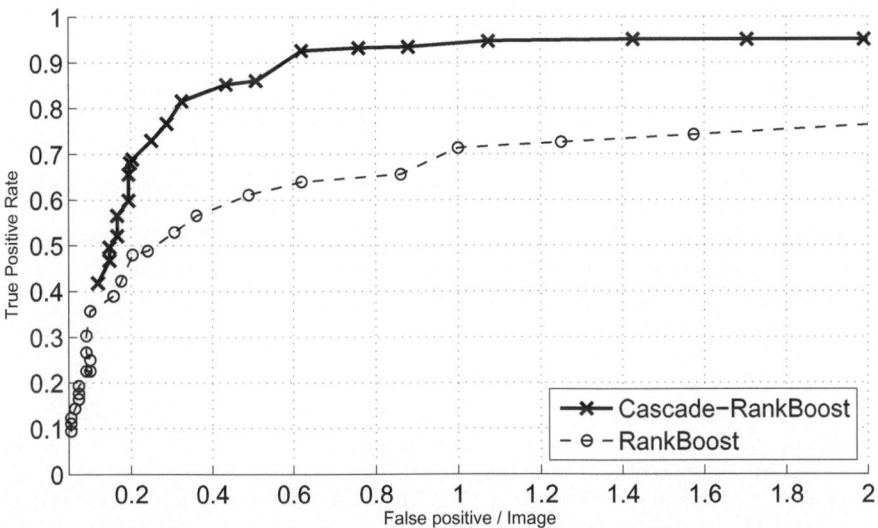

Fig. 3. The FROC curves comparing our cascade-based approach with a monolithic RankBoost classifier trained with the same data and feature set. The True Positive Rate is the number of clusters correctly detected and the False Positive per image is the number of detected non-clusters per image

4   Discussion

In this paper, we have presented a new approach for the detection of clustered microcalcifications based on a cascade architecture employing rank-based boosting classifiers. An experimental analysis accomplished on a full-field digital mammographic database demonstrated that the proposed approach is effective and computationally convenient.

The good detection performance is mainly due to the detection system that is actually made of an ensemble of classifiers, each trained on a part of the available data. In this way, during the learning phase we can use a huge number of negative samples without any drawback due to overfitting because they are distributed among the classifiers, each of them learning a training set not excessively imbalanced.

On the other hand, the cascade architecture helps in limiting the computational load of the detector because it allows to spend the right computational resource for each region to be classified: only the most difficult samples traverse all the cascade, while the easy-to-recognize background regions are discarded by the first stages. This is not possible for a monolithic detector which cannot tune its effort according to the sample to be classified.

There are some issues that need to be addressed, however. First, different types of features could be verified. Second, an alternative architecture could be considered that decouples the feature selection step from the classifier learning step. This would allow us to employ in the node classifier learning algorithms not necessarily based on boosting.

References

1. Kopans, D.B.: Breast Imaging, 3rd edn. Williams & Wilkins, Baltimore (2007)
2. El Naqa, I., Yang, Y., et al.: A support vector machine approach for detection of microcalcifications. IEEE Transactions on Medical Imaging 21(12), 1552–1563 (2002)
3. Wei, L., et al.: Relevance vector machine for automatic detection of clustered microcalcifications. IEEE Transactions on Medical Imaging 24(10), 1278–1285 (2005)
4. Singh, S., Kumar, V., Verma, H.K., Singh, D.: SVM based system for classification of microcalcifications in digital mammograms. In: Proc. 28th Annu. Int. Conf. Eng. Med. Biol. Soc., vol. 1, pp. 4747–4750 (2006)
5. Dheeba, J., Selvi, S.T.: Classification of malignant and benign microcalcification using SVM classifier. In: ICETECT 2011, pp. 686–690 (2011)
6. Zhang, X., et al.: MCs detection approach using Bagging and Boosting based twin support vector machine. Systems, Man and Cybernetics, 5000–5505 (2009)
7. Zhang, X.: A New Ensemble Learning Approach for Microcalcification Clusters Detection. Journal of Software 4(9) (2009)
8. Oliver, A., Torrent, A., Tortajada, M., Lladó, X., Peracaula, M., Tortajada, L., Sentís, M., Freixenet, J.: A Boosting Based Approach for Automatic Microcalcification Detection. In: Martí, J., Oliver, A., Freixenet, J., Martí, R. (eds.) IWDM 2010. LNCS, vol. 6136, pp. 251–258. Springer, Heidelberg (2010)
9. Viola, P., Jones, M.: Robust Real-Time Face Detection. International Journal of Computer Vision 57(2), 137–154 (2004)
10. Freund, Y., Iyer, R., Schapire, R.E., Singer, Y.: An efficient boosting algorithm for combining preferences. Journal of Machine Learning Research 4, 933–969 (2003)
11. Cortes, C., Mohri, M.: AUC optimization vs. error rate minimization. Advances in Neural Information Processing Systems 16 (2004)
12. Marrocco, C., Molinara, M., Tortorella, F.: Algorithms for Detecting Clusters of Microcalcifications in Mammograms. In: Roli, F., Vitulano, S. (eds.) ICIAP 2005. LNCS, vol. 3617, pp. 884–891. Springer, Heidelberg (2005)

Diagnostic Impact of Adjunction of Digital Breast Tomosynthesis (DBT) to Full Field Digital Mammography (FFDM) and in Comparison with Full Field Digital Mammography (FFDM)

Nachiko Uchiyama[1], Takayuki Kinoshita[2], Takashi Hojo[2],
Sota Asaga[2], Junko Suzuki[2], Shiho Gomi[1], Chieko Nagashima[1],
Yoko Kawawa[3], and Kyoichi Otsuka[4]

[1] Research Center for Cancer Prevention and Screening, National Cancer Center, Tokyo, Japan
{nuchiyam,sgomi,cnagashi}@ncc.go.jp
[2] Department of Breast Surgery, National Cancer Center, Tokyo, Japan
{Takinosh,tahojo,soasaga,jusuzuki}@ncc.go.jp
[3] Department of Radiology, National Cancer Center, Tokyo, Japan
ykawawa@ncc.go.jp
[4] Siemens Japan K.K., Tokyo, Japan
Kyoichi.otsuka@siemens.com

Abstract. According to recent reports, DBT is a useful diagnostic procedure compared to 2D mammography. In this paper, we evaluated the diagnostic impact of adjunction of DBT to FFDM and in comparison with FFDM only, in accordance with pathological findings and breast density. 303 women, having 333 lesions, (age 29-84, mean age 54.0 years old) that were recruited for this study gave informed consent. The results indicated that adjunction of DBT to FFDM was superior to FFDM only, regarding diagnostic performance.

Keywords: Digital Mammography, Tomosynthesis, DBT, FFDM, MMG.

1 Introduction

According to recent reports, DBT is a useful diagnostic procedure compared to 2D mammography because breast structures are superimposed onto a two-dimensional (2D) image [1-8] .We evaluated the diagnostic impact of adjunction of DBT to FFDM and in comparison with FFDM only, in accordance with pathological findings and breast density with reference to recent reports.

2 Materials and Methods

This study was approved by the IRB at our institute. 303 women, having 333 lesions, (age 29-84, mean age 54.0 years old) that were recruited for this study gave informed consent. The images were taken as diagnostic mammograms from October in 2009

A.D.A. Maidment, P.R. Bakic, and S. Gavenonis (Eds.): IWDM 2012, LNCS 7361, pp. 119–126, 2012.
© Springer-Verlag Berlin Heidelberg 2012

to October in 2011. 45 cases were referred from other institutions by US and 258 cases were referred by MMG or palpation. Clinical image data were acquired by an a-Se FFDM system with a spatial resolution of 85μm (MAMMOMAT Inspiration, Siemens, Germany).Two-view DBT was performed with the same rotation angle (±25°) and compression pressure as the FFDM. With one-view DBT, the radiation dose was 1.5 times compared to one-view FFDM. The radiation dose, utilizing ACR 156 phantom by FFDM, was 1.20mGy. Images were reconstructed by the shift and add method and the filtered back projection (FBP) method. FFDM and reconstructed slice images of DBT were reviewed at a dedicated workstation (MAMMO Report, Siemens, Germany). Before stating clinical evaluation, our technologists performed an evaluation of image quality utilizing an ACR156 Phantom. The thickness was changed utilizing a PMMA Plate and image quality was evaluated by counting detectable numbers of fibers, masses, and calcifications. As for the results, DBT showed better image quality compared to FFDM regarding fibers and masses. However, regarding calcifications, FFDM showed better image quality compared to DBT. According to the preliminary results, we designed clinical study how adjunction of DBT to FFDM could contribute to improve diagnostic accuracy [Fig.1.] [9]. Two radiologists and four breast surgeons evaluated and reached diagnostic consensus regarding the findings of each lesion by FFDM only and the adjunction of DBT to FFDM before surgery and in accordance with BIRADS categories; BIRADS1-2 (no findings or benign), BIRADS 3 (probably benign, but short-term follow-up or additional diagnostic procedure necessary), and BIRADS 4-5(highly suspicious or definitely malignant and a biopsy necessary). The author and the other five co-authors (two radiologists and four breast surgeons) each have over ten years' experience in reading mammograms. In addition, to read screening mammograms in our country, it is necessary to get a certificate from the committee on quality control of mammographic screening by taking a qualifying examination and the certificate must be renewed every five years. The author and the other five co-authors all passed the qualifying examination with A rank results. All the examination scores were over 90% in sensitivity and over 92% in specificity. All cases were operated on and confirmed as malignant or borderline lesions pathologically.

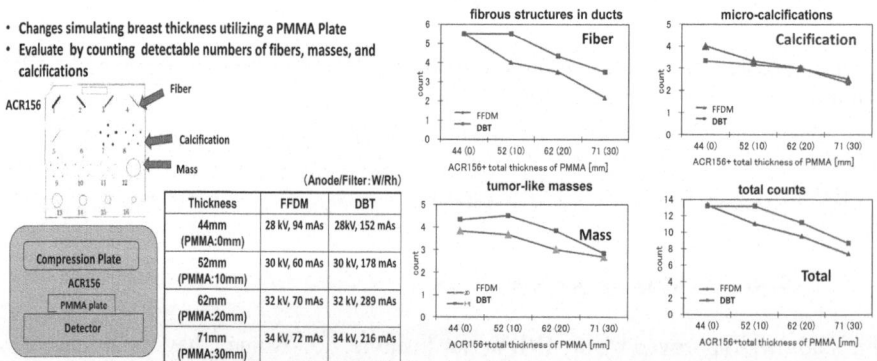

Fig. 1. Image Quality Evaluation by ACR156

3   Results

181 cases were diagnosed as fatty or scattered (BIRADS density 1-2) and 122 cases were diagnosed as inhomogeneous dense or dense (BIRADS density 3-4). Of the pathological findings, 186 lesions were diagnosed as Invasive Ductal Carcinoma(IDC), 60 lesions were diagnosed as Ductal Carcinoma in Situ(DCIS), 33 lesions were IDC predominantly Ductal Carcinoma in Situ (DCIS),16 lesions were diagnosed as Invasive Lobular Carcinoma (ILC), 7 lesions were diagnosed as Lobular Carcinoma in Situ (LCIS), 5 lesions each were diagnosed as Mucinous Carcinoma (Muc Ca) and Intra-ductal Papilloma (IDP), 4 lesions were diagnosed as Apocrine Carcinoma, 3 lesions each were diagnosed as Mixed IDC+ILC and Intracystic Papillary Tumor (ICPT), two lesions each were diagnosed as Invasive Micropapillary Carcinoma (IMPC), DCIS with LCIS, and Phyllodes Tumor, and one lesion each was diagnosed as SCC, ILC with DCIS, ILC predominantly DCIS, ILC predominantly LCIS, and Muc Ca predo-minantly DCIS (Table1.). With FFDM only, the detection rate was 88.9% (176/198) for breasts with BIRADS density 1-2 and 83.7% (113/135) for breasts with BIRADS density 3-4. The findings by FFDM only were mass (n=142; 42.6%), Focal Asymme-try (FA) (n=31; 9.3%), distortion (n=15; 4.5%), microcalcifications (n=40; 12.0%), microcalcifications with FA (n=8; 2.4%), microcalcifications with distortion (n=7; 2.1%), microcalcifications with mass (n=46; 13.8%), and none (n=44; 13.2%).

With adjunction of DBT to FFDM, the detection rate (BIRADS3-5) was 97.4% (193/198) for breasts with BIRADS density 1-2 and 94.8% (128/135) for breasts with BIRADS density 3-4. The average detection rate was 86.8% by FFDM only and 96.4% by adjunction of DBT to FFDM. There was a statistically significant difference between the FFDM only and adjunction of DBT to FFDM among BIRADS density 1-2 and BIRADS density 3-4 (P<0.05). On the other hand, there was no statistically significant difference according to breast density (FFDM only: P=0.221, 3-4; adjunc-tion of DBT to FFDM: P=0.202) (Table 1.). By BIRADS category with FFDM only, 44 lesions (13.2%) were diagnosed as BIRADS 1 or 2, 75 lesions (22.5%) were diag-nosed as BIRADS 3, 214 lesions (64.3%) were diagnosed as BIRADS 4 or 5. On the other hand, with adjunction of DBT to FFDM, 12 lesions (3.6%) were diagnosed as BIRADS 1 or 2, 21 lesions (6.3%) were diagnosed as BIRADS 3, 300 lesions (90.1%) were diagnosed as BIRADS 4 or 5 (Table 2., Fig.2.).By adjunction of DBT to FFDM, 32 more lesions were detected in comparison with FFDM only (IDC n=11, ILC n=2, ILC pred LCIS n=1, DCIS n=15, LCIS n=1, IDP n=2). In addition, regarding radio-logical findings, diagnostic accuracy was improved in 96 lesions (28.8%) in cases of BIRADS 1-2 to BIRADS 3-5 and BIRADS 3 to BIRADS 4-5. These included 93 mass-related lesions (mass, FA, or distortion) and three microcalcifications -related lesions (microcalcifications, microcalcifications and FA, or microcalcifications and distortion). However, diagnostic confidence was improved in cases of microcalcifica-tions-related lesions owing to the presence of masses or focal dense areas with micro-calcifications. In accordance with pathological subtypes, improvement of the detec-tion rate and diagnostic accuracy in invasive cancer was 4.7% and 14.1% in Sci Ca, 7.9% and 31.7% in Pap-Tub Ca, 8.2%and 35.8% in Sol-Tub Ca, and 14.3% and 43.8% in ILC. On the other hand, improvement of detection rate in non-invasive can-cer (DCIS) was 39.5% and 45.0% in diagnostic accuracy (Table 3.).

Table 1. The Detection Rate in accordance with Breast Density   (n=333)

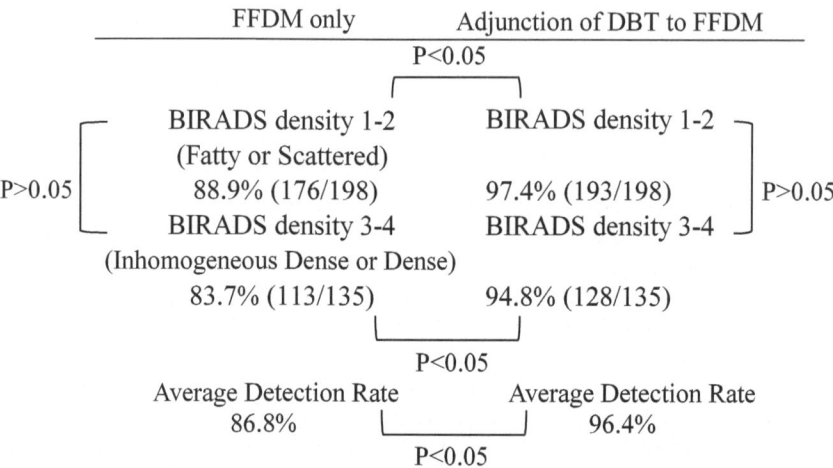

FFDM only   Adjunction of DBT to FFDM

P<0.05

BIRADS density 1-2   BIRADS density 1-2
(Fatty or Scattered)
P>0.05   88.9% (176/198)   97.4% (193/198)   P>0.05
BIRADS density 3-4   BIRADS density 3-4
(Inhomogeneous Dense or Dense)
83.7% (113/135)   94.8% (128/135)

P<0.05

Average Detection Rate   Average Detection Rate
86.8%   96.4%

P<0.05

Table 2. Category Changes of FFDM Only Vs. Adjunction of DBT to FFDM (n=333)

FFDM only		Adjunction of DBT to FFDM	
BIRADS 1 or 2	n=44	BIRADS 1 or 2	n=12
		*BIRADS 3	**n=10**
		*BIRADS 4 or 5	**n=22**
BIRADS 3	n=75	BIRADS 3	n=11
		*BIRADS 4 or 5	**n=64**
BIRADS 4 or 5	n=214	BIRADS 4 or 5	n=214

* Improved diagnostic accuracy: BIRADS 1-2 to 3-5 or 3 to 4-5 (n=96: 28.8%)

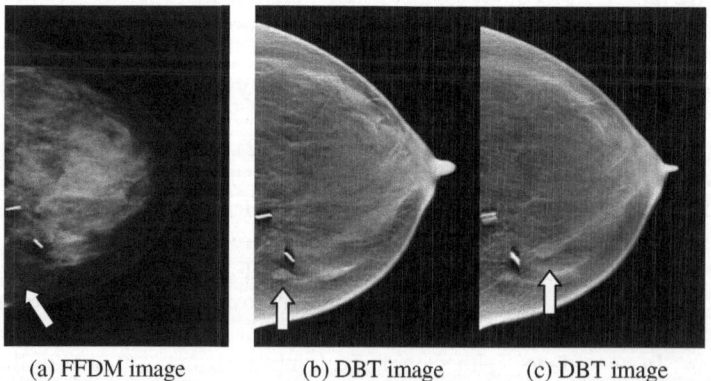

(a) FFDM image   (b) DBT image   (c) DBT image

Fig. 2. FFDM (Fig.2a) showed no abnormality in the left breast by CC view except metal clips. Corresponding to the post-operative area (white arrow), DBT (Fig.2b.-c.) showed two irregular shaped masses on different slices (white arrows). The pathological diagnosis was recurrence of IDC (Pap-Tub Ca). (Category Change: BIRADS 1 to 4)

Table 3. Radiological Findings of FFDM and Adjunction of DBT to FFDM in comparison with Pathological Findings

IDC (Sci Ca) n=92

FFDM only	Adjunction of DBT to FFDM
Mass (n=58: ***RM n=1**, IRM n=30, SPM n=27)	Mass (n=58: IRM n=4, SPM n=54)
Microcalcifications (n=4)	Microcalcifications (n=1)
	Microcalcifications with FDA (n=1)
	Microcalcifications with RM (n=1)
	Microcalcifications with SPM (n=1)
Microcalcifications with	Microcalcifications with FDA (n=1)
Focal Asymmetry or Distortion (n=6)	Microcalcifications with IRM (n=4)
	Microcalcifications with SPM (n=1)
Microcalcifications with Mass (n=10)	Microcalcifications with IRM (n=6)
	Microcalcifications with SPM (n=4)
Focal Asymmetry or Distortion (n=8)	***SPM (n=8)**
None (n=6)	***Mass (n=4: RM n=1 , IRM n=2, SPM n=1)**
	None (n=2)

Improvement of detection rate 4.7%, Improvement of diagnostic accuracy 14.1% (13/92)

IDC (Pap-Tub Ca) n=41

FFDM only	Adjunction of DBT to FFDM
Microcalcifications with IRM (n=8)	Microcalcifications with IRM (n=6)
Microcalcifications with SPM (n=1)	Microcalcifications with SPM (n=4)
**Microcalcifications with RM (n=1)	
Focal Asymmetry or Distortion (n=8)	***IRM (n=4), *SPM (n=4)**
None (n=3)	***RM (n=1), *IRM (n=1), *SPM (n=1)**
Mass (n=20:*** RM n=1**, IRM n=13, SPM n=6)	Mass (n=20: IRM n=9, SPM n=11)
Improvement of detection rate7.9%	Improvement of diagnostic accuracy 31.7% (13/40)

IDC (Sol-Tub Ca) n=53

FFDM only	Adjunction of DBT to FFDM
Microcalcifications with IRM (n=11)	Microcalcifications with IRM (n=6)
Microcalcifications with SPM (n=1)	Microcalcifications with SPM (n=6)
Focal Asymmetry or Distortion (n=9)	***IRM (n=7), *SPM (n=2)**
None (n=4)	***IRM (n=3), *SPM (n=1)**
Mass (n=27: ***RM n=6**, IRM n=15, SPM n=6)	Mass (n=27: IRM n=13, SPM n=14)
Microcalcifications (n=1)	Microcalcifications with FDA (n=1)

Improvement of detection rate 8.2%, Improvement of diagnostic accuracy 35.8% (19/53)

Table 3. *(continued)*

ILC (n=16)

FFDM only	Adjunction of DBT to FFDM
Focal Asymmetry or Distortion (n=5)	***IRM (n=1)**
	*SPM (n=4)
None (n=2)	***RM (n=2)**
Mass (n=7: SPM n=6, IRM n=1)	Mass (n=7: SPM n=7)
Microcalcifications with IRM (n=2)	Microcalcifications with IRM (n=1)
	Microcalcifications with SPM (n=1)

Improvement of detection rate14.3%, Improvement of diagnostic accuracy 43.8% (7/16)

IDC Pred DCIS (n=33)

FFDM only	Adjunction of DBT to FFDM
Microcalcifications (n=13)	Microcalcifications (n=4)
	Microcalcifications with FDA (n=5)
	Microcalcifications with RM or IRM (n=4)
Microcalcifications with	Microcalcifications with FDA
Focal Asymmetry or Distortion (n=7)	and Distortion or Spiculation (n=6)
(BIRADS 3 n=2, BIRADS 4-5 n=5)	(BIRADS 3 n=1, BIRADS 4-5 n=5)
	**Microcalcifications with IRM (n=1)
	(**BIRADS 3 to 4-5 n=1)
Microcalcifications with RM (n=3)	Microcalcifications with IRM (n=4)
or with IRM (n=2)	or with SPM (n=1)
Focal Asymmetry or Distortion (n=5)	FDA (n=1), ***IRM (n=1)**, ***SPM (n=3)**
Mass (n=3: SPM n=2, IRM n=1)	Mass (n=3: SPM n=2, IRM n=1)

Improvement of detection rate 0%, Improvement of diagnostic accuracy 15.2% (5/33)

DCIS (n=60)

FFDM only	Adjunction of DBT to FFDM
None (n=22)	None (n=7)
	*FDA with
	Distortion or Spiculation (n=5)
	*Mass (n=10; RM n=5, IRM n=2, SPM n=3)
Microcalcifications (n=14)	Microcalcifications (n=10)
	Microcalcifications with FDA
	or with Distortion or Spiculation (n=4)
Microcalcifications with	Microcalcifications with FDA or Distortion (n=4)

Table 3. *(continued)*

Focal Asymmetry or Distortion(n=5)	***Microcalcifications with Mass (n=1)**
Microcalcifications with Mass (n=1)	Microcalcifications with Mass (n=1)
Focal Asymmetry or Distortion (n=9)	FDA (n=1)
	*FDA with Distortion or Spiculation (n=2)
	*Mass (n=6; IRM n=6)
Mass (n=9: IRM n=6, ***RM=3**)	Mass (n=9: IRM n=4, SPM n=5)

Improvement of detection rate 39.5%, Improvement of diagnostic accuracy 45.0% (27/60)

FDA: Focal Dense Area   RM: Round, Oval, or Lobulated Mass
Irregular Shaped Mass (IRM): Indistinct or Microlobulated Mass   SPM: Spiculated Mass
*Improved Diagnostic Accuracy regarding Mass-related Lesions
**Improved Diagnostic Accuracy regarding Microcalcification-related Lesions

4   Discussion

According to recent reports, DBT is a useful diagnostic procedure compared to 2D mammography because breast structures are superimposed onto a two-dimensional (2D) image [1-8] .The outline of the lesion can be potentially obscured. Our preliminary results also indicated that adjunction of DBT to FFDM contributed not only to detecting the lesion, but also to clarifying the diagnostic accuracy, especially with regard to mass-related lesions. On the other hand, regarding microcalcifications-related lesions, only using DBT slice image, it is difficult to recognize the overview of the clustered microcalcifications and analyze the morphology of each microcalcification's outline at current settings for image acquisition and reconstruction. That corresponded to our preliminary phantom study and clinical study by Spangler ML, et.al. [8][9].As a result, adjunction of DBT to FFDM is the best current option. Detection rate by adjunction of DBT to FFDM was improved compared to FFDM only and especially improved in non-invasive cancer; DCIS.32 more lesions were detected by adjunction of DBT to FFDM, not only 14 invasive cancers, but also 18 non-invasive cancerous or borderline lesions. Adjunction of DBT to FFDM was useful to detect early stage breast cancer and it is not affected by breast density.

5   Conclusion

In this study, the results indicated that adjunction of DBT to FFDM was superior to FFDM only, regarding diagnostic performance. In addition, it could decrease additional other diagnostic procedures.

Acknowledgment. This study was supported by Grant-in-Aid for Scientific Research (C) (No. 23591810) in Japan.

References

1. Poplack, S.P., Tosteson, T.D., Kogel, C.A., et al.: Digital breast tomosynthesis: initial experience in 98 women with abnormal digital screening mammography. AJR 189(3), 616–623 (2007)
2. Andersson, I., Ikeda, D.M., Zackrisson, S., et al.: Breast tomosynthesis and digital mammography: a comparison of breast cancer visibility and BIRADS classification in a population of cancers with subtle mammographic findings. Eur. Radiol. 18(12), 2817–2825 (2008)
3. Good, W.F., Abrams, G.S., Catullo, V.J., et al.: Digital breast tomosynthesis: a pilot observer study. AJR 190(4), 865–869 (2008)
4. Gennaro, G., Toledano, A., di Maggio, C., et al.: Digital breast tomosynthesis versus digital mammography: a clinical performance study. Eur. Radiol. 20(7), 1545–1553 (2010)
5. Uchiyama, N., Kinoshita, T., Akashi, S., et al.: Diagnostic Performance of Combined Full Field Digital Mammography (FFDM) and Digital Breast Tomosynthesis (DBT) in comparison with Full Field Digital Mammography (FFDM). In: CARS 2011, pp. 32–33. Springer, Heidelberg (2011)
6. Förnvik, D., Zackrisson, S., Ljungberg, O., et al.: Breast tomosynthesis: Accuracy of tumor measurement compared with digital mammography and ultrasonography. Acta. Radiol. 51(3), 240–247 (2010)
7. Wallis, M.G., Moa, E., Zanca, F., Leifland, K., Danielsson, M.: Two-view and single-view tomosynthesis versus full-field digital mammography: high-resolution X-ray imaging observer study. Radiology 262(3), 788–796 (2012)
8. Spangler, M.L., Zuley, M.L., Sumkin, J.H., et al.: Detection and classification of calcifications on digital breast tomosynthesis and 2D digital mammography: a comparison. AJR 196(2), 320–324 (2011)
9. Gomi, S., Chieko, N., Taguchi, E., et al.: Clinical Utility in Digital Breast Tomosynthesis. Japan Radiology Congress (2010)

Ethnic Variation in Volumetric Breast Density

Sadaf Hashmi[1], Jamie C. Sergeant[2], Julie Morris[3], Sigrid Whiteside[3],
Paula Stavrinos[4], D. Gareth Evans[4], Tony Howell[4], Mary Wilson[4], Nicky Barr[4],
Caroline Boggis[4], and Susan M. Astley[2]

[1] Manchester Medical School, University of Manchester, Oxford Road,
Manchester M13 9PT, UK
[2] School of Cancer and Enabling Sciences,
University of Manchester, Oxford Road, Manchester M13 9PT, UK
[3] Department of Medical Statistics,
University Hospital of South Manchester, Manchester M23 9LT, UK
[4] Nightingale Centre and Genesis Prevention Centre,
University Hospital of South Manchester, Manchester M23 9LT, UK
sue.astley@manchester.ac.uk

Abstract. Volumetric breast density was determined using Quantra™ (Hologic) in 1356 women undergoing routine breast screening. Self-reported ethnicity, age, HRT use, weight and height were also available. 1038 women declared themselves to be White (British or Irish), 71 Black, 77 Asian, 91 Jewish, 31 Mixed Race and 48 Other European. Most of the Jewish group were Ashkenazi, a group in which there is a high probability of genetic susceptibility to breast cancer. Women with screen-detected or previous cancers were excluded. The only significant difference in breast density found between ethnic groups was between the Jewish women and women of White (British or Irish) ethnicity, where mean volumetric densities were 19.61% and 16.89% respectively (p=0.012), however this difference is only of borderline significance (p=0.053) once adjustments are made for age, Body Mass Index (BMI) and use of Hormone Replacement Therapy (HRT). The Jewish women had on average a lower BMI and were more likely to have used HRT.

Keywords: Breast density, ethnicity, mammography, volumetric, Quantra.

1   Introduction

Increasingly, screening programmes are looking for alternatives to the one-size-fits-all approach currently adopted for women without a family history of breast cancer. Screening could be made more effective by adapting the imaging modality and screening interval to the properties of a woman's breasts or to their individual risk of cancer. Women identified as being at high risk of developing the disease could also be offered risk-reducing interventions. An example of this is the PROCAS (Predicting Risk of Cancer At Screening) trial in the UK [1,2]. All women attending routine breast screening in the Greater Manchester Breast Screening Programme are invited to participate; those that consent undergo conventional screening mammography and

A.D.A. Maidment, P.R. Bakic, and S. Gavenonis (Eds.): IWDM 2012, LNCS 7361, pp. 127–133, 2012.

complete a questionnaire providing information about physical characteristics, life-style, family history and other factors associated with breast cancer risk. Questionnaire data are used to identify a high risk population via the Tyrer-Cuzik model [3]. Breast density is measured from the screening mammograms, and those women with a Tyrer-Cuzick 10-year risk of at least 8%, or a 10-year risk of at least 5% and area-based breast density in the top 10% among study participants, are informed of their risk and offered appropriate advice. Breast density is a key feature of PROCAS not only because it is an important risk factor for cancer; unlike many risk factors it is modifiable by lifestyle and other interventions giving the opportunity to reduce risk [4, 5], and it has become easier to quantify objectively and routinely with the advent of digital mammography.

Increased mobility of the world population has resulted in many countries having a diverse ethnic mix, now apparent in the screening age group in Greater Manchester [6]. Ethnicity affects risk of breast cancer, with women of White ethnicity having high incidence of developing this disease in comparison to other racial groups [7]. In one study, approximately 141 per 100,000 women of White ethnic origin were found to have developed breast cancer, compared to 119 for African Americans, 96 for Asian Americans, 90 for Hispanic/Latina women and 50 for American Indians/Alaskan natives [8]. Survival also differs between women from different ethnic groups [9,10] although this may in part be due to inequalities in treatment [11].

Published data on ethnicity and breast density has yielded mixed results. A UK study of 428 patients symptomatic patients using Quantra^{TM} showed significantly differences between White, Asian and Black women, but did not control for any confounding factors such as age or HRT use [12]. White, Hispanic, Asian, Native American and Black woman participated In a study of 28,501 mammograms of women enrolled on a breast-screening programme in western Washington [13]. Adjusting for age, differences in breast density were found between Native American and White women, and White and Asian women. However, when BMI, HRT use, menopausal status and parity were taken into account the difference between Native American and White women was no longer significant. More recent research in similar ethnic groups evaluated the breast density of 442 women [14]. African-Americans were found to have higher density than Asian-Americans after adjusting for BMI, family history, menstrual and reproductive factors. In this work, Asian-American and White ethnic group were found to have similar mammographic densities. In contrast with this, a British study found that Asian women had significantly lower breast density assessed using Wolfe grades than Caucasian participants [15]. However, in a study of 15,292 women of Asian, White, African-American and Other (American Indian and Caribbean) racial backgrounds no significant differences were found when confounding factors including bra size were taken into account [16]. The picture is thus unclear; previous studies have evaluated different populations using a variety of methodologies including subjective assessment of density.

The work reported here uses a fully automated, volumetric breast density measure, (Quantra^{TM}) as opposed to visual assessment or computer assisted methods as reported previously in the literature. Whilst Quantra^{TM} has not yet been validated with respect to its relationship to risk to the same extent as subjective and area-based methods of density measurement, it holds several advantages over such methods including objectivity, reproducibility, suitability for population-based studies, resolution and the ability to assess absolute, rather than relative, breast density [17]. Regardless of the degree of association with risk, the identification of women with high mammographic density is important because the detection of cancers using conventional mammography is more difficult in this case [18], and it may be appropriate to use alternative screening methodologies.

2   Methods

Data used in this study comprised image and questionnaire data for all non-White British or Irish participants recruited to PROCAS before 15th June 2011 for whom raw digital mammograms and a completed questionnaire were available, and for the first 1038 White British or Irish participants in the wider trial for whom questionnaire data had been entered in the study database and raw mammogram data were available. Women diagnosed with cancer at the time of screening and women with previous breast cancers were excluded.

The mammograms were analysed using Hologic's Quantra^{TM} (Version 1.3; Hologic Inc.) software which provided measures of breast volume, glandular volume and % density by volume for left and right breasts. These were averaged to provide a single measure of each type per women.

Questionnaire data on ethnicity, date of birth, Hormone Replacement Therapy (HRT) use, weight and height were extracted from the PROCAS study database. Body Mass Index (BMI) was calculated from the self-reported height and weight data. One way analysis of variance (ANOVA) was used to determine whether a relationship existed between the breast density measures and ethnicity. Further analysis was then completed using a General Linear Model (ANCOVA) in which adjustment was made for age, BMI and HRT use.

2.1   Ethnicities

The ethnic categories available for participants to select on the questionnaire were: Asian or Asian British – Bangladeshi, Indian, Pakistani, Chinese; Black or Black British – African or Caribbean; Jewish Origin; Jewish Ashkenazi; Mixed – White and Black African/Asian/Black Caribbean; White - British or Irish; and Other – please specify. Women were instructed 'Please tick all that apply'. In subsequent analysis, the Jewish Ashkenazi women were included in the Jewish Origin category.

3   Results

The age of participants ranged from 46 to 74 years. The mean BMI for all the ethnic groups in the study was greater than 25, in the overweight range. Mean ages and BMI for each group are tabulated in Table 1.

Table 1. Mean Body Mass Index and Age in each ethnic group studied

Ethnicity	Mean BMI (SD)	Mean Age (SD)
White British or Irish	27.36 (5.49)	58.8 (6.99)
Black or Black British	29.49 (4.60)	57.9 (7.36)
Asian or Asian British	26.24 (4.64)	57.5 (6.75)
Jewish origin	25.52 (4.22)	60.1 (6.87)
Mixed	29.75 (5.83)	56.7 (6.29)
Others	25.50 (4.66)	58.8 (6.37)
All	**27.45 (5.37)**	**58.7 (6.96)**

Just over a third of the women in the study had used HRT at some time. Usage was highest in the Jewish group and lowest in women of Black origin and those of Asian or Mixed race (Table 2). The mean age of women who reported ever using HRT (61.41 years) was significantly greater than that of women who had never used it (57.19 years) ($p<0.01$). This may relate to the menopausal status of the individuals taking part in this study.

Table 2. HRT use for women of different ethnicities

Ethnicity	Ever Used HRT (%)
White British or Irish	37.5
Black or Black British	23.5
Asian or Asian British	26.7
Jewish	42.9
Mixed	26.7
Others	35.4
All ethnicities	36.2

The volumetric breast densities of women in the different ethnic groups are presented in Table 3, and the volumetric percentage breast densitiesare shown in Table 4.

Table 3. Volumetric breast density (cm^3) for women of different ethnicities

Ethnicity	Gland volume (cm^3)		Breast volume (cm^3)	
	Mean	SD	Mean	SD
White	101.9	58.9	642.4	363.2
Black or Black British	126.4	72.2	777.8	442.5
Asian or Asian British	78.9	47.9	454.8	259.2
Jewish Origin	100.7	50.2	544.5	260.9
Mixed	117.0	45.5	694.6	293.5
Others	97.5	63.3	596.3	450.1

Table 4. Volumetric breast density (%) for women of different ethnicities

Ethnicity	Breast density (%)	
	Mean	SD
White	16.9	6.5
Black or Black British	17.1	5.9
Asian or Asian British	18.3	6.0
Jewish Origin	19.6	7.5
Mixed	17.3	3.9
Others	18.1	6.4

A one-way analysis of variance (ANOVA) was performed to determine whether a direct association existed between average breast density and ethnicity. Pairwise comparisons were carried out on each ethnic group out using Scheffe's test. Slight differences were observed in the average breast density in all ethnic groups. However, the results concluded that only women of Jewish ethnic origin had significantly higher breast density than the White British or Irish population ($p = 0.012$).

A General Linear Model was used to further investigate the link between average breast density and ethnicity whilst adjusting for HRT use, BMI and age. Univariate analysis of the variables was performed and pairwise comparisons were done using Bonferroni's test. Once adjusted for age, BMI and HRT use, the results showed that the difference between average breast density of the Jewish participants and that of the white British or Irish women was of borderline significance ($p= 0.053$).

4   Discussion

Investigation of the relationship between breast density and ethnicity, whilst facilitated by the availability of automated methods of measuring density, remains difficult because of the many confounding factors such as the possible impact of a change in lifestyle on second generation immigrants, and wide variations between definitions of ethnic groups. This study is the first that has specifically compared breast density in Jewish women with that of White British or Irish women; this comparison is particularly interesting because of the known difference in genetic susceptibility to breast cancer of Ashkenazi Jewish women [19]. The high rate of HRT use found in this group is of interest.

The population studied is unlikely to be representative of women of screening age in Greater Manchester, as attendance at screening is not uniform across all ethnic groups, with women of non-White origin less likely to present for screening [20]. Further, the sample was selected on a pragmatic basis aimed at maximizing the proportion of non-White British participants. The mobile units used for screening re-locate to facilitate access, and uptake of screening and the proportion of women consenting to take part in PROCAS vary according to location, with lower rates in less affluent areas of the city.

In this sample we found that the only ethnicities for which, after adjusting for potential confounding factors, there was some limited evidence of a difference in breast density were White British or Irish and Jewish women. This is in contrast to recently reported data from the UK which found that Asian women had lower breast density as measured by Quantra™, however that research was carried out in a symptomatic population rather than a screening population, and did not adjust for confounding factors such as age and BMI [12]. Quantra™ also provides data on volume of glandular tissue in the breast. This may be more reliable than percentage density as it is affected less by the weight of the women at the time of imaging [21]. A future line of research would be to investigate any differences in the absolute volume of gland between the ethnic groups, and to establish the impact of increased weight on breast volume.

Acknowledgements We acknowledge the support of the National Insitute for Health Research (NIHR) and the Genesis Breast Cancer Prevention Appeal for their funding of the PROCAS trial. We would like to thank the study radiologists and advanced practitioner radiographers for VAS reading. We would also like to thank the many radiographers involved in the Greater Manchester Breast Screening Programme, the study staff for recruitment and data collection, and Hologic Inc. for providing the QuantraTM software. This paper presents independent research commissioned by the National Institute for Health Research (NIHR) under its Programme Grant (Reference Number RP-PG-0707-10031). The views expressed are those of the author(s) and not necessarily those of the NHS, the NIHR or the Department of Health.

References

1. Evans, D.G., Warwick, J., Astley, S.M., et al.: Assessing individual breast cancer risk within the UK National Health Service Breast Screening Programme: a new paradigm for cancer prevention. Cancer Prevention Research (forthcoming)
2. Howell, A., Astley, S., Warwick, J., et al.: Prevention of breast cancer in the context of a national breast screening programme. Journal of Internal Medicine 271, 321–330 (2012)
3. Tyrer, J., Duffy, S.W., Cuzick, J.: A breast cancer prediction model incorporating familial and personal risk factors. Stat. Med. 23, 1111–1130 (2004)
4. Boyd, N.F., Greenberg, C., Lockwood, G., et al.: Effects at two years of a low-fat, high-carbohydrate diet on radiologic features of the breast: Results from a randomized trial. Journal of the National Cancer Institute 89(7), 488–496 (1997)
5. Cummings, S.R., Tice, J.A., et al.: Prevention of Breast Cancer in Postmenopausal Women: Approaches to Estimating and Reducing Risk. Journal of the National Cancer Institute 101(6), 384–398 (2009)
6. 2009 Ethnic Group Estimate by broad age and sex, Manchester City Council, http://www.manchester.gov.uk/downloads/download/4220/corporate_research_and_intelligence_population_publications (accessed April 16, 2012)
7. National Cancer Institute Surveillance Epidemiology and End Results, http://seer.cancer.gov/csr/1975_2009_pops09/results_merged/topic_race_ethnicity.pdf (accessed April 16, 2012)

8. Smigal, C., Jemal, A., Ward, E., et al.: Trends in Breast Cancer by Race and Ethnicity: Update 2006. Cancer J. Clin. 56(3), 169–187 (2006)

9. Li, C., Malone, K., Daling, J.: Differences in Breast Cancer Stage, Treatment, and Survival by Race and Ethnicity. Am. Med. Association (163), 49–56 (2003)

10. Jemal, A., Siegel, R., Xu, J.Q., Ward, E.: Cancer Statistics, 2010. Cancer J. Clin. 60(5), 277–300 (2010)

11. Shavers, V.L., Brown, M.L.: Racial and ethnic disparities in the receipt of cancer treatment. JNCI 94(5), 334–357 (2002)

12. Tzias, D., Wilkinson, L., Mehta, R., et al.: Correlation of Ethnicity with Breast Density as Assessed by QuantraTM. Breast Cancer Research 13(suppl. 1), O5 (2011)

13. El-Bastawissi, A.Y., White, E., Mandelson, M.T., Taplin, S.: Variation in mammographic breast density by race. Ann. Epidemiol. 11(4), 257–263 (2001)

14. Chen, Z., Wu, A.H., Gauderman, W.J., Bernstein, L., Ma, H., Pike, M.C., et al.: Does mammographic density reflect ethnic differences in breast cancer incidence rates? Am. J. Epidemiol. 159(2), 140–147 (2004)

15. Turnbull, A.E., Kapera, L., Cohen, M.E.L.: Mammographic Parenchymal Pattern in Asian and Caucasian Women Attending for Screening. Clin Radiology (48), 38–40 (1993)

16. del Carmen, M.G., Hughes, K.S., Halpern, E., Rafferty, E., Kopans, D., Parisky, Y.R., et al.: Racial differences in mammographic breast density. Cancer 98(3), 590–596 (2003)

17. Hartman, K., Highnam, R., Warren, R., Jackson, V.: Volumetric Assessment of Breast Tissue Composition from FFDM Images. In: Krupinski, E.A. (ed.) IWDM 2008. LNCS, vol. 5116, pp. 33–39. Springer, Heidelberg (2008)

18. Rosenberg, R.D., Hunt, W.C., Williamson, M.R., et al.: Effects of age, breast density, ethnicity, and estrogen replacement therapy on screening mammographic sensitivity and cancer stage at diagnosis: review of 183,134 screening mammograms in Albuquerque, New Mexico. Radiology 209, 511–518 (1998)

19. Struewing, J.P., Hartge, P., Wacholder, S., et al.: The risk of cancer associated with specific mutations of BRCA1 and BRCA2 among Ashkenazi Jews. New England Journal of Medicine 336(20), 1401–1408 (1997)

20. Goel, M.S., Wee, C.C., McCarthy, E.P., et al.: Racial and ethnic disparities in cancer screening - The importance of foreign birth as a barrier to care. Journal of General Internal Medicine 18(12), 1028–1035 (2003)

21. Patel, H.G., Astley, S.M., Hufton, A.P., Harvie, M., Hagan, K., Marchant, T.E., Hillier, V., Howell, A., Warren, R., Boggis, C.R.M.: Automated Breast Tissue Measurement of Women at Increased Risk of Breast Cancer. In: Astley, S.M., Brady, M., Rose, C., Zwiggelaar, R. (eds.) IWDM 2006. LNCS, vol. 4046, pp. 131–136. Springer, Heidelberg (2006)

Personalizing Mammographic Dosimetry Using Multilayered Anatomy-Based Breast Models

Mariela A. Porras-Chaverri[1,2], John R. Vetter[1], and Ralph Highnam[3]

[1] Department of Medical Physics, University of Wisconsin-Madison,
1111 Highland Ave., 53705 Madison, USA
{porraschaver,jrvetter}@wisc.edu
[2] School of Physics, University of Costa Rica,
San José, Costa Rica
[3] Matakina Technology Limited,
Level 6, 86 Victoria St., Wellington, New Zealand
ralph.highnam@matakina.com

Abstract. A methodology for patient-oriented calculations of mean glandular dose (MGD) is introduced in this study. The method takes into consideration the influence of the glandular tissue distribution in the MGD. The glandular tissue information was estimated from conventional mammography images using breast density assessment software followed by the Mammography-Image Based (MIB) method presented in this work. The corresponding dose conversion coefficients (D_{gN-HLB}) were determined using a Heterogeneously-Layered Breast (HLB) geometry. The effect of the glandular tissue distribution on the MGD was studied using a set of HLB models and their corresponding homogeneous model. D_{gN-HLB} values were between 48% lower and 24% larger than the value calculated using a homogeneous glandular tissue distribution, despite the current methods predicting the same coefficient for all glandular tissue distributions. The proposed methods were applied to a group of patients. For the cases analyzed, the variation in MGD was as large as 14.8% for a highly heterogeneous dense breast.

Keywords: breast imaging dosimetry, mean glandular dose, breast anatomy.

1 Introduction

The geometric model used in current dosimetric calculations approximates the breast as a homogeneous mix of adipose and glandular tissues, surrounded by skin.[2,4,11,12] This simplified breast model overlooks the heterogeneous distribution of the glandular and adipose tissues within the breast, and introduces a severe limitation in the dosimetric calculations for anatomical breasts.

This limitation has been reported by Dance *et al.*[3] who found differences as high as 48% in the conversion coefficients due to the distribution of glandular tissue. However, no changes were recommended to the current dosimetry protocols to allow for this, due to the lack of a practical method to determine the glandular tissue distribution for a large group of patients.

A.D.A. Maidment, P.R. Bakic, and S. Gavenonis (Eds.): IWDM 2012, LNCS 7361, pp. 134–140, 2012.
© Springer-Verlag Berlin Heidelberg 2012

In the present work, we introduce the Mammography-Image Based (MIB) method to estimate the glandular tissue distribution for individual patients using conventional mammography images. The MIB method is used in combination with breast density assessment software. In addition, a Heterogeneously-Layered Breast (HLB) geometry is used in the calculation of the dose conversion coefficients. The HLB geometry allows variations in the distribution of the glandular tissues. The methodology introduced in this work provides the basis for patient-oriented estimations of MGD.

2   Methods

The dose conversion coefficients were obtained using Monte Carlo techniques (MCNP5, Los Alamos, NM). The imaging geometry used in all simulations was based on the configuration described by Dance.[2] All simulations used a monoenergetic photon source with energies in the range between 0 keV and 30 keV, in 0.5 keV steps. The spectra used for these calculations were generated using methods described in detail elsewhere.[1,10] The breast geometry used in all simulations is based on the HLB model which consists of a breast core divided into layers parallel to the image receptor plane. The percent glandular composition for each layer can be modified separately and heterogeneous glandular tissue distributions can be simulated. The HLB core is surrounded by a 3.5 mm thick adipose tissue layer and a 1.5 mm thick skin layer.[8]

The particular HLB geometry used in this work had three layers of equal thickness and a semicircular breast projection with 8 cm radius (Fig. 1). The glandular fractions of the core layers were modified according to the purpose of each of the studies performed. The elemental compositions of the tissue materials used in all the simulations were based on those reported by Hammerstein et al.[5]

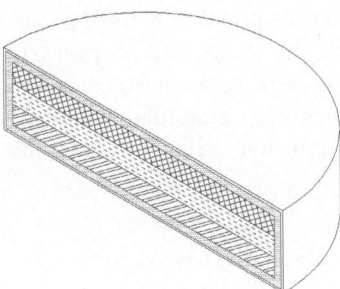

Fig. 1. Heterogeneously-layered breast (HLB) model. Each of the shaded areas corresponds to a breast core layer with different glandular composition. The breast core is wrapped in adipose tissue and skin layers.

2.1   Calculation of Dose Conversion Coefficients

The calculation of the HLB based dose conversion coefficient (D_{gN-HLB}) was performed using :

$$D_{gN-HLB} = k \sum_{E=E_{min}}^{E_{max}} \left[E \, \Phi(E) \frac{A_{ent\,surf}}{m_g} \left(\sum_{i=1}^{3} f_i(E) \, G_i \right) \right] \qquad (1)$$

where the subindex $i = 1, 2, 3$ indicates each of the breast core layers, the constant k corrects for unit conversions, E is the source energy, $\Phi(E)$ the spectrum of photons/mm^2 normalized to 1 R, $A_{ent\,surf}$ is the beam entrance plane surface area at the top of the breast, m_g is the mass of the glandular portion of the breast tissue, $f_i(E)$ corresponds to the fractional energy absorption and G_i corrects the normalized dose calculation to the glandular tissue component in the breast core as calculated by:

$$G_i = \frac{f_{g,i} \left(\frac{\mu_{en}}{\rho} \right)_{g,i}}{f_{g,i} \left(\frac{\mu_{en}}{\rho} \right)_{g,i} + (1 - f_{g,i}) \left(\frac{\mu_{en}}{\rho} \right)_{a,i}} \qquad (2)$$

where $f_{g,i}$ refers to the fraction of glandular tissue with respect to the total breast tissue, $\frac{\mu_{en}}{\rho}$ corresponds to the mass-energy absorption coefficients, and the subscripts a and g indicate adipose tissue and glandular tissue respectively. The dose conversion coefficient based on the homogeneous breast core geometry (D_{gN}) corresponds to the particular case of the HLB geometry where all the breast core layers have the same glandular composition.

2.2   Impact of Glandular Tissue Distribution Using the HLB Model

The effect of the glandular tissue distribution on the MGD was studied using a set of HLB models and their corresponding homogeneous model. The set of Monte Carlo HLB models used in this study had an average glandular composition of 25%. This value is in agreement with the mean glandular compositions found by Yaffe et al.[13] The percentage glandular composition of the individual core layers was varied to simulate four different glandular tissue configurations as shown in Table 1.

2.3   Patient-Oriented Use of HLB Model

The main obstacle to incorporating the glandular tissue distribution in the calculation of MGD is the lack of three dimensional tissue distribution information from conventional mammography images.[9] The solution proposed in this work makes use of the information provided by the mammography images through their breast density map.[6,7] This method has the advantage that it provides an approximation to the actual glandular tissue distribution within the breast using conventional mammography images.

Table 1. Heterogeneous glandular tissue distributions for HLB model

Configuration ID	Percentage glandular composition (%)		
	Layer I*	Layer II	Layer III
A	30	**35**	*10*
B	**35**	30	*10*
C	*10*	**35**	30
D	*10*	30	**35**

*Layer I is the breast core layer closest to the beam entrance surface.

The current version of the MIB algorithm divides the breast density map into three sections and calculates the amount of glandular tissue in each section of the projected breast. The MIB algorithm also segments out of the density map any chest-wall structures, such as the pectoral muscle.

Because the breast density map provides the glandular tissue information in the direction perpendicular to the plane of the image receptor, the density map for a mediolateral oblique (MLO) view approximates the glandular tissue distribution in the plane parallel to the image receptor plane for the corresponding craniocaudal (CC) image, and viceversa. An underlying assumption of this approach is that, while the breast compression may change the position of the individual breast elements, the overall glandular composition remains the same.

The resulting approximation to the actual glandular tissue distribution, can then be incorporated into the calculation of patient-oriented MGD using the corresponding HLB Monte Carlo model.

Breast density maps were generated from patient mammograms using the specialized software Volpara^{TM} (Matakina Technology, Wellington, New Zealand). The MIB method was used to determine their corresponding glandular tissue distributions. The resulting HLB geometries were used in the determination of the patient-oriented dose coefficients D_{gN-HLB} using Monte Carlo methods. In addition, the corresponding homogeneous core model was developed for each patient and the D_{gN} coefficient was determined for each case. The spectrum used in this comparison had a Rh anode, 25 μm thick Rh filter, and 28 keV with 0.40 mmAl HVL. The characteristics of the patient group and the patient-oriented HLB models are shown in Table 2.

3   Results and Discussion

3.1   Impact of Glandular Tissue Distribution Using the HLB Model

The differences found in this study were 24% lower to 48% higher than the value estimated using the homogeneous breast model. According to the current dosimetry methods, all the models in this set would have been considered to be equivalent to the 25% homogeneous model. This means that, despite the anatomical differences, the MGD would have been estimated as the same in all these cases. The full results of this study are shown in Fig. 2.

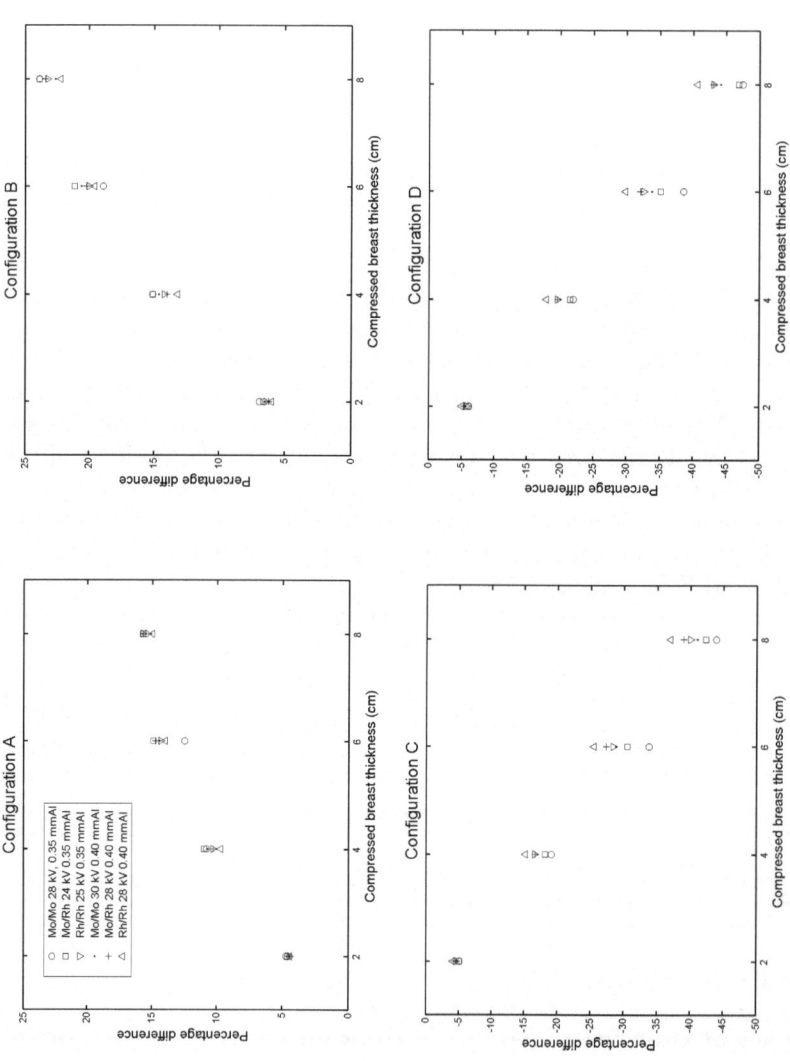

Fig. 2. Percentage difference between the D_{gN-HLB} for the HLB models from Table 1 and their equivalent homogeneous case D_{gN}. The differences arise solely from the variation in the distribution of the glandular tissue. Under the current dosimetric formalism all these glandular tissue distributions correspond to a homogeneous mix of adipose and glandular tissues with 25% glandular tissue composition.

3.2   Patient-Oriented Use of HLB Model

The D_{gN-HLB} values obtained from the patient-based HLB models were compared to the D_{gN} from the corresponding homogeneous models. The largest variation in the coefficient was found for a heterogeneously dense breast, where the D_{gN-HLB} was 14.8% higher than what was expected from the homogeneous glandular tissue distribution approximation. The complete results of this patient study are shown in Table 2.

These results suggest that the anatomical differences in patients have an effect on the dose conversion coefficients, and consequently on the value of MGD. The magnitude of this effect is dependent on the distribution of the glandular tissue within the breast of the patient and is expected to increase for thicker and more heterogeneously dense breasts.

Table 2. Comparison of D_{gN-HLB} from patient-oriented HLB models to the D_{gN} from their corresponding homogeneous breast core models

| Case ID | Compressed breast thickness (cm) | Glandular composition | | | | D_{gN} vs. D_{gN-HLB} |
		Whole breast (%)	Layer I (%)	Layer II (%)	Layer III (%)	
1a	5.8	2.6	2.4	2.9	2.5	-2.2%
1b	8.1	5.4	3.7	7.2	4.7	39.4%**
1c	5.2	3.7	4.3	4.0	2.8	6.4%
1d	8.0	3.7	6.8	3.3	0.9	39.0%**
2a	5.1	5.4	3.7	7.2	4.7	-9.1%
2b	5.2	5.6	7.1	7.0	2.6	13.8%
2c	4.8	6.7	4.0	8.1	7.4	-14.3%
2d	5.1	6.7	6.3	8.3	5.6	0.7%
3a	4.6	12.0	15.6	14.0	5.0	10.6%
3b	4.6	12.6	12.1	15.4	10.3	1.3%
3c	4.9	11.3	11.8	14.6	6.8	4.1%
3d	5.0	11.7	17.6	10.5	7.0	14.8%
4a	3.7	22.9	20.6	29.7	15.8	-1.3%
4b	4.3	23.9	16.4	32.1	23.3	-6.1%
4c	4.3	27.0	26.5	32.9	19.7	0.9%
4d	4.3	27.1	24.0	34.0	23.4	-1.0 %

a: MLO, left breast ; b: CC, left breast ; c: MLO, right breast ; d: CC, right breast
**The higher variations found for cases *1b* and *1d* can be explained due to the inclusion of additional anatomical structures that cannot be segmented out of the MLO images.

4   Conclusions

Our results suggest that the use of the homogeneous approximation to the distribution of glandular tissue leads to potentially large inaccuracies in the estimation of the MGD. The use of a breast geometry that can simulate different glandular tissue distributions, such as the HLB model, could reduce the uncertainty in the calculation of the dose conversion coefficients used for clinical dose studies. The magnitude of the uncertainty reduction depends on the particular anatomy studied, with a larger impact expected for thick, heterogeneously dense breasts.

Acknowledgments. The authors are grateful to Vikram Adhikarla, Paulina Galavis and Ivan M. Rosado-Méndez for their contributions in this study.

References

1. Boone, J.M., Chavez, A.: Comparison of x-ray cross sections for diagnostic and therapeutic medical physics. Medical Physics 23(12), 1997–2005 (1996)
2. Dance, D.R.: Monte Carlo calculation of conversion factors for the estimation of mean glandular breast dose. Physics in Medicine and Biology 35(9), 1211–1219 (1990)
3. Dance, D.R., Hunt, R.A., Bakic, P.R., Maidment, A.D.A., Sandborg, M., Ullman, G., Carlsson, C.A.: Breast dosimetry using high-resolution voxel phantoms. Radiation Protection Dosimetry 114(1-3), 359–363 (2005)
4. Dance, D.R., Skinner, C.L., Young, K.C., Beckett, J.R., Kotre, C.J.: Additional factors for the estimation of mean glandular breast dose using the UK mammography dosimetry protocol. Physics in Medicine and Biology 45, 3225–3240 (2000)
5. Hammerstein, G.R., Miller, D.W., White, D.R., Masterson, M.E., Woodard, H.Q., Laughlin, J.S.: Absorbed radiation doses in mammography. Radiation Physics 130, 485–491 (1979)
6. Highnam, R., Brady, J.M.: Mammographic Image Analysis. Kluwer Academic Publishers (1999)
7. Highnam, R., Brady, M., Shepstone, B.: A representation for mammographic image processing. Medical Image Analysis 1(1), 1–18 (1996)
8. Huang, S., Boone, J.M., Yang, K., Kwan, A.L., Packard, N.J.: The effect of skin thickness determined using breast CT on mammographic dosimetry. Medical Physics 35(4), 1199–1206 (2008)
9. Kopans, D.B.: Basic physics and doubts about relationship between mammographically determined tissue density and breast cancer risk. Radiology 246(2), 348–353 (2008)
10. Rosado-Méndez, I., Palma, B.A., Brandan, M.E.: Analytical optimization of digital subtraction mammography with contrast medium using a commercial unit. Medical Physics 35(12), 5544–5557 (2008)
11. Wu, X., Barnes, G.T., Tucker, D.M.: Spectral dependence of glandular tissue dose in screen-film mammography. Radiology 179, 143–148 (1991)
12. Wu, X.Z., Gingold, E.L., Barnes, G.T., Tucker, D.M.: Normalized average glandular dose in molybdenum target-rhodium filter and rhodium target-rhodium filter mammography. Radiology 193(1), 83–89 (1994)
13. Yaffe, M.J., Boone, J.M., Packard, N., Alonzo-Proulx, O., Huang, S.Y., Peressotti, C.L., Al-Mayah, A., Brock, K.: The myth of the 50-50 breast. Medical Physics 36(12), 5437–5443 (2009)

A Directional Small-Scale Tissue Model for an Anthropomorphic Breast Phantom

Ingrid Reiser[1,*], Beverly A. Lau[1],
Robert M. Nishikawa[1], and Predrag R. Bakic[2]

[1] Department of Radiology, The University of Chicago, Chicago, IL 60637
[2] Department of Radiology, University of Pennsylvania, Philadelphia, PA 19104
ireiser@uchicago.edu

Abstract. Mammographic tissue structure has been shown to exhibit directionality, with a preferred orientation towards the nipple. However, this property is absent in the small-scale tissue model of current breast phantoms. To improve existing breast phantoms, a model for simulating oriented breast tissue has been developed, and has been included into an existing anthropomorphic breast phantom. Within this model, directionality was introduced by filling compartments with binarized power-law noise that was oriented towards the nipple. Mammograms were simulated based on the original and the new directional phantom. Tissue orientation was measured in the simulated mammogram. Visually, the appearance of the enhanced phantom was more realistic. Further, the distribution of the orientation measure computed from the enhanced phantom was more similar to that in actual mammograms. In conclusion, the use of a directional model to simulate fibroglandular tissue greatly improves the realism of the breast phantom.

Keywords: antropomorphic breast phantom, power-law noise.

1 Introduction

X-ray breast imaging is moving toward 3D. Breast tomosynthesis and computed tomography clinical research prototypes have been developed, and, to date, a first tomosynthesis unit has received FDA approval for use in breast cancer screening and diagnosis. However, system optimization, both in terms of data acquisition and reconstruction, still needs to be performed. Since cancer detection and diagnosis are primarily limited by the complex anatomic structure of fibroglandular tissue in the breast, system optimization requires a realistic, anthropomorphic phantom to ensure that the outcome of systems optimization translates to higher quality images in clinical practice.

Several research groups have been developing statistically defined breast phantoms [2,1,4]. Our previous work in phantom development has produced a realistic-looking anthropomorphic breast phantom (Fig. 1) [6]. However recent work showed that breast structure is directional, and that it is oriented towards the nipple [7]. The previous phantom lacked the directional property of actual breast

---

* Corresponding author.

A.D.A. Maidment, P.R. Bakic, and S. Gavenonis (Eds.): IWDM 2012, LNCS 7361, pp. 141–148, 2012.

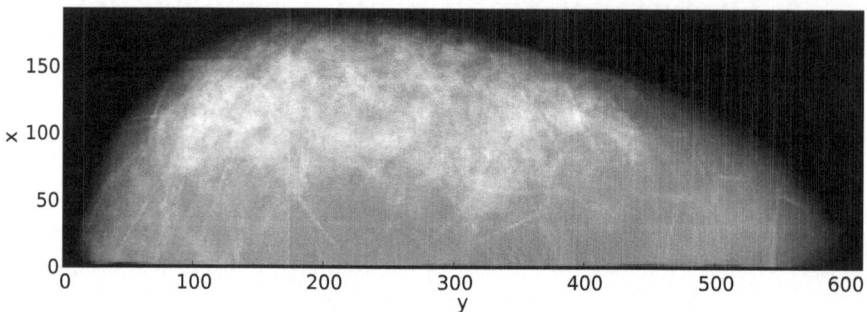

Fig. 1. Parallel projection of the original phantom, filled with isotropic power-law noise and compressed. Pixel size is 0.5 mm.

tissue. Thus the purpose of this work was to model directional breast structure, and to include this new tissue model into the phantom.

2   Method

2.1   Phantom Generation

The breast was modeled in two stages. First, the gross breast anatomy such as the overall breast shape and Cooper's ligaments were generated using Bakic's algorithm [1]. However, in this work, no dense tissue region is generated so that this base phantom only consists of skin, adipose tissue, and Cooper's ligaments. In the second stage, compartments bounded by Cooper's ligaments were filled with binarized power-law noise to mimic fibroglandular tissue. Previously, the noise had an isotropic power-spectrum, which produces noise that lacks any directionality [6]. The projection image of such a phantom is shown in Fig. 1. In this work, directionality was introduced by generating power-law noise with an ellipsoidal power spectrum $P(\boldsymbol{f})$,

$$P(\boldsymbol{f}) = \frac{c'}{(\boldsymbol{f}^T \mathbf{R}^T \mathbf{Q}^{-1} \mathbf{R} \boldsymbol{f})^{\beta'/2}} \tag{1}$$

where $\mathbf{R}$ is a matrices produced from three rotation matrices about the x and z-axes, $\mathbf{R} = R_x(\gamma)R_z(\delta)R_x(\alpha)$, and α, δ, γ are Euler angles. The angles were chosen such that the orientation of the noise field is towards the nipple. The amount of directionality is determined by $\mathbf{Q}$, a diagonal matrix with diagonal elements $q_{ii} = h$, where each element of $\boldsymbol{h}$ is the half-axis ratio of a spheroid. In this work, power spectra had a prolate symmetry.

The directional power-law noise volume was generated through an inverse Fourier transform of a complex volume with magnitude given by $\sqrt{P(\boldsymbol{f})}$ and a random phase.

2.2   Phantom Ensemble Parameters

For quantitative evaluation of the new phantom, 60 phantoms were generated from 20 empty shells. Each shell contained 150 compartments, of which 50 were filled with binarized power-law noise. The glandular fraction of each filled compartment was sampled from a uniform distribution bounded by 0.05 and 0.3. The amount of directionality was randomized by sampling the ellipsoid axis-ratio from $1/f(a,b)$ where f is a beta distribution with $a = 5, b = 5$. A cut-off value was introduced to limit the axis-ratio to 4.0 or less.

Using the same 20 empty shells and random number generator seeds, another set of 60 phantoms was generated where compartments were filled with isotropic (i.e., non-directional) binarized power-law noise.

These phantoms were compressed, upsampled and parallel-projected to produce simulated mammograms with $100\mu m \times 100\mu m$ pixel size. Blur and noise were added to the projections using a method originally proposed by Saunders *et al.* [8]. The modulation transform function (MTF) and noise-power spectrum (NPS) were those of a GE Essential mammography unit [5,6].

2.3   Quantitative Analysis

Power-law analysis was performed as described in [7]. Briefly, square regions-of-interest (ROI) were extracted from the uniform thickness region of the simulated mammograms and the periodogram was computed as the squared magnitude of the Fourier transform. A Hann window was used to prevent spectral leakage. The spatial-frequency (f) dependence of the periodogram was assumed to follow a power-law, $P(f) = c/f^\beta$. Power-law parameters β and $\log(c)$ were estimated from the periodogram assuming elliptic symmetry, and ellipse axis ratio and orientation angle were estimated as well. This analysis is described in detail in Ref. [7].

3   Results

Figure 2 shows slices through the directional phantom with $h = [4, 1, 1]$. All breast structure is oriented towards the nipple, located at ($x = 150, y = 150, z = 150$). A parallel projection of this phantom, after it has been compressed, is shown in Fig. 3. Note that the coordinates of the nipple changed due to the compression. The orientation of the breast structure can be clearly observed in the slices through the volume, as well as in the parallel projection.

The effect of the strength of the directionality, h, is shown in Fig. 4. The orientation can still be observed, but the directionality is weaker than in the phantom shown in Fig. 3.

Figure 5 shows regions of interested extracted from behind the nipple (top row), or from the upper quadrant of the breast (bottom row). With respect to Figs. 1, 3, 4, the ROI centers were located at ($x = 80, y = 190$) and ($x = 80, y = 310$), respectively. The texture in the ROIs from the original phantom is similar. In the ROIs extracted from phantoms with directionality, there is a distinct difference in the texture orientation in both ROIs, and the ROI location within the breast can be inferred from the preferred direction of the simulated tissue.

Figure 6 shows the power-law parameters β and $\log(c)$ for the ensemble of phantoms. For the isotropic and directional phantom, $(<\beta>, \sigma_\beta) = (-3.36,$

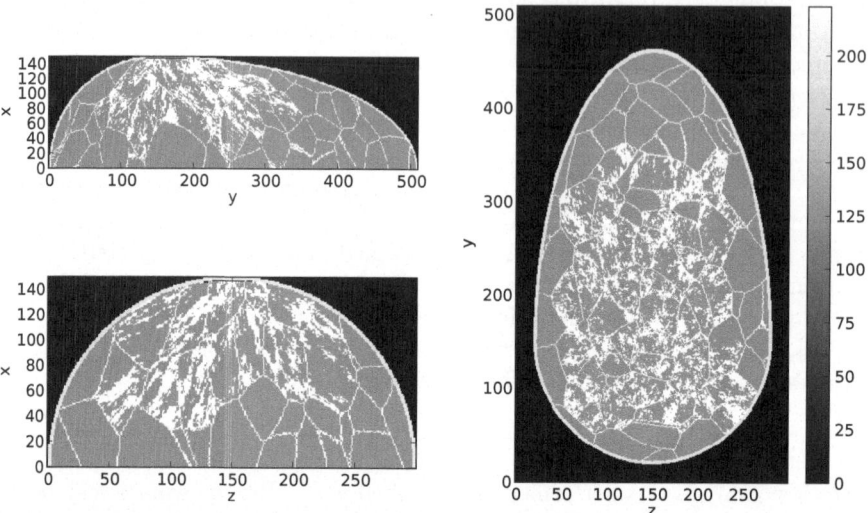

Fig. 2. Slices through the uncompressed phantom volume. For this phantom, $h = [4, 1, 1]$. Voxel size is 0.5mm isotropic.

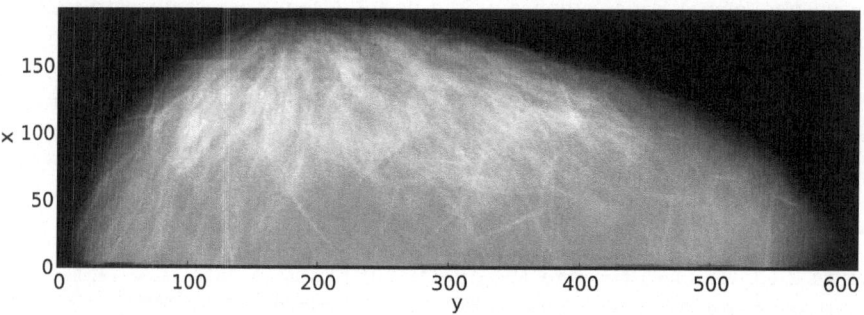

Fig. 3. Parallel projection of the compressed directional phantom. For this phantom, $h = [4, 1, 1]$. Pixel size is 0.5mm.

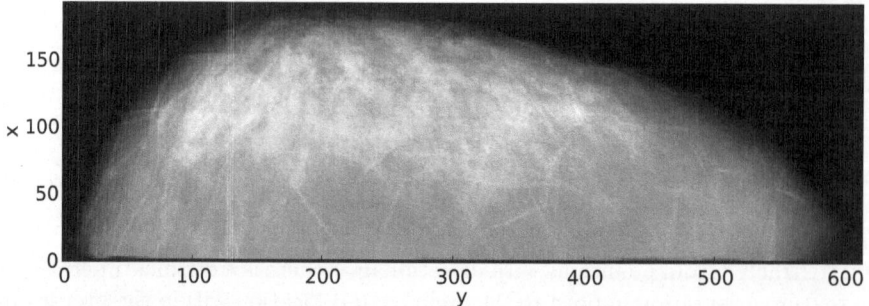

Fig. 4. Parallel projection of the directional phantom with $h = [2.1, 1, 1]$. Pixel size is 0.5mm.

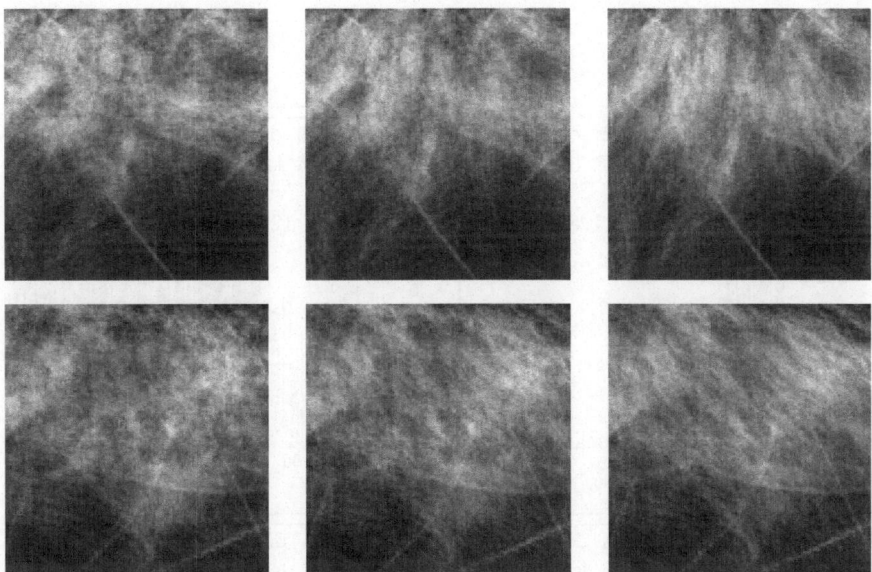

Fig. 5. Top row: ROIs extracted behind the nipple (centered on x=80, y=190 in Figs. 1, 3,4). Bottom row: ROIs extracted from the upper quadrant of the breast (centered x=80, y=310 in Figs. 1, 3,4). Left column: Original phantom, filled with isotropic power-law noise. Center column: Phantom with directional power-law noise ($h = [2.1, 1, 1]$). Right column: Phantom with directional power-law noise ($h = [4, 1, 1]$). ROI size is 6cm × 6cm.

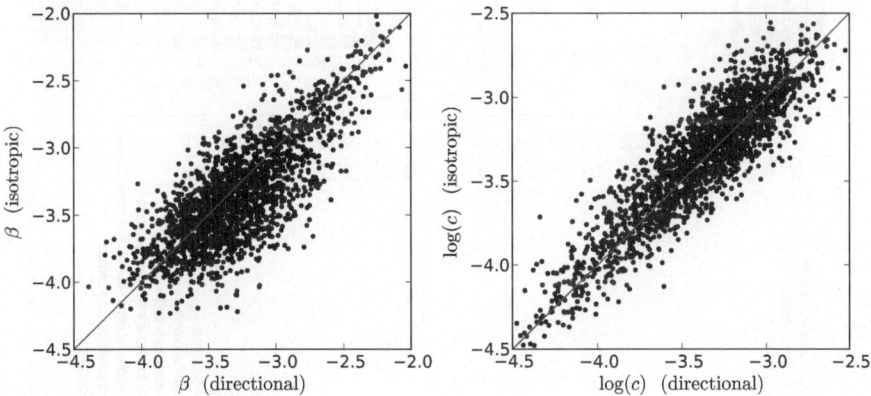

Fig. 6. Power-law parameters β and $\log(c)$, estimated from 256×256 pixel ROIs (2.56cm×2.56cm). Elliptic periodogram symmetry was assumed.

0.38) and $(< \log(c) >, \sigma_{\log(c)}) = (-3.38, 0.39)$, while for the directional phantom, $(< \beta >, \sigma_{\beta}) = (-3.29, 0.38)$ and $(< \log(c) >, \sigma_{\log(c)}) = (-3.4, 0.39)$. This is similar to what is observed in clinical mammograms [7,3]. The correlation between β and $\log(c)$ for the isotropic and directional phantom was 0.77 and 0.91, respectively.

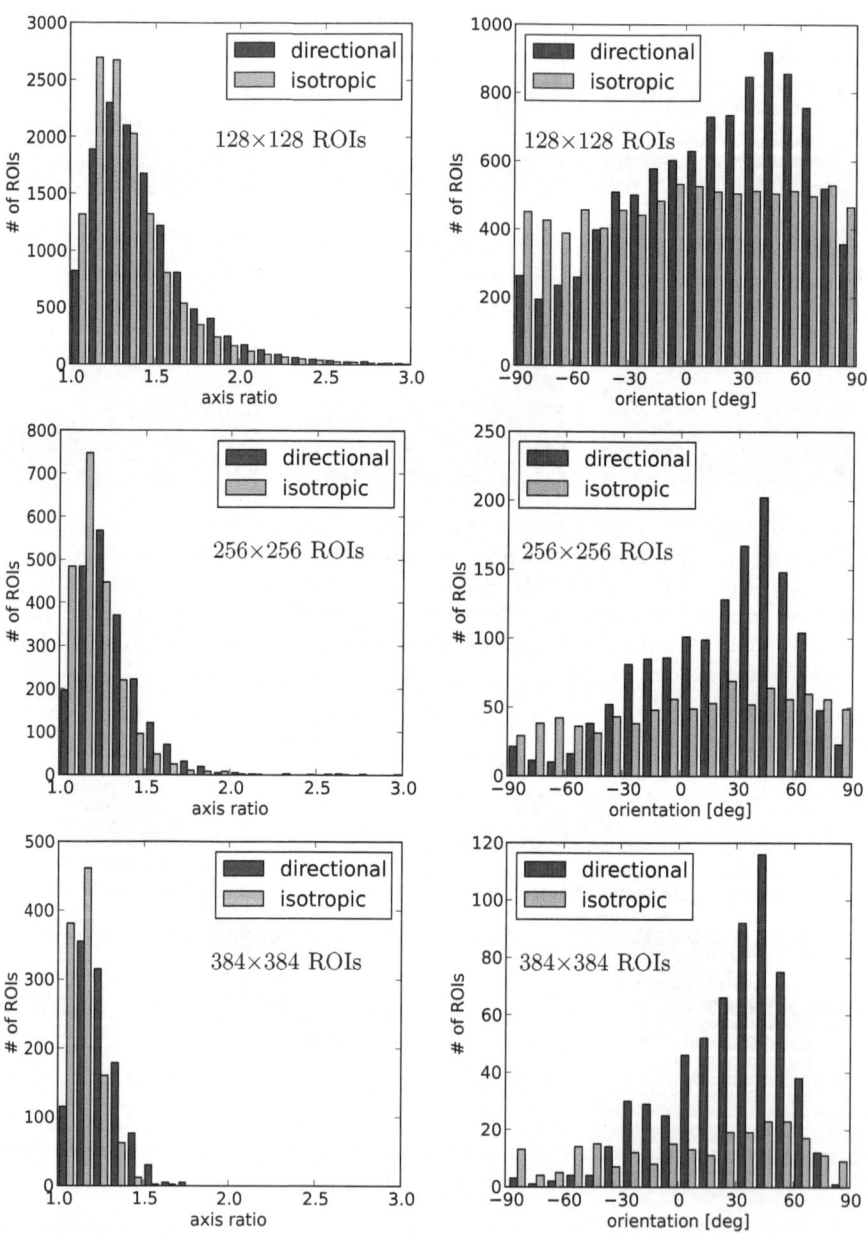

Fig. 7. Histograms of axis ratios and orientation angles. Orientation angles were included in the histogram for ROIs with an axis ratio greater than 1.2 only.

Figure 7 shows histograms of axis ratios and orientation angles for ROIs extracted from the simulated mammograms, for different ROI sizes (128^2, 256^2, 384^2). The histogram of orientation angles includes only ROIs for which the axis ratio in the periodogram was greater than 1.2 only, since an axis ratio of less than 1.2 corresponds to a periodogram that is essentially spherically symmetric. The average axis ratio decreases with decreasing ROI size, indicating that the directionality occurs on a small scale, and becomes less prominent on a larger scale. For all ROI sizes, the distribution of tissue structure orientation angles is more uniform for the isotropic phantom than it is for the directional phantom.

Table 1 lists the distribution parameters of the orientation angle for both phantoms. The average orientation angle is about 20 deg for the directional phantoms, indicating that on average, the tissue structure is pointing towards the nipple. For the istropic phantoms, average orientation angle is smaller. Thus, the average orientation for the directional phantom is more similar to what was observed for actual mammograms [7].

However the width of the angular distribution is wider for the simulated mammograms, compared to what was found for actual mammograms, and in addition, no ROI-size dependence of the axis ratio was observed in clinical images [7].

Table 1. Distribution parameters of the orientation angle θ for mammograms simulated from isotropic and directional phantoms

ROIsize	$< \theta >$ (iso)	σ_θ (iso)	$< \theta >$ (dir)	σ_θ (dir)
128	3.17	51.15	14.4	44.3
256	9.05	49.5	20.6	37.1
384	10.54	47.8	26.4	29.4

4 Discussion

The use of a directional fibroglandular tissue model visually improves the realism of the breast phantom. Quantitative comparison of power-law parameters indicate that the directional phantom produces some features observed in real mammograms, such as a preferred orientation towards the nipple, which is not observed in isotropic phantoms. On the other hand, the width of the distribution of orientation angles is larger than what is observed in real mammograms, and the amount of directionality, as measured by the axis ratio, depends on the size of ROIs that were analyzed. This may be due to the filling of individual compartments. In an actual breast, a given directionality may prevail throughout the entire breast without being disrupted at compartment borders.

5 Conclusion

A phantom with a directional tissue model has been developed, which mimics the orientation of small-scale tissue structure in clinical mammograms more closely.

Power-law parameters of this new phantom are similar to those in phantoms without directionality, and similar to what is observed in clinical images.

This phantom may be well suited for systems optimization in 3D breast imaging. Future research will include phantom validation through observer studies.

Acknowledgments. This work was funded in part by DOD W81XWH-08-1-0353, NIH grants R21 EB008801, T32 EB002103, S10 RR021039, and P30 CA14599. RM Nishikawa is a shareholder in and receives royalties from Hologic, Inc.

References

1. Bakic, P.R., Zhang, C., Maidment, A.D.A.: Development and characterization of an anthropomorphic breast software phantom based upon region-growing algorithm. Medical Physics 38(6), 3165 (2011)
2. Bliznakova, K., Bliznakov, Z., Bravou, V., Kolitsi, Z., Pallikarakis, N.: A three-dimensional breast software phantom for mammography simulation. Phys. Med. Biol. 48(22), 3699–3719 (2003)
3. Burgess, A.E., Jacobson, F.L., Judy, P.F.: Human observer detection experiments with mammograms and power-law noise. Medical Physics 28(4), 419 (2001)
4. Chen, B., Shorey, J., Saunders, R.S., Richard, S., Thompson, J., Nolte, L.W., Samei, E.: An anthropomorphic breast model for breast imaging simulation and optimization. Acad. Radiol. 18(5), 536–546 (2011)
5. Ghetti, C., Borrini, A., Ortenzia, O., Rossi, R., Ordóñez, P.L.: Physical characteristics of GE Senographe Essential and DS digital mammography detectors. Medical Physics 35(2), 456 (2008)
6. Lau, B.A., Reiser, I., Nishikawa, R.M., Bakic, P.R.: A statistically defined anthropomorphic software breast phantom. Submitted to Medical Physics (2012)
7. Reiser, I., Lee, S., Nishikawa, R.M.: On the orientation of mammographic structure. Medical Physics 38(10), 5303 (2011)
8. Saunders, R.S., Samei, E.: A method for modifying the image quality parameters of digital radiographic images. Medical Physics 30(11), 3006 (2003)

Simulation of Three Material Partial Volume Averaging in a Software Breast Phantom

Feiyu Chen[1], David D. Pokrajac[1], Xiquan Shi[1], Fengshan Liu[1],
Andrew D.A. Maidment[2], and Predrag R. Bakic[2]

[1] Delaware State University, 1200 N DuPont Hwy, Dover DE 19904
FChen09@students.desu.edu, {DPokrajac,XShi,FLiu}@desu.edu
[2] University of Pennsylvania, 3400 Spruce Street, Philadelphia, PA 19104
{Predrag.Bakic,Andrew.Maidment}@uphs.upenn.edu

Abstract. A general case for simulation of partial volume (PV) averaging in software breast phantoms is presented. PV simulation could improve the quality of phantom images by reducing quantization artifacts near borders between different materials. The validity of phantom studies depends on the realism of simulated images, which is affected by the size of phantom voxels. Large voxels may cause notable quantization artifacts; small voxels, however, extend the generation time and increase the memory requirements. An improvement in image quality without reducing voxel size is achievable by the simulation of PV averaging in voxels containing more than one simulated tissue type; the linear x-ray attenuation coefficient of such voxels is represented by a combination of attenuation coefficients proportional to voxel subvolumes occupied by different tissues. In this paper, we present results of simulated PV in the general case of voxels containing up to three materials.

Keywords: Digital mammography, computer breast phantom, partial volume simulation, computational geometry.

1   Introduction

This study is motivated by the desire to improve the quality of synthetic images generated using software breast phantoms. The partial volume (PV) averaging can help reduce the quantization artifacts on boundaries of regions with different simulated materials. The software phantoms in this study have been generated based upon the recursive partitioning of the phantom volume using octrees [1]. In this paper, we propose a solution for a general PV case with up to three simulated materials in a voxel. This work represents the first PV simulation in software phantoms generated based upon the rules for simulating anatomical structures [1-4]. PV simulation has been indirectly reported in a method for generating phantoms based upon the CT images of mastectomy specimen [5]. In that method, the values of each reconstructed breast CT image voxel were scaled and interpreted as the percentage of adipose breast tissue in the voxel.

A.D.A. Maidment, P.R. Bakic, and S. Gavenonis (Eds.): IWDM 2012, LNCS 7361, pp. 149–156, 2012.

In this paper, we present an overview of the PV simulation method including details of a planar approximation and the PV computation. The improvement of image quality is qualitatively validated. The results are shown in the form of slices and simulated X-ray projections of phantoms with and without PV.

2   Method

The effective linear x-ray attenuation in a voxel which contains more than one simulated material can be calculated as:

$$\mu_V = \frac{1}{|V|}\sum_i \mu_i |V_i| = \sum_i \mu_i p_i \; ; \; p_i = \frac{|V_i|}{|V|} \times 100\% , \tag{1}$$

where $|V|$ is the voxel volume, $|V_i|$ is the subvolume of material i with the linear x-ray attenuation μ_i, and p_i is the percentage of the material i in the voxel (Fig. 1a). One can distinguish the following cases of PV (Fig 1b):

A. *Two materials with one bounding surface*: (1) Skin and air; (2) Cooper's ligament and adipose tissue; (3) Ligament and fibroglandular dense tissue; (4) Skin and dense tissue; (5) Skin and adipose tissue, and (6) Skin and Cooper's ligament;

B. *Three materials with two bounding surfaces*: (7) Skin, ligament, and dense tissue; and (8) Skin, ligament, and adipose tissue

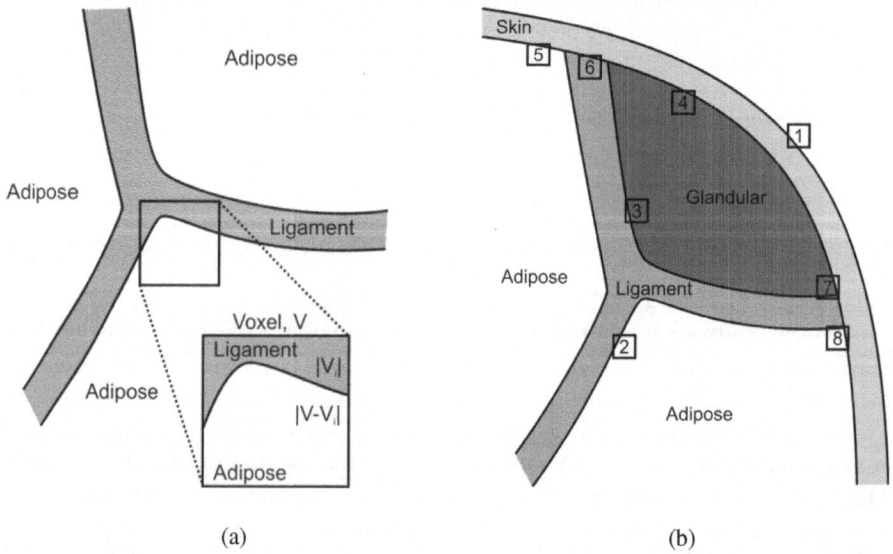

(a)   (b)

Fig. 1. (a) The concept of PV simulation; V denotes the voxel volume and V_i is the sub-volume occupied by dense tissue.(b) Different cases of material combination in a voxel.

The simulation of PV case (1) has been reported previously [6]; it can be easily extended to cases (2)-(6). In this abstract we present a general case of PV simulation based upon the planar approximation of up to two bounding surfaces in a voxel, addressing cases (7)-(8).

The planar approximation for the boundary between Cooper's ligaments and adipose tissue, as simulated in our software breast phantom [1], can be obtained as follows. Adipose compartments C_i and C_j, which may be given by shape functions f_i and f_j, determine a Cooper's ligament between them as the locus of points within a distance of D/2 from a surface $F_{ij}(\mathbf{x}) = f_i(\mathbf{x}) - f_j(\mathbf{x})$, see Fig. 2. Consider a voxel V with center $\mathbf{x}_c$. We define a planar approximation π_1 of the boundary between the Cooper's ligament and the compartment C_j as

$$\pi_1 : (\mathbf{x} - \mathbf{x}_1) \cdot sign(F_{ij}(\mathbf{x}_c)) \nabla F_{ij}(\mathbf{x}_c) = 0, \tag{2}$$

where

$$\mathbf{x}_1 = \mathbf{x}_c + sign(F_{ij}(\mathbf{x}_c)) \left(D/2 - \frac{F_{ij}(\mathbf{x}_c)}{\|\nabla F_{ij}(\mathbf{x}_c)\|} \right) \frac{\nabla F_{ij}(\mathbf{x}_c)}{\|\nabla F_{ij}(\mathbf{x}_c)\|}. \tag{3}$$

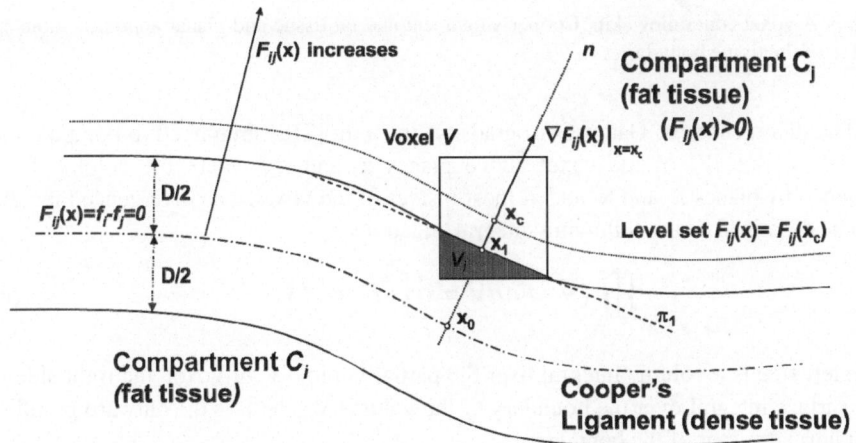

Fig. 2. Planar approximation of a boundary between Cooper's ligament and a compartment

In a general PV case with three simulated materials and two bounding surfaces in a voxel, we can construct a planar approximation for each bounding surface (Fig. 3). The result of the approximation are planes $\pi_1 : (\mathbf{x} - \mathbf{x}_1)\hat{\mathbf{n}}_1 = 0$ and $\pi_2 : (\mathbf{x} - \mathbf{x}_2)\hat{\mathbf{n}}_1 = 0$. The partial volumes $|V_i|$ of interest are subsequently calculated as the volume of a portion of the voxel V (with center $\mathbf{x}_c$) that is bellow/above the planes. For example, the PV V_i corresponding to the fat tissue in Figure 4 is computed as a volume of a part of the voxel that is both above planes π_1 and π_2.

The PV V_i in a voxel shown in Fig. 3 has been computed using planar approximations as follows. Consider a voxel of linear size Δx, with a vertex **v** located above
planes π_1 and π_2. (If no such vertex exists, the PV should be zero).

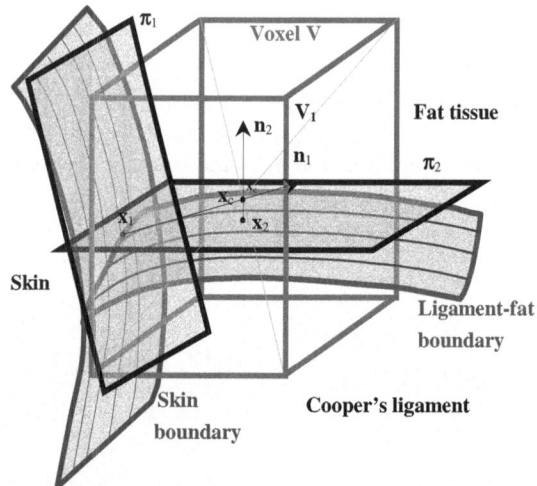

Fig. 3. A voxel containing skin, Cooper's ligament and fat tissue and planar approximations π_1
and π_2 of the tissue boundaries

The divergence (or Gauss-Ostrogradsky) theorem [7] is employed to compute the
partial volume $|V_i|$ of the voxel above planes π_1 and π_2, where the volume V_i is
bounded by planes π_1 and π_2 and at most 6 sides of the voxel. The divergence theorem
can be described as the following integral equation:

$$\iiint_{V_i} (\nabla \cdot F)dV = \oiint_{S} (F \cdot \mathbf{n})dS . \tag{4}$$

The left side is a volume integral over the partial volume V_i of voxel, the right side is
the surface integral over the boundary of the volume V_i, and n is the outward pointing
unit normal vector of the boundary.

After the appropriate choice of the vector field function inside the integral at left
side, *i.e.*, $F(\mathbf{x}) = \mathbf{x}$, the whole quantity at the left side becomes $3|V_i|$, and the right side
can be rewritten as:

$$\left(S_1 + S_2 + S_3 \right)\Delta x + A_{\pi 1}d_1 + A_{\pi 2}d_2 , \tag{5}$$

where S_i, $i=1,3$ are surface areas of the boundary formed by the voxel sides σ_1, σ_2 and
σ_3, that do not contain the vertex **v**; $A_{\pi 1}$ and $A_{\pi 2}$ are surface areas of the boundary of
V_i belonging to planes π_1 and π_2.

Subsequently, the PV can be calculated as:

$$|V_i| = \frac{(S_1 + S_2 + S_3)\Delta x + A_{\pi 1}d_1 + A_{\pi 2}d_2}{3}, \qquad (6)$$

where $d_1 = (\mathbf{v} - \mathbf{x}_1)\hat{\mathbf{n}}_1$, and $d_2 = (\mathbf{v} - \mathbf{x}_2)\hat{\mathbf{n}}_2$ are distances of the vertex $\mathbf{v}$ to planes π_1 and π_2.

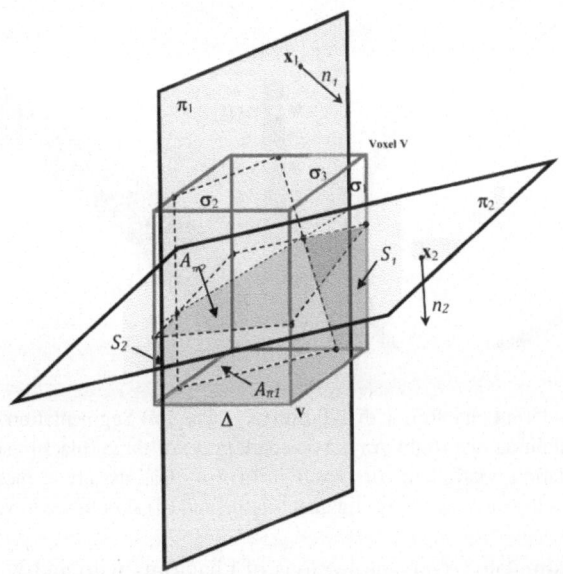

Fig. 4. Partial volume V_i of the voxel V above planes π_1 and π_2 and containing vertex $\mathbf{v}$. S_1, S_2 and S_3(here S_3=0) are surface areas of parts of the volume boundary belonging to voxel sides σ_1, σ_2 and σ_3 that do not contain the vertex $\mathbf{v}$.

3   Results and Discussion

Fig. 5 illustrates the PV simulation in a 450ml software breast phantom with 400μm voxels. Shown is the segmentation of phantom detail into air and voxels containing one, two or three materials. For the corresponding phantom detail, shown also are the equivalent linear x-ray attenuations, and percentages of ligament tissue and skin tissue.

Fig. 5 suggests that the PV simulation on the ligaments-fat boundary was qualitatively correct. The voxels containing two materials are detected at the boundaries of two materials (e.g., skin, compartment). Similarly, the three material voxels are detected where the skin meets Cooper's ligaments and a compartment. Fig. 5b indicates that the PV helped smooth the appearance of boundaries between regions with different x-ray attenuations. The computed percentages of ligament and skin tissues in a voxel (Figs. 5c, 5d) suggest the correctness of the applied algorithm. The voxels in the interior of skin/ligaments contain 100% of the corresponding tissues, while the percentages gradually decrease at the boundaries.

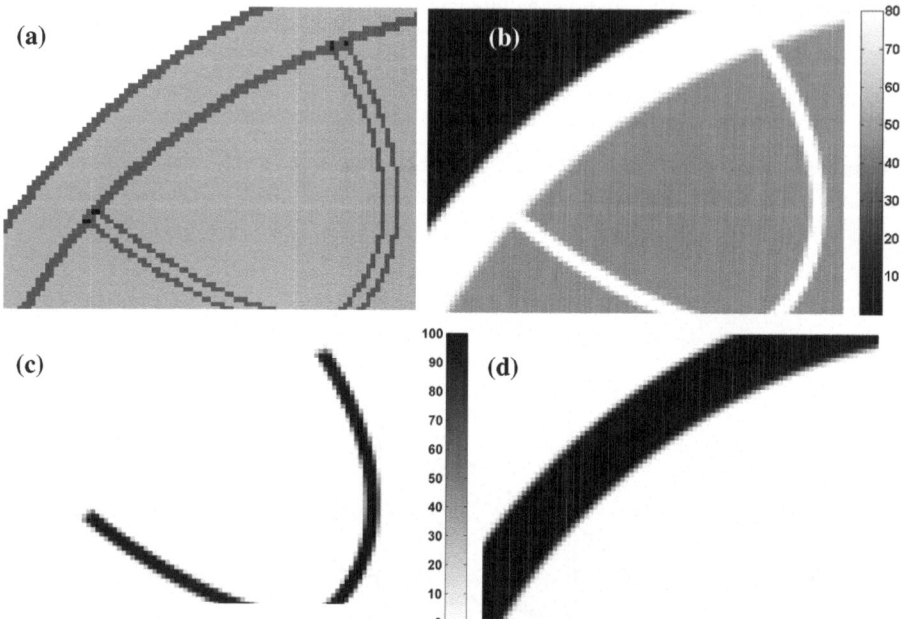

Fig. 5. Detail of a 450ml phantom with 400µm voxel size: (a) Segmentation of a phantom into air and voxels containing one (light gray), two (dark gray) or three (black) materials; (b) Simulated linear attenuation coefficients of voxels in (a) (in cm^{-1}, assuming monoenergetic x-ray beam at 20 keV); and percentage of (c) ligament tissue and (d) skin tissue in voxels from (a).

Fig. 6 shows simulated x-ray projections of phantoms with and without simulated PV. The simulated acquisition assumed a monoenergetic x-ray beam (at 20 keV) and parallel x-ray propagation, without scatter or quantum noise. The projections correspond to three phantoms with identical distributions of compartments: the phantom with 400µm voxels and no PV (Fig. 6a); the 400µm phantom with simulated PV (Fig. 6b); and the phantom with 200µm voxels and no PV (Fig. 6c). Shown also is the difference between the projections with and without simulated PV (Fig. 6d).

In a projection of the phantom with PV in Fig. 6b, the skin and Cooper's ligaments appear thinner (as compared to the phantom without PV, Fig. 6a). We believe this is caused by the reduction in the effective x-ray attenuations of voxels on the ligament/adipose tissue boundaries, which are lower than the x-ray attenuation of dense tissue (see Fig. 5b). Further, the characteristic stair-step quantization artifacts on tissue boundaries were noticeably reduced with simulated PV, as seen in the difference between PV and non PV projections (Fig 6d). Comparison of Figs. 6b and 6c indicates similar appearance of a phantom with PV simulated at a lower resolution (400µm) to a phantom simulated at a higher resolution (200µm) with no simulated PV. Hence, the application of PV may lead to an improvement in image quality without reducing voxel size.

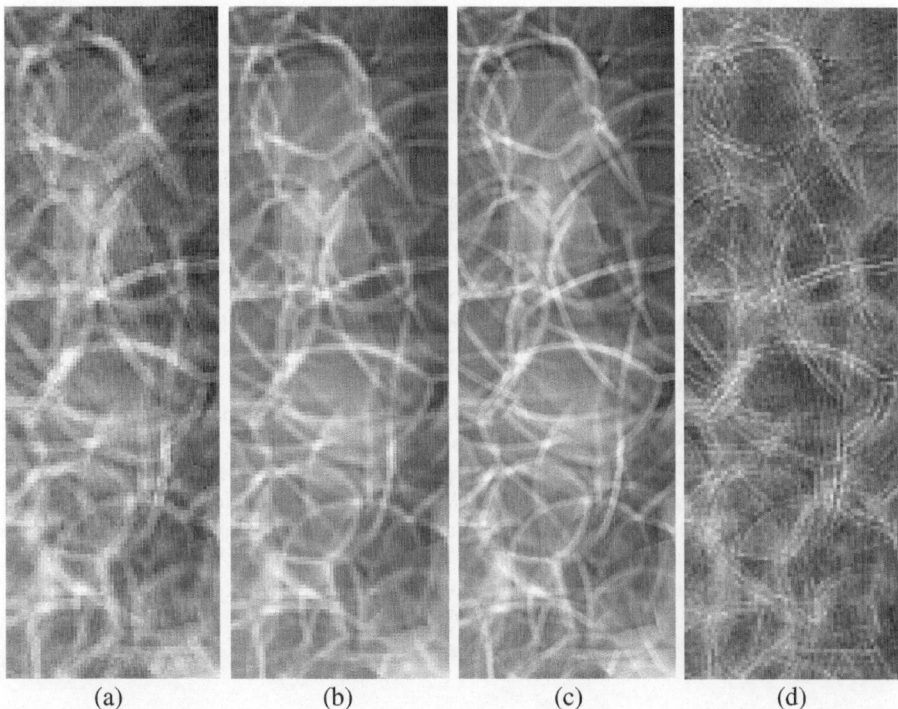

Fig. 6. Simulated projections of (a) a phantom with 400µm voxels and no PV; (b) the phantom from (a) with simulated PV; and (c) the same phantom generated at 200 µm voxels and no PV. (d) The difference between (a) and (b); the image contrast was enhanced for display purposes.

4   Conclusion

We have developed and qualitatively assessed a method for PV simulation of phantom voxels containing up to three simulated materials. The percentage of simulated tissues was estimated based upon the use of the Gauss-Ostrogradsky theorem. Cross-section and projections of phantoms with and without PV simulation were visually compared. PV simulation can improve the quality of phantom images by reducing the quantization artifacts caused by large voxel sizes.

Acknowledgements. This work was supported in part by the US Department of Defense Breast Cancer Research Program (HBCU Partnership Training Award #BC083639), the US National Institutes of Health (R01 grant #CA154444), the US National Science Foundation (CREOSA grant #HRD-0630388), and the US Department of Defense/Department of Army (45395-MA-ISP, #54412-CI-ISP). The authors would like to thank Ms. Susan Ng from Real-Time Tomography (Villanova, PA) for processing the simulated projection images.

References

1. Pokrajac, D.D., Maidment, A.D.A., Bakic, P.R.: Optimized generation of high resolution breast anthropomorphic software phantoms. Medical Physics 39, 2290–2302 (2012)
2. Bakic, P.R., Zhang, C., Maidment, A.D.A.: Development and Characterization of an Anthropomorphic Breast Software Phantom Based upon Region-Growing Algorithm. Medical Physics 38, 3165–3176 (2011)
3. Bliznakova, K., Suryanarayanan, S., Karellas, A., Paiilikarakis, N.: Evaluation of an improved algorithm for producing realistic 3D breat software phantoms: Application for mammography. Medical Physics 37, 5604–5617 (2010)
4. Chen, B., Shorey, J., Saunders, R.S.J., Richard, S., Thompson, J., Nolte, L.W., Samei, E.: An anthropomorphic breast model for breast imaging simulation and optimization. Academic Radiology 18, 536–546 (2011)
5. O'Connor, J.M., Das, M., Didier, C., Mah'D, M., Glick, S.J.: Comparison of Two Methods to Develop Breast Models for Simulation of Breast Tomosynthesis and CT. In: Krupinski, E.A. (ed.) IWDM 2008. LNCS, vol. 5116, pp. 417–425. Springer, Heidelberg (2008)
6. Chen, F., Pokrajac, D.D., Shi, X., Liu, F., Maidment, A.D.A., Bakic, P.R.: Partial Volume Simulation in Software Breast Phantoms. In: Physics of Medical Imaging. SPIE, San Diego (2012)
7. Folland, G.B.: Advanced Calculus. Prentice-Hall, Inc., Upper Saddle River (2002)

Iterative Reconstruction with Monte Carlo Based System Matrix for Dedicated Breast PET

Krishnendu Saha, Kenneth J. Straus, and Stephen J. Glick

University of Massachusetts Medical School, Department of Radiology, Worcester, MA
{krishnendu.saha,stephen.glick}@umassmed.edu,
kennethstraus@gmail.com

Abstract. Increasing sensitivity by reducing the ring diameter of breast PET system may degrade image performance at field of view periphery. In this work, the authors present a framework for computing and incorporating an accurate system model of breast PET utilizing GATE Monte Carlo simulation to compensate for this performance degradation. The system matrix (SM) generation count statistics was maximized by taking into account the geometric symmetry of the scanner. The SM was incorporated into MLEM reconstruction and compared with the Siddon ray-tracing algorithm to evaluate point source resolution and contrast recovery coefficient (CRC) of hot spheres at various radial locations. Both spatial resolution and CRC using SM based MLEM was approximately position invariant, whereas the CRC and spatial resolution with Siddon based MLEM was substantially lower for locations near the periphery of the FOV. The CRC vs noise tradeoff was markedly better with the SM based MLEM.

Keywords: System matrix, MLEM Reconstruction, Breast PET.

1 Introduction

Over the past several years it has become clear that PET imaging with fluoro-deoxyglucose (FDG) can play an important role in the detection and diagnosis of breast cancer. Many encouraging studies using whole-body PET systems to image breast cancer have been reported [1], however, it is now evident that smaller PET systems dedicated to imaging the breast have substantial advantages. A number of different dedicated breast PET systems have been proposed and developed [2-4]. To improve count statistics for dedicated breast PET, it is desirable to have high sensitivity. Improved sensitivity can also allow for reduced radiation dose to the patient, as well as minimizing acquisition time. Scanner designs that maximize geometric efficiency by placing the PET detectors close to the breast are therefore appealing. In a ring PET geometry, this means using a small bore designed to have a diameter just larger than the maximum diameter breast size to be imaged. In addition to high sensitivity, another desired goal of breast PET systems is high resolution, necessary for

A.D.A. Maidment, P.R. Bakic, and S. Gavenonis (Eds.): IWDM 2012, LNCS 7361, pp. 157–164, 2012.

accurate detection of sub-cm lesions. PET spatial resolution is degraded by various detector and radiotracer properties.

In this work, we utilized GATE Monte Carlo simulation software for estimating system matrix (SM) to address these degradation factors in MLEM reconstruction. Symmetry of the ring PET geometry is taken advantage of by using polar voxels to represent the object to be reconstructed. This results in a block-circulant SM where only one block column needs to be stored in memory. In addition, since the SM is sparse, only non-zero values are stored. This SM is then used with an iterative MLEM algorithm using data stored in LOR histograms [5]. For efficient implementation, the projector and backprojector operations used a rotator to take advantage of the polar voxel object representation.

2   Method

2.1   System Modeling

For this study, a hypothetical breast PET system is modeled, using a full ring geometry encompassing the breast with detector coverage of 360 degrees. The scanner is based on 12 detector modules with each module consisting of 32 x 96 LYSO crystals of size 2 x 2 x 20 mm. Therefore, there are 96 rings in the scanner, with a ring defined as one crystal in the axial direction. In this study, we consider 2D reconstruction, where the system matrix probabilities only describe lines-of-response (LOR) that fall within the same ring.

By geometrically limiting the acceptable LORs to those that connect a crystal within in a module to its' opposite seven modules based on maximal breast size of 18cm obtained from analyzing 23 patients breast CT images in our laboratory, there are 384 x 224 = 86016 possible LORs (this geometric constraint would allow for complete coverage of a 16.6 diameter breast). One-half of these LORs are redundant; therefore there are 43008 possible non-redundant LORs. If the 2D reconstruction matrix is defined as 200 x 200 with 1 mm voxels, then the SM will have 43008 x 200 x 200 = 1.72×10^9 elements. By using a polar voxel representation of the object, the system matrix becomes block-circulant. This means that all elements of the SM can be obtained from only one block column, thereby reducing storage by a factor of 12. This one block column represents the probabilities for LORs connecting one detector module to its opposite seven modules.

2.2   GATE Setup

The Monte Carlo simulation software package GATE [6] has been widely used to simulate PET acquisition. It can track photon interactions both through the object and within the detector including crystal penetration and scatter. In this work GATE has been used to estimate system matrix elements. The system matrix elements represent the probability of an emission at object voxel j being detected by a specific detector pair (LOR) i. These probabilities model the physics of photon transport within the detector, but not object interactions such as photon attenuation and scatter in the object. To compute the SM probability, a cylindrical activity source in air, (diameter of 18 cm - large enough to cover all possible expected object locations) is simulated using the above mentioned breast PET model. GATE allows objects to be simulated in air by using the option of back-to-back photon emission (i.e., without actually modeling positron emission). Thus positron range is not modeled in the system matrix.

2.3   Calculation Efficiency

As mentioned previously, probabilities for 1.72×10^9 elements in the SM need to be calculated for complete coverage of a 16.6 cm PET FOV. However, most of these probabilities are zero, thereby making the system matrix highly sparse. In other words, for each emission point in the object only a relatively small number of LORs can be feasibly measured. To utilize the sparseness of the SM, and thereby reduce computational burden and storage space, a linked-list LOR data structure was used. This data structure stores probabilities for only non-zero SM elements. Utilizing this linked list data format allowed for reducing the storage space by more than 99% (from 1.72×10^9 to 1.42×10^7). To further reduce storage space, a polar voxel basis function is utilized to represent the object (Fig. 1), thereby causing system matrix to be block-circulant. This means that there is substantial redundancy in the system matrix, and only elements describing the LOR probabilities from one module need to be computed and stored (these probabilities make up one block column of the system matrix).

2.4   Estimating Probabilities for the System Matrix

In forming the system matrix, simulated events producing LORs in a single module (module 0) were obtained by rotating the simulated LORs measured in other modules in such a way that one end of the LOR always resided in module 0 (Fig. 2). Upon completion of assigning all LORs in the event list, the SM probabilities represented the probability for a photon emitted from voxel j and detected at LOR i in module 0 (post-rotation). However, the desired SM element values were the probability of a photon emitted from voxel j and detected at LOR i in any module (not just module 0), i.e. before rotating all LORs to module 0 (pre-rotation). Thus an adjustment was implemented by using the following expression,

$$p(i,j) = \frac{Counts\ detected\ in\ LOR\ i\ from\ voxel\ j\ post-rotation}{Counts\ emitted\ from\ voxel\ j\ post-rotation} \times \frac{Counts\ to\ Module\ 0\ from\ voxel\ j\ pre-rotation}{Total\ counts\ from\ voxel\ j\ pre-rotation}$$

$$(1)$$

160   K. Saha, K.J. Straus, and S.J. Glick

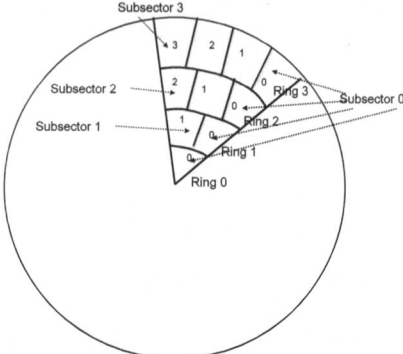

Fig. 1. The polar voxel comprises of concentric rings of equal radial dimension with each of the ring divided into number of angular subsectors corresponding to scalar multiple of number of crystals in transaxial orientation. The number of angular subsectors increases as concentric rings is farther away from center.

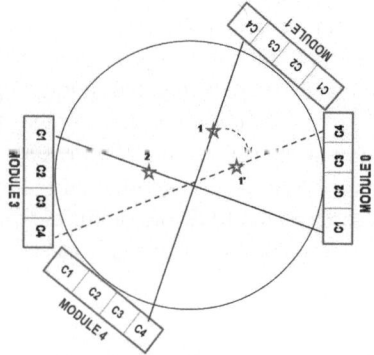

Fig. 2. LORs originating at modules other than '0' (example LOR 1 in figure) are rotated to module 0 (new LOR 1') utilizing rotational symmetry of the cylindrical scanner to improve statistics. LORs originally from module 0 (LOR 2) are not rotated.

2.5   Reconstruction Method

Reconstruction is performed using the MLEM algorithm. The measured data were binned into LOR histogram format prior to implementing reconstruction, where any LOR bins with zero events were not stored. The back projection matrix is calculated once for a unique LOR voxel pair instead of multiple times for each LOR voxel pair thus reducing computational burden by reducing the number of times the forward projection matrix is required to be calculated for a LOR.

$$\lambda_j^{m+1} = \frac{\lambda_j^m}{\sum_{i=1}^{I} p_{ij}} \sum_{k'=1}^{N'} p_{i_{k'}j} \frac{n_{k'}}{\sum_{b=1}^{J'} p_{i_{k'}b}\lambda_b^m} \quad , \tag{2}$$

where m is the iteration number, λ_j^m is the intensity in voxel j at iteration m, p_{ij} is p (detected in LOR i | emitted in voxel j), N' is the number of distinct LORs, J' is the total number of voxels lying in LOR $i_{k'}$, $\mathrm{n}_{k'}$ is the number of events detected in LOR $i_{k'}$.

2.6   Performance Evaluation

To evaluate the tomographic spatial resolution performance of reconstruction algorithms at various locations in reconstruction space (Fig. 3, left), a comparison of the resolution of reconstructed point sources at various FOV locations was performed for SM based reconstruction and Siddon line-integral based reconstruction [7]. Point sources were simulated at radial offsets of 0, 15, 25, 35, 45, 55 and 65 mm from the center in both the x and y directions (Fig. 3, left). Resolution of point sources were estimated by fitting the 2D count profile in a region surrounding the point source (10 mm×10 mm ROI with point source at the center) by a 2D Gaussian to obtain the FWHMs of the Gaussian fit.

In order to evaluate the contrast performance of spheres located in various locations as a function of noise, contrast recovery of spheres was compared with respect to background noise at various radial locations. Signal to background activity concentration was 8:1 and a 1 minute acquisition was simulated. Three spheres of 8 mm diameter located at 2, 4 and 6 cm from the center of the PET FOV are included for analysis (Fig. 3, right). In order to estimate signal counts, a region of interest (ROI) was drawn over the sphere. For the background, a ROI of same size was drawn diagonally opposite to the sphere (Fig. 3, right). The contrast recovery coefficient (CRC) and noise were estimated based on equations 3 and 4. Quantitative comparison of CRC as a function of noise was performed for SM based and Siddon line-integral based MLEM reconstruction at 10, 20, 30, 40, 60, 80 iterations.

$$CRC(\%) = \frac{S}{B} \times 100 \ , \tag{3}$$

$$Noise(\%) = \frac{\sigma_B}{B} \times 100 \ , \tag{4}$$

where S represents the mean counts in a sphere, B represents the mean counts in the background and σ_B is the standard deviation of background counts.

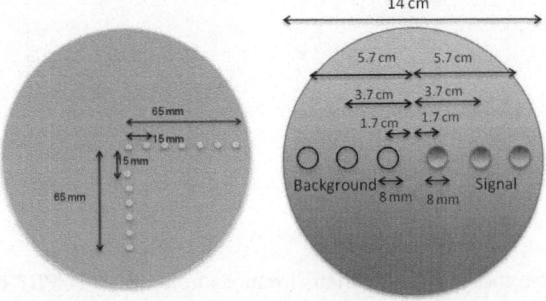

Fig. 3. Left: Point source locations for resolution phantom, Right: Modeled sphere and background locations and dimension for contrast evaluation

3   Results

3.1   Resolution Performance

The tomographic resolution of point sources as a function of x-axis and y-axis locations are shown in Fig. 4, left and right respectively. The figure illustrates overall improved resolution by the SM based MLEM method as compared to the Siddon [7] line-integral approach due to better modeling of detector response at the FOV periphery. Improvement in resolution increased as a function of distance offset from the center of the FOV with the smallest improvement at 15 mm (1.5 times) and the largest improvement at 65 mm (3 times) from center.

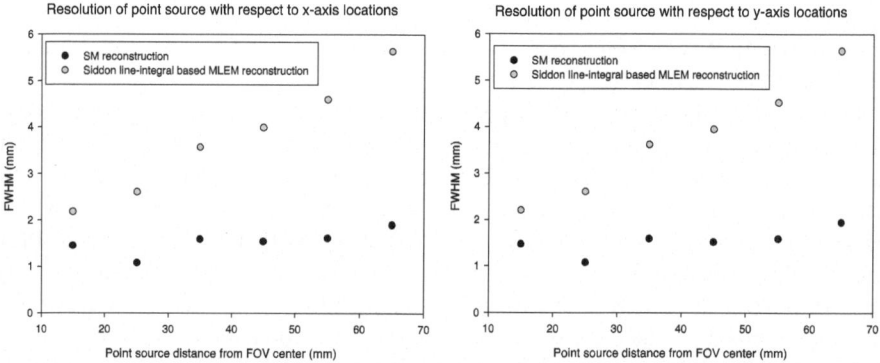

Fig. 4. Comparison of resolution of point source as function of location offset from FOV center for x-axis (left) and Y-axis (right) locations

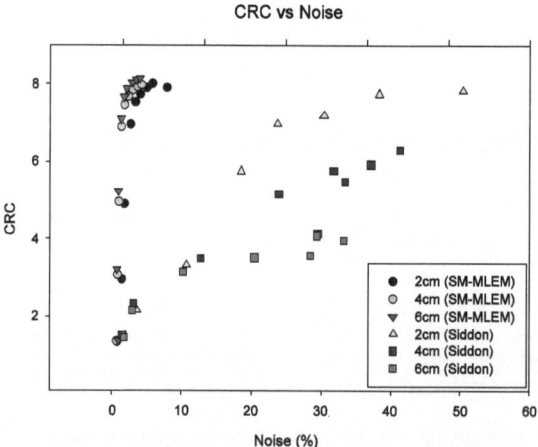

Fig. 5. CRC vs. noise for spheres at various locations from center of PET FOV (given in legend) from Siddon line-integral based MLEM and system matrix based MLEM reconstruction

3.2   Contrast Performance

For SM based MLEM reconstruction, the CRC of hot spheres (8:1) is independent of location (from the center of FOV) while location has a strong impact on CRC values for sphere reconstruction obtained with Siddon's line-integral technique (Fig. 5). The CRC value improved by a factor of 2 and 1.3 for spheres located at 4cm and 6cm respectively from the center for SM based MLEM compared to Siddon line-integral based MLEM. CRC values were similar from both techniques for sphere near to the center. Moreover, the SM based technique demonstrates reduced noise level compared to Siddon based MLEM reconstruction (Fig. 5) due to more accurate modeling of the detector physics.

4   Discussion

A novel technique for estimating the system transfer matrix using Monte Carlo simulation software that allows for modeling of photon interaction within the detector in MLEM reconstruction, unlike Siddon ray-tracing technique which estimates SM based on simple ray-tracing in image space, is presented. The technique improves various parameters of image quality such as resolution, contrast and noise as compared to that obtained using MLEM with Siddon ray tracing to model the system matrix.

The main advantage of utilizing SM based reconstruction was increased resolution by reducing noise particularly in FOV periphery. A similar reduction of noise in the sphere contrast estimate was previously observed with SM based reconstruction techniques [8]. One reason for the reduced noise may be due to accurate modeling of the detector response producing reduced mis-positioning of counts in reconstruction space. Reduced noise may allow for reduced dose to the patient.

5   Conclusions

Quantitative and qualitative evaluation illustrated the improved contrast and resolution performance of SM based MLEM reconstruction compared to Siddon line-integral based MLEM reconstruction. The technique promises to reduce reconstruction distortion at FOV periphery for smaller bore PET systems by improved modeling of the PET system response.

References

1. Champion, L., Brain, E., Giraudet, A.L., Le Stanc, E., Wartski, M., Edeline, V., Madar, O., Bellet, D., Pecking, A., Alberini, J.L.: Breast cancer recurrence diagnosis suspected on tumor marker rising: value of whole-body 18FDG-PET/CT imaging and impact on patient management. Cancer 117(8), 1621–1629 (2011)
2. Murthy, K., Aznar, M., Thompson, C.J., Loutfi, A., Lisbone, R., Gagnon, J.H.: Results of preliminary clinical trials of the positron emission mammography system PEM-I: a dedicated breast imaging system producing glucose metabolic images using FDG. J. Nucl. Med. 41, 1851–1858 (2000)

3. Zhang, Y., Ramirez, R., Li, H., Liu, S., An, S., Wang, C., Baghaei, H., Wong, W.H.: The system design, engineering architecture and preliminary results of a lower-cost high-sensitivity high-resolution Positron Emission Mammography Camera. In: IEEE NSS Conf. Rec., pp. M10–M138 (2008)
4. Bowen, S.L., Wu, Y., Chaudhari, A.J.: Initial Characterization of a dedicated breast PET/CT scanner during human imaging. JNM 50, 1401–1408 (2009)
5. Kadrmas, D.J.: LOR-OSEM: statistical PET reconstruction from raw line-of-response histograms. Phys. Med. Biol. 49, 4731–4744 (2004)
6. Staelens, S., Strul, D., Santin, G., Vandenberghe, S., Koole, M., D'Asseler, Y., Lemahieu, I., Van de Walle, R.: Monte Carlo simulations of a scintillation camera using GATE: validation and application modelling. Phys. Med. Biol. 48, 3021–3042 (2003)
7. Siddon, R.L.: Fast calculation of the exact radiological path for a three-dimensional CT array. Med. Phys. 12(2), 252–256 (1985)
8. Panin, V., Kehren, F., Michael, C., Casey, M.: Fully 3-D PET reconstruction using system matrix derived from point source measurements. IEEE Trans. Med. Imaging. 25, 907–921 (2006)

Comparison of Contact Spot Imaging on a Scanning Mammography System to Conventional Geometric Magnification Imaging

Gillian Egan[1], Elizabeth Keavey[2], and Niall Phelan[1]

[1] Breastcheck, The National Cancer Screening Service,
36 Eccles St., Dublin 7, Ireland
[2] Breastcheck, The National Cancer Screening Service,
Newcastle Rd., Galway, Ireland
{gillian.egan,elizabeth.keavey,niall.phelan}@breastcheck.ie

Abstract. The performance of contact spot imaging on a scanning photon-counting system was evaluated and compared to conventional geometric magnification imaging for the assessment of screen-detected lesions. Three digital mammography systems were compared in terms of image quality and dose; Philips MDM, Hologic Selenia, GE Essential. Assessment imaging is performed on the scanning system in contact mode by reducing the scan width in combination with increased radiation exposure. Imaging optimisation was performed prior to comparative evaluation as preliminary studies established that the current performance of conventional magnification imaging was poorly optimised. Each system was investigated in terms of its ability to image simulated masses and mircrocalcifications using breast-tissue equivalent phantoms. Contrast-to-Noise Ratio and Average Glandular Dose were measured according to the EUREF guidelines and a Performance Index was formulated to facilitate comparison of the three systems. The scanning system performed at least comparably to conventional geometric magnification and offers workflow advantages.

Keywords: Digital Mammography, Breast Imaging, Magnification, Photon-Counting, Image Quality, Image Optimisation.

1   Introduction

Conventionally, assessment of screen-detected lesions has utilised geometric magnification imaging. A magnification platform positions the breast closer to the x-ray source while the image receptor remains at a fixed distance. The inherent geometry of the scanning photon counting system renders this method of acquiring magnification views impossible. As a result users have been cautious to use the photon counting systems for assessment views. The purpose of this study was to investigate the efficacy of the photon counting systems for further investigation of screen-detected lesions as compared to standard geometric magnification.

A.D.A. Maidment, P.R. Bakic, and S. Gavenonis (Eds.): IWDM 2012, LNCS 7361, pp. 165–172, 2012.
© Springer-Verlag Berlin Heidelberg 2012

2   Method

Three different Full Field Digital Mammography (*FFDM*) systems were examined in this study; Philips MDM (Philips, Solna, Sweden) employing a *W* anode and an *Al* filter; Hologic Selenia (Hologic Bedford, MA, USA) which uses a *W* anode and a *Rh* or *Ag* filter; GE Seno Essential (GE Medical Systems, Buc, France) utilising a choice of *Mo* or *Rh* target and filter.

The study investigated the performance of each system in terms of dose and contrast for the detection of both masses and microcalcifications. CIRS (Norfolk, VA, USA) phantoms of breast equivalent material with a range of thickness and composition (glandular/adipose), 4cm (50/50), 5cm (30/70) and 6cm (20/80) were imaged. Each CIRS phantom contains a detail of 100% glandularity which was used to simulate a tumour mass. An *Al* square of 0.2mm thickness embedded in PMMA was used to simulate mircocalcifications as advocated by Zanca [1].

Conventional geometric magnification imaging is performed using a magnification table to position the breast closer to the x-ray source while the image receptor remains at a fixed distance. Table 1 below details the altered geometry for each magnification setup examined in this study. Use of the small focal spot is necessary for geometric magnification. In magnification geometry, an anti-scatter grid is not required since the increased air gap acts to reject scatter. The irradiated volume of the breast is smaller in magnification imaging as the x-ray beam is collimated to the specific area of interest. An area factor is applied to the Dance dose calculation to account for the fraction of the breast that is exposed [2]. For the Hologic and GE systems investigated, magnification factor of 1.8 and focal spot size of 0.1mm were used.

Table 1. Comparison of geometry in standard contact mode compared to MAG mode

	Focus to Breast Distance [cm]					
	Philips		Hologic		GE	
	STD	*DS*	STD	MAG	STD	MAG
4cm Breast	60	60	60	35	59.5	33.8
5cm Breast	59	59	59	34	58.5	32.8
6cm Breast	58	58	58	33	57.5	31.8

When using the Philips MDM in *Diagnostic Scan (DS)* mode, the active image reception area is reduced to approximately half width which provides coverage of the spot compression area and some additional coverage for the purpose of orientation. The collimator movement is limited corresponding to the reduced X-ray field, as seen in Figures 1 and 2 below. Exposure parameters in *Diagnostic Scan* mode are determined from the breast thickness measured under compression. The *Diagnostic Scan* function takes effect when the spot compression paddle is selected. This allows it to be used in the normal workflow for spot compression imaging without altering the modality setup. *Diagnostic Scan* images are displayed with a preset zoom on the spot compression area.

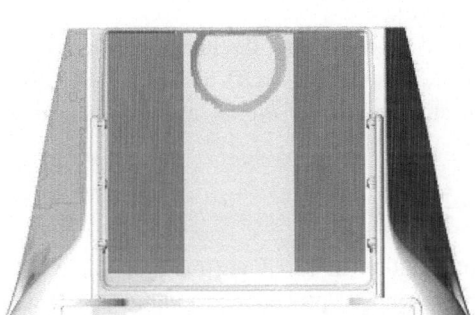

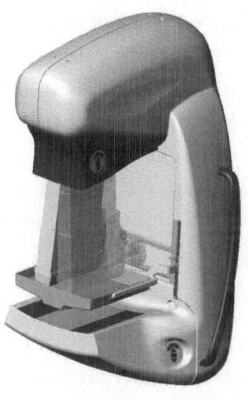

Fig. 1. *Diagnostic Scan* Image Receptor Area   **Fig. 2.** Limited Collimation

Images of all phantoms were produced in manual mode using a range of peak tube voltages from 24kV to 36kV at intervals of 2kV. The current time product (mAs) values were chosen in order to obtain a constant pixel value (*PV*) level in a reference zone of each image. This reference zone is labelled background in Figures 3 and 4.

The Contrast to Noise Ratio (*CNR*) was calculated according to the method of the European guidelines for quality assurance in mammography screening (*EUREF*) [3].

$$CNR = \frac{PV(sig) - PV(bgd)}{\sqrt{\dfrac{SD(sig)^2 + SD(bgd)^2}{2}}} \tag{1}$$

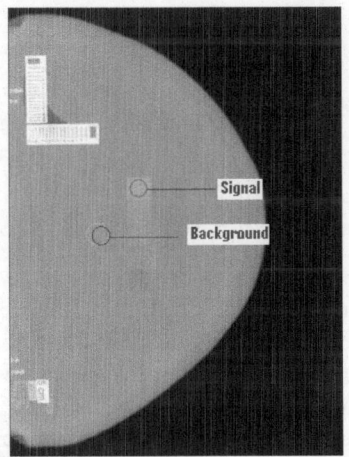

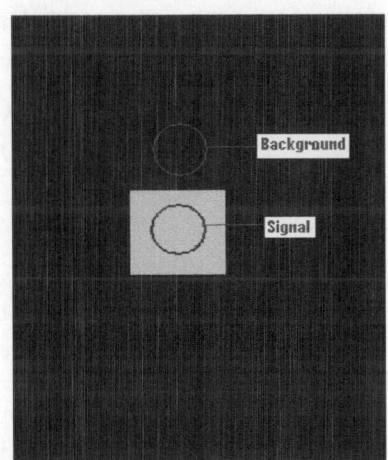

Fig. 3. CIRS Phantom – tumour simulation   **Fig. 4.** Al embedded in PMMA - microcalcification simulation

For each exposure setting, half value layer (*HVL*) and entrance surface air kerma (*ESAK*) were measured and the corresponding Average Glandular Dose (*AGD*) was calculated according to the method of Dance [2].

Overall performance results were obtained by combining the image characteristics for different exposure factor choices with corresponding AGD results. A Performance Index (*PI*) typically used for optimisation studies of digital systems was calculated for all imaging conditions examined.

$$PI = \frac{CNR^n}{AGD} \tag{2}$$

A value of $n=2$ is typically used for optimisation of screening mammography [4]. Since this study concentrates on secondary diagnostic procedures, a value of $n=4$ was used to allow additional weight to the increased importance of image quality relative to dose for the follow-up assessment imaging of screen-detected lesions. This method was suggested previously by Koutalonis [5]. Increasing the value of the exponent (*n*) in Equation 2 amplifies the difference between the systems based predominantly on their imaging ability.

Koutalonis has also recommended normalisation of the PI in order to better cross compare data between systems. As a result of this normalisation, the PI should have a value of 1 for the ideal spectral imaging conditions.

$$PI_{norm} = \frac{CNR^n{}_{norm}}{AGD_{norm}} \tag{3}$$

where;

$$CNR_{norm} = \frac{CNR}{CNR_{sys\_high}} \qquad \text{ie. CNR normalised to maximum}$$

and;

$$AGD_{norm} = \frac{AGD}{AGD_{sys\_low}} \qquad \text{ie. AGD normalised to minimum}$$

3   Results

Optimum exposure factors (*Opt*) were determined for each system using the method described above and these were compared to the standard automatic exposure control (*AEC*) factors in terms of normalised PI. The results of this comparison are shown in Figures 5 and 6, including 10% variation. Where a PI increase of more than 10% was observed, the optimisation was judged to be successful. Where the PI increase was less than 10%, the system AEC was considered to be well optimised.

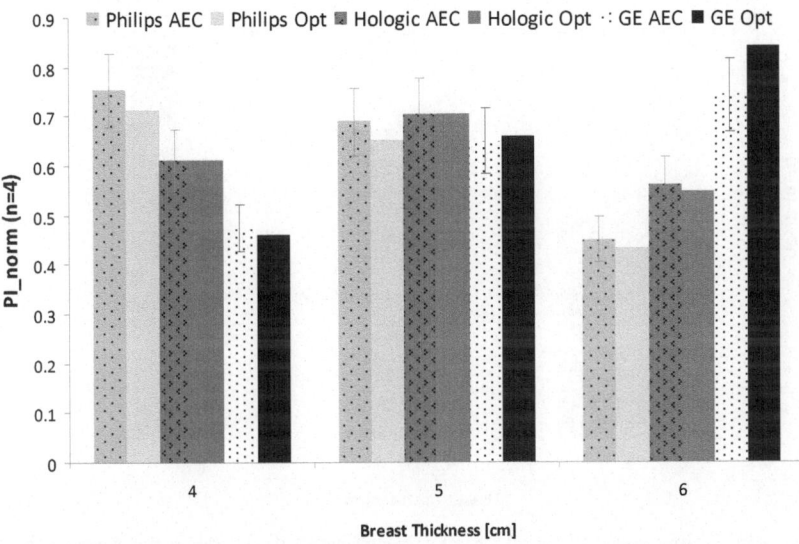

Fig. 5. Normalised PI for each system under AEC & using optimised factors for mass detection (bars indicate 10% variation)

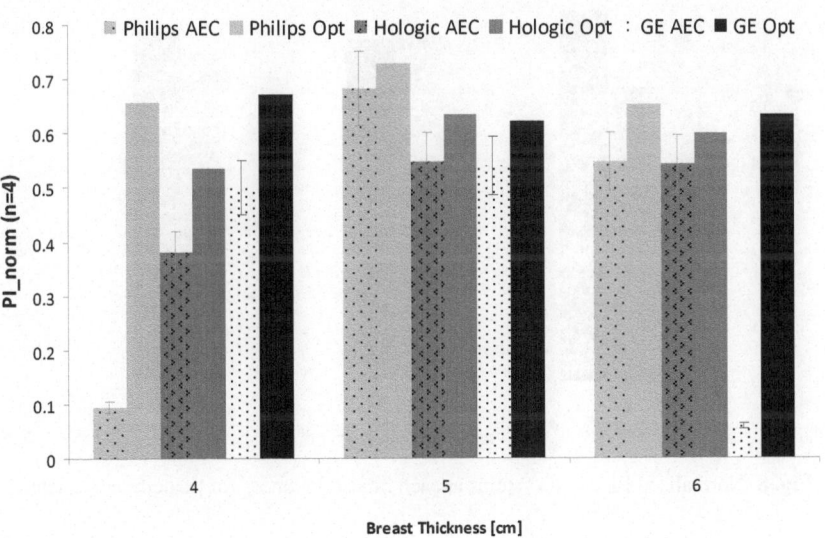

Fig. 6. Normalised PI for each system under AEC & using optimised factors for microcalcification detection (bars indicate 10% variation)

Once the optimum factors were determined for each system, for each breast type and for each detection task, the three systems were compared in terms of normalised PI. Where the system AEC yielded the best PI, these factors were then used for further analysis. These results are shown in Figures 7 and 8.

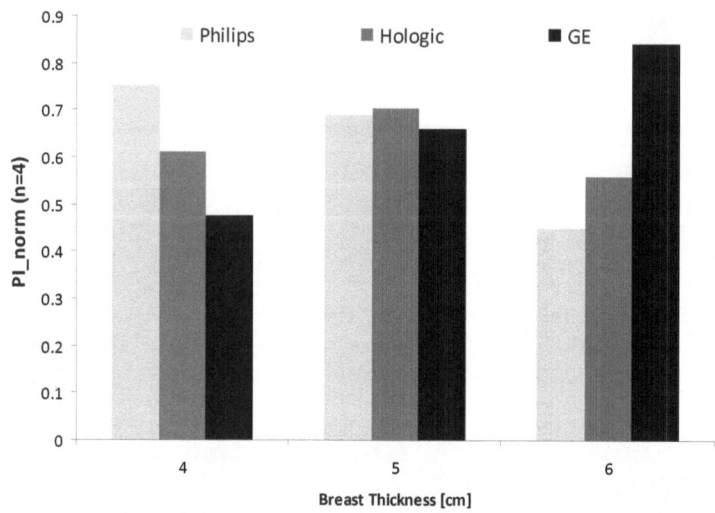

Fig. 7. Normalised PI for all systems at each breast thickness for mass detection

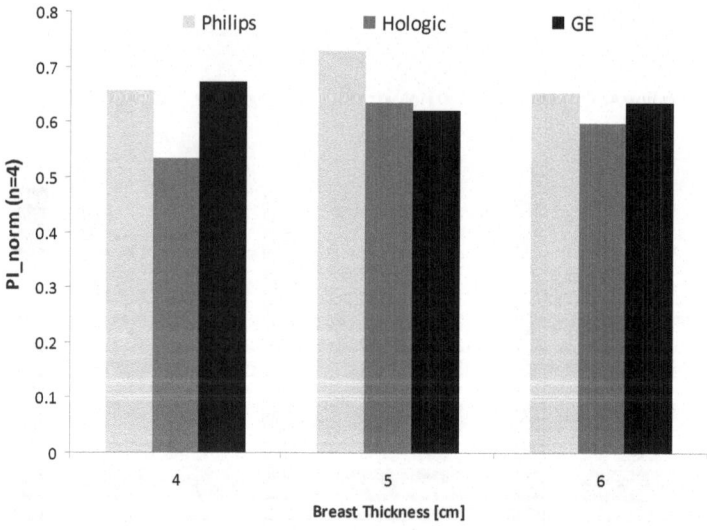

Fig. 8. Normalised PI for all systems at each breast thickness for μcalcification detection

4   Discussion

The results demonstrate that for the detection of masses, all systems in the study were well optimised with the exception of larger breasts on the GE system.

For investigation of microcalcifications, there was improved detection through use of our suggested factors for all imaging conditions considered. The benefits of our optimisation scheme for imaging microcalcifications were most significant for smaller breasts on the Philips system and for larger breasts on the GE system.

The optimum choice of factors for detection of masses was not the same as that for microcalcification detection.

The Philips system was optimal for detection of a mass in a smaller breast, while the GE system was the optimal choice for detection of a mass in a larger breast. All systems performed comparably for mass detection in an average size breast.

Regardless of breast size and composition, the Philips system performed optimally for microcalcification detection. It also offers inherent workflow advantages since modality setup was not altered for *Diagnostic Scan* views. All three systems demonstrated comparable results for microcalcification detection at larger breast sizes.

In the past it has been reported that geometric magnification mammography produced better spatial resolution and signal-to-noise ratio performance than contact mammography [6-9]. As a result, users have been reluctant to select the Philips system as it does not utilise the traditional magnification geometry. However a study by Kim et al. in 2010 illustrated that using zoom could yield similar radiologist results in the diagnosis of micorcalcifications as compared to those from geometric magnification images [10]. The conclusions of our study have validated the effectiveness of the Philips system for magnification mammography.

Previous work by Koutalonis [5], based on a Monte Carlo study of CNR and AGD in magnification mammography, outlined a simulation method for optimisation of magnification setup and comparison of same. We have applied a similar method in this experimental scenario.

In our screening programme, women are randomly assigned to a mammography machine at time of imaging - there is no preferential selection by system type. Following the practical application of the Koutalonis method, we have derived a set of guidelines for users, to recommend the best choice of system for further imaging, based on breast size and individual symptoms. Our results suggest that some selection preference may be advantageous for the acquisition of magnification mammographic views at assessment.

This study has also demonstrated that some systems might benefit from an alternative AEC setup in line with the optimal factors proposed here. However, it is noted that because the same factors are not optimum for the detection of masses and calcifications, a decision would have to be made allowing the AEC setup to favour detection criteria for the imaging task. We suggest that the AEC setup be amended to favour calcification detection since this is most typically the purpose of magnification views at assessment [6-9].

This study has shown that the scanning system performs comparably or better than conventional geometric magnification for the detection of masses and mircrocalcifications, for the range of breast sizes and compositions examined in this study, with the exception of mass detection in the larger breast, where the GE conventional geometric magnification yields a superior result.

References

1. Zanca, F., Van Ongeval, C., Marshall, N., Meylaers, T., Michielsen, K., Marchal, G., Bosmans, H.: The relationship between the attenuation properties of breast microcalcifications and aluminium. Phys. Med. Biol. 55, 1057–1068 (2010)
2. Dance, D., Young, K., Van Engen, R.: Further Factors for the estimation of mean glandular dose using the U.K., European & IAEA breast dosimetry protocols. Phys. Med. Biol. 54, 4361–4372 (2009)
3. European Commission: European guidelines for quality assurance in breast cancer screening and diagnosis, 4th edn. (2006) ISBN 92-79-01258-4
4. Nishino, L., Wu, X., Johnson Jr., F.: Thickness of molybdenum filter and squared contrast to noise ratio per dose for digital mammography. AJR 185, 960–963 (2005)
5. Koutalonis, M., Delis, H., Spyrou, G., Costaridou, L., Tzanakos, G., Panayiotakis, G.: Contrast-to-noise ratio in magnification mammography: a Monte Carlo study. Phys. Med. Biol. 52, 3185–3199 (2007)
6. Law, J.: Breast dose from magnification films in mammography. BJR 78, 816–820 (2005)
7. Sickles, E., Doi, K., Genant, H.: Magnification film mammography: image quality and clinical studies. Radiology 125, 69–76 (1977)
8. Sickles, E.: Further experience with microfocal spot magnification mammography in assessment of clustered breast microcalcifications. Radiology 137, 9–14 (1979)
9. Sickles, E.: Mircofocal spot magnification mammography using xeroradiographic and screen-film recording systems. Radiology 131, 599–607 (1979)
10. Kim, M., Youk, J., Kang, D., Choi, S., Kwak, J., Son, E., Kim, E.-K.: Zooming method of digital mammography vs digital magnification view in full field digital mammography for the diagnosis of microcaclicifications. BJR 83, 486–492 (2010)

Region Matching in the Temporal Study
of Mammograms Using Integral Invariant Scale-Space

Faraz Janan[1,*] and Sir Michael Brady[2]

[1] Department of Engineering Science, University of Oxford, UK
farazjanan@some.ox.ac.uk
[2] Department of Oncology, University of Oxford, UK
mike.brady@oncology.ox.ac.uk

Abstract. Our aim is to compare two mammograms (left-right, temporal) in an unsupervised manner. To this end, we propose a novel *region matching algorithm* (*RMA*) for mammograms based upon the non-emergence and non-enhancement of maxima and the causality principle of integral invariant scale space (in a limited sense). The algorithm has several advantages over commonly used methods for comparing segmented regions as shapes. First, it gives improved key-points alignment for optimal shape correspondence. Second, it identifies new growths and complete/partial occlusion in corresponding regions by dividing the segmented region into sub-regions based upon the extrema that persist over all scales. Third, the algorithm does not depend upon the spatial locations of mammographic features and eliminates the need for registration to identify salient changes over time. Finally, the algorithm is fast to compute and requires no human intervention.

Keywords: CAD, breast cancer, temporal study, shape analysis, region matching, integral invariants.

1 Background

The analysis of two or more mammograms in order to detect anomalies by way of clinically significant changes is a key problem in digital mammography. However, even when the two mammograms are of the same patient, the breasts may vary in size and in the way in which they are imaged. However, the internal structure is generally quite similar. Of the three pairwise comparisons most commonly made (L-R, CC-MLO, temporal), we are initially most interested in the temporal study of mammograms, since it is not only important for the detection of cancers but is also used increasingly for post-treatment care. It provides a quantitative measure of how a certain region in the breast may have evolved over time. This paper addresses temporal comparison of mammograms by employing integral invariants, in particular exploiting its scale space, for local (sub-) region matching in segmented masses. The temporal mammograms in this study are first segmented, and then the resulting regions are matched by performing shape matching. Efforts previously been made to compare two shapes regionally, for example registration techniques [6, 7]. However

A.D.A. Maidment, P.R. Bakic, and S. Gavenonis (Eds.): IWDM 2012, LNCS 7361, pp. 173–180, 2012.
© Springer-Verlag Berlin Heidelberg 2012

in most studies this phenomenon is dependent on the 'shape space' that requires a set of training data before we can do actual comparisons [5]. The best matching shapes are then divided into local /sub -regions and RMA is applied for local region matching.

Temporal images are used by the radiologist to reduce the number of false positives and corresponding suspicious lesions over time and to detect possible masses. However, changes in the breast density, positioning, and the growth and development of lesions, together with the intrinsically projective nature of mammography, mean that establishing temporal correspondences remains a challenging task. Most published algorithms use rigid or non-rigid registration to compare images, and they typically yield a dense warp map, establishing correspondences for all pixels in the mammograms. However, the appearance of a mammogram can change markedly with small changes in compression, with small changes in the imaging parameters, and any rotation of the breast prior to compression. For example, such small changes can change the textural properties of stromal tissue. Fortunately, most such changes are clinically irrelevant. Rather, correspondences are only relevant for *regions of interest*, typically locally dense regions that may (or happily, may not) be lesions. (We accept that this does not extend completely to architectural distortions; but they are a separate problem that requires a measure of (a) symmetry). That case will be addressed subsequently.

The temporal pairs mammograms that are used in this study were made available to us by Mātakina Technologies. We begin by applying a hierarchical algorithm based on iso-contours [1] to segment the breast into regions that are considered to be significant. The first reason for using this algorithm is that it is computationally very efficient, and indeed it can be the basis of a real time system, even without resorting to a GPU implementation. The algorithm segments the complete internal topography of the breast in a structured way that can subsequently be used to establish correspondences between mammograms. The shapes of the regions of interest are defined on iso-levels that give a notion of pattern and texture change in a limited sense. This is important because, in this study, image segmentation relies on the fact that pixels inside a suspected mass have different physiology than pixels in the other parts of the breast. The algorithm has worked well on the dozens of mammograms we have processed to date. An example of the segmentation of nested regions is shown in Figure 3 while the initial alignment of those regions is demonstrated in Figure 2.

We refer to each of the regions segmented in this way as a shape. Mathematically, a shape is considered to be a single closed contour that describes a solitary entity. To compare two shapes that are slightly different from each other and which may be rotated relative to each other, it is important to align them irrespective of their size and location. The algorithm that we have developed does this by using multi-scale integral invariants to describe them, as described in [4] and to align the two shapes before supplementary correspondences are established. Depending upon the sizes of the two shapes, it select various integration kernel scales for different regions segmented within a breast, thus keeping a certain relation between the number of regions within each shape.

2   Method

2.1   Integral Invariants

The core idea underlying our method is the use of circular Integral Invariants, then to take advantage of the associated scale space. Hong [2] defines the circular area integral invariants by considering a disc $B_r(p)$ of radius r applied to every point p of a closed contour C, the characteristic function is then given by,

$$\chi(B_r(p), C)\,(x) = \begin{cases} 1 \; if \; x\epsilon\{B_r(p) \cap \dot{C}\} \\ \quad 0 \; otherwise \end{cases}$$

Where $\dot{C}$ is the interior of the curve C. The local integral area $I_r(C)$ of the curve C is given by the function $I_r(p)$ at every point $p \in C$ with integral kernel χ as follows:

$$I_r(p) = \int_{\Omega} \chi(B_r(p), C)\,(x)dx$$

Where Ω is the domain of the curve C.   Two examples are shown in Figure 1. Figure 1a is a simple rectangle, showing that points of high curvature (typically detected by *differential* operators) can be found effectively, and without noise sensitivity, using integral invariants.   Figure 1c is the automatically segmented outline of a lesion and Figure 1d is its integral invariant signature at one particular scale.

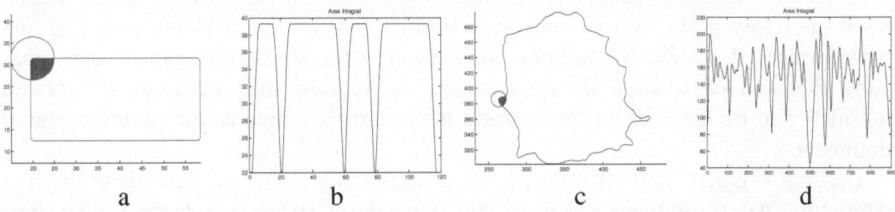

a   b   c   d

Fig. 1. a) and c) are two examples of closed polygons with integration kernels imposed on them and highlighting the integration area in red, b) and d) are the corresponding integral invariants for the complete curves. c) is the boundary of a segmented mass in *mdb010* from the Mini-MIAS mammographic database.

2.2   Scale Space and Scale Selection

Changing the size of the integral invariant kernel creates a scale space, whose lower bound defines what is meant by "fine", and whose upper bound "coarse". We note that this integral invariant scale space satisfies the established scale space properties of non-emergence, non-enhancement of maxima and the causality principle in a limited sense. Properties of scale space are given in [3].

As is often the case with scale space, a major challenge is scale selection for the integral invariant function for each segmented lesion, as these shapes may be of varying sizes with significantly large difference of ratios. Small scales can very well correspond or identify a complete occlusion in small shapes but they fail to describe large shapes. Large scales give consistent results for shape matching but do not pick small regions as distinct comparisons. Therefore a certain ratio of size of the shape and the maximum scale of integral invariant is used as described below.

Let r_{max} be the maximum scale indicator (this equates to the radius of the circular integral invariant disc at the maximum scale). Then comparing shapes (S_1, S_2) for region matching where the area of shape to integral invariant ration (SIR) is fixed, the scale indicator r_{max} is,

$$r_{max} = \lceil \min (r_{S_{1max}}, r_{S_{2max}}) \rceil,$$

$$\text{Where } r_{S_{imax}} = \sqrt{\frac{Area\ of\ S_i}{SIR * \pi}} \quad , i = [1, 2]$$

Though scale selection depends to a large extent upon the size of the shape we have observed experimenally that it also depends upon the variability in shape boundary. To date we have not established a relation between the two.

2.3   Initial Key-Points Alignment and Region Matching

The peaks of the integral invariant signature at the highest scale are considered to be salient points for being causal. Intervals between those points give the general structure of that shape. Shapes are divided into integral invariant regions (segments) based upon key points at the coarsest scale that follows the causality principle and prevail over all scales. All regions are evaluated for similarity against each other using the sum of squared differences and the regions that are most similar are considered to be the starting regions and their starting points as the points of initial alignment.

The first segment starts from the point of initial alignment and extends to the first extremum. All subsequent segments are defined by successive extrema. The last region is then selected from the point of the last extremum to the end. In this way, both shapes are divided into segments, each with a varying length. To have the best comparison, we stretch or shrink all segments to the same length using bilinear interpolation.

To compare integral invariant regions, the sum of squared differences (SD) is calculated between each pair of regions using integral invariant values along the region's boundary at all scales.

$$SD(x_1, x_2) = \sum_{n=1}^{M} (x_1(n) - x_2(n))^2 \quad where\ M\ is\ length\ (x_1, x_2)$$

The scale factor (SF) between two regions is also measured as follows,

$$SF(x_1, x_2) = \left[1 - \frac{\min\ (length(x_1,\ x_2))}{\max\ (length(x_1,\ x_2))}\right]^2$$

where (x_1, x_2) *are regions of shapes* (S_1, S_2). Then the overall discrepancy measure (DM) is

$$DM\ (x_1,\ x_2) =\ SD(x_1,\ x_2) +\ SF(x_1,\ x_2)$$

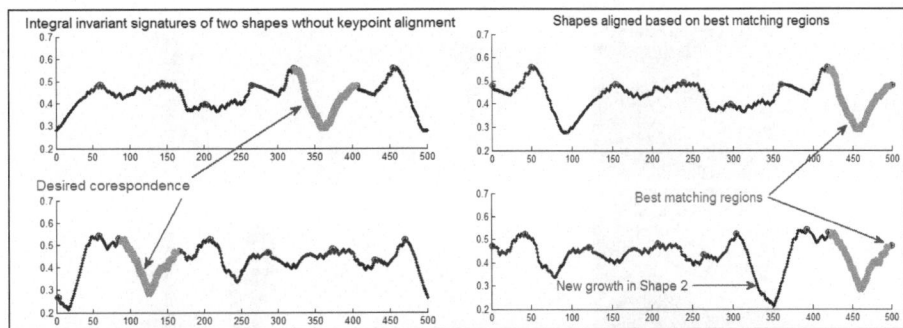

Fig. 2. Above is the scale space signature of two corresponding shapes in Figure 3 at the coarsest scale. On the left, the signatures are unaligned whereas on the right side they are aligned using *RMA*.

3   Results

Pairs of mammograms are segmented before performing shape or region matching. The segmentation algorithm develops parent-child relations in a (topographic) family tree structure, called an inclusion tree. The intensity range of an image is divided linearly into a certain number of iso-levels, and the contours are formed at those locations. Salient regions have a dense set of surrounding iso-contours. A concentric group of contours represents the diffusion of intensity in a dense pattern from the core of the object to the surrounding tissues. Regions with a higher family count or nesting depth beyond a certain threshold are selected as significant regions. A threshold of minimum family count was observed to discard regions falling beyond to reduce dense glandular structure from further analysis. The outermost iso-contour is considered boundary of that region.

Figure 3 presents the segmented regions of temporal mammograms along with their scale space, where Figure 2 gives the initial alignment of those segmented regions. Though *RMA* matches regions in shapes irrespective of their sequence however in this particular case the accuracy of matching is obvious by comparing integral invariant signature of both mammograms after initial key-point alignment.

Shape correspondence using *RMA* has been applied to the regions segmented in this way illustrated in Figure 4. The mammograms are de-noised using a Perona-Malik anisotropic diffusion filter. The lesions from pairs of temporal mammograms given are put into regional correspondences. In some cases the algorithm identifies the segments (and associated sub-regions) that correspond to new growth, while at the same time calculating the percentage change in other sub-regions. It may be noted that the number of regions in both shapes may not equal. Some obvious mismatches can also be seen where the regional differences are substantial or the non-corresponding regions are very similar. The correspondence of regions does not currently depend upon the texture or gradient information enclosed in them.

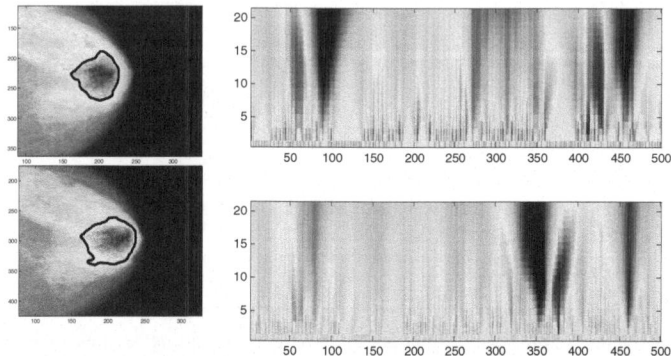

Fig. 3. Segmented regions from temporal mammograms on the left while their corresponding scale spaces is given on the right hand side

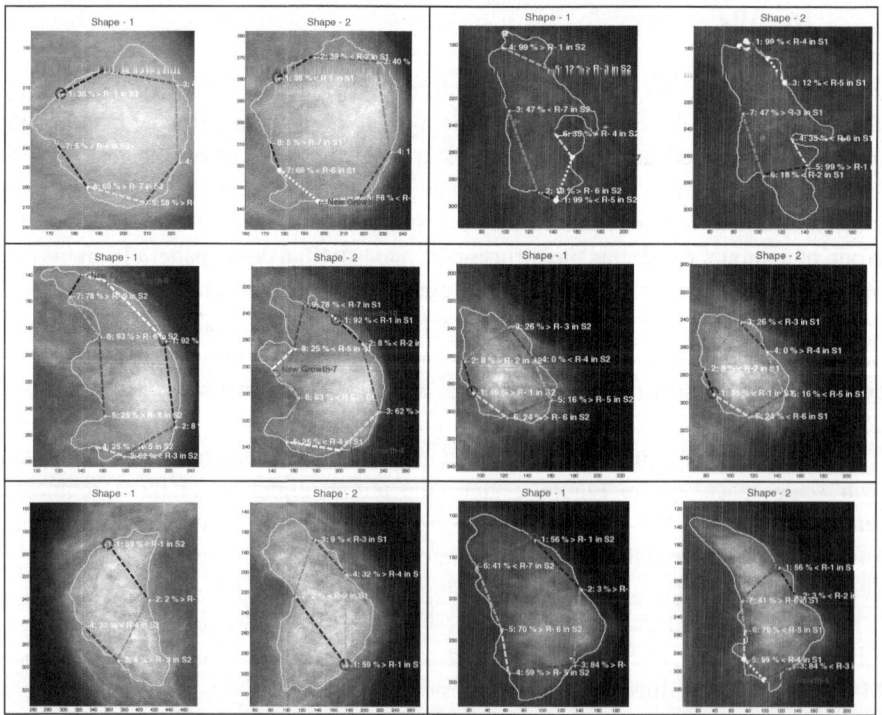

Fig. 4. Region matching of corresponding contours on the temporal mammograms. The red circles in the shapes identify points of initial alignment. Regions are color-coded and show both good and bad examples of regional correspondences.

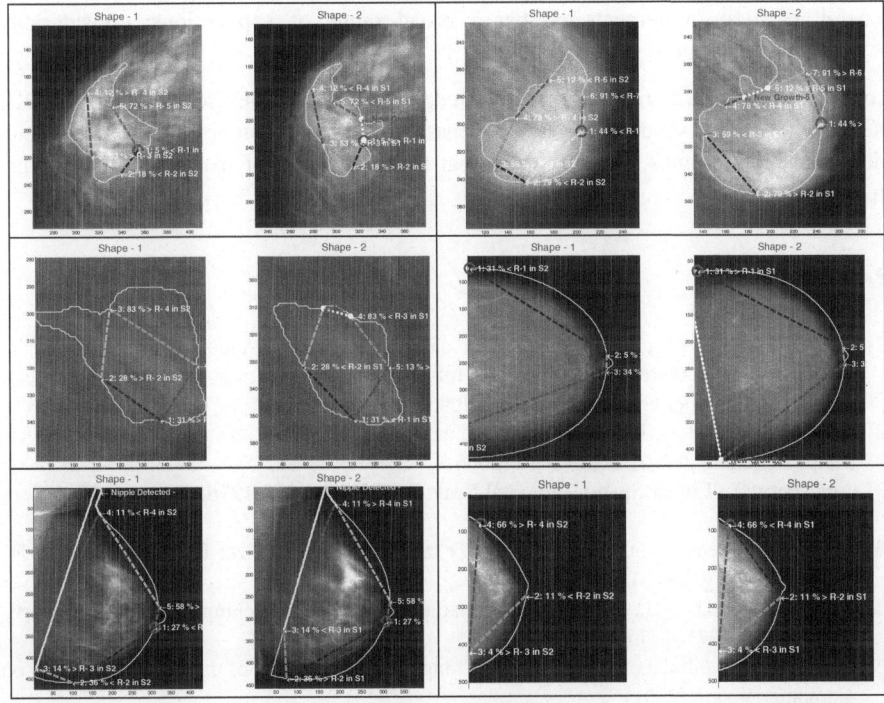

Fig.4. (*continued*)

4   Discussion

Shape matching and correspondence algorithms usually match and establish point-wise correspondences between two shapes and may even handle partial occlusion. However, they typically do not quantify partial occlusions nor identify complete occlusions or new growth.   It is important to measure regional differences quantitatively within each shape and establish correspondences based upon region matching. For masses it is vital to analyse their growth and notice the emergence or disappearance of any region. This can be helpful in detecting new growths and identifying their orientation. Following region of interest segmentation, we have introduced a method of local shape correspondence and region matching using integral invariant scale space. Integral invariant are calculate for segmented shapes from mammograms at all scales. The algorithm identifies causal peaks of this scale space as key points and breaks the shape into sub-regions based upon them. The best matching region is selected as a point of initial alignment and regions are corresponded based on a similarity measure. Though the emphasis of this paper is not on segmentation however if a better segmentation algorithm is used, RMA may produce very promising results in detecting growth of tumour and its aggressiveness with respect to shape. This region-matching technique is independent of any computational algorithms like Fast Marching or Djikstra's algorithm (Dynamic programming) and hence is very fast to compute. The proposed algorithm is quite general, easy to implement and has a broad range of applications; considerably beyond mammography.

Acknowledgments. Faraz Janan acknowledges the Islamic Development Bank (IDB) Merit scholarship scheme for their generous financial support. We also thank Mātakina Technologies, New Zealand that provided pairs of mammograms for this study.

References

[1] Hong, B.-W., Brady, M.: Segmentation of mammograms in topographic approach. In: International Conference on Visual Information Engineering (VIE 2003). Ideas, Applications, Experience, pp. 157–160 (2003)
[2] Manay, S., Cremers, D., Hong, B.-W., Yezzi Jr., A.J., Soatto, S.: Integral Invariants for Shape Matching 28(10), 1602–1618 (2006)
[3] Lindeberg, T.: Linear Spatio-Temporal Scale-Space, vol. 1252(1996). Sciences-New York (2001)
[4] Manay, S., Cremers, D., Hong, B.-W., Yezzi Jr., A.J., Soatto, S.: Integral Invariants for Shape Matching 28(10), 1602–1618 (2006)
[5] Duci, A., Yezzi, A.J., Mitter, S.K., Soatto, S.: Region matching with missing parts. Computer 24, 271–277 (2006)
[6] Belongie, S., Malik, J., Puzicha, J.: Matching shapes. In: Proc. of the IEEE Intl. Conf. on Computer Vision (2001)
[7] Veltkamp, R.C., Hagedoorn, M.: State of the art in shape matching. Technical Report UU-CS-1999-27, University of Utrecht (1999)

Characterizing Breast Phenotype with a Novel Measure of Fibroglandular Structure

John H. Hipwell[1], Lewis D. Griffin[2], Patsy J. Whelehan[3], Wenlong Song[1],
Xiying Zhang[1], Jan M. Lesniak[5], Sarah Vinnicombe[3], Andy Evans[3],
Jonathan Berg[4], and David J. Hawkes[1]

[1] Center for Medical Image Computing, UCL, Gower St., London, UK
[2] Department of Computer Science, UCL, Gower St., London, UK
[3] Dundee Cancer Centre, Ninewells Hospital, Uni. of Dundee, UK
[4] The Human Genetics Unit, Ninewells Hospital, Uni. of Dundee, UK
[5] Computer Vision Laboratory, ETH, Zürich, CH
j.hipwell@ucl.ac.uk

Abstract. Understanding, and accurately being able to predict, breast cancer risk would greatly enhance the early detection, and hence treatment, of the disease. In this paper we describe a new metric for mammographic structure, "orientated mammographic entropy", via a comprehensive classification of image pixels into one of seven basic image feature (BIF) classes. These classes are flat (zero order), slope-like (first order), and maximum, minimum, light-lines, dark-lines and saddles (second order). By computing a reference breast orientation with respect to breast shape and nipple location, these classes are further subdivided into 23 orientated BIF classes. For a given mammogram a histogram is constructed from the proportion of pixels in each of the 23 classes, and the orientated mammographic entropy, H_{om}, computed from this histogram. H_{om}, shows good correlation between left and right breasts ($r^2 = 0.76$, N=478), and is independent of both mammographic breast area, a surrogate for breast size ($r^2 = 0.07$, N=974), and breast density, as estimated using Volpara^{TM} software ($r^2 = 0.11$, N=385). We illustrate this metric by examining its relationship to familial breast cancer risk, for 118 subjects, using the BOADICEA genetic susceptibility to breast and ovarian cancer model.

1 Introduction

In the UK, for every 1000 women screened for breast cancer in the national programme, on average 16 women will present with a suspicious lesion and be recalled for further examination. Of these, two women will be correctly diagnosed with breast cancer (12%); in one woman the cancer will be missed and subsequently detected in the symptomatic clinic (6%); whilst the remaining thirteen women (81%) will have been falsely recalled; a stressful experience for the women involved and a waste of health service resources [1]. This high false positive rate

A.D.A. Maidment, P.R. Bakic, and S. Gavenonis (Eds.): IWDM 2012, LNCS 7361, pp. 181–188, 2012.
© Springer-Verlag Berlin Heidelberg 2012

is a direct consequence of the large number of normal women in the screening population, which amplifies imperfections in the specificity of the screening process. Clearly this could (and should) be improved.

Breast cancer risk is an active research field. A link with mammographic breast density, as estimated from X-ray mammograms and breast cancer risk, has been known for a number of years and has been observed in numerous studies [15,4,11]. The reason for this link is poorly understood, however, and the extent to which this risk factor is determined by genetic vs environmental factors is an on-going research topic.

The motivation for our research is to investigate whether breast cancer risk is related to the pattern of structure of the glandular tissue in an X-ray mammogram, as opposed to a global measure of breast density. There have been many publications describing mammographic texture analysis methods. These have included application of statistical, histogram based measures; grey-level co-occurrence calculations; spatial filtering; fourier analysis; wavelet decomposition and fractal analysis [8,3,10,9]. Much of this work has focussed on developing automated alternatives to manual measurements of breast density for predicting risk. In many cases the performance of these algorithms has been shown to be comparable to manual methods but an independent association with breast cancer risk has not been demonstrated [8,3,10]. For instance Manduca et al. [10] describe a comparison of a number of these methods. They found the strongest prediction of breast cancer risk for features applied at a coarse scale, reported a degree of correlation with breast density and were unable to show a significant improvement in prediction when the features were combined with percent density. However in a recent study involving 245 women diagnosed with breast cancer and 250 controls, Nielsen et al. [12] demonstrated that a computer-based texture measure (described in [13]), applied to baseline mammograms 2 to 4 years prior to diagnosis, out-performed automated and manual density measures, achieving a significant separation between cases and controls.

A distinctive characteristic of all these methods is that no prior information on the "expected" orientation of fibro-glandular tissue has been incorporated. Reiser et al. have shown that, not unexpectedly, breast structure is oriented with respect to the nipple [14]. In this paper we incorporate this information explicitly by presenting a new measure of the breast phenotype which characterizes mammographic features according to their orientation with respect to the nipple. Rather than compute an ad hoc measure of texture, however, we comprehensively classify all features in the image according to their zero, first and second order intensity characteristics. In so doing we hypothesise that mammograms which do not exhibit a regular structure of features pointing towards the nipple, indicates a higher risk of breast cancer i.e. that higher risk is associated with a more chaotic microstructure of the breast parenchyma.

In the following sections we describe our methodology and present the results of analyzing 979 digital mammograms, from 250 subjects, to determine how this measure varies within subjects (between left and right breasts). We also investigate how it relates to breast density across subjects and present initial results relating values to familial breast cancer risk as estimated using the established risk estimation software BOADICEA [2]. BOADICEA takes as input the family history of breast, ovarian, prostate and pancreatic cancer of an individual as well as the ages at which these these cancers were diagnosed. It also uses information on any BRCA1 or BRCA2 genetic testing that has been performed and the ages of unaffected family members. The software then gives an estimate of risk of breast cancer over time, using a logistic regression model derived from 22 population based studies of breast or ovarian cancer.

2   Method

All the images used in this study were "raw" full-field digital mammograms (FFDM) which were log-inverted to ensure that image intensity was linearly related to total attenuation.

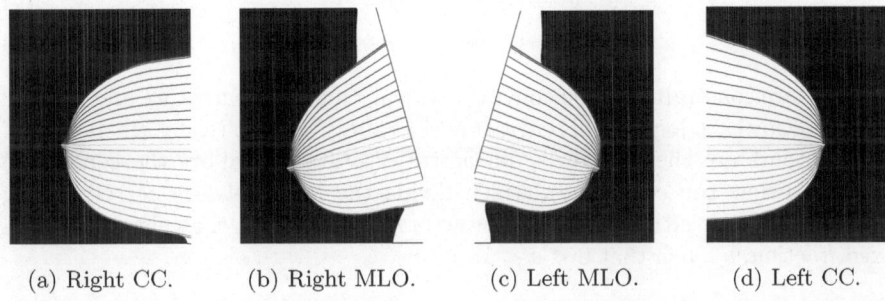

(a) Right CC.   (b) Right MLO.   (c) Left MLO.   (d) Left CC.

Fig. 1. An illustration of the reference ductal orientation result for four patient mammographic views

2.1   Breast Region, Pectoral Muscle and Nipple

In order to restrict the region of analysis in the X-ray mammogram to the breast, we first compute a binary mask to eliminate the pectoral muscle region and the background of the image, including any labels and/or annotations. We segment the pectoral muscles of all MLO view mammograms manually, to ensure accurate segmentations are obtained in all cases. The breast region is segmented from the background using a combination of breast edge detection and region growing. The nipple location is determined by estimating the most anterior point on the breast edge in CC view mammograms, and in MLO view mammograms by computing the most distal breast edge point, perpendicular to the pectoral muscle boundary. Compared to manual nipple locations identified on 1,313 mammograms by an imaging scientist, this automated approach had an accuracy of 10mm (std. dev. 11mm).

2.2   Reference Breast Structure Orientation

As described above, the hypothesis is that mammograms which exhibit a less regular pattern of structure pointing towards the nipple, represent breasts with a higher risk of developing cancer. In order to test this hypothesis, it is necessary to first compute a default or "expected" glandular orientation at each point in the breast. The reference orientation is created by generating a series of contours, emerging from the nipple, between the upper and lower breast edges and the breast centerline. The breast centerline passes through the nipple and is orthogonal to the pectoral muscle boundary (MLO views) or posterior edge of the image (CC views). In contrast to [5] we do not assume a parabolic shape of the breast but instead place n regularly spaced control points, starting at the nipple location, o, on each of (i) the breast edge above the nipple, U, (ii) the breast edge below the nipple, V, and (iii) the breast centerline, W:

$$U = \{o, u_1, \ldots, u_{n-1}\}, \tag{1}$$
$$V = \{o, v_1, \ldots, v_{n-1}\}, \tag{2}$$
$$W = \{o, w_1, \ldots, w_{n-1}\}. \tag{3}$$

U and V are constrained to be convex by calculating their curvature and linearly extrapolating each locus if this curvature rises above an empirically set threshold. The contours are then piecewise linear trajectories, C_u (above the centerline) and C_v (below the centerline), which divide the lines between corresponding control points on either upper or lower breast edges and the centerline, by a fixed fraction, a, such that $0 < a < 1$:

$$C_u = \{o, au_1 + (1-a)w_1, \ldots, au_{n-1} + (1-a)w_{n-1}\} \tag{4}$$
$$C_v = \{o, av_1 + (1-a)w_1, \ldots, av_{n-1} + (1-a)w_{n-1}\} \tag{5}$$

This creates the curved arrangement of orientations illustrated in figure 1.

2.3   Basic Image Features

The Basic Image Features (BIFs) system [7,6] classifies pixels in a 2D image into one of seven classes according to the local zero, first or second order structure. This structure is computed using a bank of six derivative of Gaussian filters (L_{00}, L_{10}, L_{01}, L_{20}, L_{11} and L_{02}) which calculate the nth (where n=0,1,2) order derivatives of the image in x and y (S_{00}, S_{10}, S_{01}, S_{20}, S_{11} and S_{02}) at a particular scale σ. By combining the outputs of these filters, any given pixel can be classified according to the largest component of:

$$\left\{ \underset{\text{flat}}{\epsilon S_{00}}, \underset{\text{slope}-\text{like}}{2\sqrt{S_{10}^2 + S_{01}^2}}, \underset{\text{maximum}}{\lambda}, \underset{\text{minimum}}{-\lambda}, \underset{\text{light line}}{\frac{\lambda+\gamma}{\sqrt{2}}}, \underset{\text{dark line}}{\frac{\lambda-\gamma}{\sqrt{2}}}, \underset{\text{saddle}}{\gamma} \right\} \tag{6}$$

given

$$\lambda = \sigma^2 \frac{(S_{20} + S_{02})}{2}; \ \gamma = \sigma^2 \sqrt{(S_{20} + S_{02})^2 + 4S_{11}^2}$$

where ϵ is a noise threshold below which regions are assumed to be flat. In addition, slopes, light lines, dark lines, and saddles can be further characterised according to their orientation. This orientation is computed with respect to the reference glandular orientation described above. We quantise this orientation into four 45-degree quadrants. This produces 23 orientated BIF classes, $B = b_0 \ldots b_{22}$. There are eight slope sub-classes (b_1 to b_8), and four sub-classes for each of light lines (b_{11} to b_{14}), dark lines (b_{15} to b_{18}) and saddles (b_{19} to b_{22}). The unorientated classifications of flat, maximum and minimum are classes b_0, b_9 and b_{10} respectively.

Once each pixel in the breast region has been classified into one of the 23 orientated BIF classes, a histogram can be generated. This is normalised by the number of pixels in the breast region, producing a 23 value feature vector, $P = p_0 \ldots p_{22}$, each element of which captures the proportion of pixels in the breast region falling into each of the 23 classes.

To obtain an overall measure of the pattern of mammographic structure, we compute the Shannon entropy of the orientated BIF histogram, and call this the orientated mammographic entropy, H_{om}.

$$H_{om} = - \sum_{i=0\ldots22} p_i \log(p_i) \tag{7}$$

This parameter quantifies the distribution of BIF classes represented by P. It will have a high value if all the orientated BIF classes are equally represented and a low value if the mammogram is dominated by a small number of classes. It therefore captures the heterogeneity of mammographic structure, orientated with respect to the nipple.

3   Results

We have applied this analysis to 979 mammograms from 250 subjects for which a complete set of data was available. We performed the BIF computation at a fine scale of $\sigma = 400\mu$mm, with the noise threshold set close to zero ($\epsilon = 1.0e^{-05}$), to capture as much information in the image as possible. The mammograms with the most extreme values of orientated mammographic entropy, H_{om}, are shown in figures 2(a) and 2(b). The mammogram with the highest value of H_{om} exhibits an irregular mammographic structure, and this is much less pronounced in the low H_{om} mammogram.

The correlation of H_{om} for 478 left and right breasts (956 mammograms) was $r^2 = 0.76$ (figure 3(a)). The area of the mammogram ROI also correlated closely between left and right breasts ($r^2 = 0.96$), however there was negligible correlation between the area of the ROI and orientated mammographic entropy ($r^2 = 0.07$, 974 mammograms). There was also little correlation between H_{om} and breast density as measured using Volpara^{TM} (Matakina Technology Ltd.) ($r^2 = 0.11$, 385 subjects) (figure 3(b)).

Finally figures 4(b) and 4(a) show initial results for orientated mammographic entropy vs familial breast cancer risk, as estimated using BOADICEA [2] (118

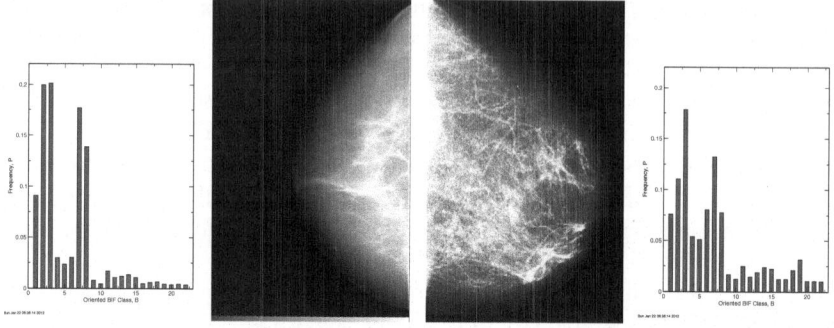

(a) Minimum entropy mammo.   (b) Maximum entropy mammo.

Fig. 2. Mammograms with extreme values of orientated mammographic entropy, H_{om}, and their corresponding BIF histograms, P. The left image is dominated by a small number of slope classes (b_2, b_3, b_7 and b_8), and a greater proportion of light line (b_{11} to b_{14}) to dark line (b_{15} to b_{18}) structures, creating a low entropy. In the right image the breast tissue is more chaotic in structure and hence pixels are more evenly distributed across all classes. This produces a high value of BIF entropy. The images have been histogram equalised for display purposes.

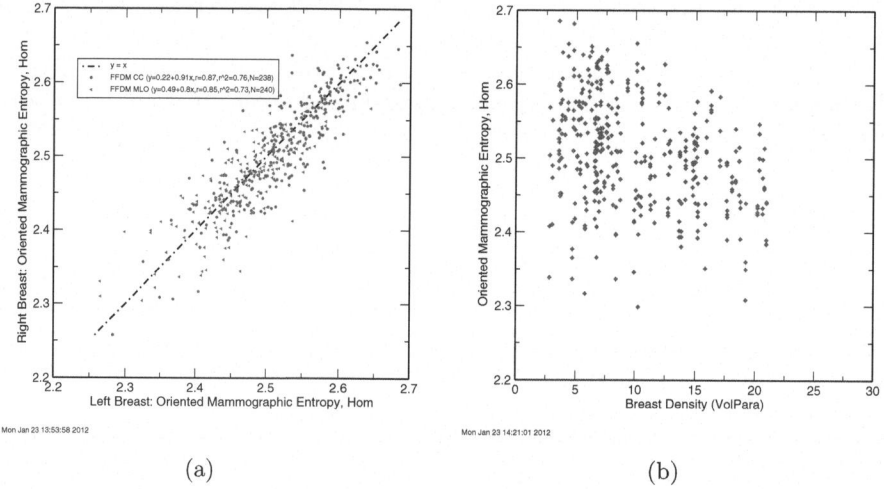

(a)   (b)

Fig. 3. (a) Orientated mammographic entropy, H_{om}, for left vs right breasts (956 mammograms). (b) Orientated mammographic entropy, H_{om}, vs breast density estimated using Volpara^{TM} (385 subjects).

subjects). Figure 4(a) appears to show a difference in the distribution of data points below a BOADICEA risk value of 0.05 compared to risk values greater than 0.05, however more data points are required to confirm or refute this. No correlation between BOADICEA risk and Volpara^{TM} was observed ($r^2 = 0.007$, 227 subjects).

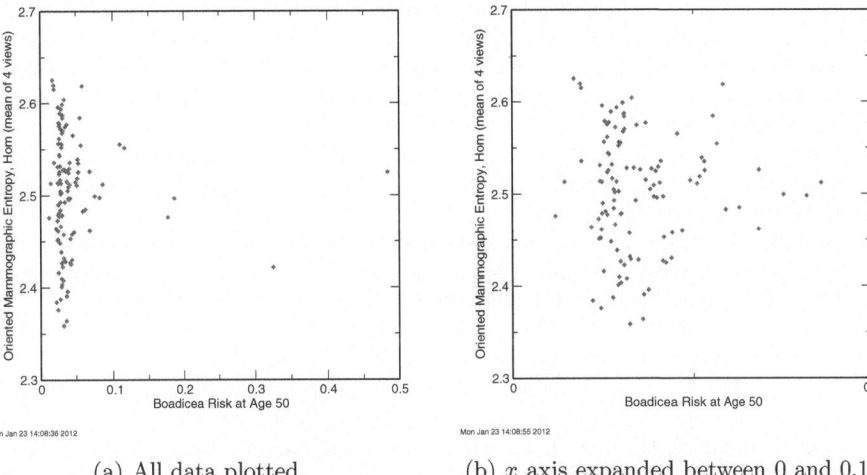

(a) All data plotted.   (b) x axis expanded between 0 and 0.1.

Fig. 4. Orientated mammographic entropy, H_{om}, vs BOADICEA risk at age 50 (118 subjects)

4   Conclusion

In this study we have developed a new metric to quantitatively characterize mammographic fibroglandular structure, according to the comprehensive analysis of zero, first and second order features orientated with respect to the breast's shape and nipple location. By calculating the correlation between left and right breasts, we have demonstrated that this parameter offers a reproducible measure of breast phenotype, exhibiting a greater variation between subjects, than between the breasts of a given subject. This parameter is independent of both the area of the ROI used in the analysis and breast density as estimated using $Volpara^{TM}$. We have also shown initial results for the distribution of the metric with familial breast cancer risk at age 50 using the BOADICEA susceptibility to breast and ovarian cancer model.

Acknowledgement. This work was funded by the European 7th Framework Program, HAMAM, ICT-2007.5.3 and EPSRC grant EP/E031579/1.

References

1. NHSBSP 61, Screening for Breast Cancer in England: Past and Future (February 2006) ISBN 1 84463 026 9, http://www.cancerscreening.nhs.uk/breastscreen/publications/nhsbsp61.pdf
2. Antoniou, A.C., Pharoah, P.P.D., Smith, P., Easton, D.F.: The boadicea model of genetic susceptibility to breast and ovarian cancer. British Journal of Cancer 91(8), 1580–1590 (2004)

3. Boehm, H.F., Schneider, T., Buhmann-Kirchhoff, S.M., Schlossbauer, T., Rjosk-Dendorfer, D., Britsch, S., Reiser, M.: Automated classification of breast parenchymal density: Topologic analysis of x-ray attenuation patterns depicted with digital mammography. American Journal of Roentgenology 191(6), W275–W282 (2008); Times Cited: 0
4. Boyd, N.F., Jensen, H.M., Cooke, G., Han, H.L.: Relationship Between Mammographic and Histological Risk- Factors For Breast-Cancer. J. National Cancer Institute 84, 1170–1179 (1992)
5. Brandt, S.S., Karemore, G., Karssemeijer, N., Nielsen, M.: An anatomically oriented breast coordinate system for mammogram analysis. IEEE Transactions on Medical Imaging 30(10), 1841–1851 (2011)
6. Crosier, M., Griffin, L.D.: Using basic image features for texture classification. International Journal of Computer Vision 88(3), 447–460 (2010)
7. Griffin, L.D.: The second order local-image-structure solid. IEEE Transactions on Pattern Analysis and Machine Intelligence 29(8), 1355–1366 (2007)
8. Jamal, N., Kg, K.H., Looi, L.M., McLean, D., Zulfiqar, A., Tan, S.P., Liew, W.F., Shantini, A., Ranganathan, S.: Quantitative assessment of breast density from digitized mammograms into tabar's patterns. Physics in Medicine and Biology 51(22), 5843–5857 (2006)
9. Li, H., Giger, M.L., Olopade, O.I., Lan, L.: Validation of Mammographic Texture Analysis for Assessment of Breast Cancer Risk. In: Martí, J., Oliver, A., Freixenet, J., Martí, R. (eds.) IWDM 2010. LNCS, vol. 6136, pp. 267–271. Springer, Heidelberg (2010)
10. Manduca, A., Carston, M.J., Heine, J.J., Scott, C.G., Pankratz, V.S., Brandt, K.R., Sellers, T.A., Vachon, C.M., Cerhan, J.R.: Texture Features from Mammographic Images and Risk of Breast Cancer. Cancer Epidemiology Biomarkers & Prevention 18, 837–845 (2009)
11. McCormack, V.A., Silva, I.D.S.: Breast density and parenchymal patterns as markers of breast cancer risk: A meta-analysis. Cancer Epidemiology Biomarkers & Prevention 15(6), 1159–1169 (2006)
12. Nielsen, M., Karemore, G., Loog, M., Raundahl, J., Karssemeijer, N., Otten, J.D.M., Karsdal, M.A., Vachon, C.M., Christiansen, C.: A novel and automatic mammographic texture resemblance marker is an independent risk factor for breast cancer. Cancer Epidemiology 35(4), 381–387 (2011)
13. Raundahl, J., Loog, M., Pettersen, P., Tanko, L.B., Nielsen, M.: Automated effect-specific mammographic pattern measures. IEEE Transactions on Medical Imaging 27(8), 1054–1060 (2008)
14. Reiser, I., Sidky, E.Y., Nishikawa, R.M., Pan, X.: Development of an Analytic Breast Phantom for Quantitative Comparison of Reconstruction Algorithms for Digital Breast Tomosynthesis. In: Astley, S.M., Brady, M., Rose, C., Zwiggelaar, R. (eds.) IWDM 2006. LNCS, vol. 4046, pp. 190–196. Springer, Heidelberg (2006)
15. Wolfe, J.N.: Breast patterns as an index of risk for developing breast-cancer. American Journal of Roentgenology 126(6), 1130–1139 (1976)

Performance of Computed Radiography and Direct Digital Radiography in a Screening Setting: Effect on the Screening Indicators

Chantal Van Ongeval[1,*], Sandra Postema[1], André van Steen[1], Gretel Vande Putte[2], Erik van Limbergen[2], Federica Zanca[1], and Hilde Bosmans[1]

[1] Department of Radiology, UZ Leuven, Belgium
{chantal.vanongeval,sandra.postema,andre.vansteen,
federica.zanca,hilde.bosmans}@uzleuven.be
[2] Leuven University Center for Cancer Prevention (LUCK), UZ Leuven, Belgium
{gretel.vandeputte,erik.vanlimbergen}@uzleuven.be

Abstract. A decentralized breast cancer screening program was started in 2002; in 2005 full-field digital mammography (FFDM) was introduced. The mammographic film-screen systems were gradually replaced by both computed radiography (CR) and direct digital mammography (DR). Quality control (QC) following the European Guidelines has been implemented for the technical aspects and for screening indicators. A previous study in our central breast unit (CBU) over the period 2005 till 2008 had shown no significant difference between the screening indicators of film-screen mammography (FSM) and FFDM. Today we are challenged with a variety of different types of mammography systems and questioned whether any difference would be present from cohorts imaged with CR versus DR. Therefore a new retrospective study over the period 2007 till 2009 has been performed, which shows no statistically significant difference in cancer detection rate (CDR), % of ductal carcinoma in situ (DCIS) and positive predictive value (PPV) between the CR and DR group, with exception of the recall rate (RR) in the subsequent round (p-value = 0,04).

Keywords: digital imaging, mammography, breast cancer screening.

1 Background

Film-screen mammography is so far the only breast imaging technique for which it has been proven that it can reduce breast cancer mortality if the quality of the whole process is well controlled [1]. Today FFDM is massively replacing FSM. For this to be justified, new performance parameters should not be inferior to what had been obtained with FSM. In selected papers this has been investigated. Most of the comparative FSM and FFDM studies in a screening setting show a higher RR, a higher CDR and a comparable to higher PPV for FFDM [2-6]. Some studies show a higher DCIS rate in the FFDM group [2], [3], [5], [6].

A.D.A. Maidment, P.R. Bakic, and S. Gavenonis (Eds.): IWDM 2012, LNCS 7361, pp. 189–196, 2012.

A diverse range of digital mammography systems and technologies is on the market. Based on the physical characteristics a distinction can be made between indirect or computed radiography systems (CR) and direct digital systems (DR). Indirect systems use a phosphor plate that stores the energy of the X-rays via the electrons of the phosphor plate; the reader is a separate device. In direct digital radiology, the conversion from X-rays to signal is 'direct' and does not require a separate reading process.

Knowing that CR systems perform worse than DR in terms of detective quantum efficiency and contrast detail analysis [7], [8], it is important to investigate the impact of this group of digital systems on the performance parameters of screening actions. Clinical studies with CR systems are rare and we are not aware of scientific papers on performance parameters of large CR based screening programs. During the Journées Françaises de Radiologie in Paris (October 2011), French data showed inferior screening performance for CR compared to DR. In some studies, the results obtained with the CR systems are part of a much larger study [9]. In an additional report of the DMIST trial, no significant difference in area under the curve (AUC), sensitivity or specificity was found between Fuji 5000 CR system, Fisher Senoscan, GE Senographe 2000D, Hologic Selenia DR systems and FSM, however large reader variations occurred with each modality [10]. A prospective paired study on the performance of CR (Fuji IP HR with Siemens 3000 Nova) and DR (GE Senographe 2000D) on BIRADS 4 and 5 lesions showed that the detection of breast lesions with calcifications is favorable with DR, but the diagnostic efficiency was identical [11]. A smaller study on 100 patients by the group of Schulz-Wendtland et al. showed no difference between CR and DR [12]. In 2009, we have also conducted a study on the effect of the introduction of digital mammography on the screening indicators in our CBU [13]. This study showed no statistically significant difference in terms of RR, CDR, PPV and detection rate of DCIS between FFDM and FSM. In that study there was only one CR system (Fuji CR system) included but the percentage of cancers in this group was too low to apply any statistics tests on the difference between CR and DR systems.

In the meantime, more mammography units have switched to FFDM, with a substantial part of them using CR technology. We have therefore decided to run a another retrospective study that we report in present text: the comparison of screening indicators for CR and DR systems. The study was performed for all mammographic units linked to our CBU during the period 2007-2009.

2   Methods and Materials

2.1   Screening Program in Flanders (Belgium)

Our screening program is based upon the European Guidelines [14] and has developed a national quality assurance manual. Acquisition of mammograms is decentralized and can take place in any radiological practice as long as the radiologist is licensed for screening and his equipment is certified. Second reading is centralized in one of the 5 central breast units.

In 2005, the use of digital mammography has been allowed and the existing quality manual was updated. There were no restrictions on the type of digital systems used as long as the system had passed first a type test procedure and then a site specific acceptance test [15], [16]. The type test protocol copies the European Guidelines for physico-technical QA and adds a radiological evaluation on 25 examinations to assess stability of processing and the global appearance of the images. Next, a set of 10 images is used to verify the data transmission of the images from the mammography center to the center for second reading and to verify the global image quality and visualization on the work station in the center for second reading. Only softcopy reading is allowed. Accreditation of a mammographic unit requires also that daily, weekly and (half)yearly physico-technical quality control of the mammography system and the viewing station is performed. In parallel to this, first and second readers have to take part in educational programs concerning theoretical concepts as well as image reading sessions.

In our Belgian screening program bilateral two-view mammography is performed. The program offers a biennial mammography screening to women aged between 50 and 69 years [15]. The participating women sign an informed consent that allows further data processing.

A total of 65 radiologists act as first reader and 6 radiologists act as second reader in our CBU. First as well as second readers are also working in a diagnostic breast center. This is deemed important seen the continuous feedback in terms of patient outcome following positive screening results. All second readers have to read a minimum of 5,000 examinations per year and are approved by the Radiological Board of the screening organization. In case of discordance between first and second reader, third reading is done by a qualified and independent second reader. All reading results are collected via an IT network.

The screening mammograms are scored with a five-point rating scale: 1 = normal finding, 2 = benign finding, 3 = probably benign finding, 4 = probably malignant finding, 5 = malignant finding.

Since 2001, a continuous and individual evaluation is done for all first and second readers in terms of RR, the number of readings and the discordance between the first and second reader. Several training courses and meetings are organized to improve possible poor results.

2.2   Image Acquisition

The period investigated was 2007-2009 and includes all screening activities with digital mammography in the CBU of Leuven. At that time, there were 13 different DR systems: 1 GE Senographe Essential system, 3 Hologic Lorad systems, 1 Siemens Novation system, 6 Siemens Inspiration systems and 2 Sectra systems. There were 9 CR systems: 8 Fuji CR systems and 1 Konica CR system. All systems had passed the European quality criteria and participated in a daily QC program for both the X-ray unit (with every day 2 flat field images and centrally supervised automatic analysis) and the monitor using the MoniQA pattern [16].

The different mean glandular doses (MGD) as calculated from automatic exposure controlled measurements of PMMA slabs of 20 mm, 40 mm and 60 mm of the different participating systems are summarized in Table 1.

Table 1. MGD as calculated from automatic exposure controlled measurements of 20 mm, 40 mm and 60 mm PMMA of the different participating systems

CR system	20 mm PMMA* (mGy)	40 mm PMMA* (mGy)	60 mm PMMA* (mGy)
Hologic Lorad Selenia + Fuji Profect CS	0.3	1.2	3.2
Siemens Mammomat 3000 Nova + Fuji Profect CS	0.4	1.3	1.7
Planmed Sophie + Fuji Profect CS	0.5	1.3	3.3
Siemens Mammomat 3000 Nova + Fuji Profect CS	0.4	1.0	2.7
Hologic M-IV + Fuji Profect CS	0.6	1.1	2.6
Siemens Mammomat 3000 Nova + Fuji Profect CS	0.5	1.6	1.9
Siemens Mammomat 3000 Nova + Fuji Profect CS	0.4	1.0	2.7
Philips Mammo Diagnost + Fuji Profect CS	0.6	1.5	3.9
GE Senographe 800T + Fuji Profect CS	0.5	1.4	2.9
Planmed Sophie + Konica CR	0.6	1.6	3.6

DR system	20 mm PMMA* (mGy)	40 mm PMMA* (mGy)	60 mm PMMA* (mGy)
Sectra (2 systems)	0.4-0.6	0.5-0.9	1.0-1.6
GE Senograph Essential	0.6	0.9	1.8
Hologic Lorad Selenia (3 systems)	0.6-0.8 (0.7)**	1.3-1.5 (1.4)**	1.5-3.5 (2.4)**
Siemens Inspiration (6 systems)	0.4-0.6 (0.5)**	0.8-1.1 (0.9)**	1.4-1.9 (1.6)**
Siemens Novation	0.5	1.0	2.0

* 20 mm PMMA → 21 mm breast; 40 mm PMMA → 45 mm breast; 60 mm PMMA → 75 mm breast
** range (mean)

2.3   Diagnostic Work Up and Data Analysis

The images and reports of cases that have to be recalled are sent back to the first reader and in parallel the CBU sends a letter to the woman with the recommendation to contact her general practitioner or other referring specialist (the woman's choice). The epidemiologist in the screening unit collects the reports of all recalls and a questionnaire to collect data on the results of the work up is sent after 3 months to the referring physician.

The following screening indicators were calculated for the period 2007-2009, for initial and subsequent round: RR, CDR, PPV and the proportion of DCIS. The RR is defined as the proportion of screened women for whom further work up was recommended (following the European Guidelines this should be < 5% in initial, < 3% in subsequent rounds). The CDR is the number of pathologically proven malignant lesions of the breast (both in situ and invasive) detected in a screening round per 1,000 women screened in that round. It should be higher than 3 times the incidence rate (IR) for initial screening examinations and 1.5 times higher than the incidence rate for subsequent screening: the background incidence of breast cancer in the absence of screening is for our country expected to be 1.25 per 1,000 women [17]. The PPV is the fraction of cancers found in the recalled women.

Results of the CR and DR group for the investigated screening parameters were compared using the chi-squared test and a value less than 0.05 was regarded as statistically significant.

3 Results

A total of 42,958 digital mammograms was evaluated. The number of digital mammograms increased significantly over the 3 year's period, with 5,578 in 2007, 10,526 in 2008 and 26,854 in 2009.

Table 2. Overview of the screening indicators for the Leuven CBU for the period 2007-2009 for CR and DR technology, initial versus subsequent rounds

Number	CR-group		DR-group		p-value	
	Initial	Subseq	Initial	Subseq	Initial	Subseq
Screened women	4,216	13,346	4,994	20,402		
Recalled women	100	122	110	235	0.59	0.04
(%)	(2.37)	(0.91)	(2.20)	(1.15)		
Cancer detection	30	69	26	107	0.24	0.92
(‰)	(7.12)	(5.17)	(5.21)	(5.24)		
DCIS	5	6	5	15	0.80	0.34
(%)	(16.67)	(8.70)	(19.23)	(14.02)		
PPV (%)	30.00	56.56	23.64	45.53	0.43	0.25

The screening indicators are summarized in Table 2. All results are conform the European Guidelines [17]. Our RR can be considered as low, but the CDR is in accordance with the European Guidelines. A consequence of these numbers is the high PPV, up to 30% for initial and 56,6% for subsequent rounds in the CR group and 23,6% for initial and 45,5% for subsequent rounds in the DR group. There was no significant difference between CR and DR in terms of CDR and PPV, but a significant difference (p = 0.04) was seen between CR and DR for the RR of subsequent rounds.

Concerning the fraction of DCIS, there was no significant difference between CR and DR. We cannot exclude that this is due to the relatively low absolute numbers.

4   Discussion

The advantage of digital mammography is the separation between acquisition, processing and display. Each of these steps can be optimized separately or changed independently. A challenge for CR technology is that plates and readers can be combined with a variety of X-ray systems, each present with their own beam qualities and preset dose levels. At acceptance, most installations of CR systems required a careful adjustment, usually in a cooperation between the manufacturer and the physicist. Notwithstanding this approach, some systems barely pass the acceptance tests. The impact of this situation, with some systems being much more critical than others, on our screening indicators could not be studied as the number of cases is too small to allow an image quality level based evaluation.

CR has economic advantages over DR systems and smaller centres have therefore chosen to implement these systems. About 54% of the German screening units are using CR technology and 34% FFDM with soft-copy reading [18]. The proportion of CR systems in France is even larger. As the number of mammography units with CR technology may be substantial (certainly when viewed on a worldwide scale), it is important to investigate the impact of this technology on the screening indicators, certainly when recent reports on the results of a lower performance of CR compared to DR appear. From 2005 onwards, our CBU supported the image acquisition and first readings of 65 certified radiologists and coped with all the European norms. A first study, reported in 2010 showed that the transition to FFDM had not changed our screening performance [13]. Present study shows that there is also no statistically significant difference in RR in the initial rounds, CDR, percentage of DCIS and PPV obtained with CR and DR systems separately. Since the start of the screening in 2001, more than 80% of all images have been read by the same group of second readers, what can be considered a strength for our studies: the group of readers is not an extra variable.

We attribute our results to (1) a strict follow up of the radiological aspects individually for all the first readers, (2) a strict control of the radiological image quality by the second readers who report to the first reader and to the physicists all artefacts or causes of quality deterioration, (3) a physico-technical QA, with daily centralized control of the quality of both X-ray system and monitor. Passing the European limiting values in terms of contrast thresholds and contrast to noise ratio requires a dose setting in which CR operates at doses that can be more than double the doses used with DR. We have no intention to allow the lowering of the CR dose setting. A more interesting study, based upon results reported in the SPIE conference 2012 [19], would be to study the performance of DR technology when operated at higher doses.

The higher recall rate in the DR group in the subsequent round may cause the somewhat higher percentage of DCIS (subsequent round: 14,02% in the DR group versus 8,70% in the CR group) in the subsequent rounds which is in line with the results of other studies in which the detection of DCIS (or microcalcifications) is higher in FFDM [2], [3], [5], [6].

The main limitation of the study is the limited number of cases in some of the groups. A larger national study is on-going. We preferred to report our data separately as this allows to exclude confounding parameters such as other second readers, other physicists controlling the systems, other epidemiologists, etc. An analysis of our CBU separately and its discussion in an international forum will face us clearly with our true situation and is considered an important aspect of our local QA goals.

Second limitation is the limited number of systems. Grouping per system is not possible due to the limited number of cases per brand. This is the result of allowing all types of systems in the screening pending a successful type test and acceptance test. Most vendors of digital mammography equipment subscribed for the type test procedure indeed.

We can conclude that CR can be implemented in a well-controlled screening organization without impact on the performance parameters. Present study did not lead to any alarming situation concerning our CR technology. We propose to continue all efforts to control its quality. Larger studies should be performed to increase the statistical confidence.

References

1. Tabar, L., Vitak, B., TonyChen, H.H., Yen, M.F., Duffy, S.W., Smith, R.A.: Beyond randomized controlled trials: organized mammographic screening substantially reduces breast carcinoma mortality. Cancer 91(9), 1724–1731 (2001)
2. Skaane, P., Skjennald, A.: Screen-film versus full-field digital mammography with soft-copy reading: randomized trial in population-based screening program – The Oslo II study. Radiology 232, 197–204 (2004)
3. Vigeland, E., Klaasen, H., Klingen, T.A., et al.: Full-field digital mammography compared to screen-film mammography in the prevalent round of a population-based screening program: the Vestfold County Study. Eur. Radiol. 18, 183–191 (2008)
4. Vinnicombe, S., Pereira, P., McCormack, F., et al.: Full-field digital versus screen-film mammography: comparison within the UK Breast Screening Program and Systematic review of published data. Radiology 251, 347–358 (2009)
5. Karssemeijer, N., Bluekens, A.M., Beijerinck, D., Deurenberg, J.J., Beekman, M., Visser, R., van Engen, R., Bartels-Kortland, A., Broeders, M.J.: Breast Cancer Screening Results 5 Years after Introduction of Digital Mammography in a Population-based Screening Program. Radiology 253(2), 353–358 (2009)
6. Del Turco, M.R., Mantellini, P., Ciatto, S., et al.: Full-field digital versus screen-film mammography: comparative accuracy in concurrent screening cohorts. AJR 189, 860–866 (2007)
7. Marshall, N.W., Monnin, P., Bosmans, H., Bochud, F.O., Verdun, F.R.: Image quality assessment in digital mammography: Part I. Technical characterization of the systems. Phys. Med. Biol. 56(14), 4201–4220 (2011)

8. Bick, U., Diekmann, F.: Digital mammography: what do we and what don't we know? Eur. Rad. 17(8), 1931–1942 (2007)
9. Heddson, B., Rönnow, K., Olsson, M., Millder, D.: Digital versus screen-film mammography: a retrospective comparison in a population-based screening program. Eur. J. Rad. 64, 419–425 (2007)
10. Hendrick, R.E., Cole, E.B., Pisano, E.D., et al.: Accuracy of Soft-Copy Digital Mammography versus that of Screen-Film Mammography according to Digital Manufacturer: ACRIN DMIST Retrospective Multireader Study. Radiology 247(1), 38–48 (2008)
11. Schueller, G., Riedl, C., Mallek, R., Eibenberger, K., Langenberger, H., Kaindl, E., Kulinna-Cosentini, C., Rudas, M., Helbich, T.: Image quality, lesion detection, and diagnostic efficacy in digital mammography: full-field digital mammography versus computed radiography-based mammography using digital storage phosphor plates. Eur. J. Radiol. 67(3), 487–496 (2008)
12. Schulz-Wendtland, R., Lell, M., Wenkel, E., Böhner, C., Dassel, M.S., Bautz, W.: DR (a-Se) versus CR (DLR) – is an improvement of the accuracy possible? A retrospective histologic analysis (n = 100). Röntgenpraxis 56(4), 129–135 (2007) (in German)
13. Van Ongeval, C., Van Steen, A., Vande Putte, G., Zanca, F., Bosmans, H., Marchal, G., Van Limbergen, E.: Does digital mammography in a decentralized breast cancer screening program lead to screening performance parameters comparable with film-screen mammography? Eur. Radiol. 20(10), 2307–2314 (2010)
14. van Engen, R., Young, K., Bosmans, H., Thijssen, M.: The European protocol for the quality control of the physical and technical aspects of mammography screening. Part B: Digital mammography. In: Fourth Edition of the European Guidelines for Breast Cancer Screening (2005), http://www.euref.org
15. Vlaams Agentschap Zorg en Gezondheid, Afdeling Preventie, Belgium. Draaiboek Vlaams bevolkingsonderzoek naar borstkanker, http://www.zorg-en-gezondheid.be
16. Thierens, H., Bosmans, H., Buls, N., De Hauwere, A., Bacher, K., Jacobs, J., Clerinx, P.: Typetesting of physical characteristics of digital mammography systems for screening within the Flemish breast cancer screening programme. Eur. J. Radiol. 70(3), 539–548 (2009)
17. Perry, N., Broeders, M., de Wolf, C., Törnberg, S., Holland, R., von Karsa, L.: European guidelines for quality assurance in mammography screening, 3rd edn. European Commission, Luxembourg (2006)
18. Skaane, P.: Digital Mammography in European population-based screening programs. In: Bick, U., Diekmann, F. (eds.) Medical Radiology – Diagnostic Imaging (2009) ISBN 978-3-540-78449-4; Baert, A.L., Reiser, M.F., Hricak, H., Knauth, M. (eds) Digital Mammography
19. Warren, L.M., Mackenzie, A., Cooke, J., Given-Wilson, R., Wallis, M.G., Chakraborty, D.P., Dance, D.R., Young, K.C.: Investigating the relationship between calcification cluster detection in digital mammography and threshold gold thickness measurements. In: Proc. SPIE Medical Imaging, vol. 8313, pp. 8313–8318 (2012)

A Quality Control Framework Using Task-Based Detectability Measurements for Digital Mammography

Aili K. Bloomquist[1], James G. Mainprize[1], Gordon E. Mawdsley[1], Martin J. Yaffe[1,2]

[1] Sunnybrook Research Institute, Toronto, Canada
{aili.bloomquist,james.mainprize,
mawdsley,martin.yaffe}@sri.utoronto.ca
[2] Department of Medical Biophysics, University of Toronto, Toronto, Canada

Abstract. Quality control for digital mammography should be objective, reproducible and applicable across different manufacturers' systems and technologies. Ideally it should be possible to set clearly defined thresholds of acceptable behaviour that can be universally applied. Other works have proposed combining measurements of detector performance with an observer model and task function to calculate the detectability index d'. This work builds on those concepts by proposing a simple phantom design for measuring system performance from a single image, allowing the calculation of NEQ and d' and including effects due to scatter and all noise sources. A second contrast-detail test-object is proposed for validation of the model using a 4AFC observer study design.

Keywords: quality control, observer model, task, detectability, NEQ.

1   Background

Current quality control protocols for digital mammography often rely heavily on subjective assessments of phantom images for overall image quality, or employ overly simplistic measures that may not reflect clinical image quality or may not reliably capture all modes of failure. Another difficulty is that many measures cannot be expressed in system-independent units, making comparisons between different manufacturers' systems difficult. Model observers have been proposed to quantify the signal to noise ratio achieved for relevant imaging tasks without the variability and subjectivity associated with the human reader by calculating the detectability index (d'). To calculate d', the system must be characterized. We present here a method for simply and reliably estimating the elements needed to calculate the system noise equivalent quanta (NEQ) of a digital mammography unit from a single phantom image. These data can then be used in the calculation of the detectability index (d') of arbitrary test objects using a non-pre-whitening model observer (NPWE) incorporating an eye-filter and internal noise. We also suggest a framework for validating the method using four alternative forced choice (4AFC) observer studies of a suitably designed contrast-detail test object.

A.D.A. Maidment, P.R. Bakic, and S. Gavenonis (Eds.): IWDM 2012, LNCS 7361, pp. 197–204, 2012.

2   Methods

2.1   QC Phantom

For the measurement of NEQ and contrast, such that detectability can be estimated, we propose imaging a 40 mm thick uniform block of polymethyl methacrylate (PMMA), on whose upper surface two strips of copper foil have been positioned, angled by approximately 5° from the sides of the block as depicted in Fig.1 (left panel). The uniform regions of the PMMA are used to evaluate the noise power spectrum (NPS) and the slanted edges of the copper foil strips are used to calculate the pre-sampled modulation transfer function (MTF) in the x and y directions. A one-mm-thick disc of PMMA with a diameter of 25 mm is used to estimate the radiological contrast of the detection tasks. The material and thickness of the contrast disc could be changed to suit the detection task being evaluated.

To validate the detectability calculations, a 4AFC observer study is being conducted using a contrast-detail test object. The test object consists of cylindrical posts of PMMA milled to have heights ranging from 0.0442 to 1.0 mm, with diameters ranging from 0.312 to 3.536 mm on top of a PMMA base with a thickness of 40 mm. Five thicknesses are used for each disc diameter, with the relevant thickness range determined from preliminary reader studies using a contrast-detail test object imaged on several digital mammography systems. This range includes the thicknesses likely to encompass discs that are just visible to just not visible under typical mammographic exposures. The thickness and diameter combinations used are described below in Table 1. For each disc diameter, a reference disc thickness that should always be visible is listed.

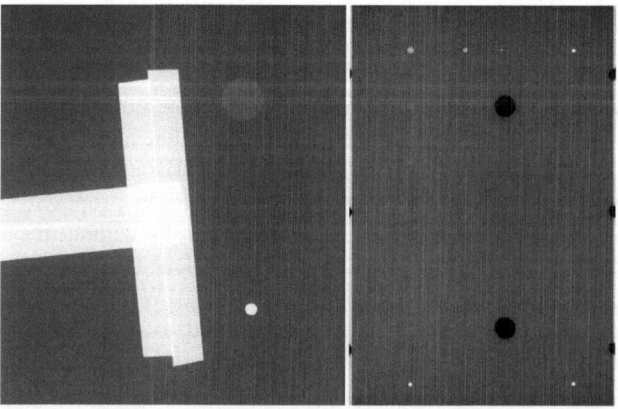

Fig. 1. Radiographs of the NEQ measurement phantom (left) and the contrast-detail test object (right) being used to validate the modeled detectability values

Table 1. Diameters and thicknesses of discs for contrast-detail test object. All measurements are in mm.

Diameter	Disc Thicknesses Reference	Test 1	Test 2	Test 3	Test 4	Test 5
0.312	1.25	1.0	0.7071	0.5	0.3536	0.25
0.625	1.0	0.5	0.3536	0.25	0.1768	0.125
1.250	1.0	0.25	0.1768	0.125	0.0884	0.0625
2.500	1.0	0.25	0.1768	0.125	0.0884	0.0625
3.536	1.0	0.1768	0.125	0.0884	0.0625	0.0442

2.2   Detectability

The detectability index (d′) for a particular detection task is calculated using a variation of the formula proposed by Burgess [1] and modified by Segui and Zhao [2] as follows:

$$d' = \Delta S \times \sqrt{\frac{O}{(N + N_i)}} \,, \tag{1}$$

where ΔS is the signal difference between the object and the background, O is the integrated signal power (perceived signal) calculated using the non-prewhitening observer (NPWE) model with eye filter described by Segui and Zhao and given in Equation (2), N is the integrated noise in the system as given in Equation (3) and Ni is the added internal noise of the viewer.

$$O = \left(\iint_{u,v} W^2(u,v) MTF^2(u,v) E^2(u,v) du dv \right)^2 \text{, and} \tag{2}$$

$$N = \iint_{u,v} W^2(u,v) NPS(u,v) MTF^2(u,v) E^4(u,v) du dv \,, \tag{3}$$

where $W(u,v)$ is the task function, $MTF(u,v)$ is the 2-dimensional (2D) MTF of the imaging system, $NPS(u,v)$ is its 2D noise power spectrum, and $E(u,v)$ is the eye filter describing the contrast sensitivity of the human visual system. Because the task explored here is detecting a disc, W is taken to be a "jinc" function (Hankel transform of a disc). Note in our formulation we calculate a single system noise rather than separating out quantum, scatter and electronic noise sources. Following the work of Burgess [3], the internal noise N_i was taken to be a scale factor, a, of the system noise N according to Equation (4).

$$N_i = a^2 \times N \tag{4}$$

The internal noise scale factor, a, was fit to be 1.5.

The pre-sampled MTF is obtained in both the x and y directions using the standard algorithm described by Fujita *et al* [4]. The relatively wide (40 mm) bands of copper foil ensure that any low-frequency drop in MTF due to off-focal radiation, scatter and/or glare in the phosphor on indirect flat panel systems can be accurately characterized. The MTF along x and y were averaged together and then radially rotated to create a 2D MTF. This is an approximation of the true 2-D MTF, which likely has non-rotationally symmetric components such as that due to the rectangular shape of the detector element.

The two-dimensional NPS is calculated using the multi-taper method (MTM), with adaptive weighting [5]. Using the MTM method results in a "cleaner" NPS with reduced low-frequency distortions, at the cost of some broadening (loss of spectral resolution) of any peaks (i.e. grid artefact) in the spectrum. Regions of interest (ROIs) are selected from the portions of the image where only PMMA was present in the beam. The ROIs are chosen such that the solid angle of the x-ray beam (θ) is less than 4.7° so changes in beam intensity across the ROI (proportional to $\cos^3(\theta)$) are kept to less than 1%.

Ideally, ΔS would be derived from the radiological subject contrast of the object being evaluated in a given task. For example, the subject contrast could be measured for a series of discs of different thicknesses in a contrast-detail test object. In this work, it is approximated using the measured image contrast for the 1 mm thick contrast disc. Over small ranges, log-relationships can be treated as linear, so assuming a linear relationship between disc thickness and induced signal difference; ΔS can be estimated for arbitrary disc thicknesses by multiplying ΔS_1 by the desired disc thickness in mm, t according to equation (5):

$$\Delta S(t) = t\Delta S_1 = t \times \left(ADU_{background} - ADU_{disc} \right). \tag{5}$$

ADU_{disc} and $ADU_{background}$ are the mean pixel values or analog-to-digital units (ADUs) measured in ROIs selected in the image of the contrast disc and nearby background areas of the phantom. For systems with limited flat-fielding (such as CR) it may be necessary to perform a manual gain correction on the image data (using images of a uniform phantom) before making this measurement.

The eye filter is modeled using the common functional form of $E(f) = f^n \exp(-cf^2)$ [6], where n and c are experimental parameters selected to match the viewing conditions of a human reader. The parameters n and c were iteratively adjusted along with the internal noise factor, a, to yield the best agreement between measured thickness thresholds and model determined thresholds. A best fit to measured data was found with $n = 0.81$, $c = 1.12$ and $a = 1.5$. This appears to hold across different systems when images are viewed at the same physical magnification.

2.3   4AFC Design

To validate the calculated detectability values, we compare them to the measured proportion correct found in a four-alternative forced choice (4AFC) observer study using a range of disc diameters and thickness. Images of the contrast-detail test object are acquired at techniques matching those used to image the NEQ phantom. Twenty-four images are acquired on each system tested to achieve sufficient different noise realizations to be able to distinguish a difference of less than 0.8 in d' with a power of 0.8 [7]. Regions of interest will be cropped from the images such that a disc appears in one of the four corners of the ROI. The selection of which corner contains the disc is randomized. A psychometric function is fit between the percent correctly detected in the 4AFC study and disc thickness for each disc diameter. Then the detectability (d') of that disc thickness and diameter can be estimated from the proportion taken from the psychometric fit and compared to the model d' determined from the QC phantom measurements. Fitting the reader data removes some of the measurement noise and avoids difficulties with infinite values resulting from test objects where the readers achieved a 100% correct detection rate. The fits were done using the "psignifit" software package and a bootstrapping technique [8].

2.4   Systems Tested

The methodology was evaluated on three different mammography units, two GE Senographe DS systems and a Planmed Nuance system. The DS detectors have 100 micron dels and a cesium-iodide scintillation layer on a photo-diode thin-film transistor array. The Planmed detector has 85 micron dels and an amorphous selenium conversion layer on an electrode array.

3   Results

In Fig. 2, we show preliminary measurements of MTF, normalized NPS (NNPS) and noise equivalent quanta (NEQ) using the proposed phantom on three different mammography systems. In Fig. 3 we show the modeled d' plotted against the d' values measured by the 4AFC.reader study. For each system the linear fits between modeled d' and measured d' for the individual readers were compared using the F test to the 95% confidence level. The results of this analysis are given in Table 2. Subsequently, the reader data were pooled and the linear fits for each system type were compared using the F test. The results of this analysis are given in Table 3.

Table 2. Test for significant differences between readers looking at the parameters of linear least-squares fits to the modeled and measured d' values for each reader and system. A 1 indicates a statistically significant difference in the parameter to the 95% confidence level.

Parameter	1 vs. 2	1 vs. 3	1 vs. 4	2 vs. 3	2 vs. 4	3 vs. 4
GE 1 m	0	0	0	0	0	0
GE 1 b	0	1	1	0	0	0
GE 2 m	0	0	0	0	1	1
GE 2 b	NA	NA	NA	NA	NA	NA
Planmed 1	0	0	0	0	0	0
Planmed 2	0	0	0	0	0	0

Table 3. Test for significant differences between systems looking at the parameters of linear least-squares fits to the modeled and measured d' values. A 1 indicates a statistically significant difference in the parameter to the 95% confidence level.

Parameter	GE 1 vs. GE 2	GE 1 vs. Planmed	GE 2 vs. Planmed
m	0	1	0
B	0	1	1

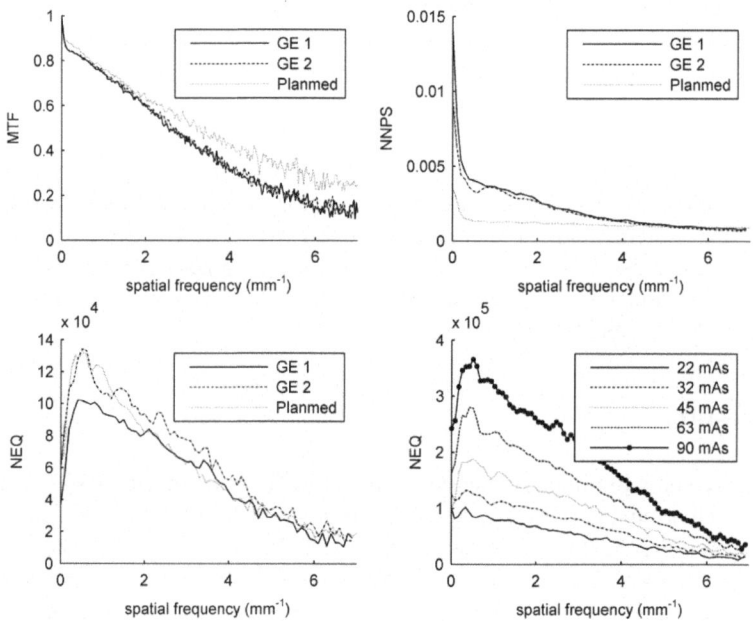

Fig. 2. Graphs of MTF (top left), NNPS (top right), and NEQ (bottom left) for three different systems at a typical exposure level and the NEQ at five different exposure levels for one system (bottom right)

4   Discussion

We have presented a framework for calculating the detectability index (d') for low contrast detection tasks that can be defined using functions in the Fourier domain. The proposed method requires only one image of one phantom to obtain the necessary measures of system performance. With a validated method of objectively measuring system performance for specific imaging tasks, it should be possible to propose broadly applicable and easily measurable standards for system performance.

One of the limitations of this study is that the ambient lighting conditions and viewing distance were not rigorously controlled. However, inter reader variability was not statistically significant most of the time.

The slopes of the linear fits between the measured and modeled d' values appear to be different for the different mammography systems. This difference was found to be statistically significant between the second GE system and the Planmed system. In addition, the intercept for the Planmed system was different than that for the GE systems. This suggests that the model used to calculate d' needs further refinement to generate completely system-independent results. Areas for improvement include a better estimation of the eye-filter parameters and inclusion of a scatter estimate in the calculation of radiographic contrast.

Future work includes extending the 4AFC study to more vendors and more readers, doing a more thorough error propagation and analysis, and extending the model and phantom used to calculate d' to predict the results of evaluating the CDMAM phantom.

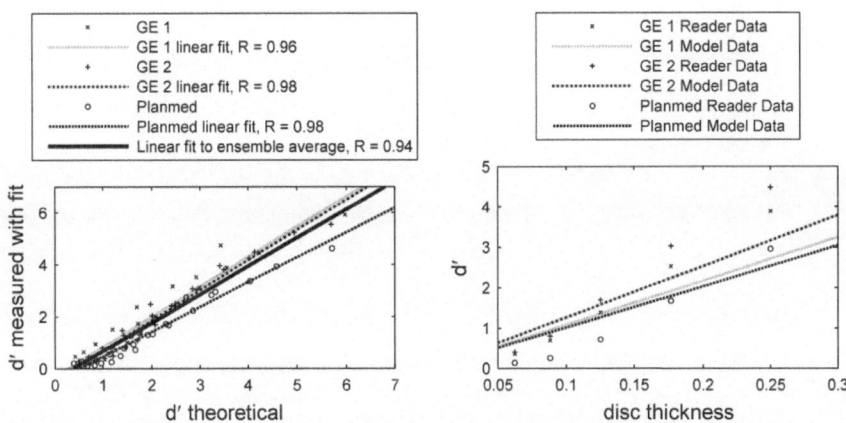

Fig. 3. Left side: Plot of modeled d' vs. measured d' values for three different mammography systems. The measured d' values are averages of the values taken from the psychometric fits made for the individual readers participating in the 4AFC study. Right side: Plot of d' values both measured from the reader study and modeled, for a disc diameter of 1.25 mm versus increasing disc thickness.

References

1. Burgess, A.E., Li, X., Abbey, C.K.: Visual signal detectability with two noise components: anomalous masking effects. J. Opt. Soc. Am. A 14(9), 2420–2442 (1997)
2. Segui, J.A., Zhao, W.: Amorphous selenium flat panel detectors for digital mammography: Validation of a NPWE model observer with CDMAM observer performance experiments. Med. Phys. 33(10), 3711–3722 (2006)
3. Burgess, A.E., Colborne, B.: Visual signal detection. IV. Observer inconsistency. J. Opt. Soc. AM. A 5(4), 617–627 (1988)
4. Fujita, H., Tsai, D.Y., Itoh, T., Doi, K., Morishita, J., Ueda, K., Ohtsuka, A.: A simple method for determining the modulation transfer function in digital radiography. IEEE Trans. Med. Im. 11(1), 34–39 (1992)

5. Wu, G., Mainprize, J.G., Yaffe, M.J.: Spectral analysis of mammographic images using a multitaper method. Med. Phys. 39(2), 801–810 (2012)
6. Burgess, A.E.: Statistically defined backgrounds: performance of a modified nonprewhitening observer model. J. Opt. Soc. Am. A 11(4), 1237–1242 (1994)
7. Bi, J., Lee, H.-S., O'Mahony, M.: d' and variance of d' for four-alternative forced choice (4-AFC). Journal of Sensory Studies 25(5), 740–750 (2010)
8. Fründ, I., Haenel, N.V., Wichmann, F.A.: Inference for psychometric functions in the presence of nonstationary behavior. J. Vision 11(6), 1–19 (2011)

Longitudinal Change in Mammographic Density and Association with Breast Cancer Risk: A Case-Control Study

Chew Ting[1], Susan M. Astley[2], Julie Morris[3], Paula Stavrinos[4], Mary Wilson[4], Nicky Barr[4], Caroline Boggis[4], and Jamie C. Sergeant[2]

[1] Manchester Medical School, University of Manchester,
Oxford Road, Manchester M13 9PT, UK
[2] School of Cancer and Enabling Sciences, University of Manchester,
Oxford Road, Manchester M13 9PT, UK
[3] Department of Medical Statistics, University Hospital of South Manchester,
Manchester M23 9LT, UK
[4] Nightingale Centre and Genesis Prevention Centre,
University Hospital of South Manchester, Manchester M23 9LT, UK
jamie.sergeant@manchester.ac.uk

Abstract. High mammographic breast density is associated with increased risk of breast cancer, but how risk varies with longitudinal change in density is less clear. To investigate, a case-control study of 30 women with screen-detected cancer and 30 women with a normal mammogram, all with two previous normal mammograms, was conducted. Percentage density for all mammograms was estimated with the thresholding software Cumulus. Mean density at first screen was not significantly different in cases and controls in contralateral (36.5 vs. 32.6, $p = 0.23$) or ipsilateral (36.0 vs. 32.9 $p = 0.37$) breasts, but mean reduction in density from first to third screen was significantly different in both contralateral (10.7 vs. 5.1, $p = 0.02$) and ipsilateral (11.7 vs. 6.2, $p = 0.04$) breasts. Using logistic regression, and controlling for age and HRT use, breast cancer risk was found to be associated with change in density from first to third screen.

Keywords: Mammographic density, breast cancer risk, case-control study, Cumulus.

1 Introduction

Mammographic breast density is the proportion of the breast occupied by radiopaque 'dense' fibroglandular tissue as opposed to radiolucent 'non-dense' adipose tissue on a mammogram. The association between high mammographic density and increased risk of developing breast cancer is well established, having been first described by Wolfe in 1976 [1-2]. A meta-analysis conducted thirty years later reported that the relative risk of developing breast cancer for women with ≥75% density compared to those with <5% density was 4.64 (95% CI: 3.64-5.91) [3]. However, the relationship

A.D.A. Maidment, P.R. Bakic, and S. Gavenonis (Eds.): IWDM 2012, LNCS 7361, pp. 205–211, 2012.
© Springer-Verlag Berlin Heidelberg 2012

between change in density over time and breast cancer risk is less well understood. While risk increases with age, and is associated with high density, density declines with age. Of the few studies examining the issue, some have found evidence of an association between change in breast density and breast cancer risk, whereas others have found no evidence of such an association. One study found that an increase (decrease) in density, as classified by the four-category American College of Radiology Breast Imaging Reporting and Data System (BI-RADS) breast composition classification [4], over a period of approximately three years was associated with an increased (decreased) rate of breast cancer relative to women whose density classification did not change during the same period [5]. A second study, where mammograms were automatically classified to one of four density categories: <5%, 5-25%, 26-75% or >75%, made similar findings over a 10 year follow-up period [6]. However, two studies found no association between longitudinal change in percentage density, as measured by computer-assisted interactive thresholding [9], and breast cancer risk [7-8]. The purpose of the current work is to further explore longitudinal change in breast density and its possible association with breast cancer risk, by examining whether such an association exists in a case-control study.

2   Method

The study population consisted of 60 women who had attended routine breast screening through the Greater Manchester Breast Screening Programme, part of the UK NHS Breast Screening Programme. Of these, 30 women had screen detected cancer in one breast, and the remainder had normal screening mammograms. The women with cancer (referred to as the cases) were drawn consecutively from those with screen detected cancer who had normal mammograms in the two previous screening rounds. The women with normal screening mammograms (referred to as the controls) were randomly selected from women with normal screening mammograms who also had normal mammograms in the two previous screening rounds. Whereas all of the mammograms from the most recent round of screening consisted of both mediolateral oblique (MLO) and craniocaudal (CC) views, some of the mammograms from the two previous rounds of screening contained only MLO views. Henceforth the most recent, diagnostic, screen will be referred to as the third screen and the two previous, prediagnostic, screens will be referred to as the first and second screens. The mean (SD) time between first and third screen was 6.5 (0.8) years for cases and 6.4 (0.9) years for controls.

Mammographic breast density was assessed for all mammograms from all three rounds of screening using the interactive thresholding software Cumulus (Version 4.0; Sunnybrook Health Sciences Centre, Toronto, Canada) [9], which has been shown to have a strong association with risk [13], and has been called the gold standard of density measurement [10]. All mammogram films were digitised, anonymised and randomised into small batches before being read by a single trained and validated Cumulus reader. The images used in Cumulus were 8-bit grayscale depth with a pixel size of 0.25 mm × 0.25 mm. Randomisation meant that the reader was blinded to the case-control status of all mammograms. The reader segmented the breast area from the background using a pixel value threshold and/or piecewise linear mask, then set a second threshold to separate the dense from the non-dense breast tissue within the breast area. The proportion of the breast area occupied by dense tissue was calculated as a percentage by the software.

As well as measurements of breast density, information on the age of the subjects at screening and whether they had ever used hormone replacement therapy (HRT) was available for inclusion in the analysis. Both age and the use of HRT are known risk factors for breast cancer and are associated with breast density. The risk of developing breast cancer increases with age and with the use of HRT. Breast density decreases with age but increases with the use of HRT [11]. Due to the possible effect on breast density measurements of the presence of breast cancer in the mammograms of cases at the third screen, separate analyses were conducted for the contralateral and ipsilateral breasts. For controls, one breast was randomly assigned to be the contralateral side and the other breast the ipsilateral side.

Two-sided independent samples t-tests were used to compare the mean age of cases and controls at first and third screen, the mean densities for cases and controls at first screen, and the mean change in density from first to third screen for cases and controls. Logistic regression was used to investigate how density at first screen and change in density from first to third screen predicted case-control status. The results presented here were produced using only the MLO views, as only the MLO views were available for every subject at all three rounds of screening.

3   Results

The mean ages of the case and control groups at the first and third screens are shown in Table 1. How many of the cases and controls had ever used HRT is shown in Table 2. Mean age was not significantly different in cases and controls at the time of first screen ($p = 0.45$) or third screen ($p = 0.40$). The two groups are similar in terms of the number of subjects who had ever used HRT, and indeed a χ^2 test with continuity correction applied found no evidence to reject the independence of HRT use and case-control status ($p = 1.00$).

Table 1. Age in years of cases and controls at first and third screen

Screen	Mean (SD) age	
	Cases	Controls
First	57.2 (4.2)	56.3 (5.0)
Third	63.7 (4.3)	62.7 (5.0)

Table 2. HRT use of cases and controls

HRT use	Cases	Controls
Ever used	18	17
Never used	12	13

The mean percentage density of the cases and controls at first, second and third screens is given in Table 3 and dot plots of the densities for the contralateral side are shown in Fig. 1. Mean density at first screen was not significantly different in cases and controls in either the contralateral side ($p = 0.23$) or the ipsilateral side ($p = 0.37$).

Mean percentage density decreased from first to third screen in both the contralateral and ipsilateral sides of cases and controls. The mean reduction in percentage density was significantly different for cases and controls in both the contralateral side (10.7 vs. 5.1, $p = 0.02$) and ipsilateral side (11.7 vs. 6.2, $p = 0.04$). To illustrate the reduction in density, a scatterplot showing the percentage density in the contralateral side at first and third screen is shown in Fig. 2.

Table 3. Percentage density at first and third screen of the contralateral and ipsilateral breasts of cases and controls

Screen	Mean (SD) percentage density			
	Cases		Controls	
	Contralateral	Ipsilateral	Contralateral	Ipsilateral
First	36.5 (13.8)	36.0 (13.4)	32.6 (11.1)	32.9 (13.5)
Second	31.4 (12.3)	31.3 (14.9)	29.2 (12.9)	29.1 (13.1)
Third	25.8 (12.8)	24.4 (12.5)	27.5 (14.2)	26.7 (12.4)

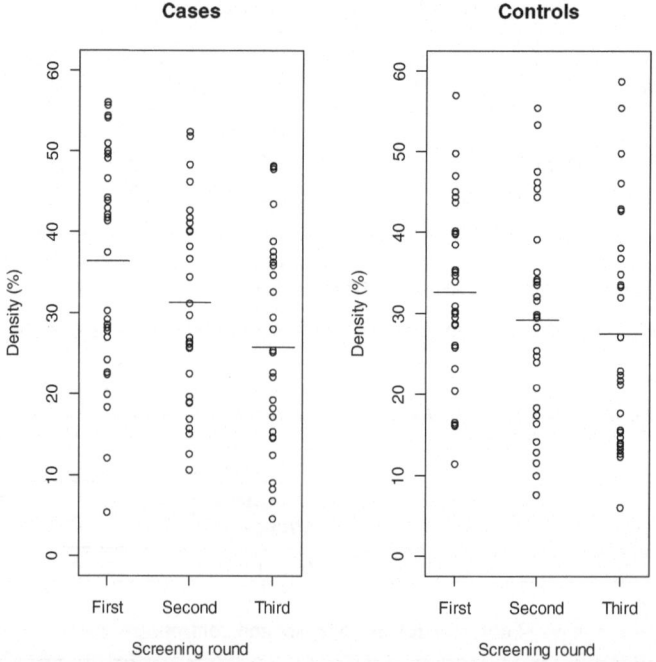

Fig. 1. Dot plots of percentage density of the contralateral breast at first, second and third screen. A horizontal line represents the mean for that plot.

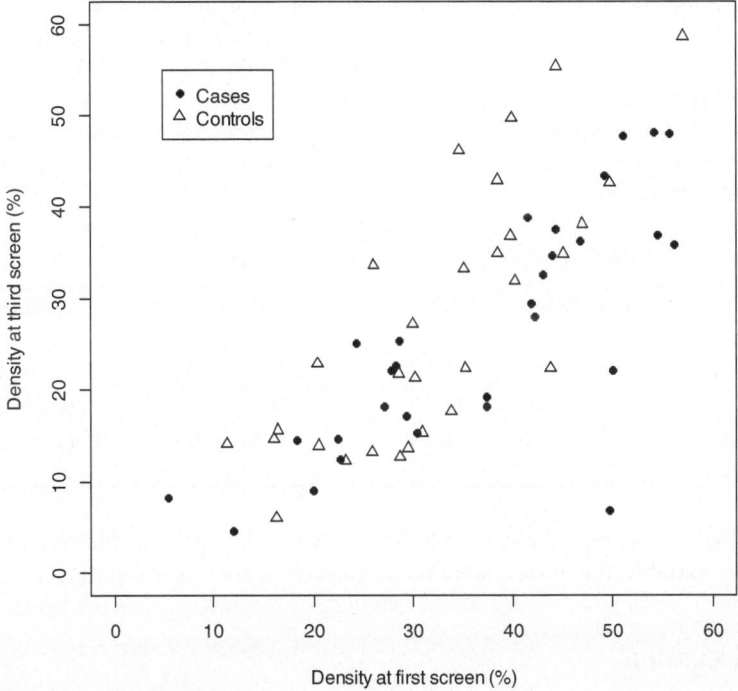

Fig. 2. Scatterplot of percentage density of the contralateral breast at first and third screen

The logistic regression model for the contralateral breast included age at third screen and HRT status alongside change in density from first to third screen as predictors of case-control status. The output from the model can be seen in Table 4. Change in density made a significant contribution to the model ($p = 0.02$) and had an odds ratio of 1.09 (95% CI: 1.01-1.17). By the Cox & Snell R^2 the model explained 11.5% of the variation in case-control status, and by the Nagelkerke R^2 it explained 15.4%. The model correctly classified 63.3% of cases, however with a χ^2 value of 14.9 and $p = 0.06$ the model only marginally escaped being rejected by the Hosmer–Lemeshow goodness-of-fit test.

Table 4. Logistic regression model for the contralateral side

Term	Coefficient	SE	Wald statistic	p	Odds ratio (95% CI)
Age	0.06	0.06	1.12	0.29	1.07 (0.95, 1.20)
HRT use	0.00	0.56	0.00	1.00	1.00 (0.33, 3.01)
Change in density	0.09	0.04	5.16	0.02	1.09 (1.01, 1.17)

A similar logistic regression model was fitted for the ipsilateral side. The output is shown in Table 5. Again the change in density from first to third screen was significant in the model ($p = 0.04$), with an odds ratio of 1.06 (95% CI: 1.00-1.12). This model performed better according to the Hosmer–Lemeshow goodness-of-fit test ($\chi^2 = 6.6$, $p = 0.57$), but explained less of the variation in case-control status as measured by the Cox & Snell R^2 (8.9%) and by the Nagelkerke R^2 (11.9%). The model correctly classified 56.7% of cases.

Table 5. Logistic regression model for the ipsilateral side

Term	Coefficient	SE	Wald statistic	p	Odds ratio (95% CI)
Age	0.06	0.06	1.07	0.30	1.07 (0.95, 1.20)
HRT use	-0.15	0.57	0.07	0.79	0.86 (0.28, 2.62)
Change in density	0.06	0.03	4.34	0.04	1.06 (1.00, 1.12)

When logistic the regression models were fitted with density at first screen as an explanatory variable, the models were found not to be statistically significant.

4   Discussion

Mammographic breast density declined from first to third screen in both the contralateral and ipsilateral breasts of cases and controls, with the mean reduction being greater for cases than controls. Furthermore, the reduction from first to third screen was associated with case-control status in a logistic regression model that included subject age and HRT use as confounding variables. No association was found between density at first screen and breast cancer risk for this group of women, even accounting for subject age and HRT use.

The primary objective of this study was to test for the presence of an association between change in density and cancer risk. Such an association was found, with the results suggesting that increased risk was associated with a greater reduction in density. This was not the result that would have been expected, as the existing literature on the subject [5-8] suggests either an association in the opposite direction or no association. However, there are several limitations to the present study that restrict firm conclusions from being drawn. The sample size was small compared to other studies of change in percentage density and breast cancer risk [7,8], cases were not matched to controls and the selection of cases was not random. It has been suggested that analyses of breast density and breast cancer risk should always take account of age and body mass index (BMI) [10]. While information on the age of the subjects at screening was available, data on BMI was not. Furthermore, the information available on subject HRT use was limited. Some variability in the results may be attributed to differences in positioning, compression and exposure of the breast in different screening rounds, as well as the subjective element in density estimation using Cumulus. The introduction of automated volumetric methods of density estimation for full-field digital mammography (FFDM) has the promise of reducing this variability, hence these technologies, once mature and once sufficient rounds of FFDM screening have been conducted, may help to further elucidate the relationship between change in breast density and breast cancer risk.

References

1. Wolfe, J.N.: Breast patterns as an index of risk for developing breast cancer. Am. J. Roentgenol. 126, 1130–1139 (1976)
2. Wolfe, J.N.: Risk for breast cancer development determined by mammographic parenchymal pattern. Cancer 37, 2486–2492 (1976)
3. McCormack, V.A., dos Santos Silva, I.: Breast density and parenchymal patterns as markers of breast cancer risk: a meta-analysis. Cancer Epidemiol. Biomarkers Prev. 15, 1159–1169 (2006)
4. D'Orsi, C.J., et al.: Breast imaging reporting and data system: ACR BI-RADS. Breast Imaging Atlas. American College of Radiology, Reston (2003)
5. Kerlikowske, K., Ichikawa, L., Miglioretti, D.L., et al.: Longitudinal measurement of clinical mammographic breast density to improve estimation of breast cancer risk. J. Natl. Cancer Inst. 99, 386–395 (2007)
6. van Gils, C.H., Hendriks, J.H., Holland, R., Karssemeijer, N., Otten, J.D., Straatman, H., Verbeek, A.L.: Changes in mammographic breast density and concomitant changes in breast cancer risk. Eur. J. Cancer Prev. 8, 509–515 (1999)
7. Maskarinec, G., Pagano, I., Lurie, G., Kolonel, L.N.: A longitudinal investigation of mammographic density: the multiethnic cohort. Cancer Epidemiol. Biomarkers Prev. 15, 732–739 (2006)
8. Vachon, C.M., Pankratz, V.S., Scott, C.G., et al.: Longitudinal trends in mammographic percent density and breast cancer risk. Cancer Epidemiol. Biomarkers Prev. 16, 921–928 (2007)
9. Byng, J.W., Boyd, N.F., Fishell, E., Jong, R.A., Yaffe, M.J.: The quantitative analysis of mammographic densities. Phys. Med. Biol. 39, 1629–1638 (1994)
10. Assi, V., et al.: Clinical and epidemiological issues in mammographic density. Nat. Rev. Clin. Oncol. 9, 33–40 (2012)
11. Vachon, C.M., Kuni, C.C., Anderson, K., Anderson, V.E., Sellers, T.A.: Association of mammographically defined percent breast density with epidemiologic risk factors for breast cancer (United States). Cancer Causes Control 11, 653–662 (2000)
12. Byrne, C., Schairer, C., Wolfe, J., et al.: Mammographic features and breast cancer risk: effects with time, age, and menopause status. J. Natl. Cancer Inst. 87, 1622–1629 (1995)
13. Boyd, N.F., Rommens, J.M., Vogt, K., Lee, V., Hopper, J.L., Yaffe, M.J., Paterson, A.D.: Mammographic breast density as an intermediate phenotype for breast cancer. Lancet Oncol. 6, 798–808 (2005)

Long-Term Stability of Image Quality Measurements for Two Digital Mammography Systems

Jennifer M. Oduko and Kenneth C. Young

NCCPM, Guildford, UK
{jenny.oduko,ken.young}@nhs.net

Abstract. Contrast-detail measurements were made at approximately weekly intervals for three months, for two full-field mammography systems with different types of detector. The measured threshold contrast values were found to be reasonably stable but with some random variation. The coefficient of variance was 8-10% for detail sizes 0.1 and 1.0mm, and 3-5% for detail sizes 0.25 and 0.5mm. The output of both X-ray sets was also monitored, and found to vary within ±1% of the mean. The variation in threshold contrast is likely to be mainly due to variation of noise in the CDMAM images. Care should be taken when setting baselines and acceptable limits, so that measured changes in threshold contrast that are of the order of ±10% of the mean are not wrongly interpreted as significant changes in performance of a digital mammography system.

Keywords. Image quality, threshold contrast, CDMAM.

1 Background

Contrast-detail measurements are widely used in Europe for the evaluation of image quality in digital mammography, as described in the European quality control protocol [1]. Under this protocol, multiple images of the CDMAM test object (Artinis, Nijmegen) are acquired and analysed using standard software available from the EUREF website, http://www.euref.org (CDMAM Analyser version 1.5.1). The errors, twice the standard error (2 SE), quoted in the output tables of the software, are based on repeated random sampling of 8, 16 or 32 images out of sets of 64 acquired on a single occasion, for each of four different full-field digital mammography systems [2]. Other previous work has also sampled large data sets acquired on one occasion [3, 4] or two occasions [5].

It is not clear whether these results give a realistic estimate of the errors of measurement for contrast-detail measurements carried out at six-monthly intervals, as is standard practice in Europe for quality control purposes. Reproducibility of the paddle and test object positioning might have some effect on the reproducibility of results. To provide a more accurate estimate of the error, measurements were repeated at weekly intervals, on the assumption that the imaging system was stable over this time and that variations were due to measurement error. The results should provide a more

A.D.A. Maidment, P.R. Bakic, and S. Gavenonis (Eds.): IWDM 2012, LNCS 7361, pp. 212–219, 2012.
© Springer-Verlag Berlin Heidelberg 2012

appropriate estimate of errors of measurement than those published previously [2-5]. It is suggested that these estimates of errors be applied to routine quality control measurements (but not that the measurements themselves be carried out at weekly intervals).

2   Method

The CDMAM phantom was positioned on the breast platform, with a 2cm thickness of polymethyl methacrylate (PMMA) above and below, and sixteen images were acquired on each of two systems, one with an amorphous selenium detector (Hologic Selenia Dimensions) and the other with caesium iodide-amorphous silicon detector (GE Essential). Measurements were repeated twelve times at weekly intervals. The same phantom was always used, and the same operator made all the measurements. The exposures were made in manual mode, with the same exposure parameters used every time. The exposure parameters were chosen by imaging a 5cm thickness of PMMA under automatic exposure control (AEC); the same kV, target and filter were used for the CDMAM images, and the nearest fixed mAs to that selected automatical-ly for 5cm PMMA. 5cm was chosen because the CDMAM phantom with 4cm PMMA is equivalent to 5cm PMMA or a 6cm average breast. The same compression paddle (size 18 x 24cm) was used every time. Both the compressed breast thickness and the initial position of the phantom on the breast support table were the same for each set of measurements. The phantom was moved by a small distance, typically 1mm, between image acquisitions, as specified in the test protocol.

After acquiring each set of CDMAM images, the air kerma at the standard position was measured with an ion chamber to detect any variation in X-ray output.

Raw images were obtained from each system for subsequent analysis. The CDMAM images were analysed using the CDMAM Analyser version 1.5.1 software. For the images of 5cm PMMA, the mean glandular dose (MGD) to a 6cm thick equivalent breast was calculated by the method of Dance et al [6].

3   Results

Figure 1a, b, c, d shows the results of weekly contrast-detail measurements on the amorphous selenium system (Hologic Selenia Dimensions), for detail sizes 0.1, 0.25, 0.5 and 1mm. Figure 1e, f, g, h shows the corresponding results for the caesium iodide-amorphous silicon system (GE Essential). There was some variation from week to week but most of the results lay within ±10% of the mean for the Dimensions and ±13% of the mean for the Essential. Variation was greater for the 0.1mm and 1.0mm detail sizes than for the other details, as shown in Table 1.

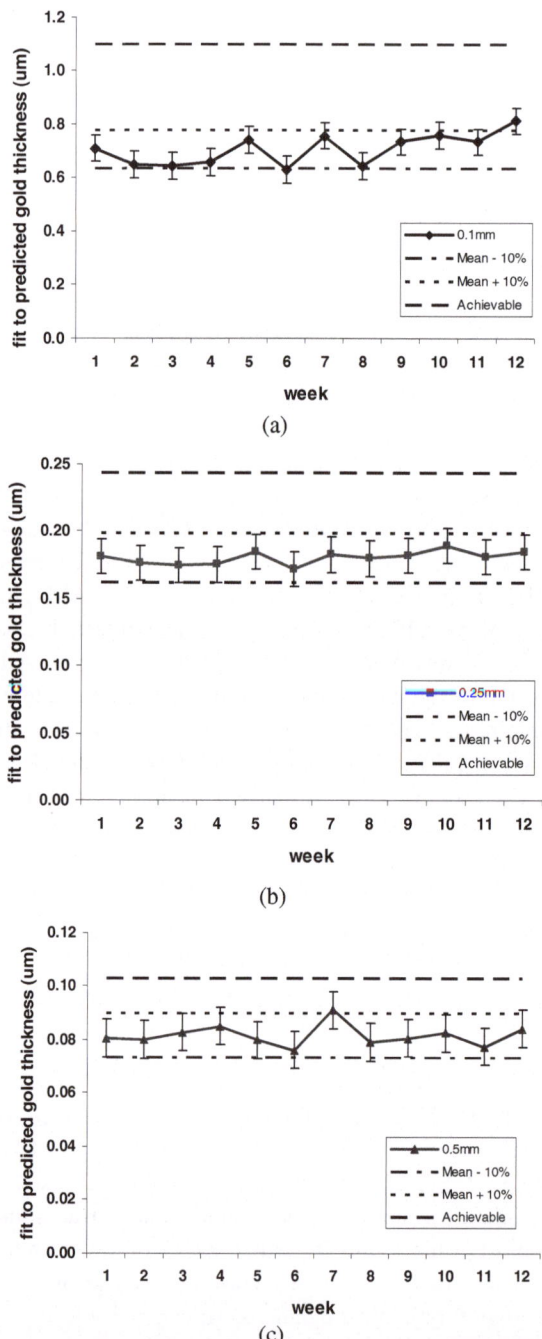

Fig. 1. Threshold-contrast measurements for the 0.1, 0.25, 0.5 and 1.0mm detail sizes, for a Hologic Selenia Dimensions (a, b, c, d) and a GE Essential (e, f, g, h). Error bars are 2 SE (standard error). The "Achievable" level is defined in the European Protocol [1].

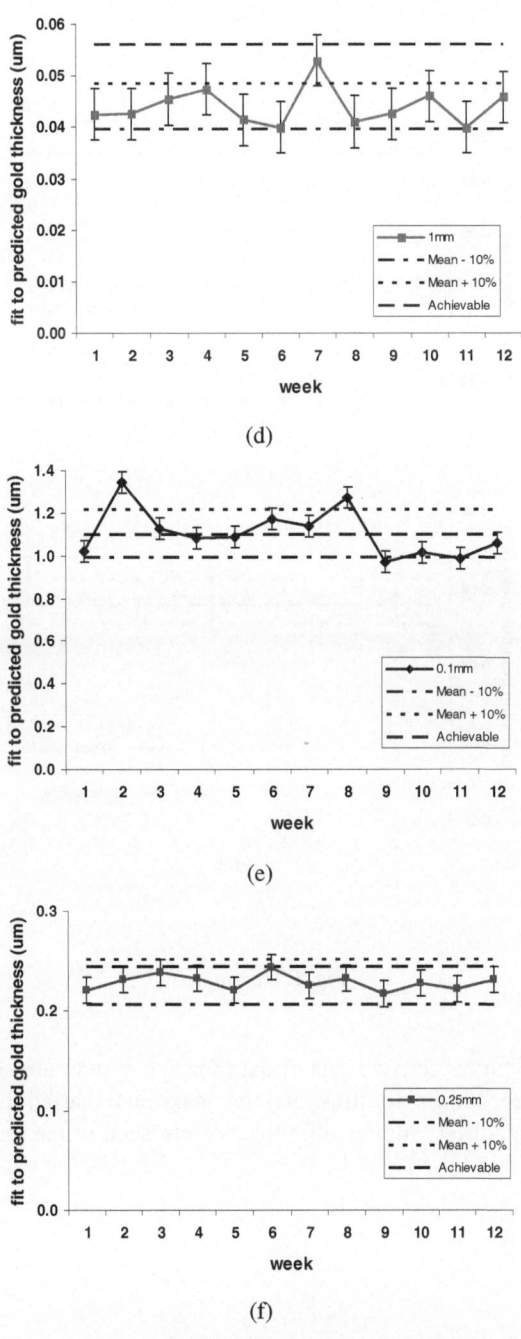

(d)

(e)

(f)

Fig. 1. (*continued*)

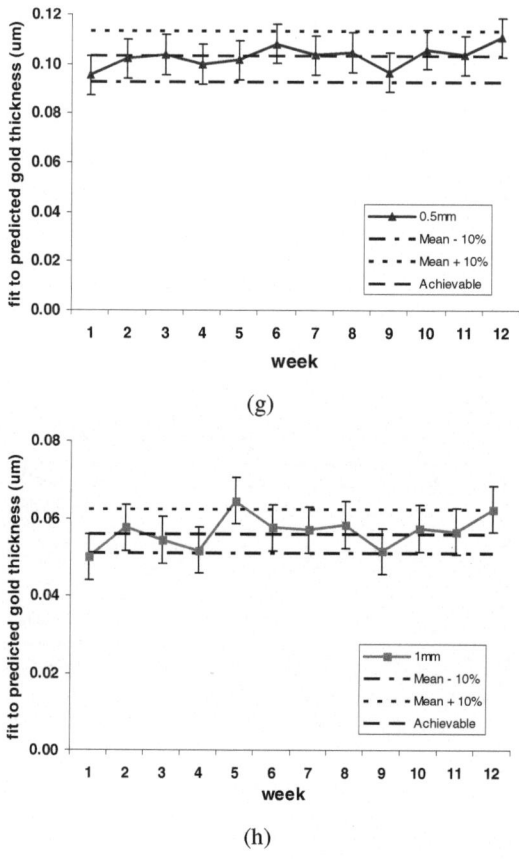

(g)

(h)

Fig. 1. (*continued*)

Contrast-detail curves for two sets of data for one system are shown in Figure 2. These curves were chosen to illustrate the maximum variation observed in the twelve data sets acquired. Similar differences were seen in the results for the other system.

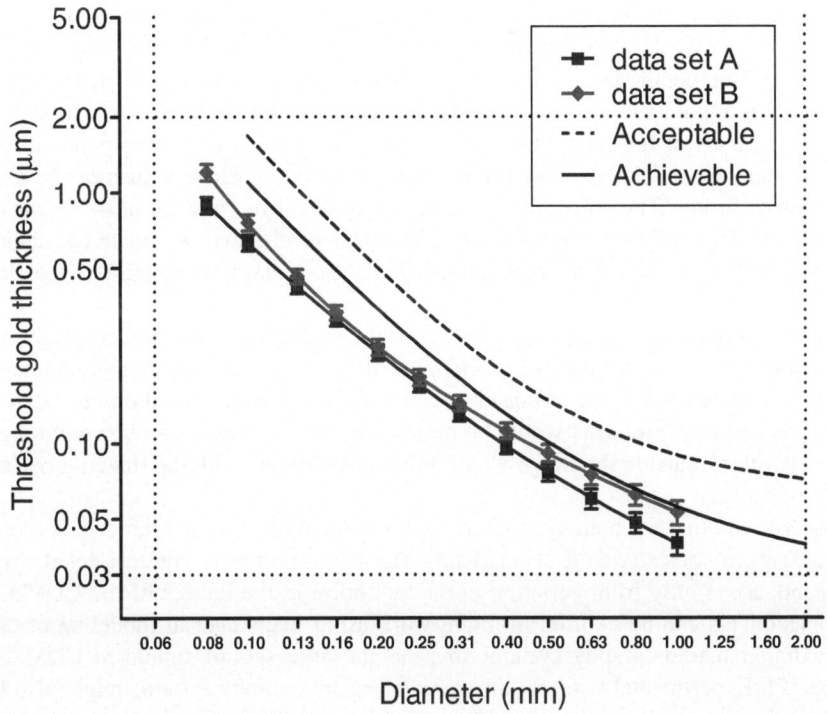

Fig. 2. Contrast-detail curves for two sets of measurements, for a Hologic Selenia Dimensions

The X-ray output showed much less variation over time. All the measured values were within ±1% of the mean.

Table 1. Coefficient of variance (CoV) estimated from the analysis software and measured values for two different digital mammography systems

Detail size (mm)	CoV estimated from analysis software	CoV measured: Hologic Selenia Dimensions	CoV measured: GE Essential
0.1	4%	8%	10%
0.25	4%	3%	4%
0.5	4%	5%	4%
1.0	5%	9%	8%

4   Discussion

Although the conditions of measurement were standardised, the threshold gold thicknesses determined by contrast-detail measurements varied from week to week. In most cases the values lay within a range of ±10% from the mean for the Hologic Selenia Dimensions and ±13% for the GE Essential. The coefficient of variance was greater (8-10%) for the smallest and largest detail sizes (0.1 and 1.0mm), than for the 0.25 and 0.5mm detail sizes (3-5%). It is clear from the contrast-detail curves shown in Figure 2 that points in the middle of the curve are likely to show less variation than those at the ends of the range. On the CDMAM test object, this corresponds to the smallest and largest details having fewer nearest neighbours whose values can be used in the curve-fitting. The software estimates a coefficient of variance of 4-5% for all detail sizes. This difference from the experimental results may be related to taking repeated smaller samples from a large pool of images, as has been suggested in earlier work [5].

Clearly an initial baseline value based on eight or sixteen measurements might not be suitable for setting a range (e.g. ±10%) within which subsequent measurements might be expected to lie, due to this observed variation. A value based on the mean of several sets of measurements would be more suitable in setting a baseline and range, such that values outside the range would indicate problems with the imaging performance of a system.

The X-ray output for both systems was stable to within ±1%, and the detector temperatures were constant, so it seems likely that the variation in contrast-detail measurements arises only from variation in random noise in the images of the CDMAM test object. This can be verified in future work using mathematical modeling of different digital mammography systems to generate large sets of simulated CDMAM images [7]. Experimental work on other digital mammography systems might also be worthwhile, as not all systems may be as stable in performance as those described here.

These results suggest a need for further development to improve the reproducibility of image quality measurements.

5   Conclusions

Over a period of about three months, contrast-detail measurements for two different digital mammography systems showed no obvious trends, but results mostly varied by up to 10% from the mean value for an amorphous selenium system and by up to ±13% for a caesium iodide-amorphous silicon system. Care should be taken when setting a baseline, and when interpreting a single set of measurements, as an increase or decrease within approximately ±10% or ±15% of the mean is unlikely to indicate a significant change in equipment performance.

References

1. European Commission (EC): European Guidelines for Quality Assurance in Breast Cancer Screening and Diagnosis, 4th edn. Office for Official Publications of the European Communities, Luxembourg (2006)

2. Young, K.C., Alsager, A., Oduko, J.M., Bosmans, H., Verbrugge, B., Geertse, T., Van Engen, R.: Evaluation of software for reading images of the CDMAM test object to assess digital mammography systems. In: Proceedings of SPIE Medical Imaging, 69131C, 1–11 (2008)

3. Young K.C., Cook J.J.H., Oduko J.M., Bosmans H.: Comparison of software and human observers in reading images of the CDMAM test object to assess digital mammography systems. In: Proceedings of SPIE Medical Imaging, vol. 614206, pp. 1–13 (2006)

4. Young, K.C., Cook, J.J.H., Oduko, J.M.: Automated and Human Determination of Threshold Contrast for Digital Mammography Systems. In: Astley, S.M., Brady, M., Rose, C., Zwiggelaar, R. (eds.) IWDM 2006. LNCS, vol. 4046, pp. 266–272. Springer, Heidelberg (2006)

5. Yang, C.-Y.J., Van Metter, R.: The variability of software scoring of the CDMAM phantom associated with a limited number of images. In: Proceedings of SPIE Medical Imaging, 65100C (2007)

6. Dance, D.R., Young, K.C., van Engen, R.E.: Further factors for the estimation of mean glandular dose using the United Kingdom, European and IAEA dosimetry protocols. Phys. Med. Biol. 54, 4361–4372 (2009)

7. Mackenzie, A., Dance, D.R., Workman, A., Yip, M., Wells, K., Young, K.C.: Development and validation of a method for converting images to appear with noise and sharpness characteristics of a different detector and X-ray system. Med. Phys. 39(5), 2721–2734 (2012)

Characterization of Spatial Luminance Noise in Stereoscopic Displays for Breast Imaging

Cecilia Marini-Bettolo*, Joel Wang, Wei-Chung Cheng,
Robert J. Jennings, and Aldo Badano

Division of Imaging and Applied Mathematics, Center for Devices and Radiological
Health, Food and Drug Administration, 10903 New Hampshire Ave, Silver Spring,
MD 20993 USA
cecilia.bettolo@fda.hhs.gov

Abstract. Stereoscopic displays are being considered for 3D breast imaging applications. Characterization of the physical properties of the display devices in terms of parameters of relevance for medical imaging tasks is needed. Among the set of relevant characteristics of stereoscopic displays, luminance noise introduced by the device has not been studied so far. We present two methods for measuring spatial noise in stereo displays, one visual and one quantitative, and report a comparison between them. We have applied both methods to a stereo-mirror display. The visual method is based on the TG18-AFC pattern. The quantitative method relies on the evaluation of the noise power spectrum (NPS) using high resolution images acquired with a photometric CCD camera. Both methods were tested on different stereo display configurations. The visual results show higher variability among observers compared to the 2D display mode. The NPS shows peaks corresponding to the pixel and sub-pixel structure.

1 Introduction

With the advent of digital imaging and the recent advancements in display technology, stereoscopic display techniques are now being reconsidered and rapidly being developed in several applications besides the medical field [1]. Stereoscopic displays have also been proposed for breast imaging. In standard 2D digital mammography lesions are hidden by underlying and overlying normal tissue, which is projected in one single 2D image. Stereoscopic digital mammography can help in unmasking lesions from normal anatomical background. This has been shown to increase sensitivity and specificity [2,3]. Similar volumetric information can be obtained with two orthogonal projections in standard 2D mammography, but it has been shown [4] that, in the case of stereo imaging, the dose delivered is lower, due to binocular summation by the human visual system. Stereoscopic display techniques can also be used for the visualization of 3D medical sets. For example in Ref. [5] stereo has been shown to improve detection performance of lung nodules in CT data sets compared to other methods.

Methods for the characterization of 2D display systems have been extensively analyzed [6,7]. However, methods for testing 3D stereo displays are only just

---

* Corresponding author.

A.D.A. Maidment, P.R. Bakic, and S. Gavenonis (Eds.): IWDM 2012, LNCS 7361, pp. 220–227, 2012.

now beginning to be developed. In particular, methods for noise and resolution have not been addressed in the literature. In this work we discuss a spatial noise characterization methodology as applied to a stereo-mirror display. Two different methods to estimate the spatial luminance noise of a stereo display system are used and compared: a visual method based on the use of the TG18-AFC pattern [8] performed by 12 observers, and a quantitative method based on the evaluation of noise power spectrum (NPS) and variance, σ^2.

2   Methods

2.1   Display

The two methods were tested on a stereo-mirror display (courtesy of A. Abileah, Planar Systems, Inc.). The system is schematized in Fig. 1. This device is based on the separation of the two stereo views using linear polarization and consists of two LCDs, a half-mirror, and passive cross-polarized glasses. The two LCDs have an angular separation of 110° and the mirror is placed on the bisect plane between the two displays. The image of the lower display is transmitted with no change in polarization, whereas the image of the upper display is reflected by the mirror. Through reflection the image gets polarized at 90° and mirrored. The right lens (RL) transmits the bottom image and blocks the upper one, whereas the left lens (LL) operates in the opposite way. Since the image of the top LCD is specular due to reflection on the mirror, the top image has to be inverted before sending it to the LCD. The images coming out of the glasses are reconstructed by the observer in one 3D image through stereopsis. The display system requires an alignment. This is done by looking at the same image on both displays (see Fig.1). The tilt of the mirror is adjusted, by means of two screws located beneath the mirror support, until the two images coincide.

The monitors are two identical 20″ displays (PL201OM-BK, Planar). The spatial noise is due to variations in luminance across the screen and to the pixel structure. Each pixel is composed of 3 sub-pixels and inactive area connecting them, as shown in Fig. 2.

2.2   Visual Method

In order to perform a visual analysis of noise in a stereo display, a visual experiment was designed that provides a numerical score for different display configurations. Using the display described above, 6 test scenarios were created (see Table 1). The user was asked to position his head at about 40 cm away from the screen. The experiments were performed in a dark laboratory. Depending on which scenario was being tested, one or both monitors were switched on, the mirror was set in place, and the user wore polarized glasses. The TG18-AFC test pattern [8], used to evaluate noise for 2D displays, was displayed. The pattern is organized into 4 quadrants each with different signal sizes. Each quadrant consists of 58 (59) squares for the top quadrants (bottom quadrants), containing

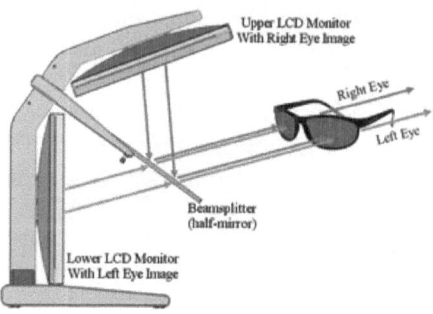

Fig. 1. Set up of stereo-mirror display: two LCD monitors placed oriented at 110°, half-mirror on the bisect-plane, and passive cross-polarized glasses. The right eye will see the mirrored 90° polarized image, whereas the left eye will perceive the image from the bottom display (Planar Systems, Inc.).

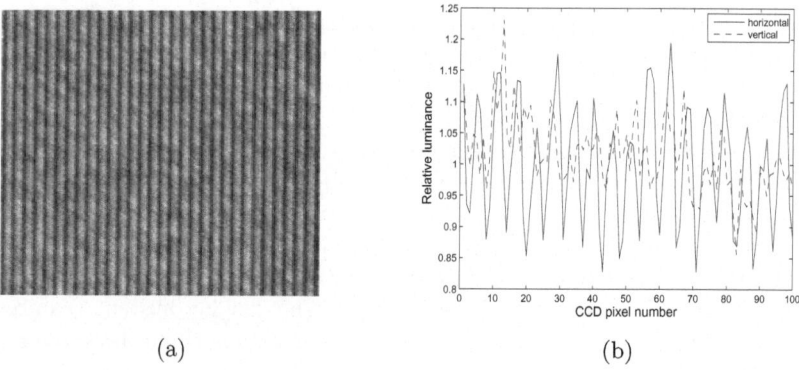

(a)   (b)

Fig. 2. a) Image of display acquired with high resolution CCD camera. b) Vertical and horizontal profiles of top image.

signals. The user was asked to label which signals were visible in each of the squares in the test pattern. After the user had finished the first 3 scenarios, the test image was rotated to prevent the user from unconsciously memorizing the signal locations, and thus skewing the results.

A total of 12 observers performed the test, 6 males and 6 females within the age of 18-30 years, 50% of whom had corrected vision. No stereo visual check was performed on the readers.

2.3   Quantitative Method

For the evaluation of NPS and σ^2, all the elements of the stereoscopic system were measured together, and left and right eye views were tested separately. The luminance noise was estimated using high-resolution images of a uniform pattern displayed on the stereo display. The images were acquired with a photometric CCD camera (Lumetrix P144F, Westboro Photonics). The grey level was set to 230, the

Table 1. Visual analysis setup configurations

Experiment	bottom screen	top screen	mirror	glasses
a	pattern	off		
b	pattern	pattern	x	x
c	pattern	off	x	x
d	pattern	uniform	x	x
e	off	pattern	x	x
f	uniform	pattern	x	x

same value as the background of the test pattern used for the visual method. The camera consisted of an array of 1392×1032 4.65 μm pixels coupled to a macro lens, Nikon AF Micro-Nikkor (60 mm f/2.8D), with aperture set to f/11. This aperture reduces the veiling glare inside the camera and maximizes the depth of field allowing objects not exactly on the true focal plane to be captured with relatively good sharpness. The camera was at a distance of 100 cm from the bottom display, on a rail parallel to the bottom display, and it could move parallel to the display, horizontally and vertically. This alignment ensured constant magnification within one image (CCD plane) and between different images (across the display plane) (see Fig. 3). A second alignment was needed to have the pixel arrays of the CCD and display aligned. The displays support was tilted slightly, until the pixel columns of the display were vertical on the CCD image.

The glasses were mounted 1 cm in front of the camera, and, in order to facilitate switching between the two lenses, they were free to move parallel to the display plane. The left lens (LL) is the one paired to the bottom screen and the right lens (RL) is the one paired to the top screen. In order to reduce cross talk between the two lenses, it is crucial that the polarization axes of the lenses be parallel and orthogonal to the polarization axes of the images. This was ensured by a level placed on the bow connecting the lenses.

Different configurations, listed in Table 2, have been used to measure the noise of the stereo display. The measurements were performed in a dark laboratory, to minimize direct illumination of the camera and reflection. The displays were switched on 20 min before acquisition. A series of dark images were taken, which were required by the software (Lumetrix RT32) supplied with the camera, to flat-field correct the images.

The optimal focus setting was determined by manually rotating the focus ring of the lens until the image appeared visually in focus. This procedure had been tested to be satisfactory for the noise evaluation measurement. The images were acquired with the same software. The corrected luminance maps were saved in ASCII format, and read with MATLAB into matrices of 1032×1392 pixels. The regions at the edge of the CCD chip (64 pixels on each side) were discarded, resulting in an image of 968×1328 pixels. For each image the variance, σ^2, was computed:

$$\sigma^2 = \sum_{i=1}^{G} \sum_{j=1}^{H} (I(i,j) - \bar{I})^2 \tag{1}$$

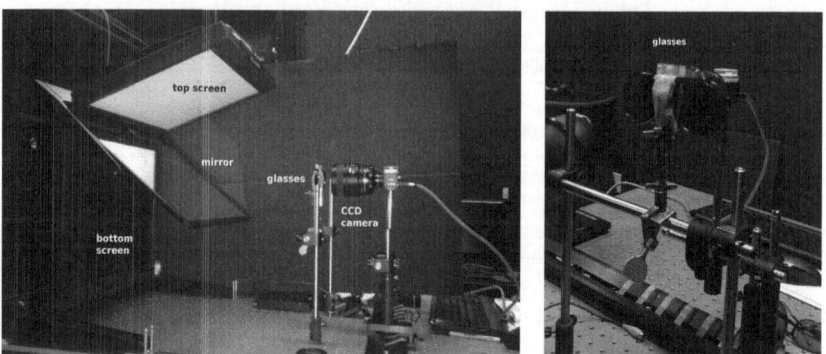

Fig. 3. Setup used to estimate noise luminance: (left) side view and (right) front view

Table 2. List of different configurations used to measure NPS of the stereo display system

Experiment	bottom screen	top screen	mirror	left lens LL	right lens RL
1	on				
2	on	on	x	x	
3	on	on	x		x
4	on		x	x	
5		on	x		x
6	on		x		x
7		on	x	x	

where G and H are the image dimensions, $I(i,j)$ the luminance value for the pixel of coordinates (i,j) and $\bar{I}$ is the mean luminance value of the image. The variance was used to calculate the coefficient of variation, COV, defined as:

$$COV = 100\sigma/\bar{I} \tag{2}$$

The noise power spectrum, NPS, was used to quantify the frequency content of the variations. The image was divided in square areas of 128×128 pixels, ROIs, and the 2-dimensional Fast Fourier Transform (FFT) was applied to each ROI:

$$nps(u_n, v_k) = \sum_{i,j=1}^{128} I(i,j)e^{-2i\pi(u_n i + v_k j)} \tag{3}$$

The NPS is defined as the average of the squared absolute value of the FFT of each ROI [9]:

$$NPS(u_n, v_k) = \frac{(\Delta x)^2}{M \cdot 128 \cdot 128} \sum_{m=1}^{M} |nps(u_n, v_k)|^2 \tag{4}$$

where Δx is the CCD camera pixel size, M is the number of ROIs and u_n, v_k are frequency components. The NPS was then normalized by dividing by the relative signal power, i.e., σ^2, and then frequency reorganized, and the 3 central columns and rows were eliminated, which correspond to the zero frequency. In order to have a lower limit for the noise measurements, the NPS of the CCD camera was measured. Images of a uniform illuminated scene, generated with an integrating sphere, were acquired. The luminance level of this had been set to the same value used for the NPS measurement of the display, and measured with a photometer.

3   Results

3.1   Visual Method

For the visual tests, the percentage of correct signal detection was calculated. Each user was given four scores per test scenario, one for each quadrant of the test pattern. Fig. 4(a) shows that in the first quadrant almost all users could see all the signals. However, in quadrant 2, most users begin to show a decline in signal detection accuracy. The results for the second quadrant show a good spread, see Fig. 4(a), separately plotted in Fig. 4(b). The overall group scores for each different scenario are shown in Fig. 4(b). The observer variability for stereo viewing increases compared to the 2D mode (configuration a in Table 1).

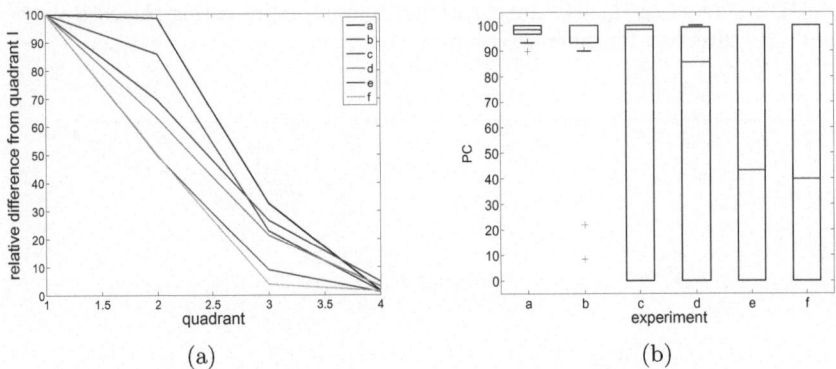

(a)   (b)

Fig. 4. a) Percentage of signal detection for each quadrant respect to the first quadrant. The different curves indicate the different setups used. b) Percentage of correct signal detection for quadrant 2 as a function of different setups. The edges of the box indicate the 25% and 75% percentage of correct detection, the whiskers extend to the most extreme data points, not considered outliers. The outliers are shown with markers.

3.2   Quantitative Method

First the σ^2 and NPS were estimated for different regions across the bottom display. Since the luminance varies across the display, each image was corrected with an offset to match one image chosen as reference.

The camera was placed in the center of the display and images of the different setups listed in Table 2 were acquired for the NPS evaluation. The results are shown as 1D traces along the 64th pixel row and column (see Fig. 5), representing the NPS in the x and y direction. The NPS peaks at a frequency values of 39 mm^{-1}, 78 mm^{-1} and 117 mm^{-1}, corresponding to the size of the pixel and subpixels of 26 μm, 13 μm and 8.5 μm. The 1D NPS traces of the CCD are shown in Fig. 6(a).

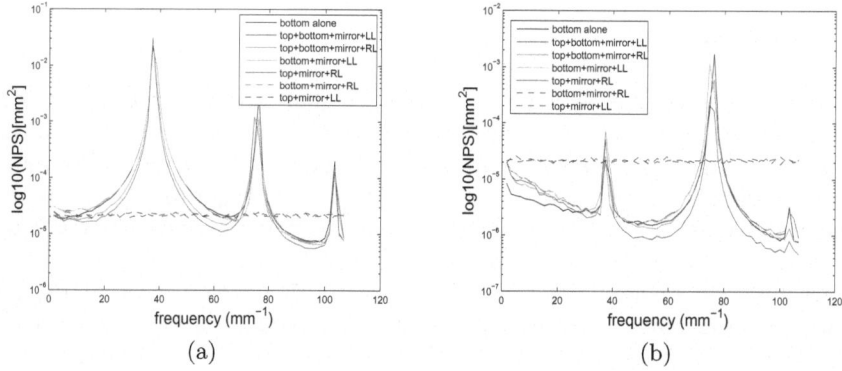

Fig. 5. 1D traces along the 64th pixel row and column, representing the NPS in the x (a) and y (b) direction for different setups

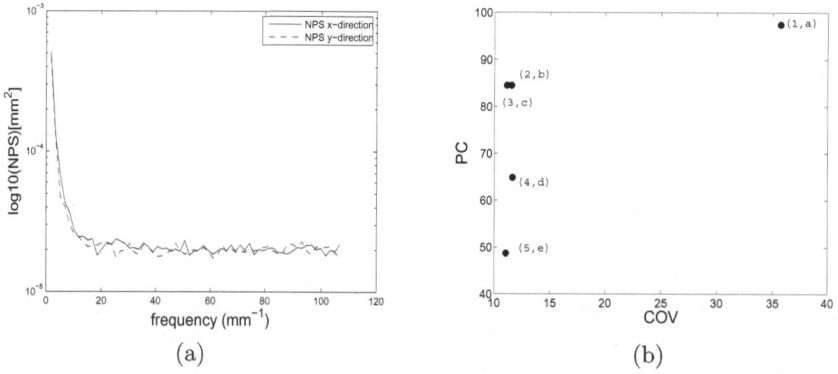

Fig. 6. a) Noise power spectrum of CCD camera. b) Comparison visual and quantitative results: on the y-axis the percentage of correct signal identification (visual), on the x-axis the coefficient of variation (quantitative).

3.3   Discussion

The visual noise results relative to quadrant 2 are compared with the quantitative results in Fig. 6(b). The data appear uncorrelated, suggesting that the visual test is not applicable to stereo-systems. We speculate that in the visual method the observer suffers from signal cross talk since the head is free to move, whereas when the camera is used, the lenses are aligned with the axes of polarization. If this holds the two methods should be correlated in the 2D mode. This could be tested with different displays. Our analysis needs to be extended to different stereo displays technologies, as well as to a range of luminance levels.

4   Conclusions

The aim of this study was to assess methodologies to estimate spatial noise in stereo display systems. Two methods, visual and quantitative, have been applied. Both methods appear to be uncorrelated, which implies that the visual method might not be applicable to stereo display systems. More research is needed to characterize noise, in particular for mammography stereo devices. In future work the noise characterization will be complemented with a study of resolution of the display and CCD system.

Acknowledgments. The authors would like to thank Rachel Wilk for the assistance during the visual tests.

References

1. Abileah, A.: Technologies and testing methods. Journal of the SID 19(11) (2011)
2. Getty, D.J., D'Orsi, C.J., Pickett, R.M.: Stereoscopic Digital Mammography: Improved Accuracy of Lesion Detection in Breast Cancer Screening. In: Krupinski, E.A. (ed.) IWDM 2008. LNCS, vol. 5116, pp. 74–79. Springer, Heidelberg (2008)
3. Webb, L.J., et al.: Comparative performance of multiview stereoscopic and mammographic display modalities for breast detection. Medical Physics (2011)
4. Maidment, A.D.A., Bakic, P.R., Albert, M.: Effects of quantum noise in binocular summation on dose requirements in stereography. Medical Physics 30 (2003)
5. Wang, X.H., et al.: Compare display schemes for lung nodule CT screening. Journal of Digital Imaging (2010)
6. Badano, A., et al.: Noise in flat-panel displays with subpixels structure. Medical Physics 31 (2004)
7. Saunders, R., Samei, E.: Resolution and noise measurements of five CRT and LCD medical displays. Medical Physics 33 (2006)
8. Assessment of display performance for medical imaging systems. AAPM on-line report no. 03 (2005)
9. IEC, IEC 62220-2-1. Medical electrical equipment - Characteristics of digital X-ray imaging devices. tech. rep., IEC (2007)

Volumetric and Area-Based Breast Density Measurement in the Predicting Risk of Cancer at Screening (PROCAS) Study

Jamie C. Sergeant[1], Jane Warwick[2], D. Gareth Evans[3], Anthony Howell[3],
Michael Berks[1], Paula Stavrinos[3], Sarah Sahin[3], Mary Wilson[3], Alan Hufton[1],
Iain Buchan[4], and Susan M. Astley[1]

[1] School of Cancer and Enabling Sciences,
University of Manchester, Oxford Road, Manchester M13 9PT, UK
[2] Imperial Clinical Trials Unit, School of Public Health,
Imperial College London, London W2 1PG, UK
[3] Nightingale Centre and Genesis Prevention Centre,
University Hospital of South Manchester,
Manchester M23 9LT, UK
[4] School of Community Based Medicine, University of Manchester, Oxford Road,
Manchester M13 9PL
jamie.sergeant@manchester.ac.uk

Abstract. Mammographic density, defined as the proportion of the breast area in a mammogram that contains fibroglandular tissue, is associated with risk of breast cancer. However, measures of mammographic density are subject to variation in the underlying imaging process and in the assessments of observers. Automatic volumetric measures of breast density remove much of this variability, but their association with risk is less well established. We present density measurements produced using area-based visual analogue scales (VAS) and by volumetric assessment software (Quantra™, Hologic Inc.) in the PROCAS study. The distributions of VAS scores (n = 22 327) and volumetric quantities (n = 11 653) are given, as are their relationships for subjects with results by both (n = 11 096), but these are not directly comparable as one is area-based and the other volumetric. Inter-observer variability in visual area-based estimation is examined by a scatter plot matrix.

Keywords: Breast density, area-based measures, volumetric measures, inter-observer variation, Quantra.

1   Introduction

The association between high mammographic breast density and increased risk of developing breast cancer is well established for area-based measures of density [1]. In such measures, density is usually defined as the proportion of the breast area, as

A.D.A. Maidment, P.R. Bakic, and S. Gavenonis (Eds.): IWDM 2012, LNCS 7361, pp. 228–235, 2012.

projected on a mammogram, that contains radiopaque fibroglandular tissue rather than radiolucent adipose tissue. Although area-based measures of breast density have been shown to be related to breast cancer risk, they do have drawbacks. Firstly, as density is measured from the two-dimensional projection of the breast on the mammogram image, measurements are subject to change if the breast is positioned or compressed differently. Secondly, many area-based methods of measuring breast density depend upon the subjective assessments of a human observer. Such area-based methods include classification schemes such as the American College of Radiology Breast Imaging Reporting and Data System (BI-RADS) breast composition categories [2], Boyd categories [4], visual assessment on a continuous percentage scale and semi-automated interactive thresholding methods such as Cumulus (Sunnybrook Health Sciences Centre, Toronto, Canada) [3].

Volumetric measures of breast density aim to improve upon area-based measures by estimating the volume of dense tissue in the breast rather than its projection on a mammogram. Such measures should provide more precise estimates of the amount of dense tissue and therefore, as breast cancer generally originates in such tissue, could more accurately describe the relationship between density and risk. However, volumetric methods are a recent development and are yet to surpass area-based density measures as predictors of breast cancer risk [16], which may be due to refinements in methodology being required, or due to the relatively small amount of follow-up data available to date. Volumetric methods can provide data on the quantity of glandular tissue independently of the quantity of fatty tissue in the breast, hence they may also prove to be a more consistent indicator of risk than area-based measures, as there is evidence that fluctuations in a woman's weight are reflected in the amount of fat in their breasts [7]. In addition, many volumetric methods are fully automated and so also eliminate observer variability from density estimates. Volumetric measures can be divided into those in which the signal from the mammography unit, in terms of the pixel values of a digitised film or unprocessed ("raw") full-field digital mammography (FFDM) image, is calibrated using differing thicknesses of tissue equivalent materials [8-12], and those where an imaging physics model is employed, such as Standard Mammogram Form [13] for screen-film mammography, and Quantra^{TM} [14] and Volpara^{TM} [15] for FFDM.

Research into the measurement of breast density for breast cancer risk prediction takes place against a backdrop of wider research into the estimation of breast cancer risk. In particular, large-scale studies such as the Predicting Risk Of Cancer At Screening (PROCAS) study [5-6], based in Manchester, UK, and the Swedish Karma study [17] are attempting to predict breast cancer risk on an individual level for patients attending breast screening. Although current risk models typically do not include breast density as a component of risk, there is some evidence that they would benefit from doing so [18-19]. In the current work preliminary density results from the PROCAS study, both area-based and volumetric, are presented.

2   Method

2.1   The PROCAS Study

The PROCAS (Predicting Risk Of breast Cancer At Screening) study is collecting risk information at the time of routine breast screening, calculating individual breast cancer risk from this information and feeding back the calculated risk to the patient, with the aim of facilitating risk-reducing interventions where appropriate. The study aims to recruit 60 000 participants from those invited to screening by the Greater Manchester Breast Screening Programme, part of the UK NHS Breast Screening Programme, and has to date recruited over 38 000. Those who consent to join the study fill in a questionnaire, from which data on their family history of breast cancer, and lifestyle and hormonal risk factors is extracted and used to estimate their risk of developing breast cancer using the Tyrer-Cuzik model [20]. Breast density data is obtained using the screening mammograms, and approximately 10% of those recruited provide a saliva sample for genetic analysis. Currently the study feeds back risk information to those women classified as high risk, defined as having a Tyrer-Cuzick 10-year risk of at least 8% or a 10-year risk of at least 5% and area-based breast density in the top 10% among study participants, and to a subset of those deemed to be at low risk, defined as having a 10-year risk of less than 1.5% and area-based density of 10% or lower.

2.2   Density Measurement in PROCAS

Area-based density estimation in PROCAS is provided by visual assessment, recorded on a visual analogue scale (VAS). Two mammogram readers from a pool of 13 radiologists and advanced practitioner radiographers independently view a subject's mammograms and mark their percentage density estimates on a set of 10cm horizontal lines labelled 0% and 100% at the ends. Each of the two readers estimates the density for the mediolateral oblique (MLO) and craniocaudal (CC) views of each breast. The VAS readings are scanned and automatically converted to percentages. Values are averaged across the four views, and the two readers' averages combined to produce a single estimate for each subject. Assignment of readers to subjects is not predetermined, and depends on workflow. Reading is blind in the sense that readers do not know the identity of the second reader and cannot see their results.

Volumetric density estimation is provided by the assessment software Quantra[TM] (Version 1.3; Hologic Inc.). Raw FFDM mammogram images from screening are retained and processed by Quantra[TM]. Breast volume, glandular tissue volume and percentage density (their ratio) are given per breast rather than per individual view, and the average of the results for the two breasts is then taken as the single Quantra[TM] percentage density estimate.

To aid the illustration of results from the methods, only VAS results for FFDM mammograms are presented here. It has been observed in the PROCAS study that VAS results for screen-film mammography tend to be lower than those for FFDM. We present the VAS results for 22 327 subjects and Quantra^{TM} results for 11 653 subjects. The distribution of these density estimates is displayed, as is the relationship between the VAS and Quantra^{TM} measures for the 11 096 subjects that have results by both methods. To illustrate the inter-reader variation present in the VAS density estimates, a scatter plot matrix of VAS estimates by individual readers is shown.

3   Results

The histograms of results produced by VAS and Quantra^{TM} displayed in Fig. 1 show that the VAS density estimates take a much larger range of values than those produced by Quantra^{TM}, with the VAS estimates tending to take lower values: the median VAS density is 21.38% (IQR: 12.12-33.38) and the median Quantra^{TM} density is 15.50% (IQR: 13.00-19.00). For Quantra^{TM} gland volume and breast volume the medians are 89.0 cm^3 (IQR: 63.0-126.0) and 556 cm^3 (IQR: 370.5-805.0) respectively.

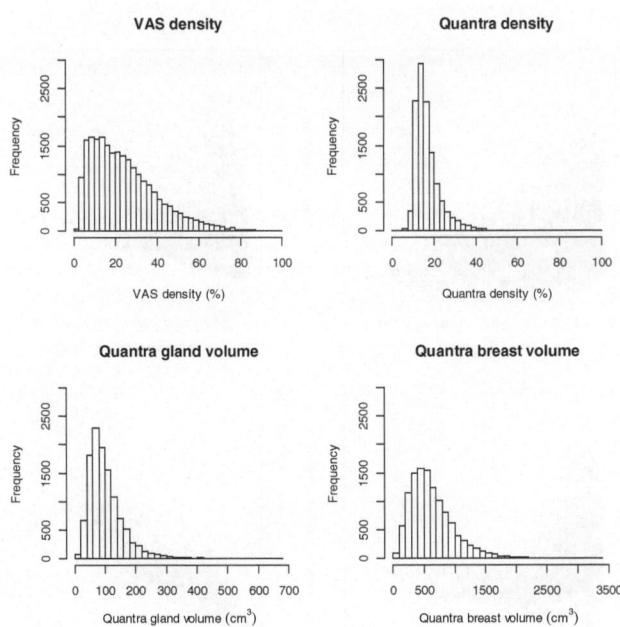

Fig. 1. Histograms of VAS density estimates and Quantra^{TM} density, breast volume and gland volume estimates

Fig. 2 contains pairwise scatterplots of the four variables from Fig. 1 for subjects with both VAS and Quantra^{TM} density results. As one would expect from volumetric and area-based measures, Quantra^{TM} density broadly increases with VAS density, and in a non-linear manner. Also in line with expectations is Quantra^{TM} gland volume increasing with breast volume, which it is of course bounded by. It is interesting to note that both the larger VAS and Quantra[TM] densities tend to occur at more moderate values of gland volume and particularly breast volume. Fig. 3 shows a scatter plot matrix for the individual VAS results produced by the 13 readers. The departures from the lines of perfect concordance show the extent of variation in the readers' opinions. In the absence of a ground truth, it not possible to assess reader accuracy with this data, only inter-reader variation.

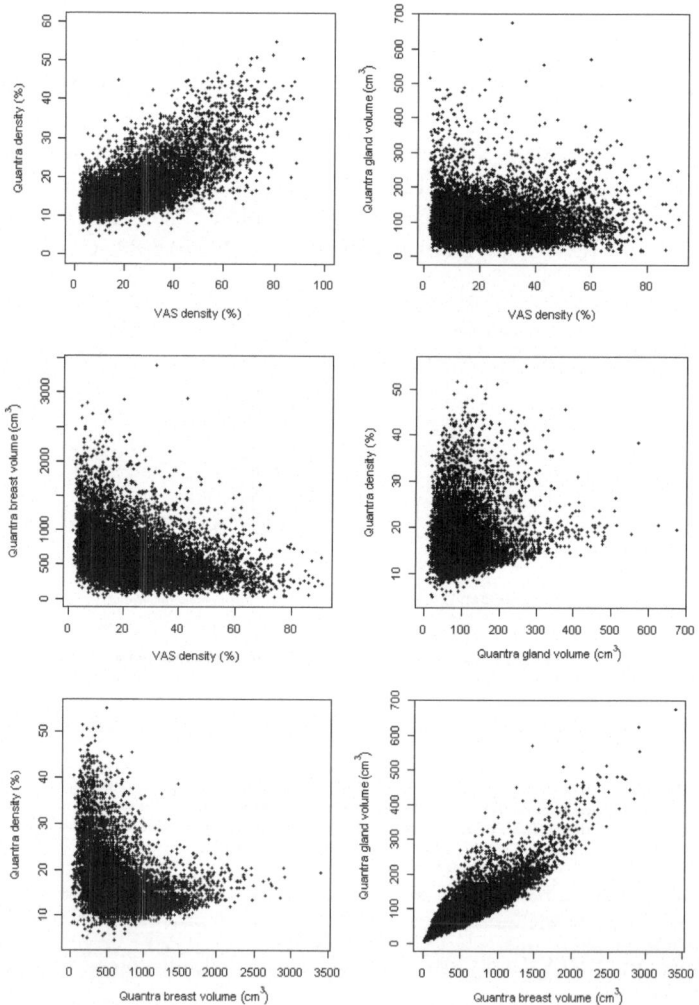

Fig. 2. Pairwise scatterplots of VAS and Quantra[TM] density variables for subjects with results by both methods

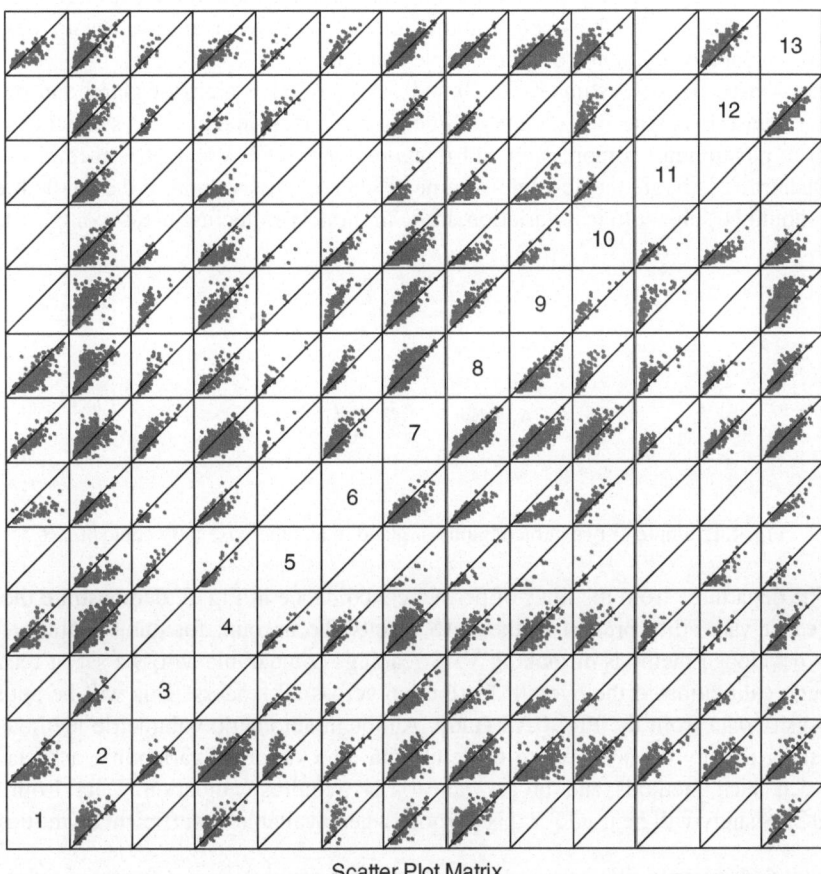

Scatter Plot Matrix

Fig. 3. Scatter plot matrix of VAS density estimates by individual readers, labelled 1 to 13. Plot (i,j) contains all subjects whose density was estimated by both Readers i and j. Each plot contains the line of perfect concordance.

4 Discussion

While the plots in Fig. 1 and Fig 2 show different distributions of breast density estimates by the area-based VAS and the volumetric Quantra^{TM}, it is our assertion that a direct comparison is inappropriate. A trivial example of the difference between area-based and volumetric density measurement is shown in Fig. 4, where the two smaller cubes represent regions of gland in an otherwise fatty breast. In a projection in which the glandular regions completely coincide (A) an area-based method will show one square unit of dense tissue, whilst in a different projection of the same breast (B), the measured area would be two square units. A volumetric measure would always yield a volume of two cubic units of glandular tissue. In reality the situation is compounded by variations in shape and density, but the limitations of attempting to derive a mathematical relationship between volumetric and area-based approaches to density measurement are apparent from this simple example.

Area-based density estimates are based on the relative areas of gland and of the whole breast in a projection on a two-dimensional image, and are thus subject to variation in positioning, compression and imaging conditions. Volumetric methods such as Quantra^{TM} estimate the absolute volume of glandular tissue and of the whole breast and should be subject to less variation, more accurately reflecting breast composition.

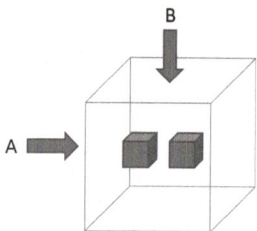

Fig. 4. Example of two cubic regions of gland in an otherwise fatty cubic breast

The departures from the lines of perfect concordance in Fig. 3, demonstrate the inter-reader variability present in the VAS results. To account for this variability, we have developed methods of making VAS readings comparable across a set of readers through calibration to the overall distribution across all readers. This will be applied to density data from the PROCAS study. Although automatic volumetric methods of assessing density do not have to contend with inter-observer variability, association between such methods and breast cancer risk requires validation. Data from the PROCAS study will be used for this purpose when available in sufficient quantities.

Acknowledgements. We acknowledge the support of the National Insitute for Health Research (NIHR) and the Genesis Breast Cancer Prevention Appeal. We would like to thank the study radiologists and advanced radiographer practitioners for VAS reading. We would also like to thank the many radiographers in the screening programme, the study centre staff for recruitment and data collection, and Hologic Inc. for providing the Quantra^{TM} software. This paper presents independent research commissioned by the National Institute for Health Research (NIHR) under its Programme Grant (Reference Number RP-PG-0707-10031). The views expressed are those of the author(s) and not necessarily those of the NHS, the NIHR or the Department of Health.

References

1. McCormack, V.A., dos Santos Silva, I.: Breast density and parenchymal patterns as markers of breast cancer risk: a meta-analysis. Cancer Epidemiol. Biomarkers Prev. 15, 1159–1169 (2006)
2. D'Orsi, C.J., et al.: Breast imaging reporting and data system: ACR BI-RADS. Breast Imaging Atlas. American College of Radiology, Reston (2003)

3. Byng, J.W., Boyd, N.F., Fishell, E., Jong, R.A., Yaffe, M.J.: The quantitative analysis of mammographic densities. Phys. Med. Biol. 39, 1629–1638 (1994)
4. Boyd, N.F., et al.: Mammographic density and the risk and detection of breast cancer. N. Engl. J. Med. 356, 227–236 (2007)
5. Evans, D.G., Warwick, J., Astley, S.M., et al.: Assessing individual breast cancer risk within the UK National Health Service Breast Screening Programme: a new paradigm for cancer prevention. Cancer Prevention Research (forthcoming)
6. Howell, A., Astley, S., Warwick, J., et al.: Prevention of breast cancer in the context of a national breast screening programme. Journal of Internal Medicine 271, 321–330 (2012)
7. Patel, H.G., Astley, S.M., Hufton, A.P., Harvie, M., Hagan, K., Marchant, T.E., Hillier, V., Howell, A., Warren, R., Boggis, C.R.M.: Automated Breast Tissue Measurement of Women at Increased Risk of Breast Cancer. In: Astley, S.M., Brady, M., Rose, C., Zwiggelaar, R. (eds.) IWDM 2006. LNCS, vol. 4046, pp. 131–136. Springer, Heidelberg (2006)
8. Kaufhold, J., Thomas, J.A., Eberhard, J.W., Galbo, C.E., Gonzalez Trotter, D.E.: A calibration approach to glandular tissue composition estimation in digital mammography. Med. Phys. 29, 1867–1880 (2002)
9. Pawluczyk, O., Augustine, B.J., Yaffe, M.J., Rico, D., Yang, J., Mawdsley, G.E.: A volumetric method for estimation of breast density in digitised screen-film mammograms. Med. Phys. 30, 352–364 (2003)
10. Diffey, J., Hufton, A., Astley, S.: A New Step-Wedge for the Volumetric Measurement of Mammographic Density. In: Astley, S.M., Brady, M., Rose, C., Zwiggelaar, R. (eds.) IWDM 2006. LNCS, vol. 4046, pp. 1–9. Springer, Heidelberg (2006)
11. Yaffe, M.J., Boone, J.M., Packard, N., et al.: The myth of the 50-50 breast. Med. Phys. 36, 5437–5443 (2009)
12. Malkov, S., Wang, J., Kerlikowske, K., Cummings, S.R., Shepherd, J.A.: Single x-ray absorptiometry method for the quantitative mammographic measure of fibroglandular tissue volume. Med. Phys. 36, 5525–5536 (2009)
13. Highnam, R.P., Pan, X., Warren, R., et al.: Breast composition measurements using retrospective SMF. Phys. Med. Biol. 51, 2695–2713 (2006)
14. Hartman, K., Highnam, R., Warren, R., Jackson, V.: Volumetric Assessment of Breast Tissue Composition from FFDM Images. In: Krupinski, E.A. (ed.) IWDM 2008. LNCS, vol. 5116, pp. 33–39. Springer, Heidelberg (2008)
15. Highnam, R., Brady, S.M., Yaffe, M.J., Karssemeijer, N., Harvey, J.: Robust Breast Composition Measurement - Volpara™. In: Martí, J., Oliver, A., Freixenet, J., Martí, R. (eds.) IWDM 2010. LNCS, vol. 6136, pp. 342–349. Springer, Heidelberg (2010)
16. Assi, V., et al.: Clinical and epidemiological issues in mammographic density. Nat. Rev. Clin. Oncol. 9, 33–40 (2012)
17. Karma: Karolinska Mammography Project for Risk Prediction of Breast Cancer, http://karmastudy.org/
18. Tice, J.A., Cummings, S.R., Ziv, E., Kerlikowske, K.: Mammographic breast density and the gail model for breast cancer risk prediction in a screening population. Breast Cancer Res. Treat. 94, 115–122 (2005)
19. Chen, J., Pee, D., Ayyagari, R., et al.: Projecting absolute invasive breast cancer risk in white women with a model that includes mammographic density. J. Natl. Cancer Inst. 98, 1215–1226 (2006)
20. Tyrer, J., Duffy, S.W., Cuzick, J.: A breast cancer prediction model incorporating familial and personal risk factors. Stat. Med. 23, 1111–1130 (2004)

Breast Cancer Risk Prediction via Area and Volumetric Estimates of Breast Density

Brad M. Keller[*], Emily F. Conant, Huen Oh, and Despina Kontos

Department of Radiology, University of Pennsylvania, Philadelphia, PA USA
Brad.Keller@uphs.upenn.edu

Abstract. We performed a study to assess the potential value of absolute and relative measures of area and volumetric breast density in predicting breast cancer risk. A case-control study was performed. The raw mediolateral-oblique (MLO) view digital mammography (DM) images of 106 women with unilateral breast cancer and 318 age-matched controls were retrospectively analyzed. The unaffected breast of the cancer cases was used as a surrogate of higher cancer risk. For each image, area and volumetric breast density measures were estimated using fully-automated software. The performance of the density metrics to distinguish between cancer cases and controls was assessed using linear discriminant and ROC curve analysis. Absolute measures of dense tissue content had stronger discriminatory capacity (AUCs=0.65-0.67) than percent density (AUCs=0.57). Shape-location features also showed modest discriminatory power (AUC=0.56-0.65). A combined area-volumetric model was able to outperform (AUC=0.70) any single-feature model. Absolute measures of fibroglandular tissue content were seen to be more discriminative than percent density estimates, indicating that total fibroglandular tissue content may be more reflective of cancer risk than relative measures of density. Our results suggest that area and volumetric breast density measures could be complementary in breast cancer risk assessment.

Keywords: Volumetric breast density, digital mammography, breast cancer risk.

1 Introduction

Breast cancer is the most commonly diagnosed cancer in women and is the second leading cause of cancer death in women in the United States [1]. Work by Gail *et al.* has shown that several factors are associated with an increased risk for developing breast cancer, such as current age, age at menarche, age at first live birth, and number of first-degree relatives with breast cancer [2], which forms the basis of the standard model presently used by the National Cancer Institute (NCI) for assessing breast cancer risk in the general population. However, while this model has been shown to work well at the population level in predicting group-wise cancer rates, it has only a modest discriminatory capacity at the individual level in identifying which women will eventually develop breast cancer, with a reported area under the receiver operating characteristic (ROC) curve (AUC) of 0.58 [3]. Increased knowledge of

---

[*] Corresponding author.

A.D.A. Maidment, P.R. Bakic, and S. Gavenonis (Eds.): IWDM 2012, LNCS 7361, pp. 236–243, 2012.

individual risk is therefore critical to the improvement of patient management with regards to appropriately personalized screening recommendations [4] and preventative strategies [5].

Beginning with work by Wolfe *et al.*, multiple studies have established that mammographic breast density, the relative amount of fibroglandular tissue in the breast as seen through mammography, is a strong, independent risk factor for breast cancer [6, 7]. Previous work investigating the incorporation of area breast percent density as a predictor of breast cancer risk to the Gail model found that addition area breast percent density lead to only a marginal improvement of discriminatory capacity [8]. However, while the majority of these studies have focused on assessing breast cancer risk as a function of the *relative* amount, or percentage, of dense tissue in the breast, recent studies have also suggested that *absolute* measures of the dense tissue content should also be assessed in addition to relative measures of breast density [9].

Breast density has been most commonly assessed subjectively through either visual categorization [10] or via semi-automated thresholding methods [11]. Research into the creation of repeatable, fully automated measures of breast density from full-field digital mammograms (FFDM) is ongoing [12, 13]. Area-based measures of breast density are effectively estimates of fibroglandular tissue content measured from a projection image of the breast, and it has been suggested that such measures may not properly measure the actual amount of fibroglandular tissue content in the breast[14]. Volumetric measures have been more recently proposed and are shown to provide orthogonal information about cancer risk when compared to the Gail risk factors [15]. Area and volumetric measures are known to have only moderately strong correlation to one another [16], further indicating the existence of a complimentary role. A recently emerging hypothesis is that volumetric measures of density may be more indicative of breast cancer risk than the area-based measures [17], as volumetric estimates may allow for more accurate assessment of the total fibroglandular tissue content of the breast [14]. Figure 1 illustrates two cases with similar volume percent density scores and different area percent density scores.

In this study we compare the potential utility of area and volumetric estimates of fibroglandular tissue content in breast cancer risk assessment. Both absolute and relative measures are considered. A retrospective case-control study is performed, using the unaffected breast of the cancer cases as a surrogate of cancer risk. The performance of the area and the volumetric density measures is assessed using linear discriminant classification and ROC curve analysis. A multivariable model using feature-selection is also assessed in order to evaluate the complimentary role, if any, of the area and the volumetric breast density estimates in assessing breast cancer risk. The results of this investigation could have significant implications on the implementation of breast density risk stratification in clinical practice.

2   Methods

The raw (i.e., "For Processing") mediolateral-oblique (MLO) digital mammography (DM) images from 106 women with unilateral breast cancer and 318 age-matched controls were retrospectively collected and analyzed under Health Insurance Portability and Accountability Act (HIPAA) guidelines and Institutional Review

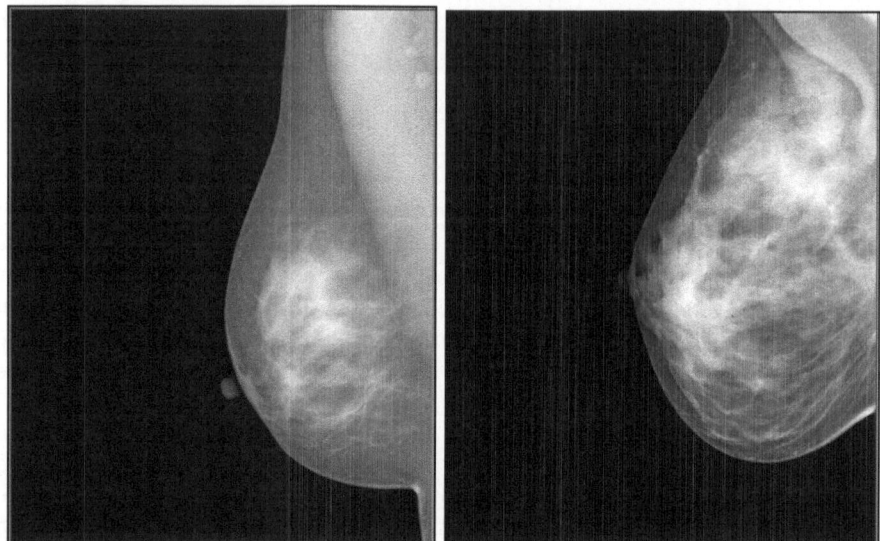

Fig. 1. Sample mammograms with similar estimates of volumetric percent density but different estimates of area percent density. Left) Mammogram with similar volumetric percent density (15%) and area percent density (20%) estimates. Right) Mammogram with a similar volumetric percent density (18%), but an increased area percent breast density (47%) estimate.

Board (IRB) approval. DM was performed with either a GE Healthcare 2000D or DS FFDM system at 0.1 mm/pixel resolution and 14 bit gray-levels. The images of the unaffected (e.g., contralateral) breast of the cancer cases were used as a surrogate of higher cancer risk and age-matched controls were subsequently side (i.e., right/left) matched to the cases.

Area-based breast density analysis was performed using a previously validated method [13] that segments the fibroglandular tissue through a combination of unsupervised and supervised machine learning techniques. Essentially, an adaptive k-class fuzzy c-means algorithm is applied which partitions the breast to into several regions based on gray-level intensity values. A linear discriminant classifier is then applied to identify and aggregate those sub-regions of the breast which are predominantly dense into a single dense tissue segmentation. The area of the dense tissue segmentation is then used to calculate the amount of absolute dense tissue and whole breast area and the corresponding breast percent density (PD%) measures. In addition, a series of standard shape descriptors of binary segmentations [18] were used to characterize the morphometry of the dense tissue segmentations acquired using the validated method described above, namely compactness, eccentricity, and center of mass location of the dense tissue area relative to the skin line. Compactness and eccentricity were used to provide global descriptors of the shape of the dense tissue area; location information was used to investigate if density locality has a predictive role in breast cancer risk assessment. Volumetric breast density analysis was performed using Quantra™ (Hologic Inc.), an FDA approved and commercially available, fully-automated software based on an extension of the Highnam & Brady

[19] method for digital mammography, which seeks to quantify a volumetric estimate of breast density from an acquired mammographic image based on the x-ray attenuation properties of fibroglandular and adipose tissue. Quantra^{TM} provides estimates of fibroglandular tissue and whole breast volume as well as a volumetric percent density score (VPD%).

As the breast density metrics tend to follow a log-normal distribution, all metrics considered in this work are log-transformed before being entered into the model. The strength of the association between the area and volumetric density measures was assessed by linear regression and Pearson's correlation, both for the absolute tissue content estimates and percent density. Student's paired t-test was used to determine if there are systematic differences between the 2D and 3D measures. The discriminatory capacity of each of the features relative to cancer status was assessed using leave-one-woman out cross-validation of a predictive, linear discriminant model (LDA) and Receiver Operating Characteristic (ROC) curve analysis. The area under the curve (AUC) was computed in order to assess LDA performance. Finally, the performance of a combined model incorporating area and volumetric density features selected via a linear stepwise feature selection [20] stage was compared to individual feature classifier performance in order to determine if area and volumetric descriptors of breast density provide complementary information and improve the discriminatory capacity of predictive models of cancer risk.

Table 1. Receiver Operating Curve (ROC) performance analysis of the area and volumetric density features in classifying cancer cases versus controls (univariate analysis). Metric names and associated area under the ROC curve (AUC) are reported. All AUCs were found to be statistically significant ($p<0.05$).

Metric	AUC
Dense Area	0.65
Breast Area	0.67
Area PD%	0.57
Compactness	0.55
Eccentricity	0.56
Distance from skin-line	0.66
Dense Volume	0.67
Breast Volume	0.64
Volume PD%	0.57

3   Results

Area and volumetric estimates of breast density were found to be significantly correlated ($p<0.001$). Area and volumetric estimates of absolute fibroglandular tissue content were found to be more strongly associated ($r=0.73$) than percent density

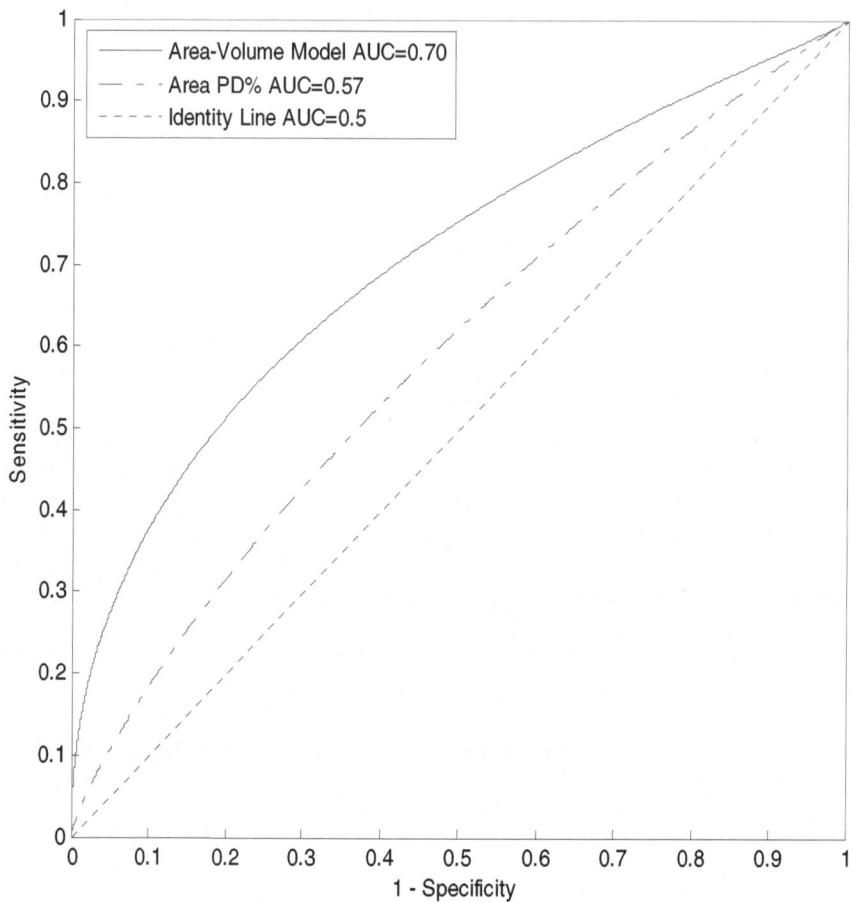

Fig. 2. ROC performance plots of the area percent density (PD%) (dash-dot), the combined area-volumetric LDA model (solid) and reference AUC=0.5 line (dotted). All AUCs were found to be statistically significant (p<0.05).

estimates (r=0.62). Paired Student's t-tests indicated that area and volume methods, both the absolute and the percent density measures, are different (p<0.001).

When comparing the performance of the univariate LDA classifiers to distinguish between cancer cases and controls, the absolute measures of dense tissue content outperformed the percent density measures for both the area and volumetric density assessment methods (Table 1), with dense tissue volume demonstrating the highest overall performance (AUC=0.67). Total breast size also was able to distinguish cancer status, regardless of whether breast area (AUC=0.67) or volume was considered (AUC=0.64). Each of the three area shape-location features considered in this work (*i.e.*, compactness, eccentricity and distance from skin-line) were able to distinguish cancer status to some degree, with the location feature, e.g., distance from skin-line, showing the strongest discriminatory capacity (AUC=0.66). When the feature-set was considered in aggregate to create a multivariable model, stepwise linear feature selection choose a total of four features from the ones in Table 1 as being statistically independent (p<0.01): Dense tissue area, dense tissue volume, compactness and distance from skin-line. Performance of the combined LDA model comprised of these four features showed improved discrimination in assessing cancer status (AUC=0.70; Figure 2) as compared to any of the single feature models.

4   Discussion and Conclusion

In this study, we have evaluated the discriminatory capacity of fully-automated area and volume-based measures of breast density in cancer risk assessment. When considered individually, area and volume measurements show comparable discriminative capacity for distinguishing cancer status, regardless of whether relative percent breast density or absolute breast density estimates. Furthermore, absolute measures of fibroglandular tissue content were seen to be more discriminative than percent density estimates, both for area and volumetric assessments of breast density. These results indicate that the total amount of fibroglandular tissue volume may be more reflective of cancer status than the relative content.

Shape-location features of the area based dense tissue segmentation were shown to have some discriminatory capacity for cancer status, in particular the distance of the dense tissue segmentation from the skin line. This implies that the spatial location of the dense tissue within the breast may play a role in overall breast cancer risk. Future work will look to further analyze this finding, as well as further in investigating and quantifying the relative individual contributions of area, volume, and morphometry in breast cancer risk prediction.

Interestingly, while there did not appear to be a difference in the performance of the area and volume based density measures when considered individually, the use of stepwise feature selection showed that a combined area-volume model considering both total fibroglandular volume and area, as well as dense tissue shape and location, outperformed any of the single-feature models, indicating that the volumetric and area descriptors of dense tissue may play complimentary roles in assessing breast cancer risk, with the combination model having an AUC of 0.70. This indicates that a combined model considering both volume and area breast density may be most beneficial in terms breast cancer risk prediction. Future work will seek to validate these findings with larger clinical studies and to incorporate these measures with other known risk factors for breast cancer into breast cancer risk prediction models.

Acknowledgements. This work was supported in part by American Cancer Society Grant RSGHP-CPHPS-119586, United States Department of Defense Breast Cancer Research Program Concept Award BC086591, and National Institutes of Health Population-Based Research Optimizing Screening through Personalized Regimens (PROSPR) Grant 1U54CA163313-01.

References

1. Jemal, A., Siegel, R., Xu, J., Ward, E.: Cancer statistics. CA Cancer J. Clin. 60, 277–300 (2010)
2. Gail, M.H., Brinton, L.A., Byar, D.P., Corle, D.K., Green, S.B., Schairer, C., Mulvihill, J.J.: Projecting individualized probabilities of developing breast cancer for white females who are being examined annually. J. Natl. Cancer Inst. 81, 1879–1886 (1989)
3. Rockhill, B., Spiegelman, D., Byrne, C., Hunter, D.J., Colditz, G.A.: Validation of the Gail et al. model of breast cancer risk prediction and implications for chemoprevention. J. Natl. Cancer Inst. 93, 358–366 (2001)
4. Lehman, C.D., Blume, J.D., Weatherall, P., Thickman, D., Hylton, N., Warner, E., Pisano, E., Schnitt, S.J., Gatsonis, C., Schnall, M., DeAngelis, G.A., Stomper, P., Rosen, E.L., O'Loughlin, M., Harms, S., Bluemke, D.A.: Screening women at high risk for breast cancer with mammography and magnetic resonance imaging. Cancer 103, 1898–1905 (2005)
5. Smith, K.L., Isaacs, C.: Management of women at increased risk for hereditary breast cancer. Breast Dis. 27, 51–67 (2006)
6. Wolfe, J.N.: Breast patterns as an index of risk for developing breast cancer. AJR Am. J. Roentgenol. 126, 1130–1137 (1976)
7. Boyd, N.F., Guo, H., Martin, L.J., Sun, L., Stone, J., Fishell, E., Jong, R.A., Hislop, G., Chiarelli, A., Minkin, S., Yaffe, M.J.: Mammographic density and the risk and detection of breast cancer. N. Engl. J. Med. 356, 227–236 (2007)
8. Tice, J.A., Cummings, S.R., Ziv, E., Kerlikowske, K.: Mammographic breast density and the Gail model for breast cancer risk prediction in a screening population. Breast Cancer Res. Treat 94, 115–122 (2005)
9. Stone, J., Warren, R.M., Pinney, E., Warwick, J., Cuzick, J.: Determinants of percentage and area measures of mammographic density. Am. J. Epidemiol. 170, 1571–1578 (2009)
10. D'Orsi, C.J., Bassett, L.W., Berg, W.A., Feig, S.A., Jackson, V.P., Kopans, D.B.: Breast imaging reporting and data system: ACR BI-RADS, Mammography 4th ed., Reston, Am. Col. of Rad. (2003)
11. Martin, K.E., Helvie, M.A., Zhou, C., Roubidoux, M.A., Bailey, J.E., Paramagul, C., Blane, C.E., Klein, K.A., Sonnad, S.S., Chan, H.P.: Mammographic density measured with quantitative computer-aided method: comparison with radiologists' estimates and BI-RADS categories. Radiology 240, 656–665 (2006)
12. Heine, J.J., Cao, K., Rollison, D.E., Tiffenberg, G., Thomas, J.A.: A quantitative description of the percentage of breast density measurement using full-field digital mammography. Acad. Radiol. 18, 556–564 (2011)
13. Keller, B., Nathan, D., Wang, Y., Zheng, Y., Gee, J., Conant, E., Kontos, D.: Adaptive multi-cluster fuzzy C-means segmentation of breast parenchymal tissue in digital mammography. Med. Image Comput. Comput. Assist. Interv. 14, 562–569 (2011)
14. Kopans, D.B.: Basic physics and doubts about relationship between mammographically determined tissue density and breast cancer risk. Radiology 246, 348–353 (2008)
15. Lokate, M.A., Kallenberg, M.G., Karssemeijer, N., van den Bosch, M.A., Peeters, P.H., van Gils, C.H.: Volumetric breast density from full-field digital mammograms and its association with breast cancer risk factors: a comparison with a threshold method. Cancer Epidemiol. Biomarkers Prev. (2010)

16. Kontos, D., Bakic, P.R., Acciavatti, R.J., Conant, E.F., Maidment, A.D.A.: A Comparative Study of Volumetric and Area-Based Breast Density Estimation in Digital Mammography: Results from a Screening Population. In: Martí, J., Oliver, A., Freixenet, J., Martí, R. (eds.) IWDM 2010. LNCS, vol. 6136, pp. 378–385. Springer, Heidelberg (2010)
17. Shepherd, J.A., Kerlikowske, K., Ma, L., Duewer, F., Fan, B., Wang, J., Malkov, S., Vittinghoff, E., Cummings, S.R.: Volume of mammographic density and risk of breast cancer. Cancer Epidemiol. Biomarkers Prev. 20, 1473–1482 (2011)
18. Sonka, M., Hlavac, V., Boyle, R.: Image processing, analysis, and machine vision. PWS Pub., Pacific Grove (1999)
19. Highnam, R., Jeffreys, M., McCormack, V., Warren, R., Davey Smith, G., Brady, M.: Comparing measurements of breast density. Phys. Med. Biol. 52, 5881–5895 (2007)
20. Draper, N., Smith, H.: Applied Regression Analysis. Wiley Series in Probability and Statistics. Wiley-Interscience (1998)

Fully-Automated Fibroglandular Tissue Segmentation in Breast MRI

Shandong Wu[1,*], Susan Weinstein[2], Brad M. Keller[1], Emily F. Conant[2], and Despina Kontos[1]

[1] Computational Breast Imaging Group, Department of Radiology,
University of Pennsylvania, Philadelphia, PA, USA
[2] Breast Imaging Section, Department of Radiology,
Hospital of the University of Pennsylvania, Philadelphia, PA, USA
{Shandong.Wu,Susan.Weinstein,Brad.Keller,
Emily.Conant,Despina.Kontos}@uphs.upenn.edu

Abstract. We propose an automated segmentation method for estimating the fibroglandular (i.e., dense) tissue in breast MRI. The first step of our method is to segment the breast as an organ from other imaged parts through an integrated edge extraction and voting algorithm. Then, we apply the nonparametric non-uniform intensity normalization (N3) algorithm to the segmented breast to correct bias field which is common in breast MRI. After that, fuzzy C-means clustering is performed to categorize the breast tissue into two clusters, i.e., fibroglandular tissue and fat. The automated segmentation results are compared to manual segmentations, verified by an experienced breast imaging radiologist, to assess the accuracy of the algorithm, where the Dice's Similarity Coefficient (DSC) shows a 0.73 agreement in our experiments. The benefit of the bias correction step is also shown through the comparison with the results obtained by excluding the bias correction step.

Keywords: Breast segmentation, fibroglandular tissue segmentation, breast MRI.

1 Introduction

Mammography has been the standard image modality for breast cancer screening, where the percentage density (PD%), which measures the relative amount of fibroglandular tissue in the breast as seen mammographically, is an established independent image-derived risk factor for breast cancer risk assessment [7, 8]. Since mammographic imaging is the 2D projection of 3D breast structures, the PD% estimation suffers from the tissue superposition problem and is also sensitive to certain imaging properties (e.g., body position, compression level, and detector settings, etc.), which may impact the resulting estimation of cancer risk [1]. Breast magnetic resonance imaging (MRI) provides 3D scanning and has emerged as an

---

* Corresponding author.

A.D.A. Maidment, P.R. Bakic, and S. Gavenonis (Eds.): IWDM 2012, LNCS 7361, pp. 244–251, 2012.
© Springer-Verlag Berlin Heidelberg 2012

effective modality for the clinical management of breast cancer [12]. Studies also indicate that the percentage of fibroglandular tissue (FT%) computed in breast MRI is correlated to mammographic breast PD% [3, 4, 5, 6], which suggests that breast MRI may also play a role in breast cancer risk prediction. To estimate the FT% in breast MRI, accurate segmentation of the fibroglandular tissue from the breast is a fundamental step.

Fibroglandular tissue segmentation in breast MRI is challenging in several aspects. First, the fibroglandular tissue appears only within the breast; hence, segmenting the breast as an organ from the remaining parts of the MR images is critical, which is done mostly by manual or semi-automated delineation method in previous work. Second, fibroglandular tissue may present anywhere over the breast with varying amounts and appearances, which is hard to model by computational segmentation algorithms. Third, within the segmented breast region in MR images there are no obvious anatomical clues associated with the fibroglandular tissue that may potentially serve as contextual information to aid identifying the fibroglandular tissue. In addition, the bias field is common in breast MRI where the intensity inhomogeneity may considerably affect the appearance of tissue properties. The problem of automated fibroglandular tissue segmentation has received little attention in the literature to date [1]. In addition to the qualitative estimation of the amount of fibroglandular tissue by visual assessment [15], most previous studies rely on semi-automated segmentation methods such as interactive thresholding [3, 5] or clustering [2, 4, 6]. Fuzzy C-means (FCM) has been used where the number of clusters is either interactively determined by users [4] or based on initial intensity range assumptions followed by interactive adjustments [2]. It is known that visual assessment produces subjective results and interactive methods introduce inter- and intra-reader variability [2, 3, 4, 5, 6]. In dealing with the intensity inhomogeneity,

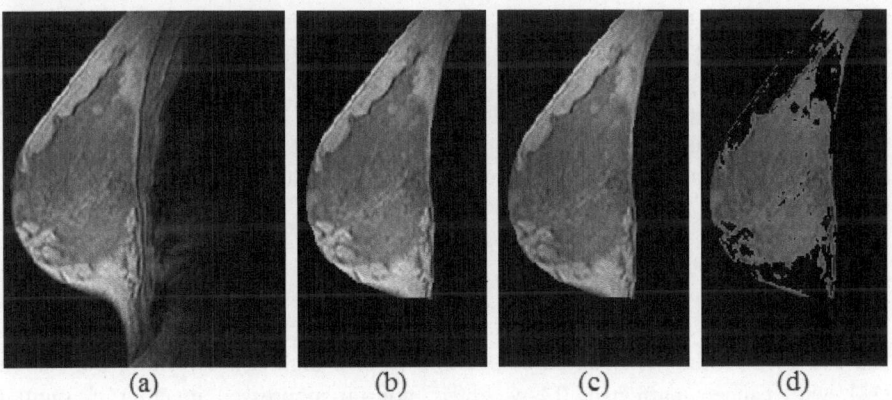

| (a) | (b) | (c) | (d) |

Fig. 1. Proposed algorithm steps for fibroglandular tissue segmentation. (a) A breast MRI slice. (b) Segmented breast. The darker regions are the fibroglandular tissue. (c) After performing bias field correction. (d) The segmented fibroglandular tissue.

FCM, N3 [9], and CLIC [10] algorithms have been recently tested for breast MR images [1], where different combinations of these algorithms yield varying performance, which is based on the visual evaluation by radiologists.

In this work, we propose a fully automated method for fibroglandular tissue segmentation. The method consists of three algorithmic steps: breast segmentation, bias field correction, and clustering-based fibroglandular segmentation, all are fully automated and no manual interaction is needed at any step of our method. In the experimental evaluation, segmentation accuracy is reported on the agreement of the algorithm- and manual-generated results from an experienced breast imaging radiologists using the Dice's Similarity Coefficient (DSC). We also compare the segmentation accuracy between applying and excluding the bias correction step, to demonstrate the importance of the bias correction step.

2   Methods

The three main steps of the proposed segmentation method are shown in Figure 1. All of the three steps are fully automated. The first step is to segment the breast as an organ from other imaged parts in breast MR images, which is implemented based on the integrated edge extraction and voting algorithm previously reported in [11]. This step is critical to the fibroglandular tissue estimation because it precludes the interferences coming from the non-breast regions [14]. Second, we further process the segmented breast by applying the nonparametric non-uniform intensity normalization (N3) algorithm [9] to correct bias filed. This way the intensity inhomogeneity is removed or reduced and as a result, there is better discrimination between the intensity ranges of the different tissues, corresponding to the fibroglandular tissue and fat, respectively. Attributed to the first two steps in breast segmentation and intensity inhomogeneity correction, we are allowed to predefine the number of clusters to be equal to two for the subsequent clustering step, where we guide the fuzzy C-means (FCM) algorithm to divide the breast into two broad intensity-based clusters: fibroglandular tissue and fat. Since fibroglandular tissue appears darker than fat in the non-fat-suppressed breast MR images, we can select the cluster that has a lower average intensity value as the segmented fibroglandular tissue from the two clusters.

3   Results

We use 10 3D bilateral MRI cases selected from a high-risk screening population [13], with cancer-unaffected, T1-weighted, non-fat-suppressed imaging in sagittal view. The 10 cases are randomly selected from the sets of ACR Breast Imaging Reporting and Data System Atlas (BI-RADS) density categories 3 and 4; hence these breasts have relatively high fibroglandular tissue density. There are 56 slices for each scan, resulting in 10x56=560 2D MRI slices used in the validation experiments.

Women in our study were imaged prone in a 1.5T scanner with dedicated surface breast coil; matrix size: 256×256; slice thickness: 2-3.5mm; flip angle: 20°. The algorithm-generated fibroglandular tissue segmentation results are compared with manually segmented results, confirmed from an experienced breast imaging radiologist, which are considered as ground truth here for validation purposes. The manual fibroglandular tissue segmentation is aided by an in-house developed interactive tool, where the operator first selects one or multiple region(s) of interest outlining the rough region of the fibroglandular tissue in the breast and then tunes an intensity threshold to determine the segmentation of fibroglandular tissue.

The segmentation accuracy is based on assessing the agreement between the algorithm- and manual-generated segmentation in terms of the Dice's Similarity Coefficient (DSC). We also compare the segmentation performance between applying and excluding bias correction (i.e., step 2) to evaluate the benefit resulting from the N3 algorithm. Table 1 lists the volumetric DSC performance for each of the 10 cases in terms of applying and excluding step 2. Overall we achieve an average segmentation accuracy of DSC=0.73 when step 2 applied and the accuracy decreases to 0.70 when step 2 is excluded. This suggests improved segmentation due to the bias correction step. To further illustrate the segmentation performance, Fig. 2 shows the slice-wise DSC for each of the 10 cases, where the accuracy is also compared between applying and excluding step 2. It is observed that in general the segmentation accuracy is relatively low for boundary slices compared to the central slices. Selected segmentation examples are shown in Fig. 3 with the comparison to corresponding manual segmentations. As can be seen, the automated segmentation results are generally accurate except for a small area near the top right corner of the breast where the intensities of some fat tissue fall in the range of fibroglandular tissue.

Table 1. Segmentation performance (DSC) for the 10 cases

Case	#1	#2	#3	#4	#5	#6	#7	#8	#9	#10	Average
FCM with Bias Correction	0.70	0.62	0.64	0.90	0.78	0.74	0.78	0.66	0.71	0.77	**0.73**
FCM without Bias Correction	0.63	0.49	0.63	0.84	0.77	0.73	0.77	0.64	0.68	0.77	**0.70**

4   Discussion and Conclusion

We propose a fully-automated method for fibroglandular tissue segmentation in breast MRI, which includes three main algorithm steps. The first two steps, namely breast area segmentation and intensity normalization, are important in the sense that they maximize the preclusion and reduction of a variety of interferences such that we can directly pre-determine the number of clusters (e.g., 2) for the subsequent FCM clustering algorithm. Our method is validated by 10 3D MRI scans, on a total of 560 2D MRI slices, and experimental results demonstrate that the proposed method is able to produce reasonable fibroglandular tissue segmentation. It is also shown that the N3 algorithm improves the segmentation accuracy from 0.70 to 0.73 for the 10 cases.

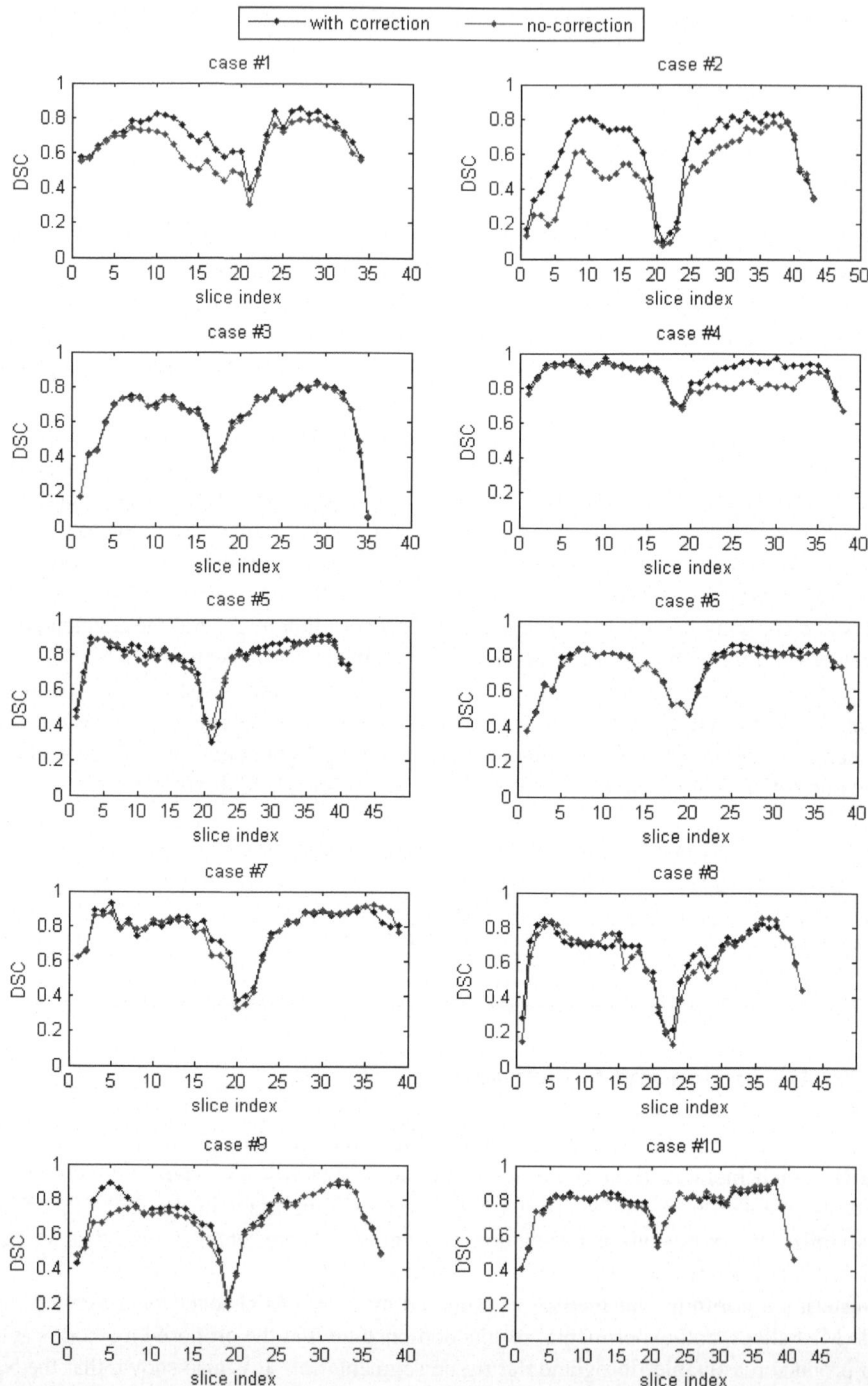

Fig. 2. Slice-wise segmentation performance (DSC) for each of the 10 cases, which is also shown in terms of applying or excluding bias correction (i.e., step 2)

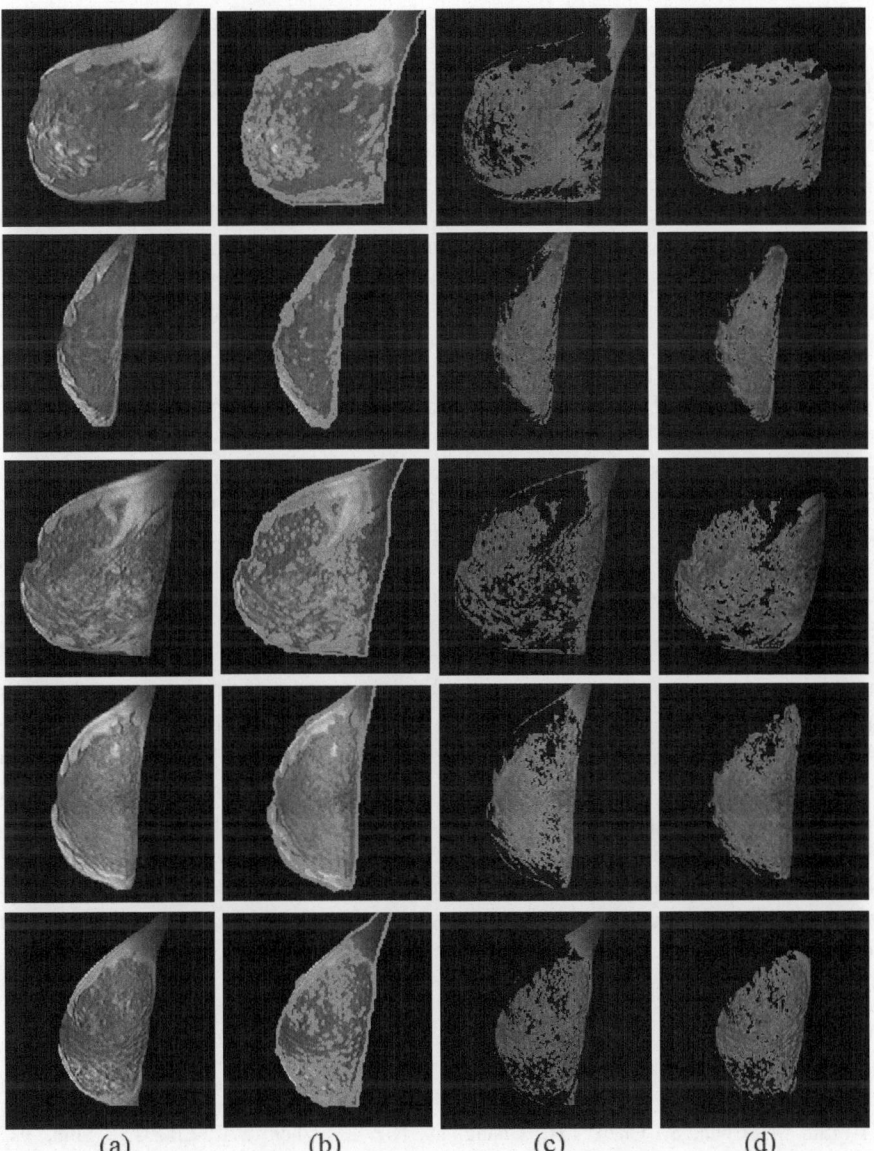

(a)   (b)   (c)   (d)

Fig. 3. Segmentation examples with the comparison to manual segmentation. Each row shows for one case example. (a) Segmented and bias corrected breast. (b) Contour (green) of the segmented fibroglandular tissue. (c) Final automated segmentation. (d) Manual segmentation.

As observed in Fig. 2, segmentation for the superior/inferior slices is relatively less accurate compared to the central slices. We attribute this result mostly to the signal attenuation and the strong noise effect in the boundary slices. Specific pre- or post-processing may be applied to those slices, as part of future work, to improve segmentation.

The current segmentation by FCM is based on intensity information. As can be seen from the examples shown in Fig. 3, some false positive segmentation results indicate that intensity information alone may not be fully adequate to sufficiently discriminative in identifying the fibroglandular tissue versus fat in breast MR images. Additional tissue/anatomical properties, such as relevant tissue priors, may be useful to become incorporated in the segmentation algorithm to improve segmentation.

Bias field is a major factor to accommodate in fibroglandular tissue segmentation for breast MRI. Bias field impact the intensity distribution in breast MR images and therefore the FCM may suffer from the consequence of the bias field. While the N3 algorithm is used in this study, we will continue to test other MRI bias correction algorithms and compare the resulting segmentation performance.

In future work, we also plan to further evaluate the performance of our algorithm in larger datasets and also compare the segmentation accuracy to readers' inter-reader variability.

Breast MRI allows for more accurate estimation of the true (e.g., 3D) amount of fibroglandular tissue in the breast and our proposed automated method is an essential step for quantitative segmentation of the fibroglandular tissue in breast MRI. Based on the segmentation results, it is straightforward to derive a volumetric percentage of fibroglandular tissue (FT%), which may ultimately aid in clinical breast cancer risk estimation.

Acknowledgment. This work was supported by NIH/NCI (1R21CA155906-01A1) and the Institute for Translational Medicine and Therapeutics (ITMAT) Transdisciplinary Program in Translational Medicine and Therapeutics (UL1RR024134) from the National Center for Research Resources. The content of this work is solely the responsibility of the authors and does not necessarily represent the official views of the National Center for Research Resources or the National Institutes of Health. We thank Ms. Kathleen Thomas, who was the research coordinator of the clinical trial from where the data originated, and Dr. Johnny Kuo for developing and maintaining the image database. We also thank Yan Wang for the assistance in running the N3 algorithm.

References

1. Lin, M., Chan, S., Chen, J.H., Chang, D., Nie, K., Chen, S.T., Lin, C.J., Shih, T.C., Nalcioglu, O., Su, M.Y.: A new bias field correction method combining N3 and FCM for improved segmentation of breast density on MRI. Medical Physics 38(1) (2011)
2. Nie, K., Chen, J.H., Chan, S., Chau, M.K., Yu, H.J., Bahri, S., Tseng, T., Nalcioglu, O., Su, M.Y.: Development of a quantitative method for analysis of breast density based on three-dimensional breast MRI. Med. Phys. 35, 5253–5262 (2008)
3. Thompson, D.J., Leach, M.O., Kwan-Lim, G., Gayther, S.A., Ramus, S.J., Warsi, I., Lennard, F., Khazen, M., Bryant, E., Reed, S., Boggis, C.R., Evans, D.G., Eeles, R.A., Easton, D.F., Warren, R.M.: Assessing the usefulness of a novel MRI-based breast density estimation algorithm in a cohort of women at high genetic risk of breast cancer: the UK MARIBS study. Breast Cancer Res. 11(6) (2009)

4. Klifa, C., Carballido-Gamio, J., Wilmes, L., Laprie, A., Shepherd, J., Gibbs, J., Fan, B., Noworolski, S., Hylton, N.: Magnetic resonance imaging for secondary assessment of breast density in a high-risk cohort. Magn. Reson. Imag. 28(1), 8–15 (2010)
5. Wei, J., Chan, H.P., Helvie, M.A., Roubidoux, M.A., Sahiner, B., Hadjiiski, L.M., Zhou, C., Paquerault, S., Chenevert, T., Goodsitt, M.M.: Correlation between mammographic density and volumetric fibroglandular tissue estimated on breast MR images. Med. Phys. 31(4), 933–942 (2004)
6. Kontos, D., Xing, Y., Bakic, P.R., Conant, E.F., Maidment, A.D.A.: A comparative study of volumetric breast density estimation in digital mammography and magnetic resonance imaging: results from a high-risk population. In: Conf. Proc. Med. Imag.: Comp.-Aid. Diag. SPIE (2010)
7. Boyd, N.F., Dite, G.S., Stone, J., Gunasekara, A., English, D.R., McCredie, M.R., Glies, G.G., Tritchler, D., Chiarelli, A., Yaffe, M.J., Hopper, J.L.: Heritability of mammographic density, a risk factor for breast cancer. N. Engl. J. Med. 347, 886–894 (2002)
8. Yaffe, M.J., Boyd, N.F., Byng, J.W., Jong, R.A., Fishell, E., Lockwood, G.A., Little, L.E., Tritchler, D.K.: Breast cancer risk and measured mammographic density. Eur. J. Cancer Prev. 7, S47–S55 (1998)
9. Sled, J.G., Zijdenbos, A.P., Evans, A.C.: A nonparametric method for automatic correction of intensity nonuniformity in MRI data. IEEE TMI 17, 87–97 (1998)
10. Li, C., Xu, C., Anderson, A.W., Gore, J.C.: MRI Tissue Classification and Bias Field Estimation Based on Coherent Local Intensity Clustering: A Unified Energy Minimization Framework. In: Prince, J.L., Pham, D.L., Myers, K.J. (eds.) IPMI 2009. LNCS, vol. 5636, pp. 288–299. Springer, Heidelberg (2009)
11. Wu, S.D., Weinstein, S.P., Conant, E.F., Localio, A.R., Schnall, M.D., Kontos, D.: Fully automated chest wall line segmentation in breast MRI by using context information. In: SPIE Medical Imaging: Computer-Aided Diagnosis, San Diego, CA (February 2012)
12. Weinstein, S., Rosen, M.: Breast MR imaging: current indications and advanced imaging techniques. Radiol. Clin. N. Am. 48(5), 1013–1042 (2010)
13. Weinstein, S.P., Localio, A.R., Conant, E.F., Rosen, M., Thomas, K.M., Schnall, M.D.: Multimodality screening of high-risk women: a prospective cohort study. J. Clin. Onco. 27(36), 6124–6128 (2009)
14. Gubern-Mérida, A., Kallenberg, M., Martí, R., Karssemeijer, N.: Multi-class Probabilistic Atlas-Based Segmentation Method in Breast MRI. In: Vitrià, J., Sanches, J.M., Hernández, M. (eds.) IbPRIA 2011. LNCS, vol. 6669, pp. 660–667. Springer, Heidelberg (2011)
15. Molleran, V., Mahoney, M.C.: The BI-RADS breast magnetic resonance imaging lexicon. Magn. Reson. Imag. Clin. N. Am. 18(2), 171–185 (2010)

Inferring the Breast Periphery from an Image When Measuring Volumetric Breast Density

Christopher Tromans[1] and Sir Michael Brady[2]

[1] Wolfson Medical Vision Laboratory, Department of Engineering Science,
University of Oxford, Parks Road, Oxford, United Kingdom, OX1 3PJ
[2] Department of Oncology, Old Road Campus Research Building,
Oxford, United Kingdom, OX3 7DQ.
cet@robots.ox.ac.uk

Abstract. Breast density is a key component of risk assessment for personalised screening, necessitating robust, repeatable measures. The Standard Attenuation Rate (SAR) enables the quantification of breast tissue radiodensity at each pixel, relative to the attenuation of a reference material, so may be used as a measure of volumetric breast density. A major complication is quantification of tissue in the periphery of the breast, the (often substantial) region between the skin boundary and the point at which the breast occupies the entire distance between the plates, since the thickness is governed by the shape of the compressed breast, rather than the separation of the plates. We present a method to measure the compressed shape from the image, hence the thickness at each point in the periphery. The method exploits the vastly different attenuation of the various breast tissues from that of air, and uses spatial smoothing to glean a signal estimating solely the underlying thickness. An iterative refinement procedure allows for variation in scatter in the periphery arising from the air boundary edge effects. The outcome of the inclusion of the periphery in breast density quantified by this method is analysed, and the importance of this region's inclusion illustrated.

Keywords: volumetric breast density, quantitative mammography, periphery equalisation.

1 Introduction

In recent years, there has been substantial progress towards personalised screening, including: when to start screening; screening frequency; and the possibility of using multiple screening modalities [1]. Breast density, together with factors such as age, biopsy results, and family history of breast cancer, have been found to be powerful indicators of who might benefit from earlier and more frequent screening, and to justify the use of modalities additional to x-ray, such as MRI and ultrasound. In order to fully exploit the clinical information captured in breast density, repeatable measures of volumetric breast density that are robust to inter and intra patient/image variations are required. The Standard Attenuation Rate (SAR) [2-3] has been developed for tissue quantification in breast density assessment and computer aided diagnosis. It incorporates a complete model of the imaging process, including photon production in the x-ray tube, explicit consideration of both absorption and scattering phenomena

A.D.A. Maidment, P.R. Bakic, and S. Gavenonis (Eds.): IWDM 2012, LNCS 7361, pp. 252–259, 2012.

within the breast, and detector signal formation; which is used to quantify relative attenuation against a reference material (analogous to the Hounsfield unit). The SAR image depends only on the attenuation of the underlying anatomy (decoupled from the x-ray characteristics used for imaging). Also, through the use of forward simulation using the image formation model, the appearance of any given tissue density/lesion may be estimated in a given surroundings. For example, a 20mm thickness of fibroglandular tissue gives a different projected attenuation when surrounded by 40mm of adipose, than when surrounded by 30mm; since it is the fibroglandular tissue that is of primary interest, it follows that by forward simulation using the two different backgrounds, the models underlying SAR enable an identical underlying feature to be ascertained between the images of varying backgrounds. Specifically, using Beer's law of attenuation and assuming a monoenergetic primary:

$$I = e^{-(\mu_{background}(H-t_{density})+\mu_{density}t_{density})}I_0$$

where the resulting image signal is I, the incident photon fluence is I_0, H is the compressed breast thickness, the background attenuation is, $\mu_{background}$, and the density is of attenuation $\mu_{density}$ and thickness $t_{density}$. It may be observed that the appearance of the density depends not only on its size and attenuation; but also on the thickness of the compressed breast and the attenuation of the tissues in the surroundings. Therefore, to make meaningful like-for-like comparison of densities between images and patients, these factors must be accounted for and normalised. Originally, this idea was developed for exploitation in computer aided detection and diagnosis applications for lesions. However, while assessing the efficacy of SAR for breast density assessment the need for "thickness normalisation" quickly became apparent. Specifically, when using a volumetric breast density measure, such as SAR, the way in which the breast deforms under compression affects the observed attenuation for a given area. For example, fibroglandular tissue is stiffer than adipose, so the deformation may force the adipose tissue surrounding a central volume of fibroglandular tissue toward the periphery, while the fibroglandular tissue itself maintains a near constant shape. The reduction in thickness of adipose results in the observed attenuation within the associated area of the projection image increasing, even though the fibroglandular volume is the same, as a forward SAR simulation would allow one to ascertain. So, when measuring the ratio of fibroglandular to adipose ("density"), it is imperative to include the entire breast since the tissue displaced to the periphery must be included to get the correct ratio. The complication arises in measuring the composition of the tissue in the periphery due to the need to know the anatomical thickness at any given pixel. This paper presents a technique to estimate this information from the acquired image.

2   Materials and Methods

The method exploits the fact that the attenuation of adipose and fibroglandular tissue are similar when compared to the vastly different attenuation of air. The radiodensity values computed in the periphery are therefore governed principally by the breast thickness; tissue composition being a second order effect. Using functions constrained to the smoothness of the shape of the compressed breast, and spatial averaging, the shape of the periphery may be estimated.

First, the breast air boundary, and the inner edge of the periphery, that is the point at which breast tissue occupies the full spacing between the compression plate, is segmented (as shown in Fig. 1).

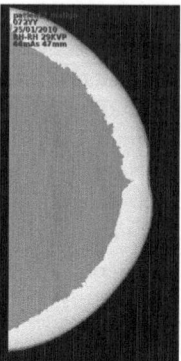

Fig. 1. The segmentation of the breast air boundary and the inner periphery edge where the breast is full thickness (magenta boundary/green fill)

Next an approximating function must be chosen that describes the intensity profile in the periphery in such a way as to approximate the variation in the signal arising from the tailing off of the thickness, rather than any changes in tissue composition (radiodensity) or image noise. To this end, we begin by assuming that the shape of the compressed breast is symmetrical about the midline and that its 3D edge shape follows a quadratic (parabola). That is, taking any section through the breast periphery perpendicular to the breast-air boundary, and plotting the thickness against the spatial distance from the boundary, will yield a parabola. Fig. 2 illustrates the geometry adopted to describe the acquisition of the mammographic image.

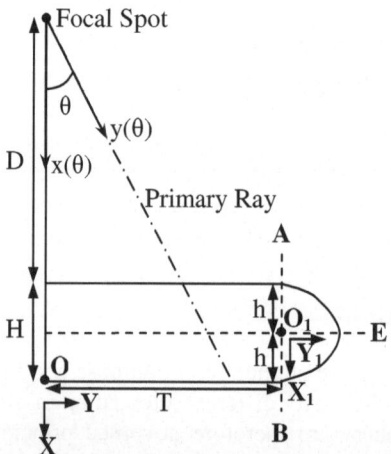

Fig. 2. The geometry used to derive the function describing pixel intensity variation arising from the change in thickness of the breast within the periphery

In Fig. 2, given the symmetry $H = 2h$ and so $|O_1A| = |O_1B| = h$, let us also suppose that $|O_1E| = d$. The ray at angle θ is shown. In the world coordinate frame OXY, the ray is $[x, x\tan\theta]$. At the top of the compression plate $x = D$, and the y displacement is $D\tan\theta$. If we denote $\tan\theta = \tau$, then in essence, since D is known, we have $y \sim \tau$, and we want to ascertain the ray traversal length through the breast is quadratic in τ, thereby following the shape we have assumed for the compressed breast. To analyse the quadratic assumption for AEB, the local coordinate frame OX_1Y_1 is established. In this coordinate frame, A and B are the points where the breast leaves the compression plates. Evidently, because of the compression, the tangent to the breast above A and B is vertical, but not of course below. The quadratic is:

$$y_1 = \frac{-d}{-h^2}(x^2 - h^2) \tag{1}$$

Translating back into the mammography world coordinate frame, gives the breast edge as:

$$\vec{v_e}(u) = (u - h)\hat{\imath} + \left(T\left(\frac{d}{h^2}\right)(u^2 - h^2)\right)\hat{\jmath} \tag{2}$$

for $-h < u < h$. Of interest in this application are two cases, as depicted in Fig. 3, the first being where the ray enters the breast outside the periphery, but exits within it (upper in the figure); and the second where the ray both enters and exits in the periphery (lower in the figure).

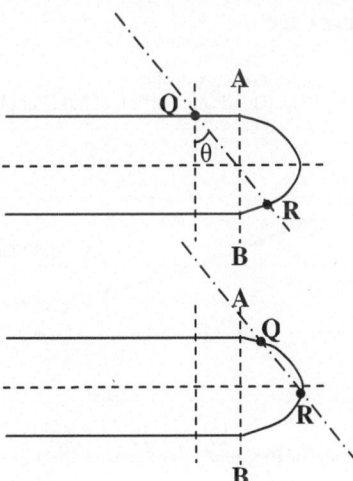

Fig. 3. The two cases of ray intersection with the tissue in the breast periphery

In the first case, the ray intersects the top compression plate at $[D, D\tau]$, and intersects the surface of the compressed breast given by equation (2) at $[u, uT]$, so:

$$uT = T - \left(\frac{d}{h^2}\right)(u^2 - h^2) \tag{3}$$

The traversal distance of interest, i.e. that over which the primary ray is attenuated leading to the image signal, is $|QR|$ and is given by:

$$QR^2 = (u - D^2)[1 + \tau^2]^{\frac{1}{2}} \tag{4}$$

It may be observed that $[1 + \tau^2]^{\frac{1}{2}}$ is at most quadratic in τ, and is in fact between linear and quadratic. For the second case, the traversal distance is given by:

$$|(u_1, \tau u_1), (u_2, \tau u_2)| = (1 + \tau^2) \left[\frac{\tau^2 + 4(d/h^2)(T+d)}{(d/h^2)} \right] \tag{5}$$

which has order $\sqrt{\tau^2(\tau^2)^{1/2}} \sim \tau^3$, though to a very good approximation is governed by τ^2.

We therefore take the pixel intensity profile of the projection of the breast edge to be at most quadratic, and allow it to vary between linear and quadratic. This is of course subject to the assumption the compressed breast shape is a symmetrical parabola: an assumption we believe to be reasonable.

A linear relation is adopted just inside the air boundary, smoothly joined to a quadratic relation for the remainder, and is fitted to the intensity profile observed perpendicular to each point on the air boundary. An example point is shown in **Fig. 4**, where the coefficient of determination being 1 to 2 significant figures shows the small effect of the tissue signal, visible as the slight undulations around the fit. This fitted function is used to describe the thickness, assuming the tissue composition to be the average of that at the periphery inner edge.

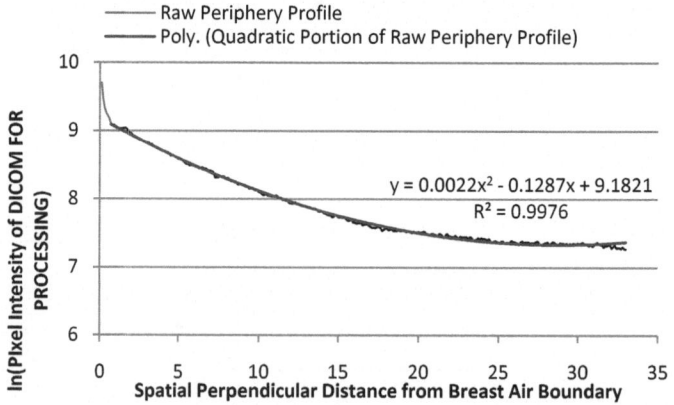

Fig. 4. The segmentation of the breast air boundary and the inner periphery edge where the breast is full thickness (left), and a periphery profile perpendicular to the air boundary (right).

Scatter complicates the problem yet further, since the image signal resulting from scatter fluctuates considerably within the periphery, as the proximity to the skin edge causes the volume of the tissue contributing scatter to vary significantly. This may be observed in Fig. 5, where the scatter signal is shown for both a periphery assumed to be a constant thickness equal to that of the rest of the breast, and for a periphery varying in thickness, as measured from a clinical image using the proposed technique. The difference is quantified for a horizontal profile across the periphery in terms of the scatter-to-primary ratio in Fig. 6.

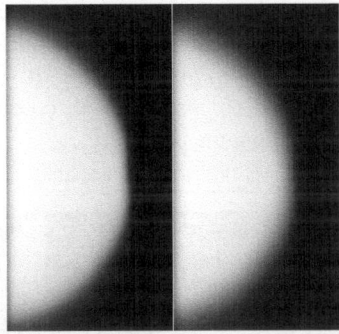

Fig. 5. The scatter image for a sample breast, adopting a constant thickness equal to that of the breast as a whole over the periphery (left), and the actual measured periphery thickness (right)

Through the explicit model of scatter that forms a part of SAR the variation in scatter is accounted for by using the current estimate of the breast shape to calculate the scatter field in the periphery, and then refining the shape estimate given the calculated scatter. These feed forward refinement cycles are repeated until convergence.

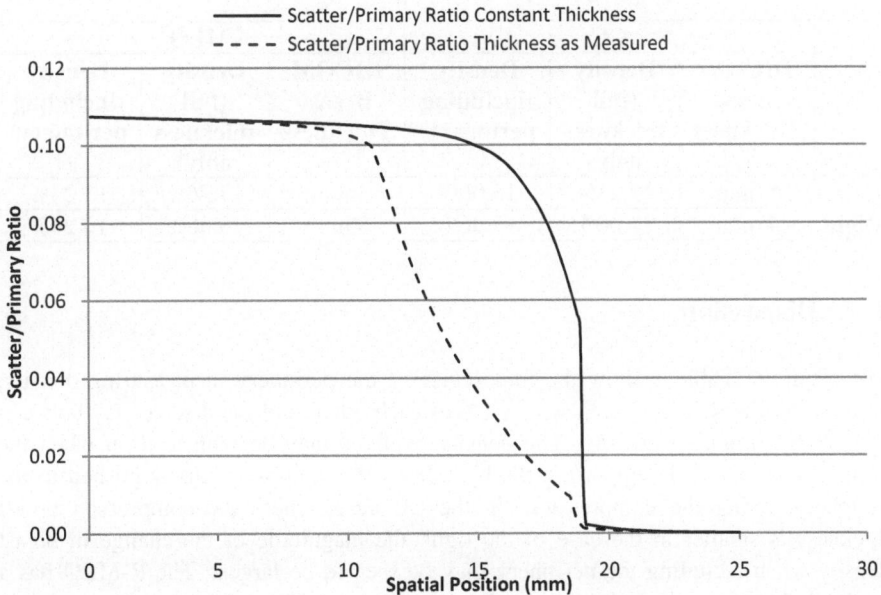

Fig. 6. The scatter/primary ratio of a profile across the periphery for the cases shown in Fig. 5

3   Results

Fig. 7 shows the thickness map, a 3D rendering of the breast shape and the SAR image computed using the breast shape computed by the proposed technique. Since each pixel intensity in a SAR image is a measure of the radiodensity of the corresponding cone of tissue above that pixel's physical detector element, breast density is measured as the mean of the SAR image pixels. Here it is converted to an adipose/fibroglandular fraction to aid comparison with other techniques. Table 1 compares breast density with and without the periphery.

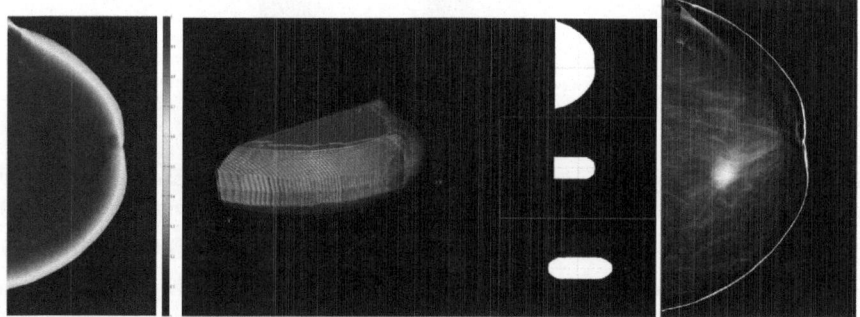

Fig. 7. A colour map of the thickness relative to the breast thickness (left) and a 3D rendering (centre), and the final SAR image including the periphery given the thickness map (right)

Table 1. Breast density readings using SAR for a typical case, with and without the periphery

	CC			MLO		
	DICOM Breast Thickness	Density (full thickness only)	Density (including periphery)	DICOM Breast Thickness	Density (full thickness only)	Density (including periphery)
Left	51mm	19.21%	13.06%	56mm	17.76%	13.24%
Right	47mm	21.20%	13.96%	55mm	13.30%	10.24%

4   Discussion

The results in Table 1 show the importance of the periphery in measuring density, with all but the R-MLO being within 1% of each other, and the discrepancy between views/sides dropping notably. The density readings may be seen to drop when the periphery is included, supporting the hypothesis that adipose tissue is pushed to the periphery during the compression. In the CC case, where the compressed breast thickness is smaller in the case of the right, the magnitude of the change in breast density when including the periphery may be seen to be largest. The R-MLO has a markedly lower density in both the measures with and without the periphery.

5   Conclusion

The breast periphery should be considered to obtain accurate breast density readings, a result of the varying deformations arising from differing breast compressions, and hence compressed breast thicknesses, between exams.

References

[1] Schousboe, J.T., et al.: Personalizing mammography by breast density and other risk factors for breast cancer: analysis of health benefits and cost-effectiveness. Ann. Intern. Med. 155, 10–20 (2011)
[2] Tromans, C.: DPhil Thesis: Measuring Breast Density from X-Ray Mammograms. DPhil Thesis, Engineering Science. Oxford University (October 2006)
[3] Tromans, C.E., Brady, S.M.: The Standard Attenuation Rate for Quantitative Mammography. In: Martí, J., Oliver, A., Freixenet, J., Martí, R. (eds.) IWDM 2010. LNCS, vol. 6136, pp. 561–568. Springer, Heidelberg (2010)

Digital Scatter Removal for Mammography and Tomosynthesis Image Acquisition

Christopher Tromans[1], Mary Cocker[2], and Sir Michael Brady[3]

[1] Wolfson Medical Vision Laboratory, Department of Engineering Science,
University of Oxford, Parks Road, Oxford, United Kingdom, OX1 3PJ
[2] Medical Physics and Clinical Engineering, Oxford University Hospitals NHS Trust,
Churchill Hospital, Oxford, United Kingdom, OX3 7LJ
[3] Department of Oncology, Old Road Campus Research Building, Oxford,
United Kingdom, OX3 7DQ
cet@robots.ox.ac.uk

Abstract. Digital x-ray acquisition allows the sophisticated processing of acquired images before display to the reader, making possible such operations as the removal in software of the systematic blurring effect of scatter. A method for analysing scatter removal is presented. The scatter model incorporated within the Standard Attenuation Rate (SAR) is used, which is a method for calculating a normalised image of tissue radiodensity. The model builds on the fundamental physical relations underlying Monte Carlo techniques; but through optimal information sampling and interpolation is able to execute in a clinically realistic time. The scatter kernel arising around each primary ray is calculated, and these are superimposed to give the scatter image. An iterative refinement procedure is used to calculate the radiodensity and scatter at each ray/pixel, cyclically feeding back to each other, to yield the scatter field. Image sharpness and contrast-to-noise (CNR) analysis is presented for two tissue equivalent phantoms. The algorithm is found to be able to match image sharpness without the grid, to that with the grid present, confirmed by residual analysis using autocorrelation plots which show the difference is almost white noise within a 95% C.I. The increased fluence in the absence of the grid is shown to allow dose to be reduced by 37-49%, whilst delivering equivalent contrast and CNR.

Keywords: scatter, dose reduction, acquisition post processing.

1   Introduction

An under-exploited benefit of digital mammography is the decoupling of the appearance of the underlying anatomy presented to the reader from how the image is acquired, facilitated by the ability to run software image processing algorithms on the digital image before presentation. Acquisition may therefore be optimised to glean the maximum signal-to-noise (SNR) ratio, where signal fundamentally means the attenuation characteristics of the underlying anatomy, as opposed to optimising contrast for human perception. Scattered photons result in a reduction in image contrast due to the

A.D.A. Maidment, P.R. Bakic, and S. Gavenonis (Eds.): IWDM 2012, LNCS 7361, pp. 260–267, 2012.

systematic low frequency blurring of the primary image, so a physical grid is usually introduced to filter a portion of them out according to their angle of incidence, though this approach is somewhat crude since the primary fluence is also attenuated. With digital post processing, it is possible to remove the effect of scatter in software, and the need for the grid is removed. This paper presents and analyses the performance of such a processing algorithm.

The Standard Attenuation Rate (SAR) [1-2] is a quantitative, normalised measure of tissue radiodensity per unit distance traversed by the primary (independent of scatter), and may be thought of as analogous to the CT Hounsfield unit. It is computed through the use of a detailed model of the physics of image acquisition, considering both primary and scattered photons, and it is the model of scatter, originally designed for quantitative analysis, that we consider here for grid replacement.

The scatter model utilises optimal information sampling and interpolation (to yield a clinical usable execution time) to calculate scattering using the molecular form factor and the coherent free electron cross section; and the incoherent scatter function and the differential Klein-Nishna collision cross section: the highly accurate fundamental physical relations underlying Monte Carlo dosimetry techniques. The scatter kernel arising around each primary ray is calculated as follows:

1. A model of the tube calculates the spectra of the photon beam of which the primary ray comprises and is incident upon the upper surface of the breast.
2. A computationally efficient ray tracer calculates the collection of tissues/materials and the traversal distance through each, that a primary ray encounters. Importantly, the spatial variation in scatter kernels, particularly prominent at the edges of the breast, are accounted for. Figure 1 shows a typical primary beam.

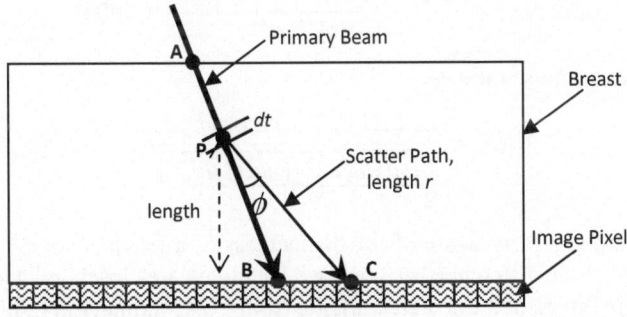

Fig. 1. The division of a primary ray into closely sampled points for scatter kernel calculation

3. The traversal path for all tissues/materials other than air is considered as a set of closely sampled points p. The scatter originating from each such p that is incident on detector pixels C near the intersection of the primary ray and the detector surface (B) is computed, using the fundamental scatter relations.
4. The scattered photons are attenuated according to photoelectric absorption that occurs along p to C. We ignore the possibility of multiple scattering. (Optionally: if there is an anti-scatter grid, both the scattered and primary photons are attenuated according to the absorption of the grid.)

A number of sampling and interpolation schemes are employed to streamline the calculation, as the above steps are highly computationally intensive. The scatter kernels for all the primary rays within the image are combined by superposition to yield the scatter image. The model may be used for both forward simulation of scatter, and in reverse, to estimate the scatter in an acquired image. However, in this case a complication arises in that the tissue radiodensity along the primary ray AB is unknown. This is resolved through the use of an iterative method that begins by approximating the scatter through the assumption of a constant scatter-to-primary ratio, and using this estimate to calculate the SAR radiodensity at each pixel. The process then begins a second iteration, feeding these values for the attenuation encountered by the primary ray back into the calculation outlined above. These iterative cycles proceed until such time as convergence is reached, and with it, the scatter arising from the homogenous tissue mix within the breast accounted for.

2   Materials and Methods

To assess the performance of any image enhancement technique the signal-to-noise ratio per unit dose is considered. In raw mammographic images the signal is taken to be contrast due to the complex relationship between the underlying radiodensity and pixel intensity. However, in a SAR image the effect of the imaging parameters are normalised, so pixel intensity only reflects radiodensity and the contrast of a given feature will always be the same. Specifically, the image quality metric adopted here is taken from Young et al [3], in which contrast is defined as:

$$Contrast = \frac{mean(bgd) - mean(fgd)}{mean(bgd)} \times 100\% \qquad (1)$$

and the contrast-to-noise ratio as:

$$CNR = \frac{mean(bgd) - mean(fgd)}{\sqrt{\frac{[sd(bgd)^2 + sd(fgd)^2]}{2}}} \qquad (2)$$

The image sharpness (a measure of the distinctness of a features edges) and contrast (the magnitude of the difference between two locations) are closely related in that in a noise-free x-ray image of a fine detail arising from a discontinuity in radiodensity: the contrast will depend on the exact location of the two points chosen to measure contrast between, and the resulting variation in contrast between slightly varying locations of the two measurement points, will be governed by the image sharpness. In a technique analogous to anisotropic diffusion, we measure image sharpness here by plotting local contrast between two points either side of, and equidistant from, the centre of an image feature (in this case the discontinuity), against the distance between the points. The shape of the resulting plot describes image sharpness.

The SAR transformation is described, at each pixel $I_{x,y}$, corrupted by noise ε:

$$SAR = m_{x,y} \log(I_{x,y} \pm \varepsilon - s_{x,y}) + c_{x,y} \qquad (3)$$

where $s_{x,y}$ is the estimated scatter signal, and $m_{x,y}$ and $c_{x,y}$ are the linear coefficients of the normalisation transform to the reference material, and hence depend on the image acquisition parameters. Since SAR is independent of scatter, and hence the presence of a grid, the contrast in the SAR image will be constant for any given feature (by definition since it reflects only the underlying radiodensity), and so attention turns to the effect of the SAR transformation on the noise term in the denominator of the CNR. Quantum noise is described by the Poisson distribution where the variance in the number of events is equal to the count (regardless of photon paths, breast thickness and tissue attenuation). Therefore, if the photon count in the without grid case is reduced to match that of the with grid case, i.e. the dose is reduced by the Bucky factor (generally around 2), then the variance in the noise arising from quantum effects will become equal, as the counts will be equal. The addition of the noiseless normalising offset, $c_{x,y}$, in the SAR transform has no effect on the variance, and the noiseless normalising coefficient $m_{x,y}$ is slightly smaller in the without grid case due to the absence of the grid interspace material, therefore the noise amplification arising from this coefficient in the SAR transform is less without the grid. The subtraction of the scatter component, $s_{x,y}$, is more complicated, since it is calculated by what amounts to a spatially varying deconvolution (of course, since the scatter kernels vary spatially, it cannot be computed by a conventional deconvolution), taking the noisy image, $I_{x,y} \pm \varepsilon$, as its input. The SAR model does not take account of stochastic noise, since no possibility exists for identifying the combination of random events that occurred during any given exposure, therefore the presence of stochastic noise will propagate through, and will result in variation in the calculated $s_{x,y}$ between exposures of the same object (when in an ideal noiseless world they'd be constant). The noisy estimate of $s_{x,y}$, when subtracted from the acquired image in equation (3), will have the effect of introducing noise into the SAR image, and hence will increasing the variance in the SAR image. The noise component in a given $s_{x,y}$ depends upon the noise component in all the surround pixel values, since scatter is contributed to any given pixel from the volume of material in the immediate surroundings. Therefore the degrading effect of noise in $s_{x,y}$ on the overall CNR of the SAR image will depend on the variation in radiodensity/composition of the object from which the image is being acquired. Were it possible to have a noise free $s_{x,y}$, the dose could be reduced by the Bucky factor in the grid's absence. In reality noise will be present, and in the next section we present an empirical analysis of the CNR for two phantoms to establish dose reductions.

3   Results and Discussion

Validation experiments have been conducted on a GE Senographe Essential, using two CIRS tissue equivalent phantoms. The first comprises of a sharp vertical discontinuity between adipose and fibroglandular tissue equivalents, 40mm thick, with a 10mm thickness of adipose placed above and below to mimic the subcutaneous fat layer just beneath the skin. The second is a BR3D phantom, which the manufacturer states was designed to "assess detectability of various size lesions within a tissue equivalent, complex, heterogeneous background" and contains an assortment of microcalcifications, fibrils and masses, and thus provides a more clinically realistic test.

Fig. 2 shows the experimental acquisitions of the discontinuity phantom with and without the grid present, and the effect of the grid on the sharpness of the discontinuity may be qualitatively assessed visually.

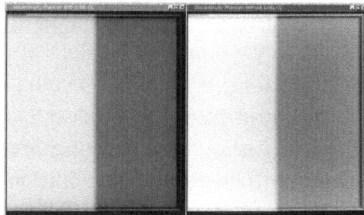

Fig. 2. Empirical image acquisitions acquired at 29kVp Mo-Rh 71mAs of the discontinuity phantom with (left) and without (right) an anti-scatter grid present

Fig. 3 shows the scatter image, $s_{x,y}$, and the primary image, $I_{x,y} - s_{x,y}$, from equation (3) calculated from the empirical acquisitions. Note the degrading of the discontinuity detail when comparing the without grid to the with grid scatter image, and the high degree of similarity in the primary images.

Fig. 3. The scatter image, in the with (far left) and without (centre left) grid case, and the primary image in the with (centre right) and without (far right) grid case calculated by SAR from the experimental acquisitions of the discontinuity phantom

Fig. 4 plots the variation in CNR with spatial distance horizontally from the discontinuity, and analogously, Fig. 5 plots the variation in image contrast (i.e. the image sharpness), for the raw and SAR empirical images of the discontinuity phantom, with and without the grid. The mean and standard deviation in equations (2) and (3) are calculated for vertical lines of 50 pixels. In the case of the raw data, the absence of the grid returns the superior CNR measure, however as may be seen from the contrast variation in Fig. 5, the presence of the grid returns the sharper image. The percentage increase in contrast between the with and without grid contrast in the raw images has a mean of 27.09%, and standard deviation 4.55. The improvement in contrast/image sharpness shown suggests the designer of this digital mammography system favours image sharpness, over CNR, and thus has included a grid. The CNR in the SAR

image remains superior in the absence of the grid, as would be expected, in fact it
may be seen that the exposure (and hence dose) may be reduced by 37% (from
71mAs to 45) before the CNR measures become approximately equal.

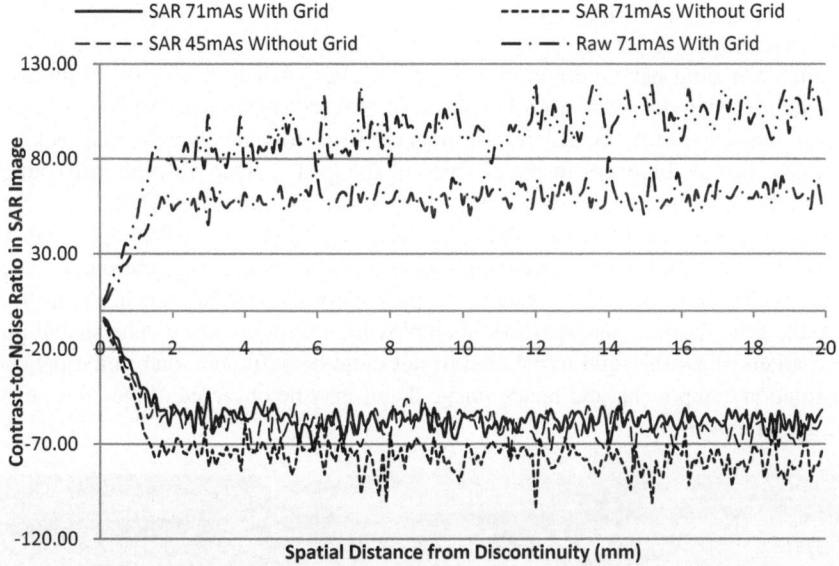

Fig. 4. The spatial variation in CNR measured around the discontinuity

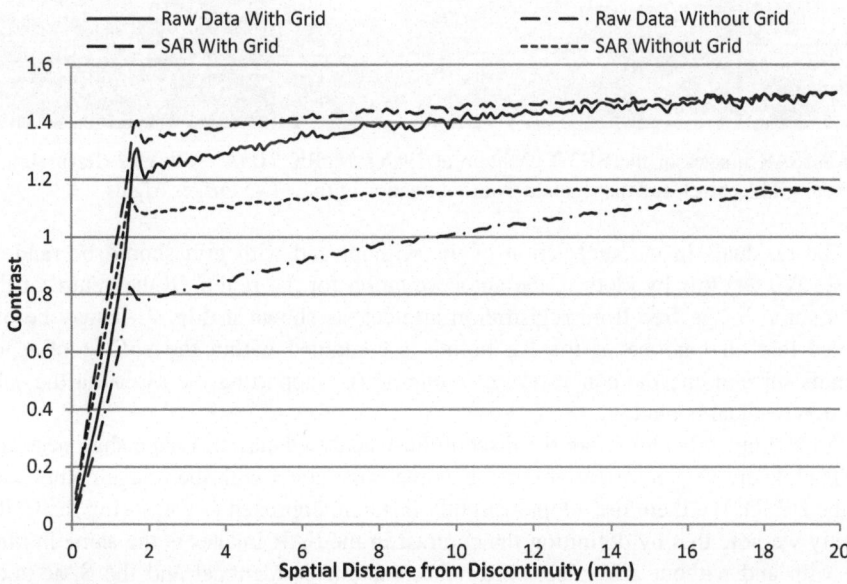

Fig. 5. Spatial variation in contrast (image sharpness) measured around the discontinuity

The shape of the contrast plots in Fig. 5 shows the improvement in image contrast/sharpness arising from the SAR processing in both the cases without and with a grid (since the grid isn't 100% efficient in filtering scatter, especially at low angles). A linear scaling, such as that used in the window and level procedure for image display has been applied to the SAR values, so the maximum contrast matches that exhibited in the raw images, factors of -5.81 with the grid, and -4.52 without. It should be noted that such a scaling has no effect on the CNR values (which as previously discussed are matched when the without grid exposure is reduced from 71 to 45mAs). The similarity in the shape of the SAR contrast plots confirms that the algorithm has achieved equivalent image sharpness in the absence of the grid, to that with the grid, but has allowed the dose to be reduced by 37%, whilst returning equivalent CNR.

Turning attention now to the BR3D phantom, Fig. 6 shows SAR images with and without the grid, and their subtraction after a rigid translation registration. The need for the registration arises from having to physically dismantling the machine to remove the grid, despite our experiments employing a positioning jig. The spatial position markers show the rigid translation to not quite be sufficient, due to the presence of a rotation component, and hence image detail may be observed at the edges of the subtraction image.

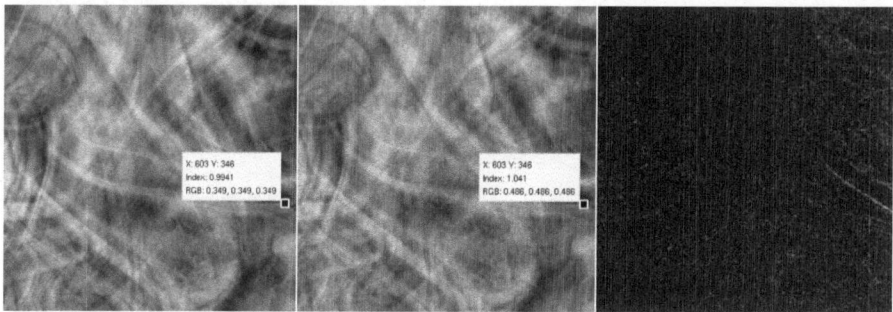

Fig. 6. SAR images of the BR3D phantom at 29kVp MoRh, 71mAs with grid (left), 36mAs without grid (centre), and the residual from subtraction of these two images (right)

The residuals in the subtraction of the without and with grid should be random noise. We test this by plotting the autocorrelation for the region in the centre of the subtraction image free from registration artefact, as shown in **Fig. 7**. It may be observed that all bar one of the lag points is contained within the 95% confidence bounds surrounding the conclusion of white noise, supporting the assertion the subtraction residual is random.

For a simple phantom, like the discontinuity analysed earlier, image sharpness and CNR plots are very informative, they become impractical with the image complexity of the BR3D. We therefore adopt a slightly different approach to measuring the CNR. Firstly we note that by definition the contrast in the SAR images is the same in both the with and without grid cases, since the phantom is identical and the SAR pixel intensity depends solely on the underlying radiodensity. This is confirmed above by subtraction, and analysis of the residual by autocorrelation to confirm randomness. To quantify the image noise, the standard deviation of the residual of subtracting two consecutive "identical" exposures is calculated, this quantifies the image noise over time, which is identical to quantifying it by measuring the standard deviation in an image of a homogenous object. The image noise quantified in this way is 0.0083 with the grid present at 71mAs, and 0.0057 without the grid at 71mAs, and 0.0081 without the grid at 36mAs, allowing a dose reduction of 49%, whilst maintaining CNR.

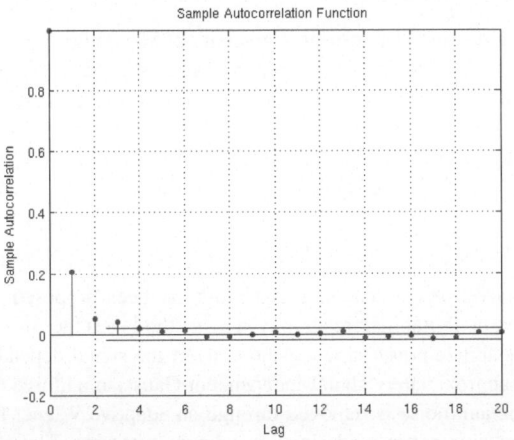

Fig. 7. The autocorrelation the region in the centre of the subtraction image (with grid - without grid) free from registration artefact

4   Conclusion

An analysis of image sharpness and CNR of SAR processed images taken with and without grid, suggest that the SAR scatter algorithm is able to restore image contrast and sharpness in the absence of a grid to that which it would be had the grid been present. Due to the increased photon fluence reaching the detector in the absence of the grid, the software scatter correction is able to facilitate dose reduction between 37 and 49%, for the phantoms tested, whilst delivering equivalent CNR.

References

[1] Tromans, C.: DPhil Thesis: Measuring Breast Density from X-Ray Mammograms. DPhil Thesis, Engineering Science. Oxford University (October 2006)
[2] Tromans, C.E., Brady, S.M.: The Standard Attenuation Rate for Quantitative Mammography. In: Martí, J., Oliver, A., Freixenet, J., Martí, R. (eds.) IWDM 2010. LNCS, vol. 6136, pp. 561–568. Springer, Heidelberg (2010)
[3] Young, K.C., et al.: Optimal beam quality selection in digital mammography. Br. J. Radiol. 79, 981–990 (2006)

Filtering of Poisson Noise in Digital Mammography Using Local Statistics and Adaptive Wiener Filter

Marcelo A.C. Vieira[1], Predrag R. Bakic[2], Andrew D.A. Maidment[2],
Homero Schiabel[1], Nelson D.A. Mascarenhas[3]

[1] Electrical Engineering Department, University of São Paulo, São Carlos, Brazil
{mvieira,homero}@sc.usp.br
[2] Department of Radiology, University of Pennsylvania, Philadelphia, USA
{predrag.bakic,andrew.maidment}@uphs.upenn.edu
[3] Computer Department, Federal University of São Carlos, São Carlos, Brazil
nelson@dc.ufscar.br

Abstract. A novel image denoising algorithm has been proposed for quantum noise reduction in digital mammography. The method uses the Anscombe transformation to stabilize noise variance and convert the signal-dependent Poisson noise into an approximately signal-independent Gaussian additive noise. In the Anscombe domain, noise is removed through an adaptive Wiener filter, whose parameters are obtained considering local image statistics. Thus, the method does not require any *a priori* knowledge about the original signal, because all the necessary parameters are estimated directly from the noisy image. The method was applied on synthetic mammograms generated based upon an anthropomorphic software breast phantom with different levels of simulated quantum noise. The evaluation of the proposed method was performed by calculating the peak signal-to-noise ratio (PSNR) and the mean structural similarity index (MSSIM) before and after denoising. Results show that the proposed algorithm improves image quality by reducing image noise without significantly affecting image sharpness.

Keywords: Digital mammography, quantum noise, image denoising, Anscombe transformation, Wiener filter.

1 Introduction

Full Field Digital Mammography (FFDM) is currently the standard tool for breast imaging and is gradually replacing screen-film mammography as the preferred tool for breast cancer screening [1]. However, mammographic interpretation is a complex task, preventing radiologists from the ideal of detecting all abnormalities visualized on mammograms. Among the lesions evaluated in mammographic reading, special attention is given to clustered microcalcifications because they may represent the only sign of malignancy [2]. Due to their small size and the confounding effects of image noise, the visibility of microcalcifications may sometimes be relatively poor. Image quality significantly influences the performance of radiologists in mammography

A.D.A. Maidment, P.R. Bakic, and S. Gavenonis (Eds.): IWDM 2012, LNCS 7361, pp. 268–275, 2012.

interpretation. Thus, high quality mammograms are required for accurate detection and characterization of suspicious lesions in breast cancer screening.

In this context, image processing algorithms have been utilized to increase the visibility of microcalcifications, with the hope of improving the performance of radiologists [3]. However, for proper use of preprocessing techniques in mammographic images, some important aspects must be considered. First, use of image processing algorithms for the enhancement of high-frequency components, such as microcalcifications, has the undesirable effect of increasing the image noise [4]. On the other hand, image processing for noise suppression typically reduces sharp transitions between pixel intensities, which results in image blurring. This could impair the detection of fine detail and small structures in the breast image.

Denoising techniques are, in general, based on the assumption that noise is additive and signal independent (that is, there is no correlation between pixel values and the values of noise components) [4]. However, mammography images are acquired using the minimum radiation dose consistent with ensuring both adequate image quality and patient safety; as such, the quantum noise should be apparent. Quantum noise is non-additive and signal-dependent (that is, noise components values are correlated with respect to the radiation intensity). A recent study has shown that quantum noise is the dominant image quality factor in mammography and exerts greater influence than spatial resolution for the tasks of detecting microcalcifications and discrimination of masses by radiologists. A failure to address noise issues can impede diagnostic performance [5].

We propose a novel image denoising algorithm for quantum noise reduction in digital mammography, aimed at improving image quality, and consequently improving radiologists' performance in clinical interpretation. The method uses the Anscombe transformation [6] to stabilize noise variance and convert the signal-dependent quantum noise into an approximately signal-independent Gaussian additive noise. In the Anscombe domain, image noise is removed through an adaptive Wiener filter, whose parameters are obtained considering local image statistics. Thus, the method does not require any *a priori* knowledge of the original signal, because all the necessary parameters are estimated directly from the noisy image.

2   Methods and Materials

The following model describes the image degradation process during acquisition [4]:

$$g(x, y) = f(x, y) * h(x, y) + n(x, y) \tag{1}$$

where $g(x,y)$ is the degraded image, $f(x,y)$ is the input image, $h(x,y)$ is the degradation function, $n(x,y)$ is the additive noise and the operator "$*$" indicates convolution.

Restoration techniques usually manipulate this equation to obtain an estimate, $\hat{f}(x, y)$, of the input image when $h(x,y)$ and $n(x,y)$ are known. The additive noise $n(x,y)$ is incorporated by the digitization process and can be modeled as signal-independent Gaussian noise. However, $f(x,y)$ cannot be considered a noise-free image because mammographic images are also corrupted by quantum noise, which is a non-additive noise and is normally modeled by a Poisson statistical distribution.

The Anscombe transformation is a variance-stabilizing transformation that converts a random variable with a Poisson distribution into a variable with an approximately additive, signal-independent Gaussian distribution with zero mean and unity variance [6,7]. Let the degraded image, $g(x,y)$, be the random variable. The Anscombe transformation of $g(x,y)$ is given by [6]:

$$z(x, y) = 2\sqrt{g(x, y) + \frac{3}{8}}. \qquad (2)$$

This equation can be represented by the following additive model [7]:

$$z(x, y) = \left(2\sqrt{u(x, y) + \frac{1}{8}}\right) + v(x, y), \qquad (3)$$

where $u(x,y)$ is the rate of the Poisson distributed image (i.e., the expected value) and $v(x,y)$ is the additive term, which is independent of the signal $s(x,y)$ and has an approximately Gaussian distribution.

After the Anscombe transformation, the additive term $v(x,y)$ includes both the quantum noise converted into Gaussian noise and the electronic white noise, originally incorporated by the digitization process. Thus, this transformation allows the use of any well-known denoising technique to reduce Gaussian additive noise by working on the image $z(x,y)$ in the Anscombe domain [7].

In this work, we use the adaptive Wiener filter to obtain an estimate, $\hat{s}(x,y)$, of the expected noise-free mammographic image in the Anscombe domain [7]. The Wiener filter calculates an estimate of a noise-free image that minimizes the mean squared error. Specifically, when $z(x,y)$ is assumed to have a Gaussian additive noise with zero mean, the Wiener filter is the optimal filter and has the following expression:

$$\hat{s}(x, y) = \bar{s} + \frac{\sigma_s^2}{\sigma_s^2 + \sigma_v^2}[z(x, y) - \bar{z}], \qquad (4)$$

where $\bar{s}$ and σ_s^2 are the mean and variance of the signal, respectively; $\bar{z}$ is the mean of the image $z(x,y)$; and σ_v^2 is the variance of the noise.

In the Anscombe domain, we can assume that σ_v^2 is equal to 1. Moreover, $\bar{z}$ is equal to $\bar{s}$ because the mean of the noise, $\bar{v}$, is equal to zero [7]. Thus, we can rewrite the equation (4) as follows:

$$\hat{s}(x, y) = \bar{s} + \frac{\sigma_s^2}{\sigma_s^2 + 1}[z(x, y) - \bar{s}]. \qquad (5)$$

Parameters $\bar{s}$ and σ_s^2 can be estimated by local statistics of a preliminary estimate of the signal in the Anscombe domain, $\hat{s}(x, y)$. We considered a square neighborhood of variable size around the pixel being processed. The preliminary estimate of the signal, $\hat{s}(x, y)$, was obtained by blurring the image $z(x,y)$ with an averaging filter mask of size 3×3 [4].

After the adaptive Wiener filtering procedure, the inverse Anscombe transformation is applied to obtain the estimate, $\hat{u}(x, y)$, of an approximately noise-free mammographic image in the spatial domain. The inverse Anscombe transformation is given by the following equation [7]:

$$\hat{u}(x,y) = \frac{1}{4}\hat{s}(x,y)^2 - \frac{1}{8}. \tag{6}$$

3   Results

The assessment of the proposed denoising algorithm was performed considering synthetic mammograms generated based upon an anthropomorphic software breast phantom [8] with a cluster of microcalcifications with 50% and 25% of normal contrast. The contrast of the microcalcifications is specified as the relative linear x-ray attenuation coefficient compared to the tabulated attenuation of hydroxyapatite. All mammograms were generated using three different levels of quantum noise, simulating the normal clinical dose, half of the normal dose and a quarter of the normal dose. All of the images were restored using the proposed filter.

In order to evaluate the performance of the proposed methodology, we calculated two widely used image quality parameters: the peak signal-to-noise ratio (PSNR) [9] and the mean structural similarity index (MSSIM) [10]. Ideal mammograms without quantum noise were also generated to provide the ground-truth reference. These parameters were measured in full mammographic images (4096 × 1792 pixels) and two regions-of-interest (ROI) of 256 × 256 pixels containing, respectively, microcalcification clusters with 50% contrast and 25% contrast.

Figure 1 shows one example of the results obtained with the denoising algorithm on the synthetic images. The image on the left shows a ROI with a cluster of microcalcification with 50% of contrast extracted from the mammogram generated with a quantum noise correspondent to a quarter of normal clinical dose. In the center is the same image after denoising and on the right is the ideal image used as reference.

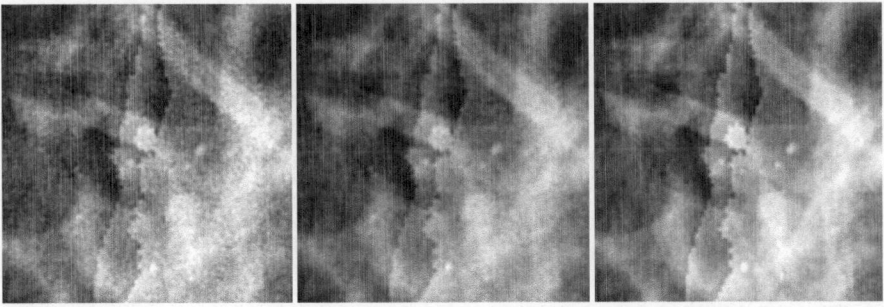

Fig. 1. ROIs (256 × 256) of a cluster of microcalcifications with 50% of contrast extracted from the mammogram generated with a quantum noise correspondent to a quarter of normal clinical dose. Left: noisy image; center: restored image; right: ideal image without noise.

Table 1 shows the PSNR and MSSIM measurements obtained with the proposed denoising algorithm for the synthetic FFDM images before and after denoising. The relative improvement of image quality achieved using the denoising methodology was also calculated. Figure 2 and Figure 3 show, respectively, the improvement in PSNR and MSSIM measurements after denoising as a function of the radiation dose.

Table 1. Results of PSNR and MSSIM measured for the proposed algorithm before and after denoising. Synthetic mammograms were generated with quantum noise corresponding to 100%, 50% and 25% of the normal clinical dose. Parameters were measured in the full mammographic images and two ROIs of 256 × 256 pixels containing, respectivelly, microcalcification clusters (MC) with 50% and 25% contrast. The relative improvement on image quality after denoising was also calculated.

Phantom Images		PSNR(dB)			MSSIM		
		Before	**After**	**Improve-ment(dB)**	**Before**	**After**	**Improve-ment (%)**
100% of the normal clinical dose	Full image	51.30	60.84	9.54	0.9921	0.9993	0.73
	ROI with 50% MC contrast	40.13	44.92	4.79	0.9329	0.9815	5.21
	ROI with 25% MC contrast	40.02	44.84	4.82	0.9317	0.9814	5.33
50% of the normal clinical dose	Full image	48.33	57.98	9.65	0.9845	0.9987	1.44
	ROI with 50% MC contrast	36.81	42.12	5.31	0.8728	0.9751	11.72
	ROI with 25% MC contrast	36.93	42.28	5.35	0.8741	0.9755	11.60
25% of the normal clinical dose	Full image	45.36	54.90	9.54	0.9702	0.9975	2.81
	ROI with 50% MC contrast	33.50	38.20	4.70	0.7776	0.9640	23.97
	ROI with 25% MC contrast	33.54	38.31	4.77	0.7771	0.9640	24.05

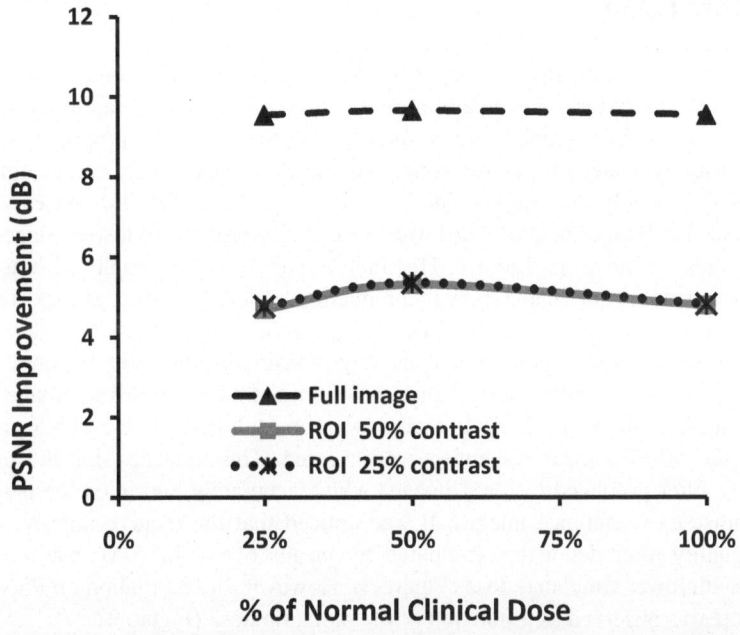

Fig. 2. Improvement in the PSNR measurements after denoising as a function of dose

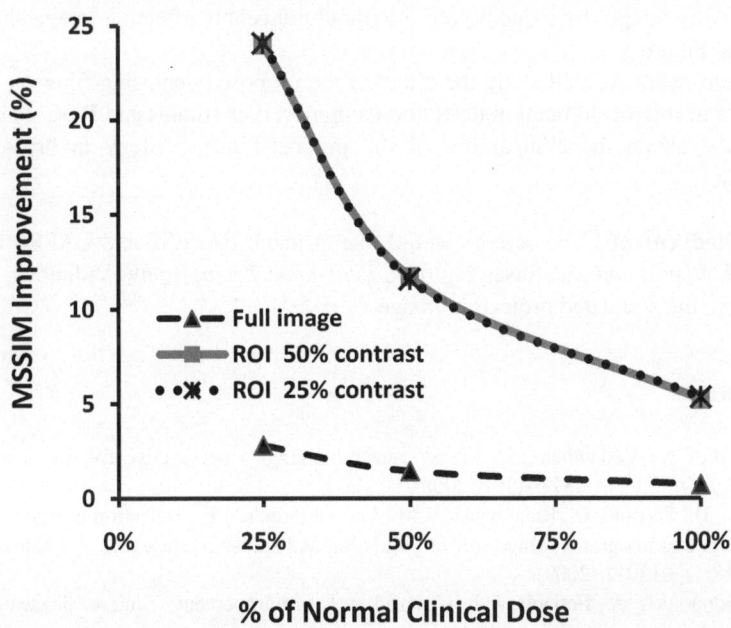

Fig. 3. Improvement in the MSSIM measurements after denoising as a function of dose

4   Discussion

In this work we investigated the use of the Anscombe transformation and the adaptive Wiener filter to reduce the quantum noise of digital mammography images. Improvement on mammographic image quality resulting from the proposed denoising method was evaluated. First, we compared the noisy and the reference images in terms of two widely used signal fidelity index: PSNR and MSSIM. As expected, it was found that images acquired at lower dose levels resulted in lower image quality index values, as shown in Table 1. This indicates that mammography quantum noise is signal-dependent and increases with a reduction in radiation dose, as expected.

In order to evaluate the proposed denoising methodology, the same image quality metrics were measured again after denoising, considering both the restored and the reference images. Results showed that the proposed filter improved image quality index values, as shown in Table 1. Increases of up to 9.65 dB in the PSNR and up to 24% in the MSSIM measurements were observed. This indicates that the proposed denoising filter produced restored images which accurately preserved the detail seen in the noise-free reference images. It was noticed that the relative improvement on image quality after denoising, evaluated by means of the MSSIM, was higher for images with lower simulated dose (Figure 3). However, little variation on PSNR measurements was observed as a function of the radiation dose (Figure 2).

Image quality assessment was also performed considering two ROIs of clustered microcalcifications extracted from the mammograms: one with 50% of contrast and one of 25% of contrast. Results suggested that the proposed methodology produced better quality images by reducing noise without noticeably affecting image sharpness, as seen at Figure 1.

In future work we will study the effect of the proposed denoising filter on the performance of microcalcification detection using observer studies and ROC analysis, in order to evaluate the clinical use of the proposed methodology in breast-cancer screening.

Acknowledgements. The authors would like to thank FAPESP and CAPES for their financial support and Ms. Susan Ng from *Real-Time Tomography* (Villanova, PA) for processing the simulated projection images.

References

1. Karellas, A., Vedantham, S.: Breast cancer imaging: a perspective for the next decade. Med. Phys. 35(11), 4878–4897 (2008)
2. Acha, B., Serrano, C., Rangayyan, R.M., Leo Desautels, J.E.: Detection of microcalcifications in mammograms using error of prediction and statistical measures. J. Electron. Imaging 18(1), 013011 (2009)
3. Papadopoulos, A., Fotiadis, D.I., Costaridou, L.: Improvement of microcalcification cluster detection in mammography utilizing image enhancement techniques. Comput. Biol. Med. 38(10), 1045–1055 (2008)

4. Gonzalez, R.C., Woods, R.E.: Digital Image Processing, 3rd edn. Prentice Hall, Upper Saddle River (2008)
5. Saunders, R.S., Baker, J.A., Delong, D.M., Johnson, J.P., Samei, E.: Does image quality matter? Impact of resolution and noise on mammographic task performance. Med. Phys. 34(10), 3971–3981 (2007)
6. Anscombe, F.J.: The transformation of Poisson, binomial and negative-binomial data. Biometrika 35, 246–254 (1948)
7. Mascarenhas, N.D.A., Santos, C.A.N., Cruvinel, P.E.: Transmission tomography under Poisson noise using the Anscombe transformation and Wiener filtering of the projections. Nucl. Instrum. Meth. A 423, 265–271 (1999)
8. Bakic, P.R., Zhang, C., Maidment, A.D.: Development and characterization of an anthropomorphic breast software phantom based upon region-growing algorithm. Med. Phys. 38(6), 3165–3176 (2011)
9. Wang, Z., Bovik, A.C.: Mean squared error: Love it or leave it? A new look at signal fidelity measures. IEEE Signal Proc. Mag. 26(1), 98–117 (2009)
10. Wang, Z., Bovik, A.C., Sheikh, H.R., Simoncelli, E.P.: Image quality assessment: from error visibility to structural similarity. IEEE T. Image Process. 13(4), 600–612 (2004)

A Novel Workflow-Centric Breast MRI Reading Prototype Utilizing Multitouch Gestures

Markus Harz[1], Felix Ritter[1], Simon Benten[1],
Kathy Schilling[2], and Heinz-Otto Peitgen[1]

[1] Fraunhofer MEVIS, 28865 Bremen, Germany
`markus.harz@mevis.fraunhofer.de`
[2] Boca Raton Regional Hospital, Boca Raton FL 33431, U.S.A.

Abstract. We propose a novel paradigm for clinical diagnostic software using a mobile multi-touch device for user interaction and dedicated monitors for image display. We show a demonstrator implementing a workflow-based breast MRI reading system tailored to multi-touch interaction. The demonstrator explores the feasibility of touch interaction for diagnostic reading of MRI patient cases. We show a patient-centric, workflow-oriented concept that is arranged around a multi-touch capable hybrid input-output device.

In this contribution we introduce clinically useful concepts of the demonstrator. Firstly, a mechanism that we dubbed location awareness takes care of security issues. Reading is supported by (1) a patient browser with graphical patient history and cancer risk factors; (2) a workflow concept using hanging protocols; (3) dedicated ROI definition, annotation, and measurement tools using multi-touch gestures. Gesture concepts and interaction paradigms are introduced for intuitive user experiences while maintaining accuracy.

1 Introduction and Prior Art

The spread of mobile devices in society is reflected by a likewise high number of radiologists owning iPhones, Android phones, iPads, and other touch display equipped personal mobile devices. Recent estimates prospectively spoke of 80% of radiologists intending to own an iPad by the end of 2012. We also note a high demand for radiology software on mobile devices, reflected in growing numbers of presentations on major conferences, and also reflected by company efforts to support their respective clinical software platforms on mobile devices. Even FDA approved iPad-based reading software is already available on the market.

There are only very few scientific publications exploring the subject of mobile device based interaction for clinical image-based diagnostic reading. We speculate that on the one hand, mobile multitouch devices are not available for long enough to be profoundly researched for this application, and on the other hand there is no clear paradigm visible how such devices should be employed to be useful and intuitive. Our contribution aims to help in both challenges. We want to provide a novel approach to integrate a mobile device in a clinical setting,

A.D.A. Maidment, P.R. Bakic, and S. Gavenonis (Eds.): IWDM 2012, LNCS 7361, pp. 276–283, 2012.
© Springer-Verlag Berlin Heidelberg 2012

and we want to present a demonstrator that implements our paradigm on a challenging clinical topic that can be explored clinically.

Prior work that we acknowledge has been presented by Lundström et al. [3], who employ multitouch gestures for interaction with medical images, and use a flexible tool selection menu. Their work, however, is aimed towards team interaction on a very large display table. A very similar approach has been presented for the application on digital pathology [4] and for medical team meetings [2,1]. A work closer to the system proposed by us has been described in the US 2011/0113329 A1 patent publication. In this work, the author proposes a static setup on the mobile device, where touch wheels and buttons are depicted and usable with two hands. BrainLab employs a wall-mounted multi-touch display for use in brain surgical interventions, and has also foreseen the integration of a multi-touch mobile device, which is, however to be attached to the main system (Pat. EP 2 031 531 A2). IBM has proposed a system in which the image data is viewed on the mobile device (Pat. US 2010/0293500 A1).

Reviewing the cited body of scientific work, patents, and available tools, we have condensed the following tachometry of concepts. It served as the outline out of which we designed and described the dedicated support we want to contribute.

Paradigm. Generally, the mobile device is foreseen to be used independently of the hospital information systems, though connected to it by WiFi. Either an App (Application, like eg. downloaded in Apples AppStore or on the Android market), or a fully web-based user interface provides the functionality.

Viewing. In particular, images are generally viewed on the device, and interaction with the images is conducted on the screen. For interaction, a reduced set of tools is offered in toolbars, emulating the interface of the corresponding workstation software.

Interaction. Usually, the tools provided follow the workstation tools, and work like those. One notable exception in some cases is the zoom/pan functionality, where eg. zooming is accomplished with a two-finger pinch gesture.

Workflow. Workflow is generally not an issue addressed by the mobile apps, since they are mostly not intended to be used for diagnostic image reading. Hence, no structured review of images is implemented, rather a random-access toolbox is provided.

Security. Login to the hospital IT is required; the device acts as a remote viewing station.

Intended use. Most applications seem to be targeting the casual user who wants to have a quick look at a specific image while away from a workstation. For example, a radiologist on call might appreciate to see a case on his mobile device to decide if he needs to drive to hospital to see the emergency patient.

In our contribution, we follow a different paradigm, propose a concept and setup that targets diagnostic reading, makes use of a different approach to security and data handling, and consequently has a different user group in mind: the radiologist doing diagnostic reading.

With our work, we want to challenge several aspects of conventional breast MRI workstations, and provide a clinically usable setup centered around a combination

of stationary display devices and a mobile device that provides ubiquitous interaction with clinical data. Most importantly, we wish to move away from the static
random access toolbox approach in current reading workstations, and introduce
workflows into breast MRI reading. In this attempt, we see the display devices
with attached IT systems and hospital IT connectivity as one unit together with
the mobile device, as opposed to the more conventional approach in which the
mobile device emulates a mouse and keyboard to pose as a better remote.

While in this contribution we will focus on the application to diagnostic reading of MRI series, other potential applications are already identified and will
shortly be mentioned in the conclusions below.

2   Material and Methods

The proposed system consists of a server side implementation that hosts the
data and displays all images on screen. It is accompanied by a client side implementation that runs as a native program on the mobile device. The two parts
are connected with a basic and efficient network protocol to exchange information and events using wireless LAN on the mobile device side, and any network
connectivity to the same network on the server side.

The software demonstrator has been implemented based on MeVisLab, an ex-
tensible medical image processing development environment, where C++-based
programming is efficiently combined with Python scripting and a powerful GUI
description language. The device demonstrator has been implemented using the
Apple inbuilt development environment, and is written for the iOS framework
in ObjectiveC. The C++ implementation of the gesture framework has been
accomplished based on the Qt framework, and not on the mobile device to allow for the easy integration of mobile devices with different operating systems,
and for arbitrary extensions without device dependencies. With application-side
interpretation and implementation of gestures, coherent interaction is guaran-
teed regardless of mobile device. Technically, for the workflow the device is only
required to send one or multiple touch points, and all intended interaction is
evaluated on the server computer.

2.1   Paradigm

In our setup, the mobile device poses as a hybrid image display and interaction
device, changing its role during the workflow. The fundamental principle is not
to show images for clinical diagnosis on the device. The major reasons are (1) the
limited screen real estate, where for example correlated viewing of orthogonal
reconstructions in sufficient size is not feasible; and (2) the fact that during
interaction the fingers will occlude a large portion of the small screen. Hence,
in our opinion image display is better left with dedicated display devices. These
can be tailored to their purpose, e.g. a defined contrast range for diagnostic
reading, or large screen sizes in a operating theater. The mobile device also
never stores data locally, which increases security, though the concept might
also include secured storage of selected key images per patient for patient visits

or interdisciplinary board meetings. In the general setting, the data is provided by a server that is typically connected to the hospital IT. The login procedure to access the data is accomplished by linking the mobile device with the display device.

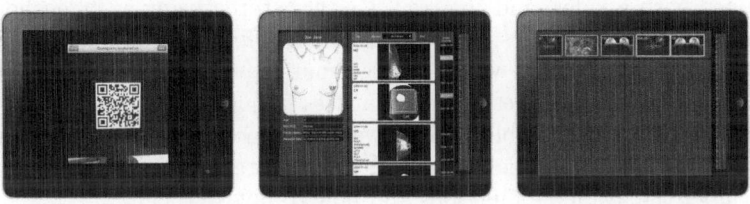

Fig. 1. iPad screens. From left: (1) Reading the QR code. (2) The patient browser interface. (3) The iPad user interface during reading. MR images are displayed on the display devices (not shown).

2.2 Authentication and Location Awareness

In our setup, we think of the mobile device as a personal item belonging to the radiologist. He will log in to his device and authenticate towards it. To connect to a display device, different mechanisms are conceivable. In our current implementation, the internal camera of the mobile device reads a QR code that is displayed on the display device and that encodes the location and capabilities of the display device. By reading in the QR code, the mobile device learns about the display device, and configures itself such that the available tools are offered, and only the applicable patient data is shown to the radiologist. In practice, in a patient room only the data pertaining to the patients in this room are offered, and diagnostic tools, annotations, and reporting functionality are not provided; in a meeting room only the data of today's tumor board meeting might be shown with annotation functionality, while in a diagnostic reading room, all functionality will be provided for all patients assigned to the doctor.

2.3 Workflow

In contrast to existing workstations for breast MRI reading, we have removed all tool bars and menus from the application. Two reasons exist for that: (1) From an assessment of several experienced breast MR readers' usage of breast MR workstations, we observed that a very small subset of available tools was frequently used. (2) With a touch-based interaction paradigm, tool bars and menus are no longer a convincing means of interaction, because they necessitate a pointing device.

Workflow analysis was carried out in a community hospital breast care center, where an above-average number of MRI exams are being read (local high-risk population). We have been trained on the same workstation by independent experts prior to the workflow analyses, such that we knew all tools that can be employed during reading. With this background, we have observed four radiologists while reading MRI exams and video-taped their work. We have interrogated the radiologists on their tool usage, and on their reasons for using or not using them. One remarkable finding was that the only annotation tool that we have seen in use was an arrow pointing to a location of interest. Sizes have been determined with a ruler, and the results either stored using a screenshot or by dictation into a reporting system. Segmentation of findings for kinetic characterization was never employed. We also noted that the tools were often selected via the menu bar and submenues of that, but less frequently using keyboard shortcuts or icons. A notable problem which was also reported by the radiologists was that the ways the mouse has to travel is rather large, and that it is impossible to remember the available functions and how to invoke them.

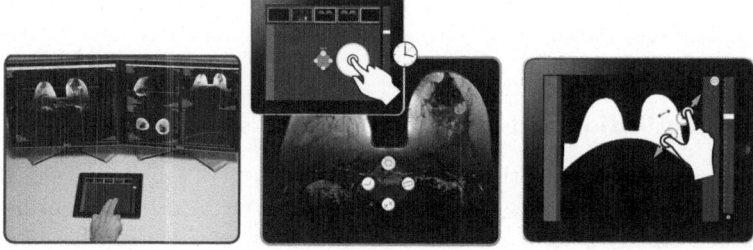

Fig. 2. Application and tools. Left: a two-monitor setup is operated by the mobile device. Middle: Bringing up the context sensitive circular menu with a tap and hold gesture. Right: The iPad screen while a measurement is performed. Breast shape shown for orientation.

From these assessments of breast MR reading workflows, we designed a novel user interface both for the mobile device and the display devices. Main driving factors were to provide intuitive usage, and to minimize the necessity of large-scale movements to access functionality. The most complex interaction is patient selection and workup of patient history, which is consequently handled on the mobile device in an intuitive patient browser that shows the patient history with clinical events and risk data (cf. Fig. 1, middle). Annotations are correlated between sketch (left), image series (middle), and time line (right) using distinctive colors.

Image series thumbnails in the middle can be previewed in larger size on the diagnostic screens together with additional information. To select a series for diagnostic reading, the series thumbnail is double-tapped, which leads into the reading workflow. The screen on the mobile device changes to the appearance in Fig. 1 (right), where the predefined workflow steps (hangings) are indicated with icons on the top, while the rest of the space is left for gesture-based interaction. Preconfigured workflow steps are then executed swipe-by-swipe.

2.4 Navigation

Breast MRI diagnostic workstations usually offer viewports to show different aspects of the data, statically arranged on one or more monitors. The user may change the layout, or zoom viewports to fullscreen and interact. This is not feasible in our system. Instead, we defined a number of viewport arrangements (hangings), where always one viewport is shown in larger size and takes all input (the master viewport), and all others support the reading with additional information. These hangings are then executed in sequence.

Navigation and interaction is done using gestures, and all gestures always apply only to the master viewport. Other viewports providing additional image data, derived data, orthogonal projections of the master view etc. are continuously updated to match the position on the master viewport.

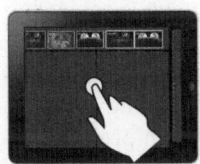 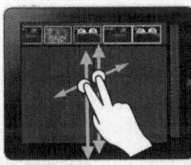 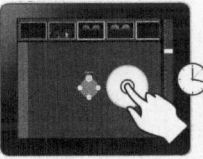 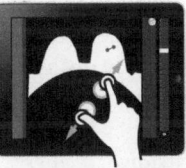

Fig. 3. Gestures. From left: (1) One finger moves selection. (2) Two fingers swipe to stack through images, move through time points, dim color overlay. (3) Three-finger swipe: previous/next workflow step. (4) Five-finger tap: back.

Gestures are composed of a number of fingers used, and a pattern of how the fingers move. We have designed the gestures such that frequently used functionality is easier to access, and that accidental triggering of harmful actions is avoided. Also, gestures are used similarly across contexts.

The following gestures are implemented currently (cf. Fig. 3):

One finger tap and move. Navigate on a master viewport.

One finger double-tap and move. Window/Level control.

One finger tap and hold. Bring up the context-sensitive circular tools menu.

Two finger swipes. Up-Down to stack through the images. In dynamic series: Left-Right to navigate through time points. In color overlays: Left-Right controls transparency.

Three finger swipes. Previous/next hanging in the workflow. Direct access of hangings: select in hanging bar.

Five finger tap. Save results, finish the session. Returns to patient selection screen.

This set of gestures can be adapted to further applications, e.g. mammography and tomosynthesis screening workflows. Regarding tool support during the workflow, all applications will share some common properties, as follows.

2.5   Tool Menu

During each workflow step, tools are only offered when they apply to the reviewed series, and to the currently selected location. Our segmentation algorithm, for example, requires a subtraction image with sufficient contrast near the seed point. Thus, the segmentation tool will be offered only if the preconditions are met.

Bringing up the tool menu is done by touching and holding a point of interest. A circular menu around the finger on the touch display, and around the selected location on the display screens will show all options that apply at this location, e.g. measurement, annotation, and segmentation tools. Once a finding is segmented, it can be annotated. In any case it will be indicated with a color mark both on the screens and the touch display. Also, it will be stored in the case database, and displayed with a graphical icon in the patient overview screen. You can always navigate to the image slices corresponding to a finding by clicking the color bar. Of course, all views are immediately synchronized.

For size measurements, we implemented a two finger scale gesture that anticipates the desired size and zooms the images automatically to enable the precise measurement even of very small structures. For reporting of finding locations, one finger interactively indicates the location of interest, and from precomputed locations of chest wall and nipples, the shortest distances are annotated and indicated.

3   Results

Our demonstrator has been presented at different major European and international radiology meetings. A formal evaluation is lacking at this point of development; the general setup and paradigm, however, was appreciated. We are currently preparing first clinical tests regarding the speed of the workflow, and detailed experiments to assess accuracy and speed of the individual tools. This answers the most critical remarks, which focussed on the speed that can be achieved by using touch interaction instead of a mouse, demanding for experimental performance figures compared with special keypads, and of course mouse and keyboard. The second most critical remark concerned the accuracy, given that fingers always touch an area rather than a point. Both criticisms will be addressed in the experiments.

4   Discussion

We propose a novel system setup utilizing a multitouch-capable mobile device to replace mouse and keyboard, where the image display is done on dedicated display devices, while auxiliary information and interaction capabilities are provided on the mobile device.

It is our intention to develop this system into a useful tool, and to evaluate it in terms of performance and user experience. Our current aim is to collect remarks and comments of the prospective users, and the breast imaging community.

Our goal for the future is to extend the applications beyond breast MRI. Since display devices exist in many places in the hospital, like e.g. in patient rooms, in meeting rooms, in dedicated diagnostic reading facilities, in the operating theater, and in recreational areas. These display devices may be of different nature: HD television in the patient room, projectors in meeting rooms, certified multi-monitor setups in the reading room and so on. The mobile device can then be utilized to provide seamless, location-specific interaction with images, always using the same general gesture-based approach, but providing task-specific tools or views on the patient data, depending on the current situation.

References

1. Avila-Garcia, M., Trefethen, A., Brady, M., Gleeson, F.: Using interactive and multi-touch technology to support decision making in multidisciplinary team meetings. In: 2010 IEEE 23rd International Symposium on Computer-Based Medical Systems (CBMS), pp. 98–103 (October 2010)
2. Avila-Garcia, M., Trefethen, A., Brady, M., Gleeson, F., Goodman, D.: Lowering the barriers to cancer imaging. In: IEEE Fourth International Conference on eScience, 2008, pp. 63–70 (December 2008)
3. Lundstrom, C., Rydell, T., Forsell, C., Persson, A., Ynnerman, A.: Multi-touch table system for medical visualization: Application to orthopedic surgery planning. IEEE Transactions on Visualization and Computer Graphics 17(12), 1775–1784 (2011)
4. Wang, Y., Williamson, K.E., Kelly, P.J., James, J.A., Hamilton, P.W.: SurfaceSlide: a multitouch digital pathology platform. PloS one 7(1), e30783 (2012)

Evaluation of Various Mammography Phantoms for Image Quality Assessment in Digital Breast Tomosynthesis

Claudia C. Brunner[1], Raymond J. Acciavatti[2], Predrag R. Bakic[2],
Andrew D.A. Maidment[2], Mark B. Williams[3], Richard Kaczmarek[1],
and Kish Chakrabarti[1,*]

[1] Center for Devices and Radiological Health, U.S. Food and Drug Administration,
Silver Spring, MD 20910
[2] Department of Radiology, University of Pennsylvania, Philadelphia, PA 19104
[3] Department of Radiology and Medical Imaging, University of Virginia,
Charlottesville, VA 22908

Abstract. We investigated the appropriateness of four different mammography phantoms for image quality evaluation in Digital Breast Tomosynthesis (DBT). We tested the CIRS BR3D phantom, the ACR Prototype FFDM Accreditation Phantom, the Penn anthropomorphic breast phantom and the Quart mam/digi EPQC phantom. This work discusses the advantages and shortcomings of each phantom and concludes that none of them, in their current form, can be considered to be adequate as an image quality evaluation phantom for DBT.

Keywords: Digital Breast Tomosynthesis, Quality evaluation, Phantoms.

1 Purpose

Digital Breast Tomosynthesis (DBT), recently approved by the FDA for screening and diagnosis of breast abnormalities, improves upon mammography by providing 3-dimensional resolution that allows depth discrimination and overcomes the problem of signal degradation by overlying anatomy. It is regulated under the Mammography Quality Standards Act (MQSA), which requires quantitative image quality evaluation with a human observer as well as objective image quality evaluation. For the quantitative evaluation, human observers have to score the visibility of specific objects in the phantom. The objective evaluation is software-based and provides information about image quality metrics such as resolution, noise and contrast-to-noise ratio (CNR). However, since image quality evaluation in DBT is currently based on quality

---

* Contact: Center for Devices and Radiological Health, U.S. Food and Drug Administration, 10903 New Hampshire Avenue, Silver Spring, MD 20993.
Email: kish.chakrabarti@fda.hhs.gov or claudia.brunner@fda.hhs.gov
"The mention of commercial products herein is not to be construed as either an actual or implied endorsement of such products by the Department of Health and Human Services."

A.D.A. Maidment, P.R. Bakic, and S. Gavenonis (Eds.): IWDM 2012, LNCS 7361, pp. 284–291, 2012.

evaluation in projection mammography, specific properties unique to DBT, such as the slice-sensitivity profile, may not be sufficiently captured. To our knowledge no study exists that would present a phantom specifically designed for DBT which can be used to perform complete quality control and acceptance tests. So far studies on quality control phantoms for DBT have only focused on single parameters of image quality such as in-plane resolution and slice thickness [1, 2].

In light of the necessity to characterize clinical image quality in DBT, the purpose of this study was to investigate the appropriateness as well as limitations of four currently available phantoms for image quality evaluation in DBT.

2   Material and Methods

For all image acquisitions, we used a Selenia Dimensions Digital Breast Tomosynthesis device (Hologic, Inc., Bedford, MA, USA) located at the Hospital of the University of Pennsylvania (Philadelphia, PA). All phantoms were scanned applying the "AutoFilter" exposure control mode of the system that automatically chooses filter, tube voltage and tube current. For each scan, 15 images were acquired at 1.07° intervals over an angle range of ±7.5°. The device reconstructs images in planes parallel to the breast support in 1 mm increments through the thickness of the phantom. We assessed the reconstructed images in the same way as DBT images are viewed under clinical conditions (i.e. slice-wise evaluation). If the phantom allowed a subjective image evaluation, it was always performed by 4 human observers. The four phantoms tested in this study were:

The **CIRS Model 020 BR3D Mammography phantom** (CIRS, Norfolk, VA, USA) consists of a set of 6 slabs made of two tissue equivalent materials mimicking 100% adipose and glandular tissues "swirled" together in an approximate 50/50 ratio by weight. One of the slabs contains an assortment of speck groups, fibers and masses; its diameters are given in Table 1. The CIRS phantom has been used in former studies for example to investigate the performance of DBT [3] or the potential of an implemented scatter correction in the image reconstruction algorithm [4].

Table 1. Diameter of the objects embedded in the target slab of the CIRS phantom

	Fibers	Specks	Masses
1	0.60 mm	0.400 mm	6.3 mm
2	0.41 mm	0.290 mm	4.7 mm
3	0.38 mm	0.230 mm	3.9 mm
4	0.28 mm	0.196 mm	3.1 mm
5	0.23 mm	0.165 mm	2.3 mm
6	0.18 mm	0.130 mm	1.8 mm
7	0.15 mm		

The **ACR Prototype FFDM Accreditation Phantom** (CIRS, Norfolk, VA, USA) is based on the well-known Mammographic Accreditation Phantom (CIRS Model 015) but with a phantom size in the range of the detector size and a finer gradation of the test objects. It contains 6 fibers, 6 speck groups and 6 masses of diameters given in Table 2. The objects are embedded in a homogeneous wax insert positioned within a PMMA block. Further, the phantom contains a cavity to calculate the CNR and large homogeneous regions to analyze the noise properties of the image.

Table 2. Diameter of the objects embedded in the ACR phantom

	Fibers	Specks	Masses
1	0.89 mm	0.33 mm	1.00 mm
2	0.75 mm	0.28 mm	0.75 mm
3	0.61 mm	0.23 mm	0.50 mm
4	0.54 mm	0.20 mm	0.38 mm
5	0.40 mm	0.17 mm	0.25 mm
6	0.30 mm	0.14 mm	0.20 mm

The **Penn anthropomorphic breast phantom** was developed at the University of Pennsylvania specifically for 3-dimensional breast x-ray imaging [5, 6]. It was designed based upon the Penn software anthropomorphic breast phantom [7]. The phantom consists of several slabs of tissue-equivalent adipose and glandular material simulating a dense fibroglandular pattern resulting in images that are qualitatively similar to clinical images with the grayscale range of adipose and fibroglandular elements approximating the pattern seen in a heterogeneously dense breast. An additional, interchangeable slab contains iodinated lesions with 5 different diameters and two different iodine concentrations. The additional slab was designed for the use with contrast enhanced digital breast tomosynthesis [6].

The **Quart mam/digi EPQC phantom** (Quart GmbH, Zorneding, Germany) is a relatively new phantom developed for mammography as well as for breast tomosynthesis [8, 9]. It consists of a PMMA body containing a wedge of 12 steps on the chest wall side to simulate different densities of breast tissue material. A titanium strip, which is equivalent to 100 μm bone material, divides each step and therefore allows the calculation of the CNR for various thicknesses. The MTF can be calculated using the edges of a brass and a lead square and a slot for a suited dosimeter detector enables performing dose measurements according to the EPQC guidelines [10]. Additionally, the phantom features so-called Landolt (broken) rings that are contained within two different layers separated by 20 mm. These rings have a gap at either of 4 different directions (top, bottom, left and right) and are sorted in groups of 6 rings of decreasing size on each step. By focusing on the planes that contain the Landolt rings, it is possible to determine the distance between planes as well as to subjectively quantify object visibility at two different heights. In order to do that, a human observer has to estimate the position of the gaps for the ring groups corresponding to the 7 thickest steps using appropriate zoom and contrast window. The number of correctly perceived gaps gives one of the imaging performance parameters. For mammography, 20 gaps have to be called correctly for the image to pass the test, but for DBT an official threshold has not yet been established.

Further, each of the 12 steps contains a low-contrast number indicating the PMMA thickness corresponding to the step. The thicker the step on which the numbers can be read, the better is the image, so that the visibility of these numbers is an additional imaging performance parameter.

The objective image analysis was done with a user-written Mathematica code, because the manufacturer's software to automatically analyze the image parameters has not yet been released. To calculate the MTF, the brass square was used, since it is further away from the step wedge and therefore suffers less from reconstruction artifacts. Both the MTF perpendicular and parallel to the breast wall were calculated. In order to estimate the noise variance, the noise power spectrum (NPS) was calculated averaging over the homogenous region in the center of the phantom of all available slices.

3   Results

Reconstructed images of each phantom under investigation are presented in Fig. 1. All images are shown with the same magnification in order to give the reader an impression about the different sizes of the phantoms and their structures.

Figure 1a shows the slice of the CIRS BR3D phantom that contains the objects. Even though the objects are hardly visible in Fig. 1, the four human observers

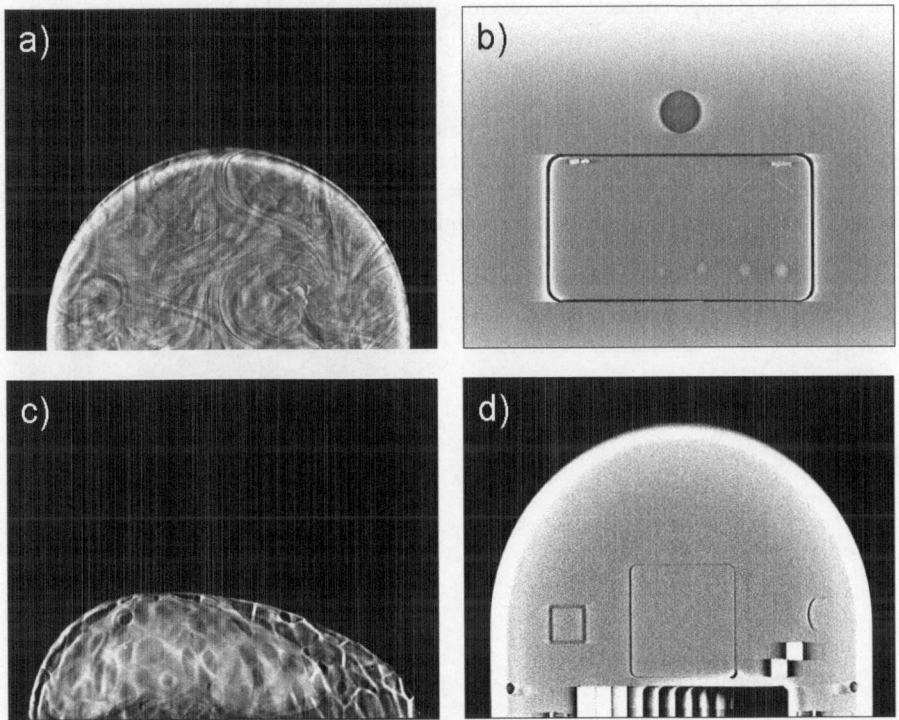

Fig. 1. Reconstructed images of the mammography phantoms under investigation: a) CIRS BR3D phantom, b) ACR FFDM phantom, c) anthropomorphic phantom and d) Quart phantom

288   C.C. Brunner et al.

detected on average 4 ½ speck groups, 5 fibers and 3 masses on a suitable screen. However, it turned out that the actual scoring depends not only on the reader, but also slightly on the order of the slabs, which is influenced by the heterogeneous background.

In the ACR phantom, shown in Fig. 1b, the objects are embedded in a homogenous background. The four human observers detected on average all 6 masses, 3 ½ speck groups and 4 ½ fibers.

Figure 1c shows that the anthropomorphic phantom is composed of dense fibroglandular tissue in the inner region in which compartments of adipose tissue are embedded. The outer region is composed of adipose tissue supported by a matrix of Cooper's ligaments. Since no objects are embedded in the phantom, it can only be stated that the phantom produces a realistic image of a breast, but neither a quantitative nor objective analysis can be performed.

The Quart phantom, shown in Figure 1d, provides means to assess image quality metrics objectively. The brass (top) and lead (bottom) squares on the right can be used to calculate the MTF and the homogeneous area in the center of the phantom allows calculating the NPS. We look at these two parameters to develop means to assess image quality as constancy testing. The MTF was calculated using the edges of the brass square perpendicular and parallel to the chest wall. The resulting MTF curves, shown in Fig. 2a, demonstrate the difference in resolution between the two directions. The 2-dimensional NPS is shown in Fig. 2b as a function of the spatial frequency. As expected, the NPS has the double-cone shape characteristic of a tomosynthesis NPS [11, 12].

The manufacturer recommends calculating the CNR using the step wedge. However, it can be seen in Fig. 1d that the step wedge affords only small ROIs which are very inhomogeneous in the reconstructed images due to edge enhancement effects. This makes it difficult to use it for CNR calculations in DBT. The CNR may be more reliably estimated using the brass and lead contrast squares. Even though they do not allow calculating a thickness specific CNR as the step wedge, they can be used for a simple CNR calculation at one specific height.

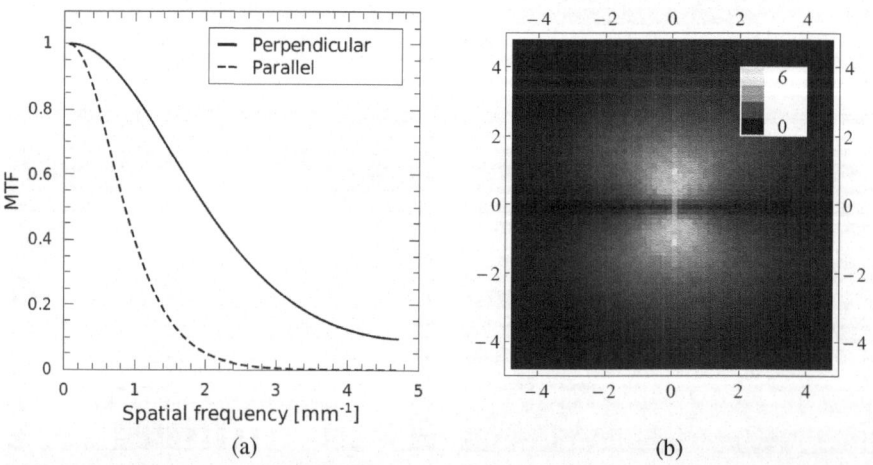

Fig. 2. MTF calculated from the brass square perpendicular and parallel to the chest wall (a) and the 2-dimensional NPS in mm² as a function of the spatial frequency in mm⁻¹ (b)

Scoring the Landolt rings turned out to be a challenging task, because finding the appropriate zoom and windowing level needs some time and experience. Further, the evaluation is quite time-consuming and wearisome for the eyes. On average the human observers were able to correctly detect 19 gaps which is slightly below the preliminary threshold for the image to pass the test. The manufacturer recommends evaluating more images in case the number of detected gaps is between 18 and 22 to have reliable results. However, since the tomosynthesis device is not on-site and our study focused on testing the phantom for its advantages and shortcomings, we did not acquire any additional images.

4   Discussion

Each phantom has its advantages and is useful for the purpose for which it was originally designed. However, we concluded that none of them by itself can be used as either a quantitative or objective phantom that provides information useful for image quality evaluation in DBT images. Further, none of these phantoms under investigation provide means to measure in-plane distance accuracy, slice-sensitivity profiles or the amount of breast tissue missed at the chest wall.

The advantages and shortcomings of each phantom can be summarized as follows:

The CIRS phantom features different objects in a heterogeneous background. It allows the qualitative evaluation of one reconstructed image slice that corresponds to the height in which the objects are positioned. Careful choice of the windowing level as well as high magnification and a trained reader are required to score the image. Also, visibility of the objects is dependent upon the ordering of the slabs, as the structures above and below the plane of reconstruction contribute to the image complexity. Therefore, it is important, in case this phantom is used for constancy tests, to always maintain the same order of slabs. Its shortcomings are that it is neither possible to check the reconstruction depth nor objective image parameters such as resolution, noise variance or CNR.

The ACR phantom allows the scoring of different objects in a homogenous background and enables the calculation of the noise variance and the CNR. However, since all masses are easily detectable, it still has to be proven that the phantom is sufficiently discriminative of differences in image quality and overall system performance for DBT. Moreover, the objects are only arranged at one specific depth so that neither the reconstruction depth nor the object visibility at different depths can be analyzed.

The Penn anthropomorphic phantom allows the evaluation of whether the scanner provides natural looking reconstruction images with breast like structures. It includes a controlled amount of dense tissue, which could be used to validate breast density estimation. Currently it only contains a limited variety of targets for a quantitative scoring of the images and no features that would enable an objective image quality evaluation. However, additional slabs containing defined objects for quantitative analysis or other features such as inserts for dosimeters (e.g., optically stimulated luminescence dosimeters) are feasible. With its realistic structure and 3-dimensional extension, this phantom has the potential to become useful for image quality analysis as well as direct dose and dose distribution measurements in DBT.

The Quart phantom is the only phantom we tested, that had features to objectively measure the image quality parameters such as MTF, NPS or CNR. Depending on the performance and user-friendliness of the upcoming software to automatically evaluate the image quality, the phantom may potentially be useful for DBT. However, since it was primarily designed for mammography, it also suffers from several shortcomings. One issue is that the step wedge affords only small ROIs which are very inhomogeneous in the reconstructed images due to edge enhancement effects. Even though the manufacturer has informed us that the upcoming software will address this issue, the results of the CNR calculation may not be reliable. Moreover, due to the straight alignment of the inserted objects in this phantom, it is not possible to calculate an oversampled MTF, as required for mammography in the IEC standard [13], from an image that has been acquired according to the manufacturer's instructions. Finally, the Landolt rings allow checking the accuracy of reconstruction depth and object visibility in tomosynthesis images. The subjective evaluation with the Landolt rings however is wearisome and time-consuming, so that this test can hardly be part of a regular quality control in the clinic. Additionally, since the human observer mostly guesses the position of the gap, it has to be investigated whether the observer's memory begins to retain the position of the gaps and therefore achieves better results after repeated scoring.

5   Conclusions

Although each phantom under study has its advantages, none of them allows a thorough quality evaluation of reconstructed tomosynthesis images. The phantoms, in their current form, may be still better suited for projection mammography. In some cases (e.g. the Penn anthropomorphic phantom) the inclusion of additional layers permitting 3-dimensional analysis is feasible; while in others (e.g. the ACR FFDM phantom) major phantom redesign would be necessary for use in DBT. For all 4 phantoms tested, neither subjective nor objective evaluations involving all the reconstructed planes are possible. Since there is no other phantom on the market, for our knowledge that includes the features to measure all image properties relevant in DBT, it is necessary to design a new phantom. In order to allow a clinical implementation the new phantom has to allow a quick subjective image evaluation or provide user-friendly software to automatically analyze the objective image parameters that optimally could be measured in only one scan.

Acknowledgement. This work was partially supported by the FDA's Critical Path Project.

References

[1] Li, B., Saunders, R., Uppaluri, R.: Measurement of slice thickness and in-plane resolution on radiographic tomosynthesis system using modulation transfer function (MTF). In: Proc. SPIE 6142, 61425D (2006)

[2] Bouwman, R., Visser, R., Young, K., Dance, D., Lazzari, B., van der Burght, R., Heide, P., van Engen, R.: Daily quality control for breast tomosynthesis. In: Proc. SPIE 7622, 762241 (2010)

[3] Vecchio, S., Albanese, A., Vignoli, P., Taibi, A.: A novel approach to digital breast tomosynthesis for simultaneous acquisition of 2D and 3D images. European Radiology 21, 1207–1213 (2011)

[4] Feng, S.S.J., Sechopoulos, I.: A software-based x-ray scatter correction method for breast tomosynthesis. Medical Physics 38, 6643–6653 (2011)

[5] Carton, A.K., Bakic, P., Ullberg, C., Derand, H., Maidment, A.D.A.: Development of a physical 3D anthropomorphic breast phantom. Medical Physics 38, 891–896 (2011)

[6] Carton, A.K., Bakic, P., Ullberg, C., Maidment, A.D.A.: Development of a 3D high-resolution physical anthropomorphic breast phantom. In: Proc. SPIE 7622, 762206-1 (2010)

[7] Bakic, P.R., Zhang, C., Maidment, A.D.A.: Development and characterization of an anthropomorphic breast software phantom based upon region-growing algorithm. Medical Physics 38, 3165–3176 (2011)

[8] de las Heras, H., Peng, R., Zeng, R., Freed, M., O'Bryan, E., Jennings, R.J.: A versatile laboratory platform for studying x-ray 3D breast imaging. In: Proceedings of IEEE Medical Imaging Conference MIC12.M-17 (2011)

[9] de las Heras, H., Schöfer, F., Tiller, B., del Río, M.C., Zwettler, G., Semturs, F.: A new method for dosimetry and image quality assurance in mammography and breast tomosynthesis. In: Proc. IRPA (2012)

[10] Perry, N., Broeders, M., de Wolf, C., Törnberg, S., Holland, R., von Karsa, L.: European guidelines for quality assurance in breast cancer screening and diagnosis - 4th (edn.) Technical report, Office for Official Publications of the European Communities (2006)

[11] Richard, S., Samei, E.: Quantitative breast tomosynthesis: From detectability to estimability. Medical Physics 37, 6157–6165 (2010)

[12] Richard, S., Samei, E.: Quantitative imaging in breast tomosynthesis and CT: Comparison of detection and estimation task performance. Medical Physics 37, 2627–2637 (2010)

[13] IEC: 62220-1-2:2007 Medical electrical equipment - Characteristics of digital X-ray imaging devices - Part 1-2: Determination of the detective quantum efficiency - Detectors used in mammography. Technical report, International Electrotechnical Commission (2007)

Effects of Medical Display Luminance, Contrast and Temporal Compensation on CHO Detection Performance at Various Browsing Speeds and on Digital Breast Tomosynthesis Images

Cédric Marchessoux[1], Ali N. Avanaki[1,*], Predrag R. Bakic[2],
Tom R.L. Kimpe[1], and Andrew D.A. Maidment[2]

[1] BARCO N.V., Healthcare Division, Kortrijk, Belgium
ali.avanaki@barco.com
[2] University of Pennsylvania, Department of Radiology, Philadelphia, PA, USA

Abstract. Prior studies have shown that temporal compensation of medical displays improve the performance in detecting lesions for digital breast tomosynthesis (DBT). This has been proven both by using computer simulations as well as clinical experiments. This paper, by using computer simulations, studies (i) the effect of the maximum luminance (L_{max}) and contrast (L_{max}/L_{min}) of the medical display on lesion detection performance, and (ii) the effect of temporal compensation of the display (by comparing displays with and without this feature) on lesion detection performance, with several slice browsing speeds using a fractional frame repeat (FFR) scheme to model displays' behavior when the refresh rate is not an integer multiple of the browsing speed.

Keywords: Medical display, digital breast tomosynthesis (DBT), clinical studies, channelized Hotelling observers (CHO), browsing speed.

1 Introduction

Digital Breast Tomosynthesis (DBT) is a three-dimensional imaging technology that involves acquiring images of a stationary compressed breast at multiple angles during a short scan. The individual images are then reconstructed into a series of thin high-resolution slices that can be displayed individually or in a dynamic mode. Because reviewing images for this modality typically is done in a dynamic mode, which was not the case with full field digital mammography, and because breast cancer screening requires the best image display quality, a display optimized for DBT modality was developed (BARCO MDMG 5221). This display was optimized with improved intrinsic key characteristics such as contrast, luminance and temporal response. This article presents the result of a follow up study reported in [1]. Additional browsing speeds and display parameters such as contrast and luminance are considered and reported. In addition, input generated by a voxelized breast model [2] is also used. This is part of

---

* Corresponding author.

A.D.A. Maidment, P.R. Bakic, and S. Gavenonis (Eds.): IWDM 2012, LNCS 7361, pp. 292–299, 2012.

virtual clinical trial (VCT) platform that is under development, with the objective to compare real DBT images in which artificial lesions were introduced and fully simulated DBT images. For fully managing a VCT, every step in the chain should be controllable. Hence, using a phantom generator in VCT simulations to provide a customized input is necessary.

1.1 Prior Work

In [1], DBT reconstructed slices were used in which single micro calcifications were inserted. We have available to us a compiled version of a commercially used DBT reconstruction engine along with anonymized and pre-processed projection data (P) from real patients and geometry information necessary to reconstruct those projections using the DBT reconstruction engine. By pre-processed projections, we mean that any vendor/device specific projection processing such as bad pixel correction and beam hardening correction have already been performed on the raw projection data and that projection data can be now used as input to a known reconstruction algorithm. The DBT reconstructed images we reviewed consist of about 50 slices, each on a 1200 x 2400 matrix. The DBT voxel size was approximately 0.1 mm x 0.1 mm x 1.0 mm. A display with improved features such as temporal response compensation was clinically evaluated with the use of a numerical observer described in [3]. The numerical observer is an extension of a Channelized Hotelling Observer (CHO) for multiple slices that can be applied for quantifying the effect of the browsing speed of a system on lesion detection performance. A multi-reader multi-case (MRMC) analysis [4] was performed with 5 readers, each trained with 500 image pairs, and all reading the same 500 test image pairs. Only integer frame repeats (FR) were used that correspond to slice browsing speeds of $F_{refresh}$/FR (50, 25, 50/3, 12.5, 10 slice per second, for $F_{refresh}$ of 50 frames per second) which is very limiting as on real displays that browsing speed is desired to be changed continuously. A sample slice and a 1-D plot (central pixel luminance over slice number) are shown in Figure 1.

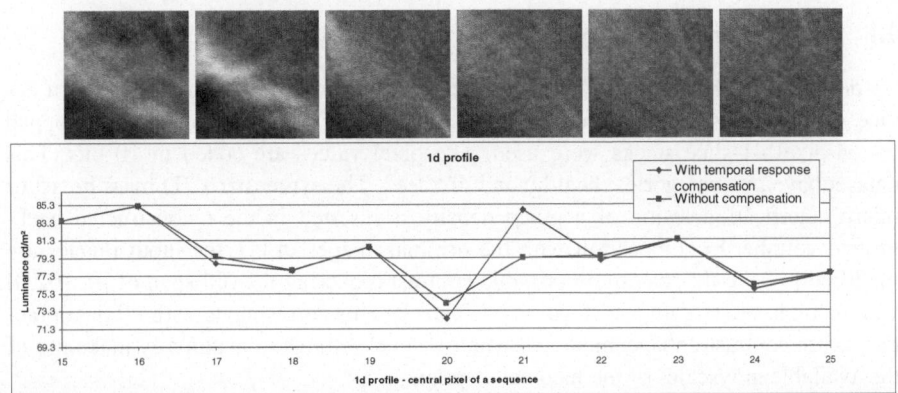

Fig. 1. Example of cropped (64 x 64 pixels) DBT slices from a 41-slice stack with a 0.4 mm lesion inserted in the center and a 1-D plot central pixels through 11 slices in cd/m² for temporal-response compensated and uncompensated displays. The signal is inserted in slice 21.

2   Methods

A key prerequisite of excellent system design in imaging systems is the control of the interplay of all its elements. Typical elements are the technology of image capture, the representation of the images as digital data, processing or enhancing of these data for a specific image display, the nature of the display technology (print or softcopy), and the psychometric judgment of the images through a human visual observer model [5]. An integrated approach, which combines a complete system model for a given imaging technology and a human visual observer model in one computational workbench, does therefore represent a great improvement for systematic image system design, optimization and even simulation of technology feasibility prior to prototypes. Engeldrum proposed a methodology named the Image Quality Circle [6], which shows the different phases to control and simulate a complete chain in the domain of vision. It also shows the links and relations between technology variables that we control from a product to the physical image parameters that we get from system modeling. The resulting image quality should be correlated to and optimized for the human perception or customer perceived preferences. From technology variables to user's preferences, the circle covers the complete chain. This methodology was used to develop and optimize a medical display for the digital breast tomosynthesis modality. A C++ simulation platform called MEVIC (Medical Virtual Imaging Chain) was used for simulating the complete chain from the image capture until the visualization of the images [7]. The virtual medical imaging chain starts with simulation of the image acquisition, over a hardware and software image processing pipeline and ends with the visualization by the medical specialist on the image display. The aforementioned chain is modeled as a cascade of three main modules: the virtual image capture, the virtual display and the virtual observer.

The key techniques that are used in MEVIC simulations for the current study are briefly described in the remainder of this section.

2.1   Simulation of DBT Images

As described in the prior work, reconstructed DBT slices from a real acquisition device were used as input images to the virtual imaging chain. In total, 6000 cropped 64x64-pixel 41-slice stacks were used. The pixel values are coded in 10 bits. This dataset have two categories: healthy and diseased. The synthesized 3D mass breast or micro calcification lesion of a given density is inserted in the reconstructed background volume. In comparison with the original images in [1], the input images are modified to have the maximum possible contrast (covering the full span of [0, 1023]) with a single offset/gain transform in each stack. This corresponds with clinical practice to use contrast-enhancement and window-level settings to maximally make use of the available grayscales of the medical display.

As the second objective to this study, we want to use the artificial backgrounds generated by anthropomorphic software breast phantom developed at the University of Pennsylvania [8]. It simulates the breast anatomy based upon the detailed analysis of histological and radiological images. The arrangement of breast tissues at the large and medium spatial scales is realistically simulated using a region growing approach. Synthetic x-ray images of the phantom are generated by simulating the breast deformation during the mammographic compression using a finite element model proposed in [9], followed by a model of the x-ray projections of the compressed phantom, assuming mono-energetic x-rays without scatter. 1648 stacks, each consisting of 32 64x64-pixel slices of phantom were used. The lesions are inserted using the procedure described in [1] to make the diseased stacks. The stacks are then randomly re-ordered to make it less likely that corresponding healthy and diseased images fall into the same training or test sets.

2.2   Display Simulation Chain

2.2.1   Contrast and Luminance

The native curve of the display is used for factoring in the effect of contrast and luminance of the display in MEVIC. Native curve value for a certain digital drive level (DDL) is the measured luminance of the display when a certain DDL is applied at the input for a long time. L_{max}, the maximum luminance of the display, is reached when the largest DDL (e.g. 1023, for a 10-bit display) is applied. L_{max} / L_{min} is the contrast with L_{min} being the minimum luminance of the display, reached for DDL of 0 ($L_{min}=1.05cd/m^2$ and $L_{max}=1000cd/m^2$). The luminance values correspond to a BARCO MDMG 5221 medical display.

2.2.2   Temporal Compensation of Display

The temporal response improvement is a proprietary solution from Barco (US Patent Application No: 2010/0207,960, 'devices and methods for reducing artifacts in display devices by the use of overdrive'). This solution allows the display to reach gray intensity values within one frame time without enhancing temporal noise or introducing artifacts. This technology was integrated in a FDA approved display optimized for digital breast tomosynthesis.

2.2.3   Fractional Frame Repeat (FFR)

The ability to continuously adjust the browsing speed is a desirable feature. Using integer frame repeats, simulations will be limited as described below. Let F_{browse} show the slice browsing speed, $F_{refresh}$ show the frame refresh rate (a display property in Hz), and FR show frame repeat. $F_{browse} = F_{refresh}/FR$. For example, at $F_{refresh}$ of 50 frame per second (fps), if each slice is fed twice to the display at consecutive refreshes (FR = 2), the apparent slice browsing speed is 50/2 = 25 slice per second (sps). In other words, FR = $F_{refresh}/F_{browse}$ = 50/25 = 2. Hence, the browsing speeds that can be simulated with integer FRs are very limited.

By allowing a fractional frame repeat, one can have arbitrary browsing speeds as follows. As an example, F_{browse} of 40 sps can be achieved if we make 5 frames out of every 4 slices. In this case FR = $F_{refresh}/F_{browse}$ = 50/40 = 5/4. To that end, we use an error accumulation method to find out which slices should be repeated: starting from the beginning of the stack (the residue is initially set to zero), each slice is copied floor(FR+residue) times, generating that many frames, and the residue is updated to

FR+residue-floor(FR+residue). This way, when the residue goes above one, an extra frame with a copy of the current slice is inserted. To have a slice browsing speed of 40 sps, on a 41-slice stack (comprised of slices 1, 2, ..., 41), when $F_{refresh}$ is 50 fps, the following slices are written to the frame buffer: 1 2 3 4 4 5 6 7 8 8 9 10 11 12 12 13 14 15 16 16 17 18 19 20 20 21 22 23 24 24 25 26 27 28 28 29 30 31 32 32 33 34 35 36 36 37 38 39 40 40 41. In this example, slice n is copied twice if mod(n, 4) = 0, and all other slices are copied only once.

2.3   Multi-slice Channelized Hotelling Observer (msCHO)

The multi-slice Channelized Hotelling model Observer (msCHO) described in [1, 3] is used with 10 LG channels of spread 15 for both real and artificial background data. The msCHO performance is computed for the pixel values achieved at the end of each refresh cycle during the T_{browse}. For example, when the frame repeat FR = 3 (see Tables 1 and 2), the detection performance is computed for image content at the end of each $1 \times T_{refresh}$, $2 \times T_{refresh}$ and $3 \times T_{refresh}$. Our observer only uses the three central slices of each stack as the other slices are lesion-free.

3   Results

3.1   Results on Real DBT Reconstructed Slices

The results on real DBT background slices are reported in Table 1. They show that FFR is working as expected since the AUCs for the FFR-generated browsing speed are similar to AUCs for speeds generated by regular (integer) frame repeating. Table 2, reports the same for a display without temporal compensation.

Table 1. Detection performance on real DBT reconstructed slices for 2 FFRs (30 & 40 sps) and three integer frame repeats (16.67, 25 & 50 sps) for a temporally compensated display on contrast-stretched data. The computations are performed in an MRMC study with N_{rd} = 5 readers, each trained with an independent subset of N_{tr} = 500 image pairs and all reading the same test set of N_{ts} = 500 test image pairs. The size of the ROI is 3. The AUCs and standard deviations are calculated using the one-shot method [4].

	Which after LCD frame is used to train 2D-CHO?	FR=1	FR= 50/40	FR= 50/30	FR=2	FR=3
AUC ± std	Frame 1	0.800 ±0.014	0.801 ±0.014	0.800 ±0.014	0.800 ±0.014	0.800 ±0.014
	Frame 2	N/A	N/A	N/A	0.801 ±0.014	0.801 ±0.014
	Frame 3	N/A	N/A	N/A	N/A	0.801 ±0.014
	Average	**0.800 ±0.014**	**0.800 ±0.014**	**0.800 ±0.014**	**0.801 ±0.014**	**0.801 ±0.014**

To study the effect of luminance and contrast on detection performance, we simulated two displays: (i) a low-contrast (LC) display with the same L_{max} as that of MDMG 5221 but a 50% lower contrast, and (ii) a low-luminance (LL) display with the same L_{max}/L_{min} as that of MDMG 5221 but a 50% lower L_{max}. The simulated detection performance of these displays at FR=1 are both less than 1% different than MDMG 5221.

Table 2. Detection performance on real DBT reconstructed slices for 2 FFRs (30 & 40 sps) and three integer frame repeats (16.67, 25 & 50 sps) for a display without temporal compensation. The settings are given in Table 1 caption.

	Which after LCD frame is used to train 2D-CHO?	FR=1	FR= 50/40	FR= 50/30	FR=2	FR=3
AUC ± std	Frame 1	0.607 ±0.026	0.607 ±0.026	0.656 ±0.022	0.608 ±0.026	0.607 ±0.026
	Frame 2	N/A	N/A	N/A	0.800± 0.014	0.801 ± 0.014
	Frame 3	N/A	N/A	N/A	N/A	0.801 ± 0.014
	Average	**0.607 ±0.026**	**0.607 ±0.026**	**0.656 ±0.022**	**0.704 ±0.020**	**0.736 ±0.018**

3.2   Results on Artificial DBT Reconstructed Slices

In Table 3, results of our preliminary experiments with the dataset generated from a sample simulated breast phantom [8] are presented: the detection performance with its standard deviation is listed for a temporally compensated display at four browsing speeds.

When a small (3%) subset of stacks with non-stationary background is added to the dataset, the AUCs drop by about 2%.

Table 3. Detection performance on artificial DBT reconstructed slices for 2 FFRs (30 & 35 sps) and two integer frame repeats (25 & 50 sps) for a temporally compensated display. The computations are performed in an MRMC study with $N_{rd} = 3$ readers [4], each trained with an independent subset of $N_{tr} = 412$ image pairs and all reading the same test set of $N_{ts} = 412$ test image pairs. The size of the ROI is 3. The AUCs and standard deviations are calculated using the one-shot method.

	Which afterLCD frame is used to train 2D-CHO?	FR=1	FR=50/35	FR=50/30	FR=2
AUC ± std	Frame 1	0.833 ±0.014	0.827 ±0.015	0.854 ±0.013	0.835 ±0.023
	Frame 2	N/A	N/A	N/A	0.853 ±0.013

4   Discussion

The insertion of single micro calcifications lesions is not completely accurate. Mimicking the x-ray absorption and generating anisotropic 3D shapes is, however, more realistic than simply inserting a simple 3D Gaussian sphere as a signal such as it is done in numerous model observer studies. The former was successfully used several times in past studies [1]. In future, within the VCT framework, lesions will be generated during the creation of the phantom.

The display MDMG 5221 used in this study features temporal response compensation. The target luminance values are reached within one frame whereas for a display without this feature, such as MDMG 5121, two to three frames are needed for final luminance values to be reached. This can be also observed in Table 1: the detection performance remains the same (within the double standard deviation range) no matter which refresh is fed to the observer. On the other hand, for an uncompensated display (Table 2), when the first frame of the slice is fed to the observer the detection performance is significantly lower. Also, as observed in Table 1 and Table 2, with the current model observer, one cannot achieve a higher AUC just by increasing the frame repeat. That is because the frames fed to the observer become almost the same after the second refresh in the display with or without temporal compensation.

In this paper and in [1], a multi slice CHO is used by computing scores for image content at the end of each $1 \times T_{refresh}$, $2 \times T_{refresh}$ and $3 \times T_{refresh}$. An alternative to this is feeding all ROI frames (those that may have part of lesion in them) to the model observer. This approach will generate results that are less consistent with those reported in [1]. Nevertheless, the average of AUCs from different refresh values mimics, in a sense, the visualization of the different frames by the observer. Further investigation will take into account the continuous light transition instead of discrete luminance values that are currently used, as well as properties of the human visual system (e.g., temporal contrast sensitivity function) in the observer model.

Detection must be performed in JND domain rather than luminance. Typically, the AUCs calculated in luminance domain are slightly lower (about 1%) than the results reported in Section 3-table 3.

Larger fluctuations in the AUC values for the experiment with the artificial dataset (Section 3.2, Table 3), as compared to the corresponding results for real data (Table 1), may be attributed to the facts that (i) fewer images are used in the experiment and/or (ii) the source of all images used in the experiment is the same phantom; thus the images have less variety. Also note that there is no significance in the fact that AUC values in Table 3 are generally larger than those in Table 1 and Table 2. This difference is a undesired side effect of the lesion insertion process: the insertion density is changed until the AUC becomes around 80%, making the classification of the set an average task (not too difficult or too easy).

We observed that the effect of temporal compensation is considerably higher than those of increasing luminance or contrast. This observation is against clinical studies with human observers and is another indication that the model observer must be improved to be a better representative of human observers. Such improvements may be achieved, as mentioned earlier, by integrating the properties of human visual system with the model observer.

5 Conclusion

In this study we gained a better understanding of current capabilities and limitations of channelized Hotelling observers to be used in virtual clinical trial framework.

Acknowledgments. This work is supported by the US National Institutes of Health (R01 grant #CA154444). Special thanks goes to Ljiljana Platiša from the University of Ghent for her support.

References

1. Platisa, L., Marchessoux, C., Goossens, B., Philips, W.: Performance evaluation of medical LCD displays using 3D channelized Hotelling observers. In: Proc. SPIE Medical Imaging (2011)
2. Bakic, P.R., Zhang, C., Maidment, A.D.A.: Development and Characterization of an Anthropomorphic Breast Software Phantom Based upon Region-Growing Algorithm. Medical Physics 38, 3165–3176 (2011)
3. Platisa, L., Goossens, B., Vansteenkiste, E., Badano, A., Philips, W.: Using channelized hotelling observers to quantify temporal effect of medical liquid crystal displays on detection performance. In: Proc. SPIE Medical Imaging (2010)
4. Gallas, B.: One-shot estimate of MRMC Variance: AUC. Academic Radiology 13, 353–362 (2006)
5. Marchessoux, C., Jung, J.: A virtual image chain for perceived image quality of medical display. In: Proc. SPIE Medical Imaging (2006)
6. Engeldrum, P.: Image quality modeling: Where are we? In: Proc. of PICS 1999: Image Processing, Image Quality, Image Capture, Systems Conference, pp. 251–255 (1999)
7. Marchessoux, C., Kimpe, T., Bert, T.: A virtual image chain for perceived and clinical image quality of medical display. J. of Display Technology 4, 356–368 (2008)
8. Zhang, C., Bakic, P.R., Maidment, A.D.A.: Development of an anthropomorphic breast software phantom based on region growing algorithm. In: Proc. SPIE Medical Imaging (2008)
9. Ruiter, N.V., Zhang, C., Bakic, P.R., Carton, A.-K., Kuo, J., Maidment, A.D.A.: Simulation of tomosynthesis images based on an anthropomorphic software breast tissue phantom. In: Proc. SPIE Medical Imaging (2008)

The Impact of Reduced Injected Radioactivity on Image Quality of Molecular Breast Imaging Tomosynthesis

Olivia Sullivan[1], Zongyi Gong[1], Kelly Klanian[2], Tushita Patel[1], and Mark B. Williams[1,2]

[1] University of Virginia Department of Physics, Charlottesville, Virginia, USA
[2] University of Virginia Department of Biomedical Engineering Charlottesville, Virginia, USA
mbwilliams@virginia.edu

Abstract. This study's objective is to compare image quality in 3-D molecular breast imaging tomosynthesis (MBIT) with that in planar molecular breast imaging (MBI) over a range of breast radioactivity concentrations. Using gelatin and point source phantoms lesion contrast, lesion signal-to-noise ratio (SNR) and spatial resolution were compared for a range of lesion sizes and depths. For both MBI and MBIT, lesion contrast is essentially constant with changing activity while SNR decreases by a factor of $1.5 - 2$ between 100% and 25% activity levels. For nearly all lesion sizes and locations contrast and SNR are significantly higher for MBIT than MBI, potentially permitting greater reductions in injected dose. Spatial resolution in MBI is dependent on lesion depth but independent of lesion location with MBIT. Reconstructed MBIT spatial resolution is substantially better than that in the projection images, suggesting future use of higher sensitivity collimators for even further reductions in injected activity.

Keywords: tomosynthesis, molecular breast imaging, radiation dose.

1 Introduction

Breast cancer is one of the most commonly diagnosed cancers among US women. In 2011, an estimated 230,480 new cases of invasive and 57,650 cases of non-invasive (in situ) breast cancer are expected to be diagnosed [1]. Nevertheless, breast cancer death rates have been steadily declining since 1991 and this is thought to be partially a result of earlier detection through screening.

The current gold standard for breast cancer screening is x-ray mammography. However, the sensitivity of mammography is significantly reduced among the $40 - 60$ % of women with radiodense breasts. The recent advent of x-ray tomosynthesis, in which multiple views of the breast are taken at different angles and then combined to form a 3-dimensional image, has shown promise for reducing the masking effect of radiodense breast tissue by providing some resolution along the direction of breast compression.

At the same time, new imaging modalities are being investigated as functional imaging adjuncts to the anatomical images of x-ray mammography and x-ray tomosynthesis. Breast scintigraphy using small field of view, dedicated breast gamma

A.D.A. Maidment, P.R. Bakic, and S. Gavenonis (Eds.): IWDM 2012, LNCS 7361, pp. 300–307, 2012.

cameras and the radiopharmaceutical ^{99m}Tc-sestamibi, referred to as Molecular Breast Imaging (MBI) or Breast Specific Gamma Imaging (BSGI), is a relatively new functional imaging modality and has entered clinical practice. Although MBI provides functional information complementary to the anatomical information of mammography [3][5], with currently recommended tracer injected activity (740 – 1110 MBq) it results in an effective whole body radiation dose of ~6 – 9 mSv. Although the additional radiation dose to the breast from MBI is comparable to that of a single mammographic view, other organs also receive dose, resulting in the larger effective dose for MBI compared to screening mammography (0.7–1.0 mSv)[5]. While this dose is comparable to that of many nuclear medicine scans, it may be more than is necessary for good quality MBI, especially given the improving imaging technologies becoming available. Thus efforts are underway to investigate the impact on MBI image quality of lowering the amount of injected radiotracer [4].

Our group is developing a dual modality tomosynthesis (DMT) scanner in which x-ray breast tomosynthesis (XBT) and molecular breast imaging tomosynthesis (MBIT) images are obtained with the breast in a single configuration under mild compression. Like XBT, in MBIT multiple gamma emission views are obtained over a range of viewing angles. Both modalities are mounted on a common upright mammography-style gantry. Following XBT the gamma camera is positioned above the breast and rotated through a range of viewing angles. For each view linear translation stages are used to position the camera as closely as possible to the breast surface. Following reconstruction the resulting 3-D tracer map can then be readily co-registered with the volumetric XBT image.

The objective of this phantom study is to compare image quality in MBIT with that in MBI over a range of radioactivity concentrations in the breast. The image metrics of lesion contrast, lesion signal-to-noise ratio (SNR) and spatial resolution are compared for a range of lesion sizes and depths under conditions of equal total number of detected counts, using a single gamma camera operated in either MBIT mode or MBI mode.

2   Methods

2.1   Experimental Setup

For simplicity rather than using the full DMT system a bench-top setup was constructed to perform the phantom MBIT study. To permit adjustable camera-to-axis of rotation (AOR) separation in addition to varying viewing angle an apparatus was built consisting of a motor-controlled rotation stage mounted on a linear translation stage (Figure 1). In this setup the y-axis is defined to coincide with the AOR, the z-axis is defined to point along the short dimension of the phantom, and the x-axis is defined to result in a right-handed coordinate system.   The dose study experiments were done by fabricating gelatin breast phantoms containing spherical simulated lesions. The gamma camera, built at the Jefferson Lab, has a 15 cm x 20 cm field of view and is equipped with a high resolution parallel hole collimator. The overall camera sensitivity is 110.4 cps/MBq (absolute efficiency of 1.1 x 10^{-4}). The phantom volume was 840 mL, which was the average breast volume of the subjects partici- pating in our pilot study of DMT [7]. The background activity concentra- tion of the phan- toms was 0.33

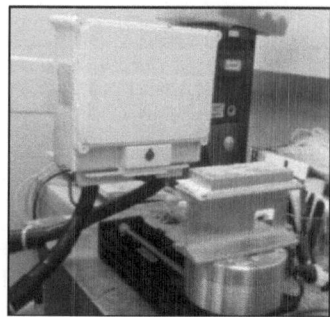 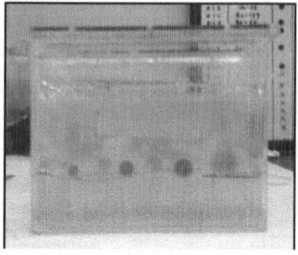

Fig. 1. Gamma camera (top left) and vertical axis rotation stage (lower right), mounted atop the linear translation stage. For clarity the phantom is not shown.

Fig. 2. Lesion phantom containing a series of simulated lesions with various sizes, placed at two different z locations (depths) within the phantom. In the photo the z-dimension is into the page.

μCi/mL, corresponding to an injected activity of approximately 25 mCi [8]. As the gelatin hardened as it was refrigerated, hollow, spherical, thin-walled acrylic lesions filled with 10x the background radioactivity concentration (3.3 μCi/mL) were placed in the phantom [2] (see Figure 2). The phantom was contained in a 6.3 cm (z-dimension) x 12 cm (x-dimension) x 7.1 cm (y-dimension) acrylic box to simulate compression to a thickness of 6.3 cm. The box containing the phantom was then mounted on the rotation stage for imaging. The resulting counting rate into the images was approximately 450 cps.

2.2   Image Acquisition

For the study described here 9 evenly spaced views were obtained over 135 degrees. For each view the phantom was positioned as close to the camera as possible, resulting in a maximum camera-to-AOR distance of 13.5 cm (for views 67.5 degrees away from the z-axis) and a minimum camera-to-AOR distance of 6.23 cm (for the view along the z-axis).

In order to evaluate the impact of reduction in injected activity, for each view projection images were obtained over 120 s, 90 s, 60 s, and 30 s to simulate injection of 100%, 75%, 50%, and 25% of the full 25 mCi activity, respectively. Times were adjusted slightly during the course of scanning to take into account radioactive decay. The volumetric MBIT images were reconstructed using an expectation maximization (EM) algorithm developed specifically for MBIT at UVa, which includes resolution recovery and attenuation correction.

In addition to the MBIT projection images, planar MBI images were obtained in which the number of detected counts equaled the total number of counts in the MBIT scans. For example, for the 50% dose acquisition, a 9 minute single-view acquisition time was used for MBI and 9 views x 60 seconds per view for MBIT. For the MBI images the phantom was positioned for viewing along the z-axis and as close as possible to the camera (camera-to-AOR distance of 6.23 cm).

The spatial resolution of planar MBI and MBIT was compared by imaging a point source phantom containing four acrylic posts, each with a 1 mm diameter, 1 mm deep well drilled in its top surface (see Figure 3). A small drop of ^{99m}Tc solution was placed in each well to create four point-like sources in air. MBIT data was obtained using a circular orbit with camera-to-AOR distance of 12.5 cm and 9 views over 135 degrees. The MBI image was taken at 0 degree view. Total acquisition time was 120 seconds for both.

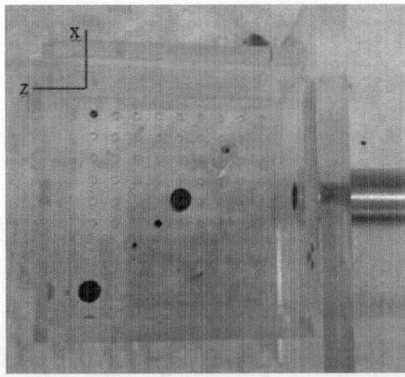

Fig. 3. Point source phantom. Drops of ^{99m}Tc solution were added to each of four wells of varying heights in y and depths in z and imaged using MBIT and planar MBI

Table 1. Size of ROIs drawn for MBIT contrast and SNR analysis

Lesion Location	Lesion Inner Diameter	Area of Circular ROI (pixels)
5 cm (Deep)	1.5 cm	16
	1.2 cm	20
	0.9 cm	9
	0.76 cm	9
	Background	416
1 cm (Shallow)	1.5cm	12
	1.2cm	12
	0.9cm	9
	0.76cm	3
	Background	544

2.3   Image Analysis

Lesion contrast and signal-to-noise ratio (SNR) was calculated for MBIT by constructing regions of interest (ROIs) in the MBIT slices intersecting the lesion centers. Lesion contrast was calculated by taking the mean pixel value of an ROI centered on the lesion and dividing it by the mean pixel value of a nearby background

Table 2. Size of ROIs drawn for planar MBI contrast and SNR analysis

Lesion Location	Lesion Inner Diameter	Area of Circular ROI (pixels)
5 cm (Deep)	1.5 cm	60
	1.2 cm	44
	0.9 cm	34
	0.76 cm	11
1 cm (Shallow)	1.5 cm	52
	1.2 cm	34
	0.9 cm	31
	0.76 cm	34
	Background	1647

ROI. SNR was calculated by subtracting the mean pixel value of the background ROI from that of the lesion ROI and dividing the result by the standard deviation of the background ROI. Similar ROI analysis was performed on the MBI images. ROI sizes for MBIT analysis and MBI analysis are listed in Tables 1 and 2, respectively. The projection images are 150 x 110 pixels with 1.4 mm x 1.4 mm pixel size and the reconstructed MBIT slices are 94 x 69 with a 2.24 mm x 2.24 mm pixel size.

Spatial resolution was calculated by finding the full width at half maximum (FWHM) of 1-D profiles through the center of the point source images along the x, y, z directions for MBIT and along the y direction for MBI.

3   Results

For the study described here the gelatin phantom contained two each of four sizes of lesion: 1.5 cm, 1.2 cm, 0.9 cm, and 0.76 cm inner diameter. One lesion of each size was placed 1 cm from the side of the phantom closest to the camera (shallow lesions) and the other four lesions were placed 5 cm from the side of the camera closest to the camera (deep lesions).

Figure 4 shows the lesion contrasts and SNR for both MBIT and MBI plotted versus the percent of the current clinical radiotracer dose. Each graph shows the results for a given lesion type (diameter and depth). Error bars signify the standard deviations in 4 repeat trials of nominally identical scans.

Figure 5 compares the spatial resolutions of MBIT and MBI obtained from scans of the point source phantom. For reference, Figure 6 shows the results of a capillary measurement of the gamma camera FWHM spatial resolution over a range of source-to-collimator distances. Given the 12.5 cm AOR-to-detector distance used for the scans of Figure 5, and the fact that the AOR was approximately centered within the phantom, the source-to-collimator distances for the four sources were 8.5, 10.5, 12.5 and 14.5 cm, respectively. Thus the FWHM resolution results for MBI are in substantial agreement with those predicted from the capillary assessment.

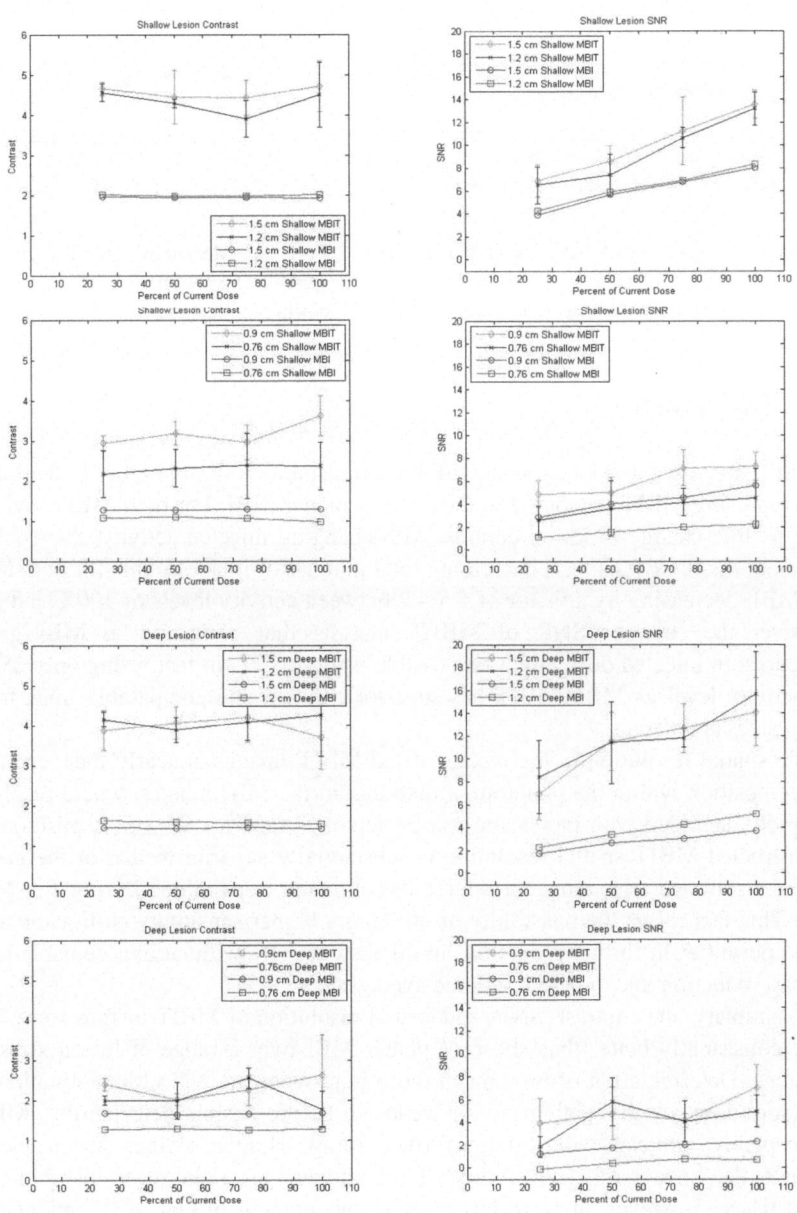

Fig. 4. Plots of lesion contrast and SNR verse the percent of the current clinical radiotracer dose

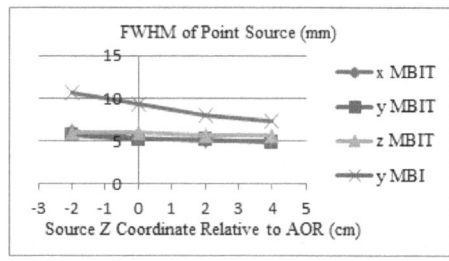
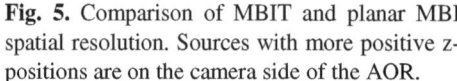
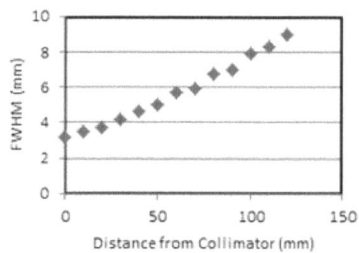

Fig. 5. Comparison of MBIT and planar MBI spatial resolution. Sources with more positive z-positions are on the camera side of the AOR.

Fig. 6. Measured gamma camera spatial resolution versus source-to-collimator separation

4   Discussion

For all lesion sizes and locations tested the contrast and SNR are higher in the images acquired using MBIT compared to those using planar MBI. For both MBIT and MBI there is little change in lesion contrast with changing injected activity. As would be expected, the SNR falls with decreasing total number of image counts for both MBIT and MBI, decreasing by a factor of 1.5 – 2 between activity levels of 100% and 25%. However the superior SNR of MBIT suggests that compared to MBI greater reductions in injected dose might be possible using MBIT. In fact, using only 25% of the activity level as MBI, MBIT has superior contrast and comparable SNR for all lesion sizes and depths.

The spatial resolution in the reconstructed MBIT images is nearly independent of source position within the phantom, unlike that in the MBI images, where resolution is rapidly degraded with increasing source depth. In fact, for all source positions the reconstructed MBIT spatial resolution is substantially superior to that of the gamma camera itself over the range of source-to-collimator separations during the MBIT scan. This fact raises the possibility of utilizing a higher sensitivity collimator which would permit even further reductions in injected activity without unacceptable lesion contrast reduction due to partial volume averaging.

In summary, the contrast, SNR, and spatial resolution of MBIT images were found to be consistently better than those of planar MBI over a range of lesion sizes and locations. Determination of how much these improvements will ultimately allow the radiation dose to the patient to be reduced before lesion detectability will be unacceptably reduced will require further study. Human studies are needed to evaluate the impact on detectability of inhomogeneous radiotracer distribution in breast tissue. However, these results provide encouragement that MBIT might make substantially lower doses possible than would be possible with planar imaging.

Acknowledgements. This work was supported by the National Institutes of Health (R01 CA149130) and Susan G. Komen for the Cure (KG100479).

References

1. Breast Cancer Statistics (October 15, 2011),
   http://www.breastcancer.org/symptoms/
   understand_bc/statistics.jsp
2. Maublant, J., De Latour, M., Mestas, D., Clemenson, A., Charrier, S., Feillel, V., Le Bouedec, G., Kaufmann, P., Dauplat, J., Veyre, A.: Technetium-99m-sestamibi uptake in breast tumor and associated lymph nodes. J. Nucl. Med. 37, 922–925 (1996)
3. O'Connor, M., Rhodes, D., Hruska, C.: Molecular breast imaging. Expert Review of Anticancer Therapy 9, 1073–1080 (2009) [Review] [37 refs]
4. O'Connor, M.K., Li, H., Rhodes, D.J., Hruska, C.B., Clancy, C.B., Vetter, R.J.: Comparison of radiation exposure and associated radiation-induced cancer risks from mammography and molecular imaging of the breast. Med. Phys. 37, 6187–6198 (2010)
5. Rhodes, D.J., Hruska, C.B., Phillips, S.W., Whaley, D.H., O'Connor, M.K.: Dedicated dual-head gamma imaging for breast cancer screening in women with mammographically dense breasts. Radiology 258, 106–118 (2011)
6. Wackers, F.J.T., Berman, D.S., Maddahi, J., Watson, D.D., Beller, G.A., Stauss, H.W.B.C.A., Picard, M., Holman, B.L., Fridrich, R., Inglese, E., Deslaloye, B., Bischof-Delaloye, A., Camin, L.M.K.: Technetium-99m hexakis 2-methoxyisobutyl isonitrile: Human biodistribution, dosimetry, safety, and preliminary comparison to thallium-201 for myocardial perfusion imaging. J. Nucl. Med. 30, 301–311 (1989)
7. Williams, M.B., Judy, P.G., Gunn, S., Majewski, S.: Dual modality breast tomosynthesis. Radiology 255, 191–198 (2010)
8. Williams, M.B., Narayanan, D., More, M.J., Goodale, P.J., Majewski, S., Kieper, D.A.: Analysis of position-dependent compton scatter in scintimammography with mild compression. IEEE Transactions on Nuclear Science 50, 1643–1649 (2003)

Automatic Seed Placement for Breast Lesion Segmentation on US Images

Joan Massich[1,*], Fabrice Meriaudeau[2], Melcior Sentís[3], Sergi Ganau[3], Elsa Pérez[4], Robert Martí[1], Arnau Oliver[1], and Joan Martí[1]

[1] Computer Vision and Robotics Group, University of Girona, Spain
jmassich@atc.udg.edu
[2] Laboratoire Le2i-UMR CNRS, University of Burgundy, Le Creusot, France
[3] Department of Breast and Gynecological Radiology, UDIAT-Diagnostic Center, Parc Taulí Corporation, Sabadell, Spain
[4] Department of Radiology, Hospital Josep Trueta of Girona, Spain

Abstract. Breast lesion boundaries have been mostly extracted by using conventional approaches as a previous step in the development of computer-aided diagnosis systems. Among these, region growing is a frequently used segmentation method. To make the segmentation completely automatic, most of the region growing methods incorporate automatic selection of the seed points. This paper proposes a new automatic seed placement algorithm for breast lesion segmentation on ultrasound images by means of assigning the probability of belonging to a lesion for every pixel depending on intensity, texture and geometrical constraints. The proposal has been evaluated using a set of sonographic breast images with accompanying expert-provided ground truth, and successfully compared to other existing algorithms.

Keywords: seed placement, ultrasound, segmentation, breast cancer.

1 Introduction

Breast cancer constitutes a leading cause of death for women in developed countries, and is most effectively treated when diagnosed at an early stage [8]. Digital Mammography is currently the most powerful screening tool for breast cancer [5], although ultrasound images can provide useful complementary information in cases where a tumor presence can be shielded due to dense glandular breast tissue [9]. Despite ultrasound imaging is a non-expensive and non-invasive technique with no side effects, its use in CAD systems is still under development. A feasible explanation is that performing automatic segmentation in US images is currently a challenge because they often suffer from poor quality and tend to generate artifacts: weak edges due to acoustic similarity between adjacent tissues, shadows as a consequence of the signal attenuation preventing to screen

---

* This work was partially supported by the Spanish Science and Innovation grant nb. TIN2011-23704, the Regional Council of Burgundy and the University of Girona BR grant nb. 09/22.

A.D.A. Maidment, P.R. Bakic, and S. Gavenonis (Eds.): IWDM 2012, LNCS 7361, pp. 308–315, 2012.

any further, low contrast when the ultrasound wave is attenuated by the tissue media, or, speckle which is an unwanted collateral artifact produced by coherent interface of scatterers that appear as a granular structure superimposed on the image.

Among the reported techniques proposals for both guided and automatic segmentation of lesions in ultrasound images, region growing procedures that expand a seed accordingly to some criteria are widely used [6]. However, a proper selection of the seeds highly determines the final segmentation results.

The goal of this work is to compare three well known automatic procedures for selecting seed points [3,7,1] with a novel seed region selection methodology that makes use of texture and intensity features with geometric constraints. The experimental results have been obtained using a set of sonographic images with expert-provided ground truth, which have been tested using an already existing framework for segmenting breast lesions in ultrasound images [4].

2   Background

Given the noisy nature of the ultrasound images and the presence of other structures rather than lesions with similar acoustic properties, placing seed points on an ultrasound image with the aim to segment breast lesions is not a trivial task at all. Thus, an automatic seed placement procedure is usually required when dealing with fully automatic segmentation procedures. Three existing automatic seed placement procedures have been analyzed and tested according to their ability to later produce reliable segmented regions that match lesions:

- Pixel Rewarding (PR)[3]. To avoid manual delineation of the tumor boundaries, this proposal combines texture, intensity, gradient and a deformable model along with empirically determined domain specific knowledge to automatically find lesion margins in ultrasound images. Each pixel of the image is rewarded according to an assessment function using its position, intensity and texture. A recursive refinement stage removes outliers and provides a close estimate of the true boundary to a deformable model which produces the final segmentation. The deformable model operates on the directional gradient, making it more robust to noise. Its main advantage is its spatially constrained seed rewarding along with the fact that the lesion's appearance is obtained by means of a learning step. On the other hand, its major disadvantage remains in choosing an appropriated neighborhood for the term representing the probability mean of the surrounding pixels when calculating the pixel reward. If the neighborhood used is too small, it might incorrectly reward a noisy region; otherwise, if the used neighborhood is too large, a proper seed can be hidden due to its neighbors' low recall.
- Intensity Binarized Ranked Regions (IBRR) [7]. A score function to rank the regions not connected with the boundary or having intersection with the image center window is used, with no need of prior information of training

process. The function takes into account both the homogeneous texture features and the spatial features of the breast lesions.

- Gradient-Based (GB)[1]. After initial Radial Gradient Index [2] filtering, the lesion candidates are segmented from the background by maximizing an Average Radial Gradient (ARD) index for regions grown from the detected points. A round robin analysis to assess the quality of the classification of lesion candidates into actual lesions and false-positives by a Bayesian neural network is used, yielding to a good overall performance. The main drawback of this seed selection procedure is its associated computational cost, which has been partially solved by means of subsampling techniques. However, due to the comprehensive nature of the seed determination, the method remains unadvisable for online applications.

3   ITG: A Novel Seed Placement Methodology for Region Selection

Characterizing breast lesions by means of image analysis techniques usually combines intensity and texture as high specificity features [9]. Besides, it is a fact that radiologists tend to center the lesions when acquiring the images [3]. Thus, the proposed methodology makes use of Intensity, Texture and Geometric constraints (ITG) and takes advantage of the mentioned statements in order to select a seed region for further region growing expansion, as is shown in Figure 1. The proposal evaluates the probability of a pixel being part of a lesion depending on its intensity, texture and position to generate a joint probability or total probability plane.

Afterwards, the largest region composed by connected pixels with a posterior probability that satisfies the imposed confidence level of being a lesion is selected. In order to compute the posterior probability, a Bayesian framework is assumed accordingly to equation 1.

$$P(Lesion|I,T) = \frac{P(I,T|Lesion) \cdot P(Lesion)}{P(I,T)} \tag{1}$$

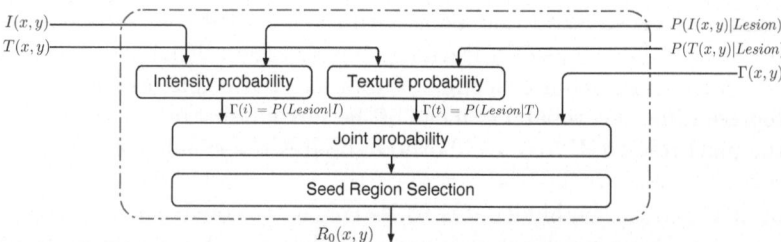

Fig. 1. Block diagram describing the seed region selection proposal

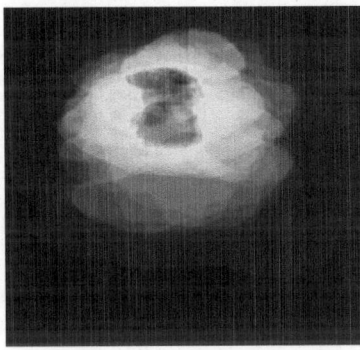

Fig. 2. Lesion occurrence on a normalized grid, where the probability is represented according to a color code, from blue (lowest) to red (highest)

Where Intensity (I) and Texture (T) are two Independent and Identically Distributed (IID) features, and $P(Lesion)$ is assumed to be a centered multivariate Gaussian distribution proportional to the image. This is a reasonable assumption, since most of the lesions are centered as corroborates the probability map obtained from the dataset ground truth delineations (see fig. 2). Notice that the denominator $P(I, T)$ can be ignored since is common for the two classes $\{Lesion, \overline{Lesion}\}$ and cancels out. Thus, the final posterior probability can be calculated accordingly to equation 2 where $P(I|Lesion)$ and $P(T|Lesion)$ are the Intensity and Texture Probability Density Function (pdf) determined during the training step.

$$P(Lesion|I, T) = P(I|Lesion) \cdot P(T|Lesion) \cdot P(Lesion|x, y) \qquad (2)$$

The used texture measure is given by the Equation 3 and corresponds to the difference between the pixel intensity value $I(x, y)$ and the mean intensity value of its N nearest neighbors (here, 8-pixel neighborhood has been used).

$$T(x, y) = I(x, y) - \frac{1}{N} \sum_{\delta=0}^{N-1} I_\delta(x, y) \qquad (3)$$

Once determined the posterior probability, the probability plane is thresholded and the largest area from the foreground is selected as the seed region. The threshold has been empirically set at 0.8 as a good tradeoff between large foreground regions and low lesion belonging recall.

In summary, the proposed seed placement methodology makes use of five inputs to automatically determine a seed region: the intensity image, the texture image, the intensity and texture Probability Density Functions, and the seed location prior; along with a fixed parameter to split the probability plane into foreground and background.

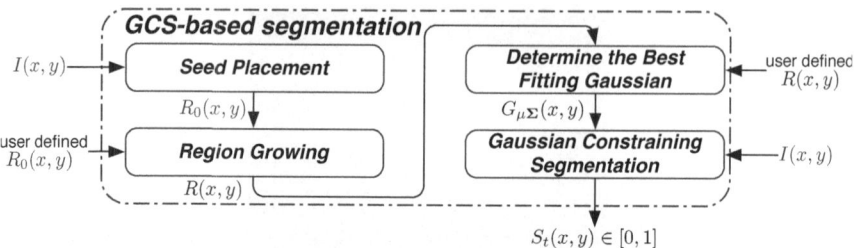

Fig. 3. Block diagram for the Gaussian Constraining Segmentation framework used to evaluate the proposal

4   Results

4.1   Experimental Setup

In order to evaluate the performance of the proposed methodology, a dataset of 25 sonographic images acquired at the *Hospital Dr. Josep Trueta* of Girona and the *UDIAT-Diagnostic Center* of Sabadell has been used. Since each image was annotated by seven radiology experts who provided the lesion delineations, the Simultaneous Truth and Performance Level Estimation (STAPLE) algorithm [10] to obtain the Hidden Ground Truth (HGT) has been used. The μ-coefficient proposed as a variance of the True-Positive Ratio (TPR) or Jaccard coefficient was then used in order to take into account the experts agreement by means of the HGT. The proposed ITG methodology along with the GB, PR, and IBRR procedures have been tested through the Gaussian Constraining Segmentation framework proposed by Massich et al. [4]. Figure 3 states the basic operations for such GCS-based segmentation framework: after an initial region $R_0(x, y)$ is determined, it is converted into a preliminary lesion delineation $R(x, y)$ by means of a region growing algorithm. Such lesion delineation is used to obtain a multivariate Gaussian function describing the shape, position and orientation of the lesion $(G_{\mu\Sigma}(x, y))$. Finally, the Gaussian Constraining Segmentation (GCS) procedure refines the segmentation by thresholding an intensity dependent function $\Psi(x, y)$ constrained by the multivariate Gaussian describing the lesion.

Figure 4 shows the segmentation results obtained for two clinical cases depending on the seed placement procedure. The blue delineation indicates the obtained seed region, while the red delineation indicates the Ground Truth, and the green delineation the obtained segmentation through the different region growing methods.

4.2   Seed Region Location

The effect of the initial seed position cannot be neglected when evaluating the performance of the proposed methodology. Thus, Figure 5a illustrates the ten Areas-of-Interest to test the influence of the lesion center distance and orientation

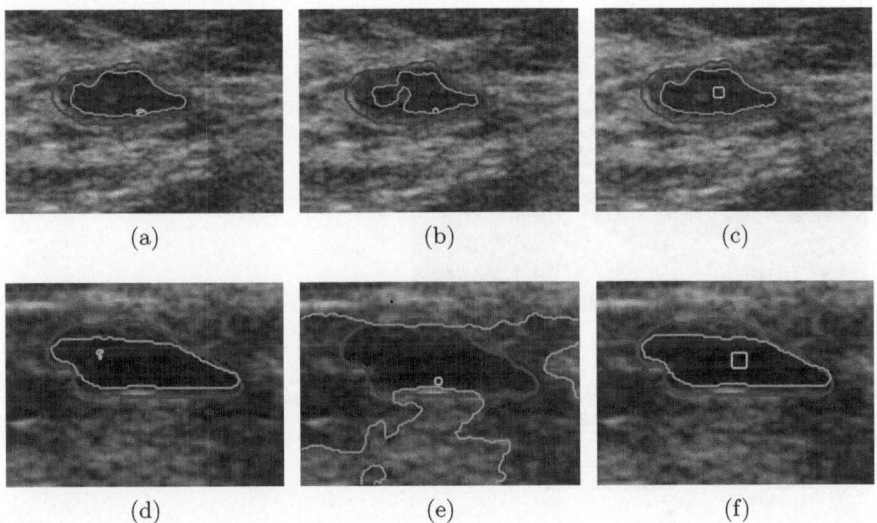

Fig. 4. Segmentation results: each row contains a clinical case (a-c,d-f), while each column corresponds to a different seed placement method: ITG (a,d), PR (b,e), and IBRR (c,f)

when seeding. The Areas-of-Interest have been selected as belonging to four different classes: out of the lesion (area 1), inside the lesion close to the boundaries (areas 2 to 5), inside the lesion but slightly shifted from the central part (areas 6 to 9), and central part of the lesion (area 10). For evaluation purposes, the region growing algorithm has been applied to each of the ten Areas-of-Interest using 15 randomly sampled seed regions for every area of interest. Figure 5b shows the segmentation results for each Area-of-Interest according to the μ value. It clearly shows that to achieve good segmentation results highly depends on the location of the seed regions within the lesion (the best segmentation results are achieved when placing the seed in the areas 6 to 10). The figure also indicates that three main classes a to c can be identified: (a) Areas-of-Interest 6 to 10 that correspond to the inner lesion area, (b) Areas-of-Interest 2 to 5 that correspond to the boundary area, and (c) Area-of-Interest 1 that corresponds to anywhere outside the lesion. The results indicates that the better segmentation results are achieved when the seed is placed in the (a) Areas-of-Interest (the inner lesion area, away from the boundaries), but not necessarily in the innest region.

4.3 Methodology Evaluation

Besides determining the role of the seed region location in terms of the achieved segmentation results, the performance of the proposed methodology has been also evaluated by comparing to the methods referred in section 2 (Pixel Rewarding, Intensity Binarized Ranked Regions, and Gradient-Based), as is shown in Figure 6: the first plot (Figure 6a) shows the ability of each methodology to place

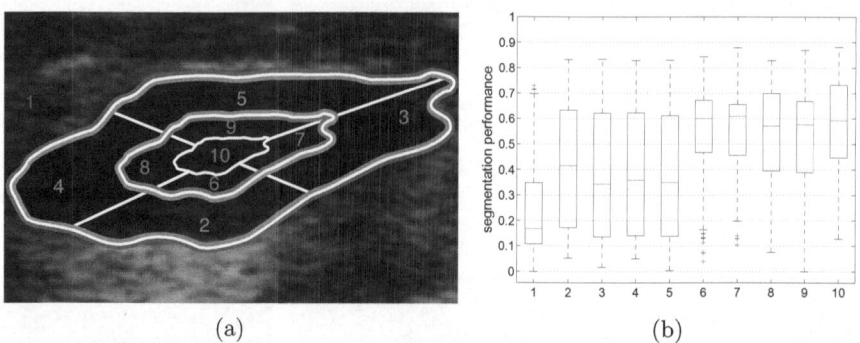

(a)   (b)

Fig. 5. (a) The 10 Areas-of-Interest to place seed regions, and (b) segmentation results for each Area-of-Interest in terms of the μ-coefficient

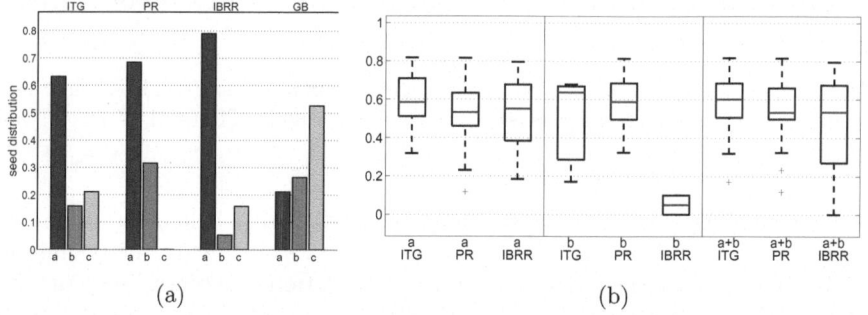

(a)   (b)

Fig. 6. Comparison between the proposed method ITG and the PR, IBRR, and GB methods: (a) distributions of seed region location, and (b) final segmentation performance depending on the seed location

the selected seed regions along the three main classes a to c for the Areas-of-Interest, while the boxplot (Figure 6b) indicates the mean and standard variation of the final segmentation results for each methodology. Although the PR and IBRR methods place more seeds in the central area than the ITG method, this new proposed method has the highest performance in terms of final segmentation results, as can be observed in Figure 6b.

5   Conclusions

The importance of a good seed placement for a region growing-based segmentation procedure has been stated. A new automatic seed placement algorithm for breast lesion segmentation on ultrasound images has been proposed. The proposal makes use of the intensity, texture and geometrical constraints to evaluate the probability of a pixel being part of the lesion. Performance of the new proposal has been successfully evaluated in terms of segmentation results on a dataset of 25 sonographic images, and compared to three existing automatic procedures. Future work includes to assess the robustness of the new proposed methodology using a larger database.

References

1. Drukker, K., Giger, M.L., Kupinski, K.M.A., Vyborny, C.J., Mendelson, E.B.: Computerized lesion detection on breast ultrasound. Medical Physics 29(7), 1438–1446 (2002)
2. Kupinski, M.A., Giger, M.L.: Automated seeded lesion segmentation on digital mammograms. IEEE Transactions on Medical Imaging 17(4), 510–517 (1998)
3. Madabhushi, A., Metaxas, D.: Automatic boundary extraction of ultrasonic breast lesions. In: Proceedings of IEEE International Symposium on Biomedical Imaging, pp. 601–604 (2002)
4. Massich, J., Meriaudeau, F., Pérez, E., Martí, R., Oliver, A., Martí, J.: Lesion Segmentation in Breast Sonography. In: Martí, J., Oliver, A., Freixenet, J., Martí, R. (eds.) IWDM 2010. LNCS, vol. 6136, pp. 39–45. Springer, Heidelberg (2010)
5. Moore, S.K.: Better breast cancer detection. IEEE Spectrum 38(5), 50–54 (2001)
6. Noble, J.A., Boukerroui, D.: Ultrasound image segmentation: A survey. IEEE Transactions on Medical Imaging 25(8), 987–1010 (2006)
7. Shan, J., Cheng, H.D., Wang, Y.: A novel automatic seed point selection algorithm for breast ultrasound images. In: 19th International Conference on Pattern Recognition (2008)
8. Sivaramakrishna, R., Powell, K.A., Lieber, M.L., Chilcote, W.A., Shekhar, R.: Texture analysis of lesions in breast ultrasound images. Computerized Medical Imaging and Graphics 26(5), 303–307 (2002)
9. Stavros, A.T., Rapp, C.L., Parker, S.H.: Breast ultrasound. Lippincott Williams & Wilkins (2004)
10. Warfield, S.K., Zou, K.H., Wells, W.M.: Simultaneous truth and performance level estimation (STAPLE): an algorithm for the validation of image segmentation. IEEE Transactions on Medical Imaging 23(7), 903–921 (2004)

Comparison of Breast Doses for Digital Tomosynthesis Estimated from Patient Exposures and Using PMMA Breast Phantoms

David R. Dance[1,2], Celia J. Strudley[1], Kenneth C. Young[1,2], Jennifer M. Oduko[1], Patsy J. Whelehan[3], and E.H. Lindsay Mungutroy[4]

[1] National Co-ordinating Centre for the Physics of Mammography,
Royal Surrey County Hospital NHS Foundation Trust, Guildford, GU2 7XX, UK
[2] Department of Physics, Faculty of Engineering and Physical Sciences,
University of Surrey, Guildford, GU2 7XH, UK
[3] Division of Cancer Research, Medical Research Institute, University of Dundee,
Dundee, DD1 9SY, UK
[4] Jarvis Breast Screening and Diagnostic Centre, Guildford, GU1 1LJ, UK
daviddance@nhs.net

Abstract. A proposed European protocol for dosimetry in digital breast tomo-synthesis (DBT) has been applied to estimate the average glandular breast dose (AGD) for two different DBT units. AGD was measured for the examination of series of women and for breast-simulating polymethyl methacrylate (PMMA) phantoms, thus assessing the suitability of the phantoms used for dosimetry in 2D mammography for DBT dosimetry. For the first system the mean values of the AGD for breast thicknesses of 21mm, 53mm and 90mm, were 1.21±0.06 (2 s.e.m), 2.12±0.07 and 4.90±0.11 mGy respectively. The corresponding values for the equivalent PMMA thicknesses of 20mm, 45mm and 70mm were 0.92, 2.08 and 4.65 mGy respectively. Similar agreement was found for the second system. It is concluded that the use of standard PMMA phantoms of appropriate thicknesses (as used for 2D dosimetry) to simulate the breast in DBT provides a reasonable estimate of the AGD.

Keywords: digital breast tomosynthesis, average glandular dose, PMMA phantoms, breast dosimetry.

1 Background

The estimation of the average dose to the glandular tissues within the breast (AGD) is an essential part of mammographic quality control, and knowledge of this dose is necessary for the optimisation of any breast imaging system which uses X-rays. In the European quality control protocol [1] for 2D mammographic imaging, breast dose is estimated both for series of patients, and using polymethyl methacrylate (PMMA) phantoms which simulate the breast. For digital breast tomosynthesis (DBT), a proto-col has recently been developed for breast dosimetry [2], which is a straightforward extension of the method used for 2D imaging, and is under consideration for use as a

A.D.A. Maidment, P.R. Bakic, and S. Gavenonis (Eds.): IWDM 2012, LNCS 7361, pp. 316–321, 2012.

European protocol for DBT. In this paper we present the results of applying this protocol to surveys of patient doses for two DBT units with very different imaging geometries, and show for each system how the dose varies with the thickness of the compressed breast. Because of the beam angulations used for DBT and the absence of an anti-scatter grid, it is not clear that breast equivalent phantoms designed for use in 2D imaging can also be used in 3D imaging to represent the same compressed breast thickness. The variation of DBT dose with breast equivalent thickness has therefore also been determined for the PMMA phantoms used for 2D imaging to validate the use of these phantoms for breast dosimetry in DBT. For comparison purposes, results are also presented for 2D imaging using the same two X-ray units.

2   Method

In the proposed European protocol for breast dosimetry in DBT, the average glandular dose (D_G) is estimated using:

$$D_G = KgcsT$$

where K is the incident air kerma at the upper surface of the breast, the factor g is a conversion factor giving the AGD for a breast of average glandularity 50%, the factor c corrects for the composition of the breast, the factor s corrects for the particular X-ray spectrum used and the factor T is a correction factor for DBT. The factors g, c, s and T have all been estimated using a Monte Carlo model of the breast and imaging system [2-5], and the first three are also the factors used in the European protocol for breast dosimetry for 2D mammography [1]. The factor T has to be determined by integrating angular dependent tomography conversion factors, t, over the angles used for the DBT exposure, and factors are given in [2] as a function of breast thickness for the two DBT systems used in this study.

The patient doses for DBT have been determined for a Hologic Selenia Dimensions unit, which acquires 15 projections in the angular range -7.5° to +7.5° and a Siemens Inspiration unit, which acquires 25 projections in the angular range -24° to +24°. For the former unit, the tomo factor T was in the range 0.992 to 0.997, and for the latter unit, it was in the range 0.960 to 0.980, so that for the same exposure factors, the AGD would be very similar to that for 2D imaging. For the Hologic unit the patient sample comprised 357 exposures (cranio-caudal and oblique views) of women aged 40-75y attending for screening or assessment, with compressed breast thicknesses in the range 20mm to 98mm. For the Siemens unit, the sample comprised 184 exposures (cranio-caudal and oblique views) of women aged 36-66y attending for symptomatic mammography with compressed breast thicknesses in the range 26mm to 103mm. For the Hologic unit, the target/filter combination of the X-ray tube was W/Al for tomosynthesis and the tube voltage range 26 kV to 43 kV, and these parameters for the Siemens unit were W/Rh and 26 kV to 32 kV.

Both systems were used in a mode which made a combined 2D and tomosynthesis acquisition so that all patients had both 2D and tomosynthesis for each view taken. For the Hologic unit the target/filter combination of the X-ray tube for 2D imaging was W/Rh and the tube voltage range 25 kV to 32 kV, or W/Ag with a tube voltage range from 30 kV to 35 kV, depending on breast thickness. These parameters for 2D imaging with the Siemens unit were W/Rh target/filter combination and tube voltage range 26 kV to 32 kV.

The equivalence used in 2D imaging between breasts of various thicknesses and PMMA [1] is based on Monte Carlo simulations, and is for women attending for breast screening in the UK in the age range 50-64. Tables 1 and 2 give the corresponding equivalent breast thicknesses and glandularities. For both systems the DBT and 2D AGDs were determined for PMMA slabs in the thickness range 20 mm to 70 mm using automatic exposure control. An air gap was used on top of the PMMA to increase the compressed thickness to that of the equivalent breast.

3   Results

Patient doses at different breast thickness are compared to phantom dose estimates in tables 1 and 2. The patient doses shown are the average of exposures where the breast thickness is within 5mm of the equivalent breast thicknesses shown in column 2 of the tables. Figures 1 and 2 show the individual 2D and DBT patient doses and the PMMA phantom doses for the Hologic Selenia Dimensions system and the Siemens Inspiration system respectively.

The ratios of the mean patient AGD values for DBT to that for 2D imaging for the two systems were 1.2 and 1.5.

Table 1. Dose measurement using Hologic Selenia Dimensions system

PMMA thickness (mm)	Equiv. breast thickness (mm)	Glandu- larity (%)	Conventional		Tomosynthesis	
			Phantom AGD mGy	Patient AGD mGy (± 2sem)	Phantom AGD mGy	Patient AGD mGy (± 2sem)
20	21	97	0.60	0.87 ± 0.06	0.92	1.21 ± 0.06
30	32	67	0.84	0.98 ± 0.08	1.13	1.23 ± 0.06
40	45	41	1.19	1.53 ± 0.11	1.58	1.78 ± 0.06
45	53	29	1.44	1.76 ± 0.12	2.08	2.12 ± 0.07
50	60	20	2.03	2.26 ± 0.18	2.52	2.60 ± 0.11
60	75	9	2.74	3.02 ± 0.17	3.77	3.79 ± 0.06
70	90	4	3.12	3.98 ± 0.96	4.65	4.90 ± 0.11

Table 2. Dose measurement using the Siemens Inspiration system

PMMA thickness (mm)	Equiv. breast thickness (mm)	Glandu-larity (%)	Conventional		Tomosynthesis	
			Phantom AGD mGy	Patient AGD mGy (± 2sem)	Phantom AGD mGy	Patient AGD mGy (± 2sem)
20	21	97	0.47	0.51 ± n/a	0.91	1.02 ± 0.08
30	32	67	0.63	0.75 ± 0.19	1.20	1.38 ± 0.32
40	45	41	0.90	1.15 ± 0.09	1.63	1.88 ± 0.15
45	53	29	1.03	1.39 ± 0.12	1.86	2.13 ± 0.17
50	60	20	1.28	1.56 ± 0.19	2.13	2.26 ± 0.21
60	75	9	1.70	1.91 ± 0.16	2.80	2.73 ± 0.22
70	90	4	2.17	2.55 ± 0.90	3.46	3.37 ± 0.77

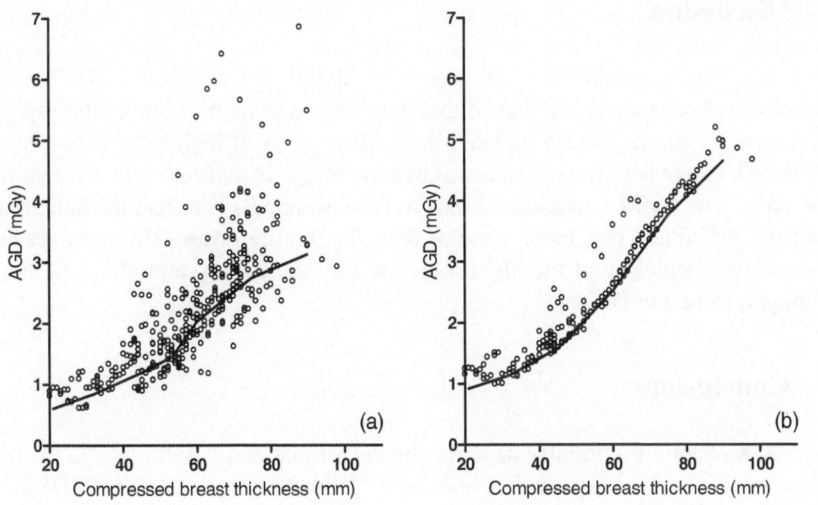

Fig. 1. AGD for patient and phantom measurements for the Hologic Selenia Dimensions system (a) doses for 2D digital mammography and (b) doses for DBT. The open symbols represent the patient doses and the solid line the doses estimated using PMMA phantoms.

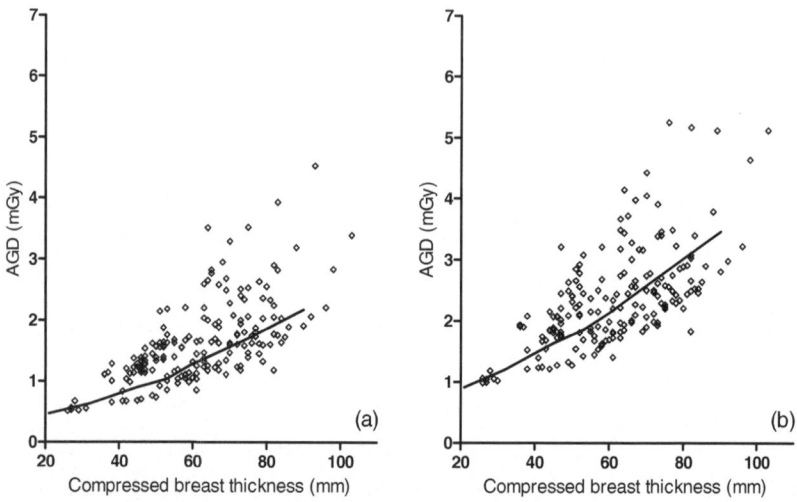

Fig. 2. AGD for patient and phantom measurements for the Siemens Inspiration system (a) doses for 2D digital mammography and (b) doses for DBT. The open symbols represent the patient doses and the solid line the doses estimated using PMMA phantoms.

4   Discussion

Overall the phantom estimates of 2D dose were slightly lower than the 2D doses calculated for real patients. It is believed that this is because modern automatic exposure control (AEC) systems tend to increase dose where areas of high local breast density are detected, whereas for phantom exposures the image is uniform over the area used by the AEC. The PMMA-measured doses in DBT were also less than the patient doses, but the difference was much smaller than for the 2D doses. This may reflect a difference in complexity of the algorithms used by the two systems for AEC in 2D mammography and in DBT.

5   Conclusions

The PMMA phantoms currently used for the determination of AGD for 2D mammography can also be used to provide a reasonable estimate of patient doses in DBT, and are therefore recommended for use in routine quality control of DBT systems. For the two systems investigated the differences between the average patient-measured values of the AGD for DBT and phantom-measured values of the AGD were no more than 24% and 13% respectively, and on average 8% and 7% respectively, of the patient AGD over the breast (phantom) thickness range 21 mm - 90 mm (20 mm – 70 mm). These differences are much smaller than the patient-to-patient variation for a given breast thickness.

For the two systems investigated, the AGD values for a single DBT view were on average factors of 1.2 and 1.5 higher than those for a single 2D mammogram. The significance of this dose increase must be assessed in relation to the clinical performance and future role of DBT systems.

Acknowledgement. This work is part of the OPTIMAM project supported by Cancer Research-UK & EPSRC Cancer Imaging Programme in Surrey, in association with the MRC and Department of Health (England).

References

1. European Commission (EC): European Guidelines for Quality Assurance in Breast Cancer Screening and Diagnosis 4th (edn.). Office for Official Publications of the European Communities, Luxembourg (2006)
2. Dance, D.R., Young, K.C., van Engen, R.E.: Estimation of mean glandular dose for breast tomosynthesis: factors for use with the UK, European and IAEA breast dosimetry protocols. Phys. Med. Biol. 56, 453–471 (2011)
3. Dance, D.R.: Monte Carlo calculation of conversion factors for the estimation of mean glandular breast dose. Phys. Med. Biol. 35, 1211–1219 (1990)
4. Dance, D.R., Skinner, C.L., Young, K.C., Beckett, J.R., Kotre, C.J.: Additional factors for the estimation of mean glandular breast dose using the UK mammography dosimetry protocol. Phys. Med. Biol. 45, 3225–3240 (2000)
5. Dance, D.R., Young, K.C., van Engen, R.E.: Further factors for the estimation of mean glandular dose using the United Kingdom, European and IAEA dosimetry protocols. Phys. Med. Biol. 54, 4361–4372 (2009)

Phantoms for Quality Control Procedures of Digital Breast Tomosynthesis

Ramona W. Bouwman[1], Oliver Diaz[2], Kenneth C. Young[3], Ruben E. van Engen[1], Wouter J.H. Veldkamp[1,4], and David R. Dance[3]

[1] National Expert and Training Centre for Breast Cancer Screening, Radboud University Nijmegen Medical Centre (LRCB), P.O. Box 6873, 6503 GJ Nijmegen, NL
r.bouwman@lrcb.nl
[2] Centre for Vision, Speech and Signal Processing,
Faculty of Engineering and Physical Scienes,
University of Surrey, Guildford, GU2 7XH, UK
[3] National Coordinating Centre for the Physics of Mammography (NCCPM),
Royal Surrey County Hospital, Guildford, GU2 7XX, UK and Department of Physics,
University of Surrey, Guildford, GU2 7XH, UK
[4] Department of Radiology, Leiden University Medical Centre,
Albunisdreef 2, 2333 ZA Leiden, NL

Abstract. For quality control (QC) protocols in full field digital mammography polymethyl methacrylate (PMMA) phantoms are generally used. The possibility of using alternative materials has been investigated for digital breast tomosynthesis (DBT) because of the increased importance of scatter and more complex imaging geometries. We have investigated the use of PMMA in combination with polyethylene (PE) to simulate a range of typical breasts using a computation model of the imaging system. The scatter-to-primary ratios (SPRs) of both breast and phantom were also investigated and a difference up to 18% is found. Neglecting this difference in SPR in designing phantoms for DBT may lead to dosimetry errors. Taking into account estimated SPR values and relevant X-ray spectra, a combination of PMMA-PE slabs has been proposed to simulate typical breasts of thicknesses 30, 60 and 90 mm. The dosimetric error associated with using these phantoms for relevant X-ray spectra is less than 10%.

Keywords: Quality control, digital breast tomosynthesis, phantoms, scatter-to-primary ratio.

1 Background

Currently, different digital breast tomosynthesis (DBT) systems are available for clinical use. Although most DBT systems are based on full field digital mammography (FFDM) platforms, or even suited for both FFDM and DBT imaging, there are significant differences. For instance, most FFDM systems use an anti-scatter grid, unlike DBT systems. Consequently, when designing breast equivalent phantoms, the scatter properties of the breast and phantom need to be taken into account for DBT,

A.D.A. Maidment, P.R. Bakic, and S. Gavenonis (Eds.): IWDM 2012, LNCS 7361, pp. 322–329, 2012.

whereas this is known not to be important for FFDM systems [1]. Similar to FFDM systems, DBT systems are equipped with an automatic exposure control (AEC) system to determine the appropriate exposure settings to obtain images of sufficient image quality. In the European Guidelines for quality assurance in breast cancer screening and diagnosis [2], polymethyl methacrylate (PMMA) slabs are used to simulate typical breasts for both image quality and breast dosimetry assessments in FFDM. For this purpose, the thicknesses of PMMA required to simulate typical breasts for a range of thicknesses were established using a combination of measurements and Monte Carlo simulations. Typical compressed breasts from 20 to 110 mm thick can be simulated by PMMA slabs 19 to 86 mm thick [3]. Thus, the thicknesses of typical breasts and the corresponding phantoms do not match. For the mammography systems in use at that time, this difference was of minor importance as the AEC system responses were solely based on the absorbed energy in the image receptor. However, as AEC systems became more advanced, the difference in thickness became more important as it could influence the exposure settings selected. For instance, advanced AEC systems may use information of the height of the compression paddle, the applied compression force and/or a pre-exposure to determine the exposure. This means that this difference in thickness needs to be corrected. For FFDM, spacers are used for this purpose. Currently, the method of operation of AEC systems for DBT (which varies by manufacturer) is not known exactly. However, it is expected that their functionality is comparable with AEC systems used for FFDM. Switching towards 3D techniques requires that the whole imaged volume is evaluated instead of only the projection of this volume. Therefore the thicknesses of breast and phantom should be more consistent, which means that spacers can no longer be used.

Evaluating the AEC in terms of image quality and dosimetry is an important part in quality control protocols like the European Guidelines. In this study, we have investigated whether a combination of two materials, PMMA and polyethylene (PE), can be used to simulate typical breasts for dosimetry measurements in DBT. For this evaluation we have determined the breast equivalence of PMMA and PE and calculated the scatter-to-primary ratio (SPR) of both the breast model and phantom in absence of an anti scatter grid. So we can assess the impact of SPR on the PMMA-PE breast equivalence.

2   Method

The typical breast compositions used in this work are described in the papers of Dance et al [3]. These are the compositions used in the European Protocol for dosimetry of FFDM [2] and are a representation of woman attending for breast cancer screening in the UK. To design phantoms which simulate typical breasts in thickness and produce the same absorbed energy per unit area at the image receptor, combinations of plastics slabs needs to be investigated which have a linear attenuation coefficient of appropriate magnitude. As can be seen from fig. 1 in the mammographic energy range, PMMA and PE are suitable materials for this purpose.

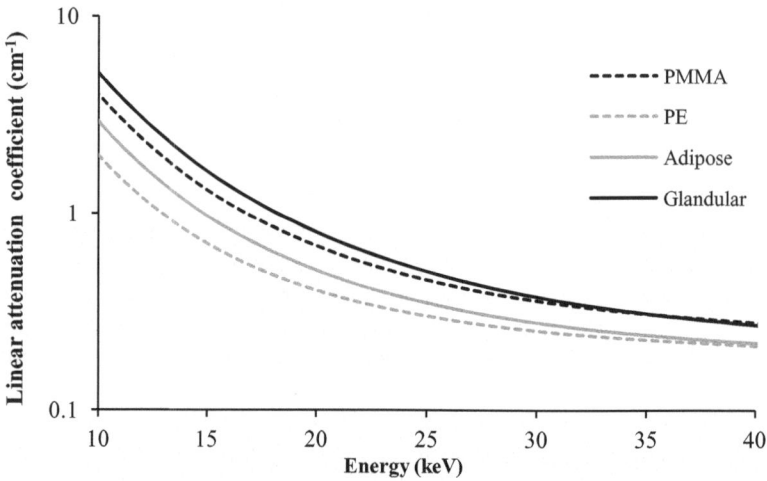

Fig. 1. Linear attenuation coefficient of PMMA, PE, adipose and glandular tissue [4]

Using a combination of PMMA and PE allows changing the standard set-up as used in FFDM towards a configuration that simulates typical breasts in both attenuation and thickness (fig. 2).

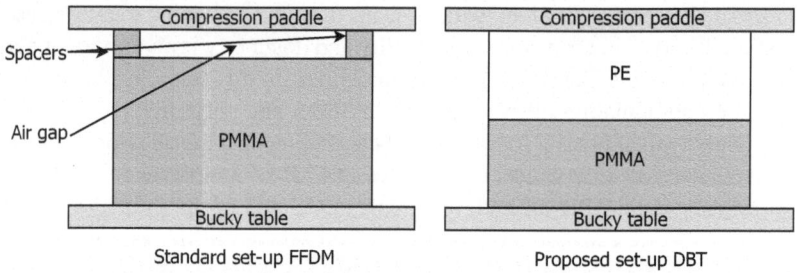

Fig. 2. (a) Standard set-up for assessing breast dose in FFDM (b) the proposed set-up for tomosynthesis. Note the air gap between the PMMA and the compression paddle in (a).

To determine the required slab thicknesses for each material, the energy absorption (X) in the image receptor is matched for both phantom and breast using:

$$X = \sum EN(E)\Delta E \cdot e^{\sum -\mu_i \cdot t_i} f(E)(1 + SPR) \qquad (1)$$

where E is the photon energy, N(E) is the number of X-ray photons of energy E and ΔE is the bin width of the X-ray spectrum. The μ_i and t_i are respectively the linear attenuation coefficients and thicknesses of all the materials along the path of the primary X-ray beam. The scatter-to-primary ratio, SPR, is the ratio of the energies absorbed per unit area of the detector from scattered and primary photons and f(E) is the energy absorption efficiency of the image receptor. Earlier work by Dance et al [1] has shown that f(E) has a minor influence on phantom thickness, and initial calculations were therefore done assuming an ideal detector (f(E)=1 for all energies, E), and equal phantom and breast SPR. This approach is appropriate when SPR is small (e.g. for FFDM or scanning DBT systems which uses a narrow X-ray beam). Combinations of PMMA and PE were found that satisfy equation 1 for these conditions for three simulated breast thicknesses (30, 60 and 90 mm) and three X-ray spectra (28 kV Mo/Mo, 32 kV W/Rh and 40 kV W/Al). The X-ray spectra from Boone et al. [5] were used for this purpose.

Full field DBT systems do not use an anti-scatter grid, and therefore it cannot be assumed that the SPR will be the similar for phantom and breast. A second series of calculations were therefore made in which a Monte Carlo model of the imaging system was used to estimate the SPR. The Monte Carlo simulations were based on the Geant4 toolkit [6, 7] using a model that was developed previously [8]. The X-ray tube was simulated as a point source 66 cm above the image receptor in a stationary position which produces 10^{10} photons per simulation. The compression paddle and bucky table were assumed to be 2.4 mm polycarbonate and 1.2 mm carbon fibre respectively. The image receptor was positioned 1.5 cm below the bucky table. During the simulation only photons reaching the image receptor in an ROI of area 10 x 10 mm^2, centred 6 cm from chest wall were recorded. The PMMA-PE slabs can be arranged in different ways, we have investigated whether the arrangement of the slabs will affect the SPR for two configurations (fig. 3).

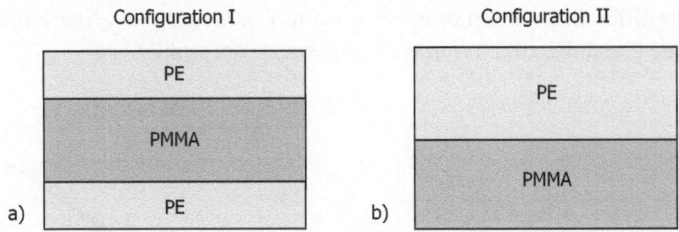

Fig. 3. Phantom configurations used to assess the effect of the arrangement of the plastic blocks on the SPR. The total amount of PMMA and PE are the same in both configurations. a) configuration I: PE slabs of equal thickness on the top and bottom of the PMMA and b) configuration II: PMMA positioned on the bucky table with the PE slab on top.

Besides the effect of the slab order, the SPR was calculated for two phantom shapes: a rectangular phantom with constant cross section of 180 x 240 mm^2 (similar to practical phantoms) and a cylinder with semi-circular cross section for which the radius increases with phantom thickness (similar to the breast model used), see table 1.

Table 1. Radii of the cylinder used for different thicknesses

Thickness [mm]	Radius [mm]
30	80
60	120
90	150

3   Results

Table 2 gives the PMMA and PE slab thicknesses corresponding to the different simulated breast thicknesses and X-ray spectra, calculated on the assumption that the breast and phantom SPR is constant and f(E) equals 1 for all energies (ideal detector). These PMMA-PE thicknesses were used in the Monte Carlo program to calculate phantom SPR. PMMA-PE breast equivalences are only given for clinical relevant X-ray spectra.

Table 2. PMMA and PE thicknesses corresponding to typical breasts assuming constant SPR and f(E)=1 for all energies

Breast thickness [mm] (Glandularity)	30 [mm] (72%)	60 [mm] (21%)	90 [mm] (4.0%)
28 kV Mo/Mo (30 µm) HVL = 0.366 mm Al	PMMA:27.0 PE: 3.0	PMMA: 33.7 PE: 26.3	
32 kV W/Rh (50 µm) HVL = 0.569 mm Al	PMMA:25.6 PE: 4.4	PMMA: 31.4 PE: 28.6	PMMA: 34.7 PE: 55.3
40 kV W/Al (700 µm) HVL = 0.778 mm Al		PMMA: 25.4 PE: 34.6	PMMA: 26.1 PE: 63.9

The calculated phantom SPR for the different slab arrangements is shown in fig. 4(a) and for different phantom cross sections in fig. 4(b). In this figure results for 32 kV W/Rh are given. Results for other X-ray spectra are similar.

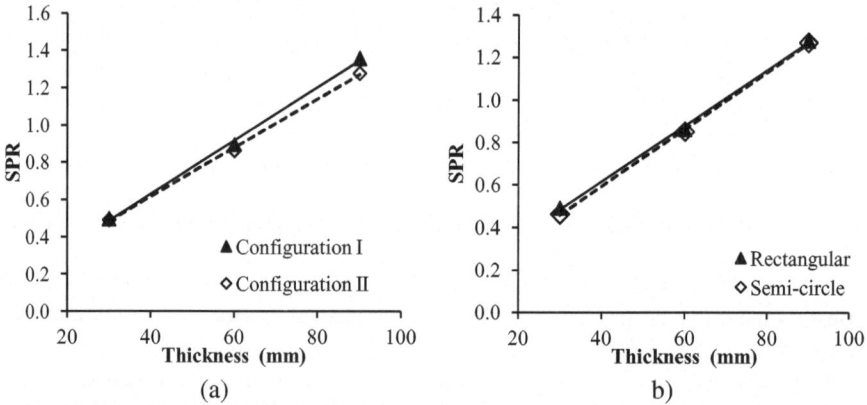

(a)   b)

Fig. 4. Phantom SPR using 32 kV W/Rh for a) phantom configurations I and II and rectangular cross sections b) two different phantom cross sections and configuration II

From those figures we can conclude that the arrangement of the slabs has a small effect on the phantom SPR. The maximum difference in SPR was found for a 90 mm breast and was less than 10%. For practical reasons all additional Monte Carlo simulations will be performed using configuration II unless stated differently. Likewise, we found small differences in phantom SPR using different cross sectional areas and shapes. The largest differences are found for a 30 mm breast and can go up to 6% for the relevant X-ray spectra. Again, for practical reasons we decided to continue using rectangular cross sections.

In fig. 5 the calculated breast and phantom SPR are plotted against breast thickness for 32 kV W/Rh. This figure shows that compared to the breast SPR, the phantom SPR is larger. The maximum difference between phantom and breast SPR is 18%. The observed difference between phantom and breast SPR seems to depend slightly on the X-ray spectra used and therefore only the results for 32 kV W/Rh is shown.

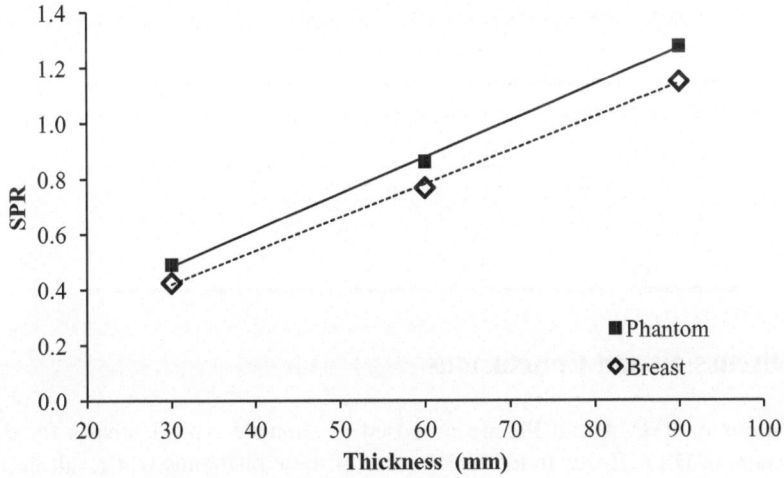

Fig. 5. Breast and phantom SPR calculated using Monte Carlo simulations using an energy spectrum of 32 kV W/Rh

Inclusion of the SPR (for full field images without an anti-scatter grid) in the calculation of the PMMA-PE breast equivalence resulted in different slab thickness as shown in table 3. From this table it is concluded that due to the SPR the amount of PMMA needed to achieve the equivalence increased. From equation 1, it is evident that neglecting this difference in SPR results in underestimation of the energy accumulated in the image receptor.

Table 3. PMMA and PE thicknesses corresponding to typical breasts assuming f(E)=1 for all energies and using the breast and phantom SPRs calculated using the Monte Carlo simulations

Breast thickness [mm]	30 [mm]	60 [mm]	90 [mm]
28 kV Mo/Mo (30 μm)	PMMA: 29.4 PE: 0.6	PMMA: 34.9 PE: 25.1	
32 kV W/Rh (50 μm)	PMMA: 27.5 PE: 2.5	PMMA: 33.9 PE: 26.1	PMMA: 37.6 PE: 51.5
40 kV W/Al (700 μm)		PMMA: 31.4 PE: 28.6	PMMA: 32.1 PE: 57.9

For QC purposes it is practical to use a single PMMA-PE combination, per thickness, to simulate typical breasts. For each thickness, an optimal set of PMMA and PE slabs was selected using clinical relevant X-ray spectra with the restriction that individual slab thicknesses are multiples of 2.5 mm. The chosen thicknesses with the corresponding maximum error in accumulated energy for a 30, 60 and 90 mm breasts are given in table 4. This table shows that the error in accumulated energy at the image receptor is less than 10%. This error is sufficiently small and comparable with errors using current dose evaluations using PMMA phantoms for FFDM.

Table 4. Selected PMMA-PE slab thicknesses for simulating typical breast with corresponding maximum error in accumulated energy in the image receptor

Breast thickness [mm]	Slab thickness [mm]		Max error (%)
	PMMA	PE	
30	27.5	2.5	7
60	32.5	27.5	9
90	32.5	57.5	9

4   Discussion and Conclusions

Combinations of PMMA and PE are proposed to simulate typical breasts for dose measurement in DBT. It was found that the use of these phantoms will result in estimated doses for typical breasts with an error of less than 10%.

In order to design PMMA-PE combinations for simulating typical breasts, the PMMA-PE breast equivalence was determined by matching primary energy deposition and thickness. The PMMA-PE equivalence that was found is used to determine and compare breast and phantom SPR. It was found that phantom SPR is larger (maximum 18%) than the breast SPR depending slightly on the X-ray spectrum. This means that SPR affects the PMMA-PE breast equivalence. Including the SPR in determining the breast equivalence resulted in using more PMMA. In general, neglecting the influence of SPR will result in an underestimation of the breast dose. Furthermore the effect of the phantom cross sectional areas and the arrangement of slabs were investigated. It was found that different configuration and cross sections had a small effect on SPR. For practical reasons it was decided to position the PMMA slabs on the bucky with the PE slab on top and to use slabs with a rectangular cross section.

Further work is required to implement the proposed phantoms in QC-procedures. There is a need to evaluate the effects of image receptors and the effect of the angled radiation on the PMMA-PE breast equivalence. Furthermore a validation survey needs to be performed to compare patient doses with doses measured with the proposed phantoms.

Acknowledgement. The authors gratefully acknowledge Roeland van der Burght from Artinis Medical Systems (Zetten, NL) who provided the phantoms. This work was partially funded by the HighRex project within the EU Sixth Framework Programme, Life Science, Genomics and Biotechnology for Health.

References

1. Dance, D.R., Young, K.C., van Engen, R.E.: Further factors for the estimation of mean glandular dose using the United Kingdom, European and IAEA breast dosimetry protocols. Phys. Med. Biol. 54, 4361 (2009)
2. Perry, N., Broeders, M., Wolf de, C., Törnberg, S., Holland, R., Karsa von, L.: European guidelines for quality assurance in breast cancer screening and diagnosis. 92-79-01258-4 (European Commission) (2006)
3. Dance, D.R., Skinner, C.L., Young, K.C., Beckett, J.R., Kotre, C.J.: Additional factors for the estimation of mean glandular breast dose using the UK mammography dosimetry protocol. Phys. Med. Biol. 45, 3225 (2000)
4. Berger, M.J., Hubbell, J.H., Seltzer, S.M., Chang, J., Coursey, J.S., Sukumar, R., Zucker, D.S., Olsen, K.: NIST Standard Reference Database, vol. 2011 (1987)
5. Boone, J.M., Fewell, T.R., Jennings, R.J.: Molybdenum, rhodium, and tungsten anode spectral models using interpolating polynomials with application to mammography. Med. Phys. 24, 1863 (1997)
6. Agostinelli, S., et al.: GEANT4 - A simulation toolkit. Nuclear Instruments and Methods in Physics Research, Section A: Accelerators, Spectrometers, Detectors and Associated Equipment 506, 250 (2003)
7. Allison, J., et al.: Geant4 developments and applications. IEEE Transactions on Nuclear Science 53, 270 (2006)
8. Díaz, O., Yip, M., Cabello, J., Dance, D.R., Young, K.C., Wells, K.: Monte Carlo Simulation of Scatter Field for Calculation of Contrast of Discs in Synthetic CDMAM Images. In: Martí, J., Oliver, A., Freixenet, J., Martí, R. (eds.) IWDM 2010. LNCS, vol. 6136, pp. 628–635. Springer, Heidelberg (2010)

Development of a Quality Control Protocol for Digital Breast Tomosynthesis Systems in the TOMMY Trial

Celia J. Strudley[1], Kenneth C. Young[1], Jennifer M. Oduko[1], Padraig Looney[1], Annabel Barnard[1], and Fiona J. Gilbert[2]

[1] NCCPM, Guildford, UK
celia.strudley@nhs.net
[2] University of Cambridge, UK

Abstract. Seven Hologic Dimensions digital breast tomosynthesis (DBT) systems have been installed for the TOMMY trial, a UK based multi-centre trial comparing conventional 2D digital mammography with DBT. In the absence of established guidelines for DBT quality control, a specific protocol was developed and applied. Physics tests of 2D and DBT performance were conducted at baseline and are repeated every 6 months, and include dose to the European standard breast model, tomosynthesis contrast to noise ratio, geometric distortion, z-resolution and threshold contrast detail detection. In addition routine performance checks (daily, weekly and monthly) are conducted on each system and reviewed centrally. Doses delivered under automatic exposure control by the systems were found to be well matched, with a mean glandular dose for the standard breast model (53mm equivalent breast thickness) of 1.89 mGy (range 1.79 to 2.00 mGy) for DBT and 1.41 mGy (range 1.36 to 1.48 mGy) for 2D imaging. Detector performance and image quality measurements were also well matched. All the systems exceeded the achievable image quality standard in the European guidelines for conventional digital mammography.

Keywords. Digital breast tomosynthesis, QC, mean glandular dose, contrast noise ratio, geometric distortion, z-resolution, threshold contrast detail detectability.

1   Introduction

The TOMMY trial is a UK trial comparing conventional 2D digital mammography with digital breast tomosynthesis (DBT). Seven Hologic Dimensions systems with tomosynthesis capability have been installed at six sites. Prior to starting the trial the technical performance of each of these systems in conventional and DBT imaging was assessed during the second half of 2011. The protocol for tomosynthesis quality control was based upon a draft protocol for the Highrex project, development work for which has been published [1] and [2]. The tests described in the Highrex protocol were adapted for the TOMMY trial following our experience in testing Hologic Dimensions tomosynthesis systems. Physics tests will be repeated at six month intervals during the trial and radiographers are carrying out additional performance tests daily,

A.D.A. Maidment, P.R. Bakic, and S. Gavenonis (Eds.): IWDM 2012, LNCS 7361, pp. 330–337, 2012.
© Springer-Verlag Berlin Heidelberg 2012

weekly and monthly. The expected duration of the clinical image collection period of the trial is fifteen to eighteen months. This paper outlines the methods used and presents results from the initial physics tests and the regular radiographer tests covering a period of from three to seven months following commissioning.

2   Method

Dose. The mean glandular dose (MGD) to the European standard breast model was measured using a range of PMMA thicknesses for both conventional and tomosynthesis images acquired under AEC control using the method described for conventional mammography in the European protocol [3]. For DBT the method of dose calculation was as described by Dance et al [4].

CNR. Contrast to noise ratio (CNR) measurements were made in conventional mode using 0.2mm thick aluminium foil, as described in the European protocol . Tomosynthesis CNR measurements were made in a similar manner, using the same aluminium foil. To reduce the effect of the non-uniformity of the tomosynthesis images on CNR measurement, the 5mm x 5mm regions of interest (ROIs) used were subdivided into 1mm x1mm elements as shown in Figure 1. The tomosynthesis CNR was averaged over measurements made in 5 focal planes closest to the plane representing the actual height of the aluminium foil above the breast support table.

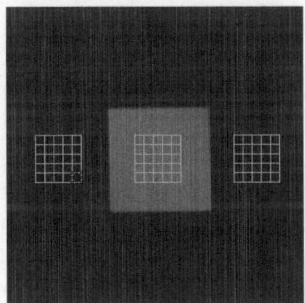

Fig. 1. Positioning of ROIs used for tomosynthesis CNR

Tomosynthesis Geometric Distortion. A 2mm thick sheet of polymethylmethacrylate (PMMA), engraved and painted with a diagonal grid of lines at 1cm intervals, was successively sandwiched at heights of 5, 30 and 55mm above the breast support table between plain slabs of PMMA making up a total thickness of 57mm PMMA. Tomosynthesis images were visually assessed to find the plane for which the image of the lines appeared to be best in focus. This was repeated at several positions within the image and the apparent vertical distortion at each position given in terms of apparent height of best focus relative to that at the centre of the chest wall edge of the image.

Tomosynthesis z-Resolution. A 5mm thickness of PMMA containing six 1mm diameter aluminium spheres was imaged successively at three heights within a total thickness of 55mm PMMA as described above for geometric distortion. Polynomial spline curves were fitted to line profiles taken in the vertical direction through the centre of each sphere, as shown in Figure 2, in order to assess the full width half maximum for each.

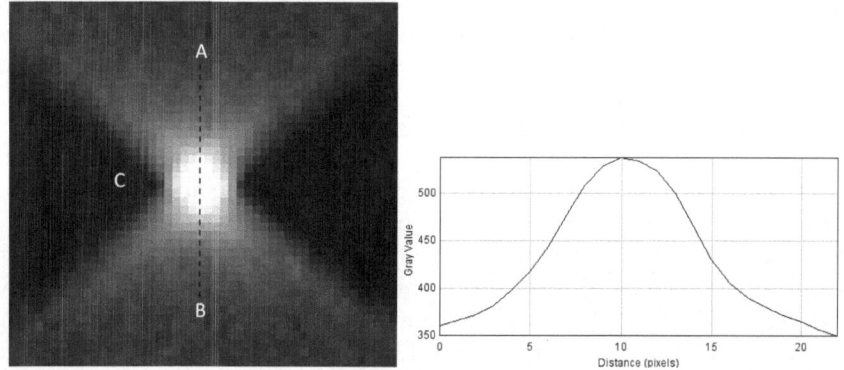

Fig. 2. A vertical reslice through a stack of focal planes showing the appearance of the 1mm aluminium sphere, and a line profile taken vertically through the centre. The line AB indicates from where the line profile is taken and the letter C indicates the region from which the minimum is taken to calculate the FWHM.

Detector MTF. The method described in the IEC protocol [5] was used.

Threshold Contrast Detail Visibility. This was assessed using the CDMAM test object as described in the European protocol. Sixteen images were acquired in conventional mode and in tomosynthesis mode. Each reconstructed tomosynthesis image was split (using a Hologic proprietary tool) into a set of two dimensional images representing focal planes at 1mm interval heights above the breast support table. From each set one image was selected, which represented the height of the CDMAM and in which the CDMAM was best in focus. The sixteen conventional images and the sixteen selected tomosynthesis images were analysed using CDCOM [6] and CDMAM [7] analysis software. Where CDMAM images are not flat, CDCOM can either fail to read or inaccurately read CDMAM images, and so it was found to be necessary to apply a flattening algorithm to the tomosynthesis focal planes.

Radiographer QC. Tomosynthesis tests are carried out in addition to the usual digital mammography quality control. Each day a tomosynthesis image of a 45mm PMMA block is acquired and each month tomosynthesis images of PMMA blocks with thicknesses of 2cm and 7cm are also acquired, all under AEC control. These images are checked for artefacts and the exposure factors compared against baseline values. Each week a conventional and a tomosynthesis image of a plain 45mm PMMA block and a tomosynthesis image of a 50mm PMMA block containing a single 1mm diameter aluminium ball are sent for analysis at our centre.

3 Results

Dose. Under AEC control, the MGD to the standard breast model (53mm equivalent breast thickness) was 1.89 mGy (range 1.79 to 2.00 mGy) for DBT and 1.41 mGy (range 1.36 to 1.48 mGy) for conventional imaging. Figure 3 and Table 1 show the average MGDs for the seven systems for conventional imaging and DBT for a range of equivalent breast thicknesses. The European dose limits for conventional digital mammography are also shown in Figure 3.

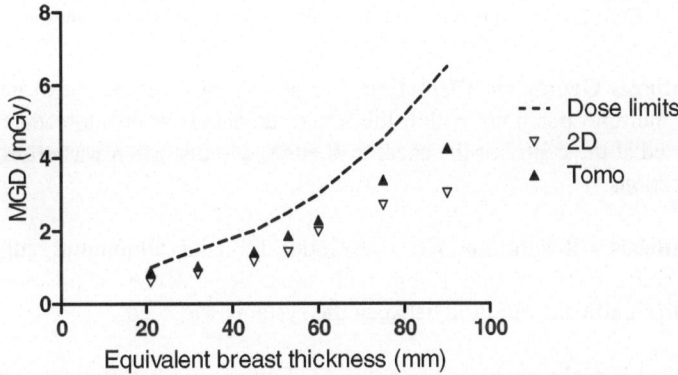

Fig. 3. MGD to the standard breast averaged over the seven systems, for conventional and tomosynthesis images

Table 1. MGD to the standard breast and CNR, averaged over the seven systems and coefficient of variation (CoV), for conventional and tomosynthesis images

Equivalent breast thickness (mm)	MGD for 2D images (mGy)		Average MGD for tomo images (mGy)		Average CNR for 2D images		Average CNR for tomo images	
	Average	CoV	Average	CoV	Average	CoV	Average	CoV
21	0.60	3.4%	0.89	3.1%	10.9	2.9%	29.1	2.5%
32	0.84	2.4%	1.04	3.5%	9.9	2.3%	22.2	2.8%
45	1.17	2.4%	1.43	3.9%	9.0	3.5%	18.9	2.8%
53	1.41	3.2%	1.87	4.2%	8.4	3.4%	18.5	3.5%
60	1.98	1.6%	2.29	3.8%	8.6	3.3%	17.2	3.7%
75	2.69	2.1%	3.39	4.3%	8.3	3.0%	14.8	4.7%
90	3.03	2.5%	4.25	3.6%	6.7	4.7%	11.3	4.3%

CNR. Average CNR measurements in conventional and tomosynthesis modes for the seven systems involved in the trial are shown in Figure 4 and Table 1. The limiting values derived from the European standard for conventional mammography are also shown in Figure 4.

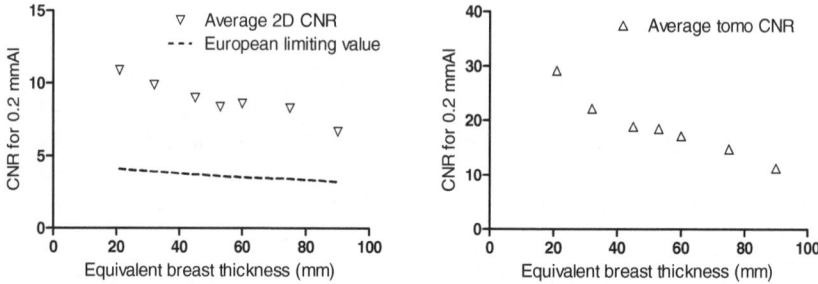

Fig. 4. CNR for conventional exposures (left) and tomosynthesis exposures (right)

Tomosynthesis Geometric Distortion. For all systems, the height of best focus assessed at multiple positions within the image deviated by no more than 1mm from that assessed at the centre of the chest wall edge. No distortion was observed in the x and y directions.

Tomosynthesis z-Resolution. The z-resolution for 1mm aluminium balls was found to range between 10mm and 12mm with some dependence on position within the image. No significant variation between the systems was seen.

Detector MTF. Only small differences in MTF were seen between the seven systems. The MTF measurements are shown in Figure 5 and Table 2.

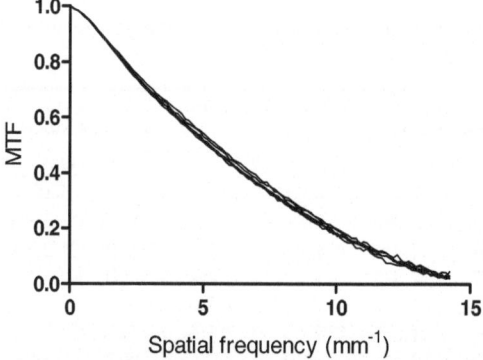

Fig. 5. The MTF measured for the seven systems

Table 2. Average MTF measurements for the seven systems

Spatial frequency (mm-1)	Average MTF	Standard deviation in MTF	Coefficient of variation
2.0	0.804	0.005	0.7%
4.0	0.605	0.010	1.7%
6.0	0.444	0.012	2.6%
8.0	0.308	0.010	3.3%
10.0	0.187	0.009	4.8%
12.0	0.093	0.009	9.7%

Threshold Contrast Detail Visibility. Figure 6 and Table 3 below show the threshold gold thickness for a range of detail diameters for conventional and tomosynthesis images of a CDMAM test object. The results from all systems are shown and compared against the minimum acceptable and achievable values for conventional mammography as defined in the European protocol.

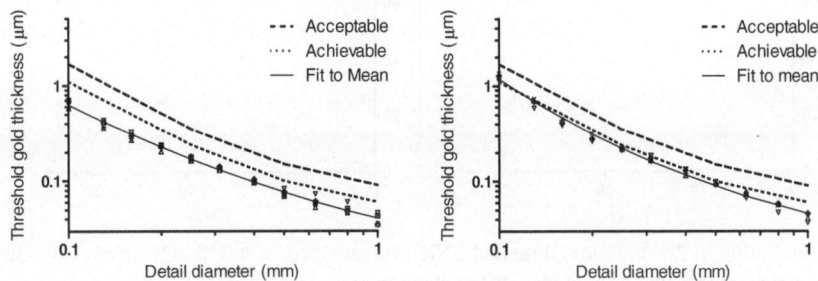

Fig. 6. Contrast detail curves from each of the systems for 2D (left) and DBT (right) images

Table 3. Average threshold gold thickness and coefficient of variation for 2D and tomo CDMAM images

Detail size (mm)	2D Threshold gold thickness (μm)	CoV	Tomo Threshold gold thickness (μm)	CoV	European limiting values for 2D mammography Minimum acceptable	Achievable
0.10	0.655	8.3%	1.277	6.7%	1.680	1.100
0.25	0.175	4.0%	0.218	2.3%	0.352	0.244
0.50	0.075	6.8%	0.095	2.3%	0.150	0.103
1.00	0.040	12.3%	0.043	8.9%	0.091	0.056

Radiographer QC. Analysis of routine QC images acquired by radiographers has shown that dose and SNR in both conventional and tomosynthesis images have remained stable and no clinically significant artefacts have been seen. The variation in dose and SNR measurements for each system over time are shown in Figure 7.

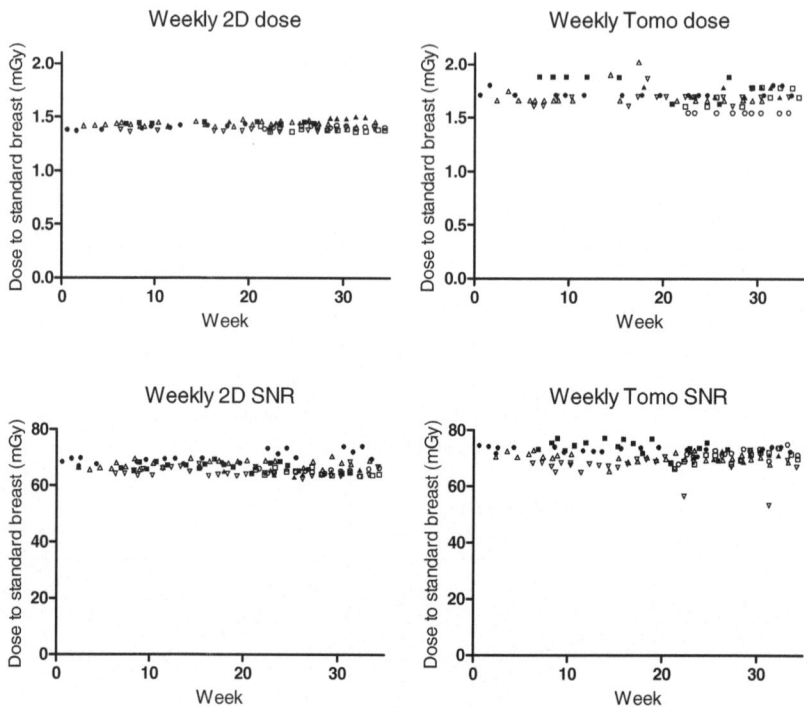

Fig. 7. Variation in 2D and tomo dose and SNR from analysis of weekly QC images of 45mm PMMA (each system represented by a different symbol)

4   Discussion

The initial technical performance measurements demonstrated that the seven systems are well matched and routine quality control tests show that performance has remained stable during the three to seven months since commissioning.

The results of analysis of tomosynthesis CDMAM images show that detection of a range of contrast detail sizes is not quite as good as for conventional mammography, but close to the achievable level defined in the European standard. In clinical practice the substantial advantage that tomosynthesis gains by reducing obscuration by overlying breast structure will tend to compensate for this difference.

The QA protocol described will be further developed and applied to tomosynthesis systems from other manufacturers. Additions are likely to include measurements of spatial resolution within tomosynthesis planes and more sophisticated methods of assessing geometric distortion and Z-resolution. Some initial measurements on a Siemens tomosynthesis system have demonstrated that the methods detailed above could be successfully applied. In testing the performance of tomosynthesis systems from other manufacturers account needs to be taken of differences in reconstruction algorithms and rotation geometry which may affect tomosynthesis uniformity, geometric distortion and reconstruction artefacts, which in turn may affect details of the method used to quantify image quality. The ability to download DICOM reconstructed tomosynthesis images with minimal post reconstruction processing applied is critical in allowing assessment of tomosynthesis imaging performance.

Acknowledgements. This work was carried out as part of the TOMMY Trial, which is funded by the NIHR Health Technology Assessment programme (www.hta.ac.uk/2296). The views and opinions expressed are those of the authors and do not necessarily reflect those of the Department of Health. The role of the TOMMY Trial Management Group[1] in the development and support of the project is acknowledged. Radiographers and physicists at each of the sites involved in the trial have also contributed to this work by assisting in the gathering of QC data.

References

1. van Engen, R.E., Bouwman, R., van der Burght, R., Lazzari, B., Dance, D.R., Heid, P., Aslund, M., Young, K.C.: Image Quality Measurements in Breast Tomosynthesis. In: Krupinski, E.A. (ed.) IWDM 2008. LNCS, vol. 5116, pp. 696–702. Springer, Heidelberg (2008)
2. Bouwman, R.W., Visser, R., Young, K.C., Dance, D.R., Lazzari, B., van der Burght, R., Heid, P., van Engen, R.E.: Daily quality control for breast tomosynthesis. In: Hsieh, J., Samei, E. (eds.) Medical Imaging 2010: The Physics of Medical Imaging (2010)
3. European Commission (EC): European Guidelines for Quality Assurance in Breast Cancer Screening and Diagnosis, 4th edn. Office for Official Publications of the European Communities, Luxembourg (2006)
4. Dance, D.R., Young, K.C., van Engen, R.E.: Estimation of mean glandular dose for breast tomosynthesis: factors for use with the UK, European and IAEA breast dosimetry protocols. Phys. Med. Biol. 56, 453–471 (2011)
5. IEC 62220-1-2: Medical electrical equipment – Characteristics of digital X-ray imaging devices – Part 1.2: Determination of the detective quantum efficiency – Detectors used in mammography (2007)
6. CDCOM version 1.6 available from EUREF website, euref.org
7. CDMAM analysis UK v1.4, NCCPM, Guildford, UK

---

[1] FJ Gilbert, MGC Gillan, SW Duffy, SM Astley, KC Young, M Michell, YY Lim, H Dobson, J Cooke, H Puroshothaman, K Duncan.

A Modelling Framework for Evaluation of 2D-Mammography and Breast Tomosynthesis Systems

Premkumar Elangovan[1], Alistair Mackenzie[2,3], Oliver Diaz[1], Alaleh Rashidnasab[1],
David R. Dance[2,3], Kenneth C. Young[2,3], Lucy M. Warren[2,3], Eman Shaheen[4],
Hilde Bosmans[4], Predrag R. Bakic[5], and Kevin Wells[1]

[1] Centre for Vision, Speech and Signal Processing, University of Surrey,
Guildford, GU2 7XH, UK
[2] NCCPM, Royal Surrey County Hospital,
Guildford, Surrey, GU2 7XX, UK
[3] Department of Physics, University of Surrey,
Guildford, GU2 7XH, UK
[4] Department of Radiology, University Hospitals Leuven,
Herestraat 49, 3000 Leuven, Belgium
[5] Department of Radiology, University of Pennsylvania,
Philadelphia, PA 19104, USA
p.elangovan@surrey.ac.uk

Abstract. Planar 2D X-ray mammography is the most common screening technique used for breast cancer detection. Digital breast tomosynthesis (DBT) is a new and emerging technology that overcomes some of the limitations of conventional planar imaging. However, it is important to understand the impact of these two modalities on cancer detection rates and patient recall. Since it is difficult to adequately evaluate different modalities clinically, a collection of modeling tools is introduced in this paper that can be used to emulate the image acquisition process for both modalities. In this paper, we discuss image simulation chains that can be used for the evaluation of 2D-mammography and DBT systems in terms of both technical factors and observer studies.

Keywords: Digital breast tomosynthesis, 2D-mammography, modeling, simulation.

1   Introduction

Breast cancer is one of the major causes of mortality in women in North America and Western Europe [1]. As a result breast screening programmes have been introduced in many western countries [2]. Mammography is the accepted radiological imaging technique for this purpose that uses low energy X-rays to image internal structures of the breast. An ideal mammogram is one in which the normal breast tissues such as adipose and glandular tissues can be differentiated from lesions and calcifications that are the signatures of malignancy. In reality, the quality and interpretation of a

A.D.A. Maidment, P.R. Bakic, and S. Gavenonis (Eds.): IWDM 2012, LNCS 7361, pp. 338–345, 2012.
© Springer-Verlag Berlin Heidelberg 2012

mammogram are affected by factors, such as overlapping tissues, dose, image processing and system characteristics.

One of the most promising advances in the field of breast cancer imaging is digital breast tomosynthesis (DBT) - a technique that uses low dose projections acquired at different angles to construct tomographic planes parallel to the detector. A commonly used reconstruction algorithm is the filtered back projection [3] because of its rapid execution time, but the 3D reconstruction is not perfect due to the limited number of projections. Further, tomosynthesis also suffers from similar quality degradation issues as a conventional 2D mammogram. However, tomosynthesis is considered to be a step forward in the field of breast imaging because clinical studies [4] have shown that a better visualization of lesions and calcifications can be achieved by blurring the appearance of overlapping tissues in the image.

It is important to understand the impact of tomosynthesis on the detection and recall rates of the patients who are invited for screening before considering this new modality for routine breast screening. Performing a comparison clinically is particularly time consuming and expensive, and some evaluations could be conducted more easily using mathematical modeling tools.

In this paper, we address this issue by introducing a modeling framework which includes a collection of simulation tools that can be used to represent the image acquisition process for planar mammography and for DBT. With this framework, it is possible to perform a comparison of 2D mammography and DBT systems. A brief introduction to the modeling tools is given in Section 2 and some selected simulation results are presented in Section 3.

2   Materials and Methods

For the initial development of the model, we have simulated 2D and DBT systems manufactured by Hologic (Bedford, Massachusetts, USA), as such systems are available in our centre, though the methodology can in principle be applied to any mammographic imaging system. The Hologic Selenia Dimensions 3D system is equipped with an a-Se (amorphous selenium) detector with a pixel pitch of 70 µm. The system can operate in both 2D mammography and 3D tomosynthesis mode. The dimensions of the detector are 24x29 cm^2 and an anti-scatter grid can be positioned above the detector to reduce the scatter during the acquisition of 2D mammograms. When operating in tomosynthesis mode, the X-ray source moves continuously over the angular range +7.5° to -7.5°, and 15 projections are acquired during this process. The center of rotation of the X-ray tube is directly above the a-Se layer of the detector. After acquisition, the pixels are resampled to a pitch of 140µm. No anti-scatter grid is used during tomosynthesis acquisition and the projections are reconstructed into breast planes of 1mm thickness.

Figure 1 shows the flowcharts of the modeling framework. A brief description of each module is given in section 2.1 followed by the methodology in section 2.2.

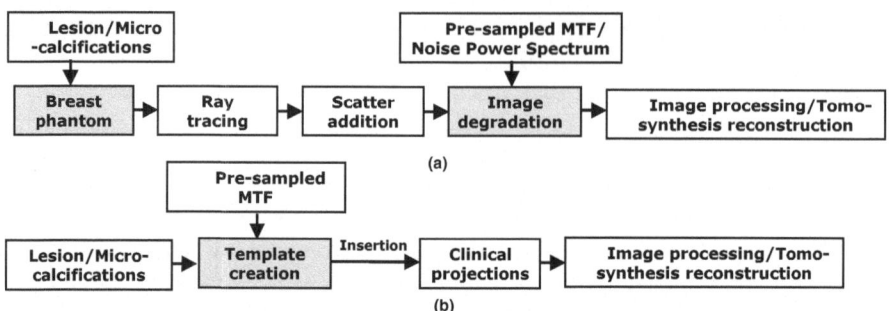

Fig. 1. Flowcharts illustrating the simulation chains described in Section 2.2, (a) using breast phantom and (b) using clinical projections

2.1   Modeling Tools

Breast Phantom. We used the software breast phantoms developed by Bakic *et al* [5]. These phantoms include all the primary breast tissues such as adipose tissue, fibroglandular tissue, Cooper's ligaments and skin. The simulation parameters of the breast model can be modified to account for variations in the breast anatomy such as thickness and glandularity.

Lesion Simulation Model. We used lesion simulation tool proposed by Rashidnasab *et al* [6-7], which uses fractal growth methods such as DLA (diffusion limited aggregation) and Random walk, to grow lesions in a 3D space. The model parameters can be varied to control the simulated mass structure and size. The DLA approach generates lesions that have porous interior and irregular boundaries, whereas Random walk approach generates lesions with relatively symmetric appearance. The dataset used here included both benign and malignant simulated masses. The methods had been validated by means of observer studies and found to provide realistic lesions.

Micro-calcification Simulation Model. We used the validated built 3D models of micro-calcification clusters developed by Shaheen *et al* [8]. The authors scanned biopsy specimen containing micro-calcifications using a micro-CT scanner, and subsequently segmented the calcifications from the background using thresholding techniques. The dataset used here included mainly malignant micro-calcification clusters, and their realistic appearance had been validated by means of observer studies.

Ray Tracing Tool. We used a ray tracing tool based on the Siddon algorithm [9] which computes the path traveled by an X-ray photon inside a voxelized phantom. The tool stores an individual record of each unique tissue and its path length traversed by a ray. This information was used to create a primary image using Beer's law and attenuation coefficients [10] corresponding to the appropriate mammographic X-ray spectrum [11].

Scatter Addition Tool. We used the scatter kernels proposed by Diaz *et al* [12], as a replacement for Monte Carlo simulations, to model scatter in mammography and tomosynthesis systems. Scatter kernels, whose coefficients depend on the breast thickness, glandularity and air gap at each pixel point, were convolved with the primary image to generate the scatter map. The model also accounted for the scatter from the compression paddle and the incident angle of the x-ray photons.

Conversion of Image Quality Tool. We used the methods of Mackenzie *et al* [13], which use measurements of the signal transfer properties, pre-sampled MTF (Modulation Transfer Function) and NPS (Noise Power Spectrum) performed on a tomosynthesis imaging system, to adapt the image quality of acquired images or simulated images. These measurements were used to blur the projection images and then add noise corresponding to a specific detector pixel size and specific exposure parameters respectively. The image was first scaled such that the pixel value was equivalent to the detector air kerma. The blurring process involved convolving a pre-sampled MTF and movement blur of the system being modeled with the projection images as shown in equation 1, where I_0 is the projection image and $H(u,v)$ is MTF of the system.

$$I_{blur} = FFT^{-1}\left\{ FFT\{I_0(x, y)\} \cdot MTF(u, v) \right\}$$ (1)

Subsequently, addition of noise to the blurred images involved creation of three flat field images, one for each major noise source (structure, electronic, quantum) from the NPS coefficients calculated for a detector air kerma of 1 μGy. The noise coefficients were then converted into real images (I_e: electronic noise, I_q: quantum noise and I_s: structure noise) equivalent to the noise at 1 μGy. The noise was added as shown in equation 2 using the knowledge of the dose to the detector and its response to electronic, quantum and structure noise.

$$I_{blur+noise} = I_e(x, y) + I_q(x, y)\sqrt{I_{blur}(x, y)} + I_s(x, y)I_{blur}(x, y) + I_{blur}(x, y)$$ (2)

Image Processing Tool. The Selenia V4.7.3 FFDM image processing package was used to convert the raw image thus calculated into an image for presentation to the radiologists.

Tomosynthesis Reconstruction Tool. The Hologic reconstruction software was used to reconstruct the tomographic breast image planes from the projection images.

2.2   Methodology

An initial experiment was conducted whereby the masses [6-7] and micro-calcifications [8] were inserted into the breast phantom [5] by replacing the tissue voxels with lesion/micro-calcification voxels at appropriate locations. One mammogram and 15 tomosynthesis primary projections were acquired using the ray tracing tool [9], Beer's law and attenuation coefficients [10] corresponding to the appropriate X-ray spectrum [11], at different angles in accord with the Hologic specification. The information such as thickness, glandularity, and air gap that is required for the selection of appropriate scatter kernels [12] was extracted from the ray tracing results and fed into the tool, for addition of scatter to the primary images. Using the MTF and noise model [13], a system MTF was applied to the projections corresponding to the detector and system, and noise was added to the projections corresponding to a specific dose. The effect of projection angle on the pre-sampled MTF and NPS were also taken into account. Each 2D-mammogram was post-processed using the Selenia V4.7.3 FFDM image processing package. The remaining 15 tomosynthesis projections were processed using the Hologic tomosynthesis reconstruction tool.

In a second experiment, the aforementioned methodology was adapted as follows: instead of a phantom, lesions and micro calcifications were inserted into clinical 2D-mammograms and individual tomosynthesis projections. The method of insertion into 2D-mammogram was adopted from Rashidnasab *et al* [6-7], and the method of insertion into tomosynthesis projections was adopted from Shaheen *et al* [8]. A series of templates were created from the projections of the lesion or micro-calcifications. At the desired location of insertion, each pixel in the template was multiplied by the corresponding pixel in each of the raw projection images. Prior to insertion, the scatter was removed from the insertion site, and after modification of the transmission factors by multiplication of the template, the scatter was added back.

Further, the model was validated by simulating a phantom that is used for routine quality control of mammography equipments, and comparing the modeled outcome with the ground truth data. The phantom comprised a 4.5cm polymethyl methacrylate (PMMA) block resting on the breast support, and an aluminum foil of dimension $10x10x0.2$ mm^3 placed 1 cm above the breast support. Since this setup is representative of a 5.3cm breast, which is typically used for exposure measurements, an airgap of 8mm is allowed between the compression paddle and the top of the PMMA block for geometrical and exposure consistency. Other modeling parameters included: 23μGy average detector entrance air kerma per projection; tungsten target and aluminum filter (0.7mm) at 31kVp; and SPR (scatter to primary ratio) of 0.5. The average detector entrance air kerma for the modeled projections, for the sake of noise addition, was estimated from the known signal transfer properties of the detector and the average pixel value in the actual projections. Both actual and modeled projections were reconstructed using the same version of the reconstruction software for consistency.

3   Results

Figure 2 shows the actual and modeled projections along with the corresponding reconstructed tomographic planes. CNR (contrast to noise ratio) measurements were performed on the in focus plane at which the aluminum foil was located. The CNR measurement for the actual and modeled planes had a reasonably good agreement; the percentage error was approximately 15%. Discrepancy in the CNR may have been due to error in the detector air kerma approximation and also possibly due to reconstruction artifacts. Other contributing factors could have been the effect of phase lag and blurring due to finite size of the focal spot, which were not accounted for.

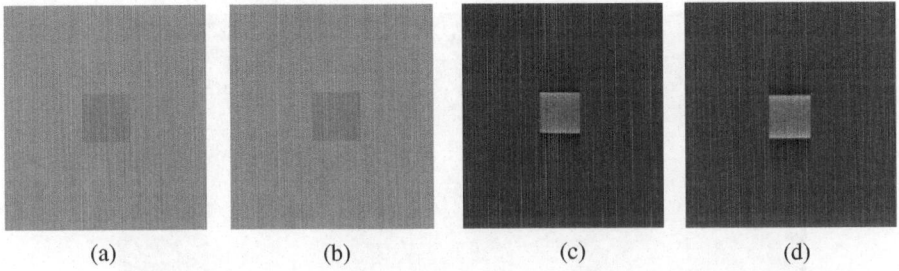

Fig. 2. (a) Actual projection; (b) modeled projection; (c) actual plane; (d) modeled plane

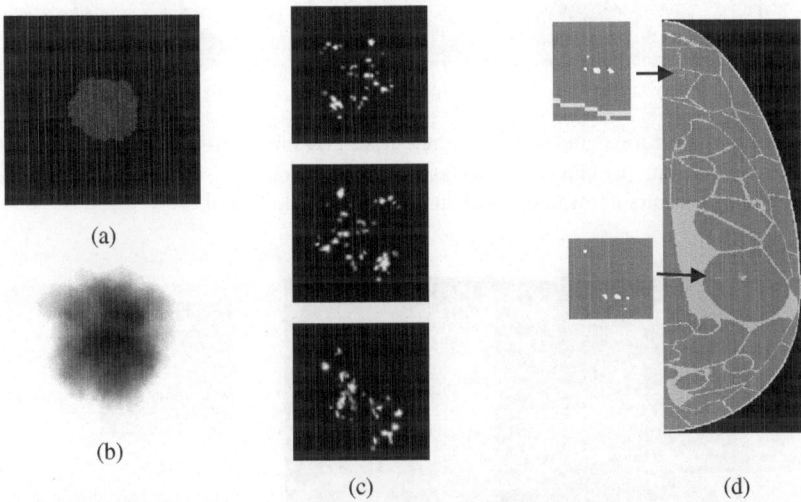

Fig. 3. (a) Simulated lesion rendered in 3D; (b) 2D projection of the lesion; (c) micro-calcifications; (d) breast phantom with micro-calcifications inserted into an adipose region to highlight visibility

Figure 3 shows the results of insertion of a micro-calcification cluster (cluster size: 5mmx4mmx4mm; >30 calcifications) into the breast phantom (thickness: 65mm; dense tissue: 25%) alongside an example of a simulated mass and micro-calcification cluster. Figure 4 shows the results of insertion of a relatively large (~12mm) conspicuous lesion (method: random walk; fractal dimension:2.82) into clinical projections followed by the application of the reconstruction software. Figure 5 shows a processed 2D mammogram and reconstructed tomographic plane of a breast with a small (~5mm) subtle simulated lesion (method: DLA; fractal dimension: 2.54). It is obvious from Figure 5 that there are significant variations in the lesion appearance between both modalities. Impact of this distinction on the cancer detection can be determined by conducting further studies using the proposed framework.

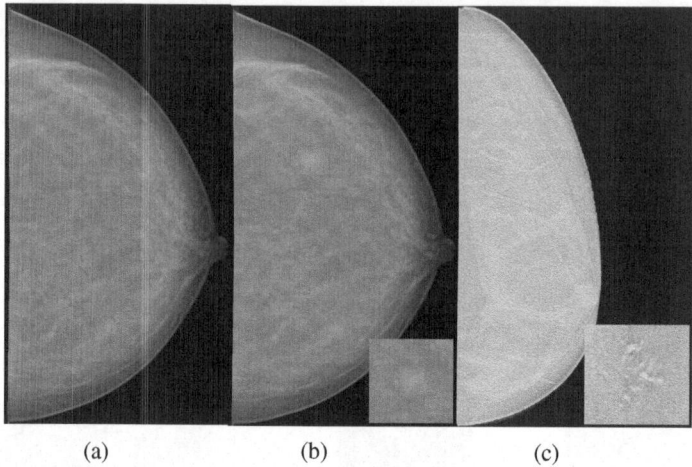

(a)   (b)   (c)

Fig. 4. Reconstructed tomographic breast plane from (a) clinical projections prior to insertion of a simulated lesion; (b) clinical projections after insertion of a 12mm obvious simulated lesion; (c) breast phantom projections with inserted micro-calcifications

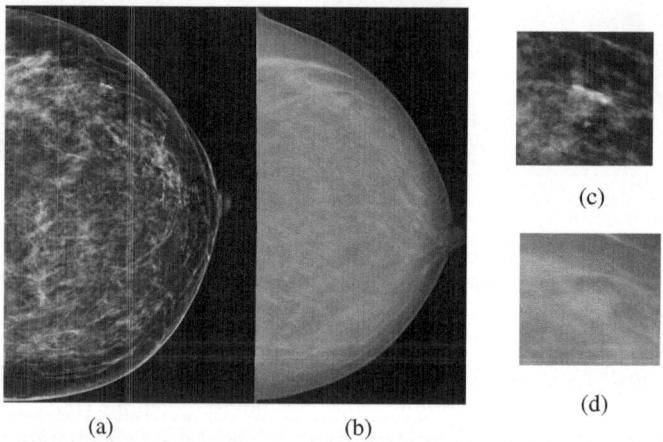

(a)   (b)

Fig. 5. (a) Processed 2D mammogram of a breast with a 5mm subtle simulated lesion; (b) reconstructed tomographic plane of the same breast; (c-d) thumbnail insets showing inserted regions in detail

4   Discussions and Conclusions

A modeling framework to simulate 2D-mammography and digital breast tomosynthesis systems has been proposed to allow comparative studies. The simulation chain using breast phantoms demonstrated its use for studying the impact of technical factors on the image formation and image quality. The other simulation chain using clinical images demonstrated that this is useful for conducting observer performance studies to investigate the detectability of lesions in 2D and DBT.

Acknowledgements. This work is part of the OPTIMAM project and is supported by Cancer Research-UK & EPSRC Cancer Imaging Programme in Surrey, in association with the MRC and Department of Health (England). We would like to thank Celia Strudley at NCCPM, RSCH for her timely help and support for this work. We are grateful for the help and support of staff from the Jarvis Breast Screening Unit, Guildford. Also, we would like to thank Hologic for providing us with the reconstruction tool and image processing software.

References

1. Parkin, D.M., Fernandez, L.M.G.: Use of statistics to assess the global burden of breast cancer. The Breast Journal 12, 70–80 (2006)
2. NHS Breast Screening Programme, Annual Review (2009),
   http://www.cancerscreening.nhs.uk/breastscreen/publications
3. Mertelmeier, T., Orman, J., Haerer, W., Dudam, M.K.: Optimizing filtered backprojection reconstruction for a breast tomosynthesis prototype device. In: Proc. SPIE, vol. 6142, pp. 61420F1-61420F12 (2006)
4. Teertstra, H.J., Loo, H.J., Van den Bosch, M.A., Van Tinteren, H., Rutgers, E.J., Muller, S.H., Gilhuijs, K.S.: Breast tomosynthesis in clinical practice: initial results. Eur. Radiol. 20, 16–24 (2010)
5. Bakic, R.B., Zhang, C., Maidment, A.D.A.: Development and characterization of an anthropomorphic breast software phantom based upon region-growing algorithm. Med. Phys. 38, 3165–3176 (2011)
6. Rashidnasab, A., Elangovan, P., Dance, D.R., Young, K.C., Diaz, O., Wells, K.: Modeling realistic breast lesions using diffusion limited aggregation. In: Proc. SPIE, vol. 8313, p. 83134L (2012)
7. Rashidnasab, A., Elangovan, P., Dance, D.R., Young, K.C., Yip, M., Diaz, O., Wells, K.: Realistic simulation of breast mass appearance using random walk. In: Proc. SPIE, vol. 8313, p. 83130L (2012)
8. Shaheen, E., Ongeval, C.V., Zanca, F., Cockmartin, L., Marshall, N., Jacobs, J., Young, K.C., Dance, D.R., Bosmans, H.: The simulation of 3D microcalcification clusters in 2D digital mammography and breast tomosynthesis. Med. Phys. 38, 6659 (2011)
9. Siddon, R.L.: "Fast calculation of the exact radiological path for a three-dimensional CT array. Med. Phys. 12, 252–255 (1985)
10. Berger, M.J., Hubbell, J.H., Seltzer, S.M., Chang, J., Coursey, J.S., Sukumar, R., Zucker, D.S.: XCOM: Photon cross sections database. NIST Standard Reference Database 8, 87-3597 (1998)
11. Boone, J.M., Fewell, T.R., Jennings, R.J.: Molybdenum, Rhodium and Tungsten anode spectral models using interpolating polynomials with application to mammography. Med. Phys. 24, 1863–1874 (1997)
12. Diaz, O., Dance, D.R., Young, K.C., Elangovan, P., Bakic, P.R., Wells, K.: A fast scatter field estimator for digital breast tomosynthesis. In: Proc. SPIE, vol. 8313, p. 831305 (2012)
13. Mackenzie, A., Workman, A., Dance, D.R., Yip, M., Wells, K., Young, K.C.: Development and validation of a method for converting images to appear with noise and sharpness characteristics of a different detector and X-ray system. Med. Phys. 39 (in press, 2012)

Is the Outcome of Optimizing the System Acquisition Parameters Sensitive to the Reconstruction Algorithm in Digital Breast Tomosynthesis?

Rongping Zeng[1], Subok Park[1], Predrag R. Bakic[2], and Kyle J. Myers[1]

[1] Office of Science and Engineering Laboratories, Center for Devices and Radiological Health, Food and Drug Administration, Silver Spring, USA
{rongping.zeng,subok.park,kyle.myers}@fda.hhs.gov
[2] Department of Radiology, The University of Pennsylvania, Philadelphia, USA
Predrag.Bakic@uphs.upenn.edu

Abstract. There exist various reconstruction algorithms for digital breast tomosynthesis (DBT). However, when optimizing the data acquisition parameters for better image quality in terms of a specific task, researchers usually pick one of their favorite or available reconstruction algorithms. It is unclear whether using a different reconstruction algorithm would yield a different conclusion in the system optimization, thereby yielding a different optimized acquisition configuration. We look into this problem through simulation and present our preliminary results in this report.

Keywords: Digital Breast Tomosynthesis, Reconstruction Algorithms, System Optimization.

1 Introduction

In DBT, the x-ray tube travels over a limited angular range and radiates the object at a certain number of locations along its trajectory to generate multiple projection views. The reconstruction algorithms then take the projection views and reconstruct a 3D volume of the scanned object. Such reconstructed 3D volumes can help reveal the structures that are usually overlapped in traditional 2-view mammographic images, potentially leading to improved decisions on breast cancer malignancy [1, 2]. Different from traditional CT, projection views in DBT are collected within a limited angular span. They are insufficient for volume reconstruction. It is necessary to optimize the system geometry, such as the angular span, angular sampling and x-ray exposure, for improved image quality.

Research has been conducted to investigate the problem of optimizing data acquisition parameters for DBT. Although there exist various reconstruction algorithms for DBT, researchers usually pick one of their favorite or available reconstruction methods when trying to optimize the data acquisition parameters, such as in the studies using the filtered back projection (FBP) method [3], the maximum-likelihood (ML) method [4] or the simultaneous algebraic reconstruction technique (SART) [5].

A.D.A. Maidment, P.R. Bakic, and S. Gavenonis (Eds.): IWDM 2012, LNCS 7361, pp. 346–353, 2012.

While the data acquisition condition determines how much information is collected about the object, the different reconstruction methods likely provide reconstructed DBT volumes with different properties. Therefore a natural question arises on the optimization of the DBT scanning geometry: will the use of different reconstruction algorithms yield very different outcomes?

In this work, we present our initial attempt to address this question using images generated through a simulated DBT system. The simulation includes modeling the DBT system data acquisition process, utilizing realistic breast phantoms, applying various image reconstruction algorithms including FBP and iterative methods, and performing a task-based image-quality evaluation with model observers. The method and results are described in the following report.

2   Methods

2.1   System Simulation

The simulated DBT system had an ideal detector and a point x-ray source traveling along an arc trajectory. The distance from the x-ray source to the detector was 65 cm and the rotation center of the x-ray tube was located 4.5 cm above the detector. The detector element size was 500 x 500 μm^2 and the detector was large enough to cover the projections of the object from all the angles within the angular spans simulated in this work. The photon scatter was ignored in the simulated x-ray transport process. Only quantum noise was considered, with a uniform photon flux of $3x10^4$ counts and 20 keV energy across the detector elements.

To simulate the breast, we used the Bakic voxelized breast phantom software [6] to generate a set of digital breast phantoms of 500 µm resolution along each of the three dimensions. Specifically, we set the breast phantoms to be of cup size B, compressed thickness of 5 cm and glandular density of 25%. With these parameter values, the software created a set of 3D breast phantoms of 409x130x103 voxels with random tissue structures. We assigned the glandular and adipose tissues to have attenuations of 0.0802 /mm and 0.0456 /mm, respectively, according to the values measured at 20 keV in [7]. To simulate lesion-present breasts, we embedded six oblate spheroids in the digital breast phantoms. The spheroids had a major axis of 8 mm and a minor axis of 4 mm. They were all located in the center plane of the object, about 26 mm above the detector. The six lesions were well separated from each other in that plane. Figure 1a shows an example image of the middle plane of a lesion-present breast phantom.

To generate projection views, we used the forward projector developed by Long et al [8], the MATLAB implementation of which is available in the online reconstruction package: http://web.eecs.umich.edu/~fessler/code/index.html. For reconstruction, we set the slice interval to be 2 mm and the in-slice resolution to be 500 µm, the same as that of the breast phantom. Details of the reconstruction methods are described next.

2.2   Reconstruction Algorithms

The purpose of this work is to evaluate the effect of different reconstruction algorithms on system optimization. We picked four types of reconstruction algorithms for this purpose: the filtered back projection (FBP)[9], the simultaneous algebraic reconstruction technique (SART) [10], the maximum-likelihood (ML) method [9, 10]and the total-variation regularized least-square reconstruction method (TVLS) [10, 11]. The first three are extensions of reconstruction algorithms for conventional full-view computed tomography. They have been applied to tomosynthesis since the origination of such systems. While FBP is an analytical reconstruction method, the other three are iterative reconstruction methods. SART finds a solution to a group of linear equations associated with the integrals of attenuation along the rays received at the detector elements. It aims to purely match the data without considering the noise in the measured data. ML is a statistical reconstruction method. It estimates the image by maximizing a likelihood function of the data under an assumed probability density function. The TVLS, on the other hand, attempts to find a solution that minimizes a cost function containing a disagreement measure between the estimate and the data and a total-variation based smoothness constraint function on the estimate. We chose to include these four types of reconstruction algorithms because we believe together they are fairly representative of the categories of methods that are currently actively applied to the DBT systems.

Each of the reconstruction algorithms has its tunable parameters. To limit the reconstruction space, we fixed the parameters so that the computation was efficient and the reconstructed images had reasonably good image quality. The image quality we considered in this work was lesion detectability using a Channelized Hotelling model observer (CHO), which will be described in Section 2.3.

For FBP, the ramp filter is usually modified to have smooth roll-offs at the high-frequency ends by multiplying with a window function. There are various choices on the window function that can result in different tradeoffs between the image resolution and noise level. However, due to the linearity of the filtering process, the various window functions may not significantly affect the lesion detectability of a Hotelling (optimal linear) model observer [12]. Therefore we selected a commonly-used Hann filter for the FBP reconstruction.

For the other three types of iterative algorithms, the step size and the total number of iterations need to be determined. Step size usually affects the convergence rate of the cost function. To achieve a fast convergence speed, we manually tuned the step size to be as large as possible, while still keeping the optimization process stable and hence able to reach an optimal solution. Usually an iterative process terminates when the cost function starts to converge. However, due to the limited number of views and the measurement noise, we note that iterating until a full convergence may not yield pleasing final images. Since we considered lesion detectability to be the image quality metric, we picked the number of iterations for each algorithm to have approximately the best lesion detectability in an ensemble of breast phantoms. Specifically, we generated a small set of breast phantoms, with half of them containing lesions, and passed them into the simulated DBT system; we then reconstructed and saved the DBT volumes at each iteration from the 1st up to the 12th iteration; afterward, we estimated and compared the lesion detectability of the DBT volumes obtained at each iteration to find the optimal iteration number for each iterative reconstruction algorithm.

Besides the step size and the number of iterations, the TVLS algorithm has another special parameters that controls the trade-off between the data agreement term and the regularization term. We did not optimize the trade-off parameter. Instead, we selected two parameter values, one having stronger regularization and one milder regularization, which we will call TVLS-strong and TVLS-mild, respectively.

To summarize, five reconstruction algorithms were evaluated in this work, namely, FBP, SART, ML, TVLS-strong and TVLS-mild.

2.3   Image Quality Assessment

To assess image quality, we considered the task of detecting lesions that were embedded in digital breast phantoms, i.e., a binary decision problem of discriminating whether an image contains a certain signal. We used a channelized Hotelling model observer (CHO) to detect the lesions. The detectability signal-to-noise ratio (SNR) was considered to be the figure of merit.

The CHO builds upon the Hotelling model observer [13]. It works as follows. Given a reconstructed image f, the CHO calculates the decision variable as the matrix product of the channelized signal template s_u, the inverse of the noise covariance K_{f_u} and the channelized image f_u as follows,

$$t = s_u^T K_{f_u}^{-1} f_u, \tag{1}$$

where the $(.)_u$ indicates a channelization is applied to the variable. The purpose of channelization is to reduce the data dimensionality while maintaining the observer's ability to extract useful information from the data. By comparing the value of t to a certain threshold value, the observer determines whether the image contains a lesion or not. Therefore, the better the distributions of t are separated under the signal-present and signal-absent cases, the more likely the CHO arrives at a correct decision. This separability can be quantified by the signal to noise ratio (SNR) of t, as defined below in Eq. (2), to summarize the lesion-detection based image quality:

$$SNR_t = |\bar{t}_1 - \bar{t}_0| / \sqrt{(\sigma_1^2 + \sigma_0^2)/2}, \tag{2}$$

where $\bar{t}_1$ and $\bar{t}_0$ are the means, and σ_1^2 and σ_0^2 are the variances of the decision variable t in the lesion-present (subscript of 1) and lesion-absent (subscript of 0) cases, respectively.

The Laguerre-Gauss (LG) functions were used as the channel functions [14] as they are efficient to describe rotationally symmetric functions, such as a Hotelling template estimated using stationary backgrounds and rotationally symmetric signals. As the signal diameter was about 8 mm, we set the width of the LG functions to be 4 mm and utilized 12 channels. The CHO was applied to a set of 2D subimages (31x31 pixels) that surrounded the expected lesion location at the focal slice of the lesion. The lesion-present subimages were cropped from the lesion-present DBT volume and the lesion-absent subimages from the lesion-absent DBT volumes. Among the extracted subimages, a subset of them was used to train the observer (i.e., estimate the covariance) and the rest was used as a testing set to estimate the SNR_t. Because the background structure was not uniform, the signal templates were obtained by subtracting the reconstructed lesion-absent from the lesion-present mean background DBT images, where the mean background was an average over multiple breast phantoms.

With the image quality as defined above, we may investigate the effect of reconstruction methods on ranking system acquisition parameters. Suppose we are trying to optimize the angular span for lesion detectability; we may simulate projection data across a set of angular span with a fixed number of views. Each set of projection data is reconstructed by each of the selected reconstruction algorithms. For each reconstruction algorithm, the system acquisition parameters can be ranked based on the image quality of the reconstructed volumes. If the rankings agree despite the use of different reconstruction algorithms, we may be able to conclude that optimization of the system acquisition parameters are not sensitive to the reconstruction algorithms; otherwise, the findings of optimal data acquisition parameters would be expected to vary based on the reconstruction algorithm being used in the DBT system.

3   Results and Discussion

To determine the optimal number of iterations for each iterative algorithm, we used 30 lesion-present and 30 lesion-absent breast phantoms. For each of the 30 lesion-present breast phantoms, six lesions were inserted in the middle of the breast phantoms. Nine views and a $50°$ angular span were used as the system acquisition parameters to generate the projection views. Figure 1 shows the slice of one digital breast phantom that contains the lesion centers, along with its DBT slices reconstructed using the aforementioned reconstruction algorithms. Figure 2 shows the curves of lesion detectability vs. the iteration number. Based on those curves, we determined the total numbers of iterations to be 1 for SART and 5 for ML, TVLS-strong and TVLS-mild.

With the reconstruction parameters having been determined, we then examined the effect of the reconstruction algorithms on the optimization of angular span in the DBT system. For this purpose, we generated another set of 80 breast phantoms. Lesions of the same size and shape were inserted into 40 of breasts at the same locations. We fixed the number of views at 9 but varied the angular span from 10 to 60 degrees to generate projection views. The lesion detectability SNR of the reconstructed DBT volumes was estimated using the method described in Sect 2.2. Figure 3 shows the curves of lesion detectability vs. angular span for the five reconstruction algorithms. It can be seen that the curves present similar trends: lesion detectability increases as the scan angle increases, reaches a peak at the 50 degree span and drops afterward. The consistent trends among reconstruction algorithms suggest that the DBT system optimization may not be very sensitive to the reconstruction algorithm being used.

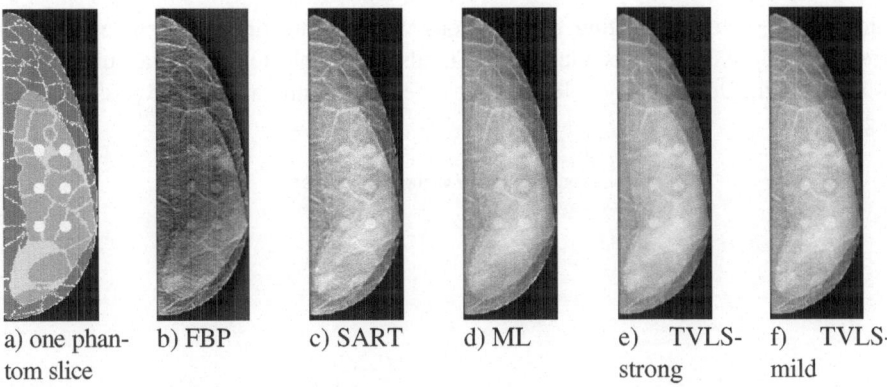

a) one phan-   b) FBP   c) SART   d) ML   e)   TVLS-   f)   TVLS-
tom slice   strong   mild

Fig. 1. a) One slice of a 3D breast phantom that contain the spherical lesion centers and the corresponding DBT slices reconstructed using b) FBP, c) SART, d) ML e) TVLS-strong and f) TVLS-mild from 9 noisy projection views in a 50 degree angular span. The window level of the FBP slice is [-0.2 0.6] and the window level for the other four is [0 0.8].

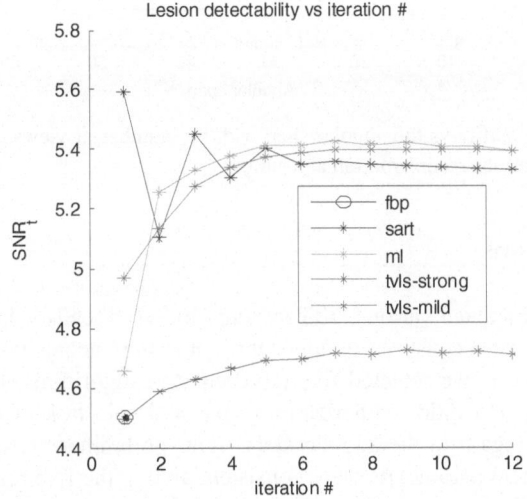

Fig. 2. Lesion detectability vs iteration number of the reconstruction algorithms at the acquisition of 9 views within 50 degrees. FBP is an analytical method, so there is only one iteration. SART has the best performance at the 1st iteration; the other three reach their optimum at about the 5th iteration.

The major goal of this work is to evaluate how the reconstruction algorithm may affect DBT system optimization. The preliminary results reported in this paper show that the choice of which algorithm to use may not be critical for optimizing the angular span. Future work is needed to see how the other acquisition parameters may be affected by the reconstruction algorithms. As the simulated scenario in this work was limited to a detection task of a simple-shaped lesion, further evaluation based on other tasks, such as detecting calcifications or discriminating between regular and irregular shapes, will be conducted. It is also desirable to include an uncertainty estimate on the detectability SNR in order to test the significance of the possible findings.

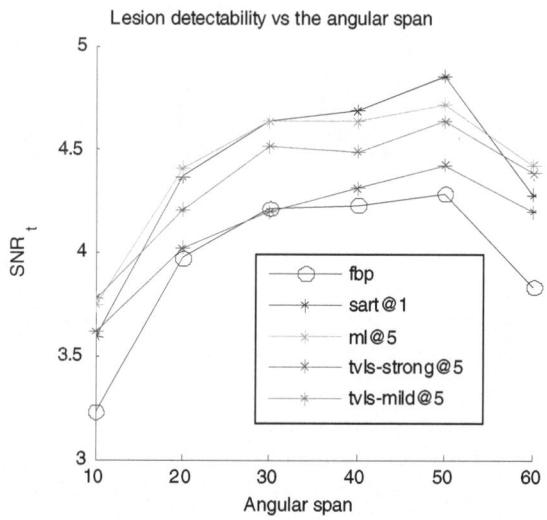

Fig. 3. Lesion detectability vs the angular span with the number of views of 9. The trends are similar among the various reconstruction algorithms.

4   Conclusions

In this work, we simulated various DBT systems and used realistic breast phantoms to examine the effect of reconstruction algorithm on system acquisition parameter optimization. Specifically, we selected five representative algorithms (FBP, SART, ML, TVLS with strong and mild regularizations) and a simple task of optimizing lesion detectability with regard to the angular span. Our preliminary results show that the ranking of the system parameters were consistent among the five reconstruction algorithms. This suggests that optimizing the system acquisition parameters, in particular angular span, may not be sensitive to the reconstruction algorithm for the detection of simple spherical lesions. However, a particular reconstruction algorithm may be preferred based on other factors like the computation time and memory requirements. Future work on validating this finding on a larger optimization space, a larger phantom set and for other clinically relevant tasks will be conducted. It will also be interesting to investigate how the ranking may change with a 3D model observer which incorporates 3D spatial correlation using multiple reconstruction slices, or when directly using the projection data rather than the reconstructed images in the image quality assessment stage.

Acknowledgement. The authors would like to thank Stefano Young's support for creating and sharing the breast phantoms for this work.

References

1. Andersson, I., et al.: Breast tomosynthesis and digital mammography: a comparison of breast cancer visibility and BIRADS classification in a population of cancers with subtle mammographic findings. European Radiology 18, 2817–2825 (2008)
2. Gur, D., et al.: Digital Breast Tomosynthesis: Observer Performance Study. American Journal of Roentgenology 193, 586–591 (2009)
3. Richard, S., Samei, E.: Quantitative imaging in breast tomosynthesis and CT: Comparison of detection and estimation task performance. Medical Physics 37, 2627–2637 (2010)
4. Reiser, I., Nishikawa, R.M.: Task-based assessment of breast tomosynthesis: Effect of acquisition parameters and quantum noise. Medical Physics 37, 1591–1600 (2010)
5. Zhang, Y., Chan, H.-P., Goodsitt, M.M., Schmitz, A., Eberhard, J.W., Claus, B.E.H.: Investigation of Different PV Distributions in Digital Breast Tomosynthesis (DBT) Mammography. In: Krupinski, E.A. (ed.) IWDM 2008. LNCS, vol. 5116, pp. 593–600. Springer, Heidelberg (2008)
6. Bakic, P.R., et al.: Development and characterization of an anthropomorphic breast software phantom based upon region-growing algorithm. Medical Physics 38, 3165–3176 (2011)
7. Johns, P.C., Yaffe, M.J.: X-ray characterisation of normal and neoplastic breast tissues. Physics in Medicine and Biology 32, 675 (1987)
8. Long, Y., et al.: 3D Forward and Back-Projection for X-Ray CT Using Separable Footprints. IEEE Transactions on Medical Imaging 29, 1839–1850 (2010)
9. Wu, T., et al.: A comparison of reconstruction algorithms for breast tomosynthesis. Medical Physics 31, 2636–2647 (2004)
10. Zhang, Y., et al.: A comparative study of limited-angle cone-beam reconstruction methods for breast tomosynthesis. Medical Physics 33, 3781–3795 (2006)
11. Sidky, E.Y., et al.: Enhanced imaging of microcalcifications in digital breast tomosynthesis through improved image-reconstruction algorithms. Medical Physics 36, 4920–4932 (2009)
12. Abbey, K., Barrett, H.H.: Human- and model-observer performance in ramp-spectrum noise: effects of regularization and object variability. J. Opt. Soc. Am. A 18, 473–488 (2001)
13. Barrett, H.H., Myers, K.J.: Foundations of Image Science. Wiley Interscience, New Jersey (2004)
14. Gallas, B.D., Barrett, H.H.: Validating the use of channels to estimate the ideal linear observer. J. Opt. Soc. Am. A 20, 1725–1738 (2003)

Usefulness of Adjunction of Digital Breast Tomosynthesis (DBT) to Full-Field Digital Mammography (FFDM) in Evaluation of Pathological Response after Neoadjuvant Chemotherapy (NAC) for Breast Cancer

Nachiko Uchiyama[1], Takayuki Kinoshita[2], Takashi Hojo[2], Sota Asaga[2],
Junko Suzuki[2], Yoko Kawawa[3], and Kyoichi Otsuka[4]

[1] Research Center for Cancer Prevention and Screening, National Cancer Center, Tokyo, Japan
nuchiyam@ncc.go.jp
[2] Department of Breast Surgery, National Cancer Center, Tokyo, Japan
{Takinosh,tahojo,soasaga,jusuzuki}@ncc.go.jp
[3] Department of Radiology, National Cancer Center, Tokyo, Japan
ykawawa@ncc.go.jp
[4] Siemens Japan K.K., Tokyo, Japan
Kyoichi.otsuka@siemens.com

Abstract. We assessed the radiological findings and capability of DBT in adjunction to FFDM to predict response to NAC in comparison with other diagnostic modalities. 25 women (ages 29-73, mean age, 53.0 years old) having 26
lesions were recruited for this study and gave informed consent. In accordance with   this preliminary study, the adjunction of DBT to FFDM combined
with other diagnostic modalities will contribute to more accurate assessment of
pathological response to NAC.

Keywords: Digital Mammography, Tomosyntthesis, Neoadjuvant Chemotherapy, DBT, US, FFDM.

1   Introduction

Neoadjuvant chemotherapy (NAC) is performed to reduce tumor size prior to surgery
in women with breast cancer. The imaging methods that have been used until now to
assess tumor response to neoadjuvant chemotherapy have serious limitations; for
example, mammography alone cannot identify mass lesions in very dense breasts or
distinguish viable residual lesions from the surrounding fibrous reaction after NAC
[1]-[8]. Digital breast tomosynthesis has been only recently applied clinically. The
diagnostic advantages in comparison to mammography have been reported on, including the fact that the slice images can be evaluated because tomosynthesis decreases
the overlap in breast tissue [9]-[14]. In this study, we assessed the radiological findings and capability of DBT in adjunction to FFDM to predict response to NAC in
comparison with other diagnostic modalities.

A.D.A. Maidment, P.R. Bakic, and S. Gavenonis (Eds.): IWDM 2012, LNCS 7361, pp. 354–361, 2012.

2   Materials and Methods

This study was approved by the IRB at our institute. 25 women (ages 29-73, mean age, 53.0 years old) having 26 lesions were recruited for this study and gave informed consent. Images utilizing adjunction of DBT to FFDM were taken for diagnosis from December, 2009 to October, 2011. Pathological diagnosis was confirmed by Core Needle Biopsy (CNB) and the pathological subtypes were Invasive Ductal Carcinoma (n=20), Invasive Lobular Carcinoma (n=3), Invasive Micropapillary Carcinoma (n=2), and Mucinous Carcinoma (n=1). The diagnostic procedures were performed within one month prior to surgery. For each patient, MMG and US were both performed on the same day, but not always in the order and were evaluated independently. Examination utilizing other modalitieswere carried out later.

Contrast-enhanced MRI was performed on 15 patients, and contrast-enhanced CT was performed on 10 patients both before NAC and after NAC. Imaging utilizing adjunction of DBT to FFDM was performed before and after NAC in 10 out of 25 cases. In 15 out of 25 cases, imaging utilizing adjunction of DBT to FFDM was performed only after NAC. Whole-breast US was performed with an 8 MHz wide-band high-resolution transducer (aplio^{TM} XV, Toshiba Medical Systems, Japan). Transverse and longitudinal scans were acquired. Breast MRI was performed with a 3-Tesla system (Magnetom Trio, Siemens, Germany).Patients were studied in the prone position with a dedicated breast surface coil. The entire breast was imaged once before and four times after intravenous injection of 0.1mmol of Gd-DTPA/Kg of body weight (Magnevist; Schering, Germany). The post-processing procedures included digital image subtraction, Maximum Intensity Projection (MIP) and Multiplanar Reconstruction (MPR) by slices of 3mm thickness. Breast CT was performed with multi-detector raw CT (MDCT) (Aquilion64, Toshiba Medical Systems, Japan). The images were acquired before injection of an iodine contrast medium, and 60 seconds after, and 3 minutes after injection of the total amount of 100ml, at the rate of 3ml/second (Iopamidol 300, Bayer AG, Germany). The images were reconstructed as slices of 2mm thickness and evaluated.

With regard to DBT and FFDM, clinical image data were acquired by an a-Se FFDM system with a spatial resolution of 85μm (MAMMOMAT Inspiration, Siemens, Germany).Two-view DBT was performed with the same compression angle and compression pressure as the FFDM. With one-view DBT, the radiation dose was 1.5 times compared to one-view FFDM. The radiation dose with ACR 156 was 1.2mGy with FFDM. FFDM and reconstructed 1mm slice images from DBT were reviewed at a dedicated workstation.

The author and the other five co-authors (two radiologists and four breast surgeons) each have over ten years' experience in reading mammograms. In addition, to read screening mammograms in our country, it is necessary to get a certificate from the committee on quality control of mammographic screening by taking a qualifying examination and the certificate must be renewed every five years. The author and the other five co-authors all passed the qualifying examination with A rank results. All the examination scores were over 90% in sensitivity and over 92% in specificity. In addition, the two radiologists and four breast surgeons are experienced not only with regard to mammography, but also with regard to US, MRI, and CT.

The clinical response to chemotherapy was classified into the following categories, based on the "response evaluation criteria in solid tumors" (RECIST), using the measurements obtained with the different imaging methods: 1) Complete Response (CR): no clinical evidence of residual tumor, 2) Partial Response (PR): reduction in size of the tumor by more than 30%; 3) Non-Responders : a: Stable disease (SD): reduction in size of the tumor by less than 30%, 4) Progressive disease (PD): increase in size of tumor or presence of new lesions. Pathological response to chemotherapy was classified into four categories: Grade 0 (No Response), Grade 1(Slight Response), Grade 2 (Fair Response), and Grade 3 (Complete Response) [15]. The clinical stages of the patients before NAC were II or III. All patients underwent surgery based on their response to NAC and residual tumor size estimated by diagnostic imaging was compared with the residual tumor size determined by surgical pathology.

3   Results

Pathological responses of the lesions to NAC were Grade 0 (n=1), Grade 1 or Grade 2 (n=21), and Grade 3 (n=4).MMG findings of pathological Grade 3 were microcalcifications only (n=1), scar only (n=1), and microcalcifications with reduced mass lesion (n=2). Two out of four (50.0%) lesions demonstrated CR, and two out of four lesions demonstrated PR (50.0%). Regarding the Grades 1-2 cases, lesions were diagnosed as reduced mass with or without microcalcifications (n=19) demonstrated   PR (19/21, 90.5%) and 2 lesions diagnosed as only distortion or scar demonstrated CR (2/21, 9.5%). Regarding the Grade 0 case, the lesion detected as an enlarged mass (n=1) was diagnosed as PD (1/1, 100.0%). Adjunction of DBT to FFDM findings of pathological Grade 3 were microcalcifications only (n=1), Scar only (n=1), and microcalcifications with scar without any density (n=2) that suggest CR (Fig.1). Regarding pathological Grades 1-2, the lesions were detected as reduced masses with or without microcalcifications (n=20) that suggested 20 cases were PR (20/21, 95.2%), and 1 case of only distortion or scar (n=1) that suggested CR (1/21, 4.8%). Regarding the Grade 0 case, the lesion was detected as an enlarged mass (n=1) that suggested PD (1/1, 100.0%). US findings of pathological Grade 3 (n=4) were diagnosed as CR (n=2, 50.0%), SD (n=1, 25.0%) and PR (n=1, 25.0%).

US findings of pathological Grades 1-2 (n=21) were diagnosed as PR (n=17, 81.0%), SD (n=3, 14.3%) and CR (n=1, 4.8%). In the case of US findings of pathological Grade 0 (n=1), the lesion was diagnosed as PD (n=1, 100.0%).

MRI (n=15) findings of pathological Grade 3 (3 lesions) were diagnosed as CR (n=2, 66.7%) and PR (n=1, 33.3%). MRI (n=15) findings of pathological Grades 1-2

(11 lesions) were diagnosed as PR (n=10, 90.5%) and CR (n=1, 9.5%). In the case of MRI findings of Grade 0(n=1), the lesion was diagnosed as PD (n=1, 100.0%).

CT (10 cases with 11 lesions) findings of pathological Grade 3 (n=1) were diagnosed as CR (n=1, 100.0%). CT findings of pathological Grades 1-2 (n=10) were diagnosed as PR (n=10, 100.0%).

MMG only resulted in two under-diagnosed lesions (2/26, 7.7%) and two over-diagnosed lesions (2/26, 7.7%).US resulted in one under-diagnosed lesion (1/26, 3.8%) and five over-diagnosed lesions (5/26, 19.2%). MRI resulted in one under-diagnosed lesion (1/15, 6.7%) and one over-diagnosed lesion (1/15, 6.7%). Compared to MMG, US showed no statistically significant difference (P>0.08), while CT, MRI and adjunction of DBT to FFDM showed statistically significant differences; 0.02, 0.04 and 0.04, respectively (Table1).

Table 1. Comparison of NAC Response by Diagnostic Evaluation and Pathological Evaluation

*Pathological Response	MMG (n=26)	US (n=26)	CT (n=11)	MRI (n=15)	*** DBTFFDM (n=26)
Grade 0	PD: 1/1	PD: 1/1		PD: 1/1	PD: 1/1
	100.0%	100.0%		100.0%	100.0%
Grades 1-2	PR: 19/21	PR: 17/21	PR: 10/10	PR: 10 /11	PR: 20/21
	90.5%	81.0%	100.0%	90.9%	95.2%
	CR: 2/21	SD: 3/21		CR: 1/11	CR: 1/21
	9.5%	14.3%		9.1%	4.8%
		CR: 1/21			
		4.80%			
Grade3	CR: 2/4	CR: 2/4	CR: 1/1	CR: 2/3	CR: 4/4
	50.0%	50.0%	100.0%	66.7%	100.0%
	PR: 2/4	PR: 1/4		PR: 1/3	
	50.0%	25.0%		33.3%	
		SD: 1/4			
		25.0%			
		**P=0.08	P=0.02	P=0.04	P=0.04

* The clinical response to chemotherapy was classified in accordance with RECIST
Analyzed by t-Test   * DBTFFDM: Adjunction of DBT to FFDM

4   Discussion

Accurate evaluation of tumor response to NAC is necessary for optimization of preoperative planning. MRI and CT have recently developed the potential to assist the other traditional imaging methods in the evaluation of response to NAC [4]-[8]. By mammography, it is difficult to identify a mass lesion in dense breasts or to distinguish a viable lesion from a fibrous reaction owing to NAC. Using US only can result in over-diagnosis of chemotherapy-induced fibrosis, because in the case of a hypo-echoic lesion, it is difficult to differentiate between a fibrotic change induced by neoplastic change and a reduction in the tumor by NAC. In addition, it is difficult to measure by hand-held probe the overview of a large mass lesion or multi-centric lesions, such as locally advanced tumors that could be treated by NAC (Fig.1).

On the other hand, adjunction of DBT to FFDM has potential diagnostic advantages. In accordance with our study, compared to FFDM only, adjunction of DBT to FFDM can evaluate the inside of and the outline of the lesion. Compared to US, adjunction of DBT to FFDM can evaluate the overview of the lesion objectively.

Accurate evaluation of tumor response to the pharmacological treatment is fundamental for optimal surgical planning. CE-MRI and CE-CT have recently developed the potential to assist the other traditional imaging methods in the evaluation of response to chemotherapy. These are able to discriminate between neoplastic and fibrotic tissue, based on the rate of contrast media enhancement. In addition, the higher sensitivity of MRI can detect non-invasive lesions as enhanced lesions that can be over-diagnosed as residual invasive components (Fig.2). According to our study, compared to CE-CT or CE-MRI, with adjunction of DBT to FFDM, it is possible to correlate the macroscopic evaluation with the pathological diagnosis without utilizing a contrast medium.

The combination of adjunction of DBT to FFDM with other diagnostic modalities will contribute to improved diagnostic accuracy with regard to NAC response to locally advanced breast cancer. According to our preliminary results, adjunction of DBT to FFDM could have a possibility for alternative diagnostic procedure of CE-CT and CE-MRI.

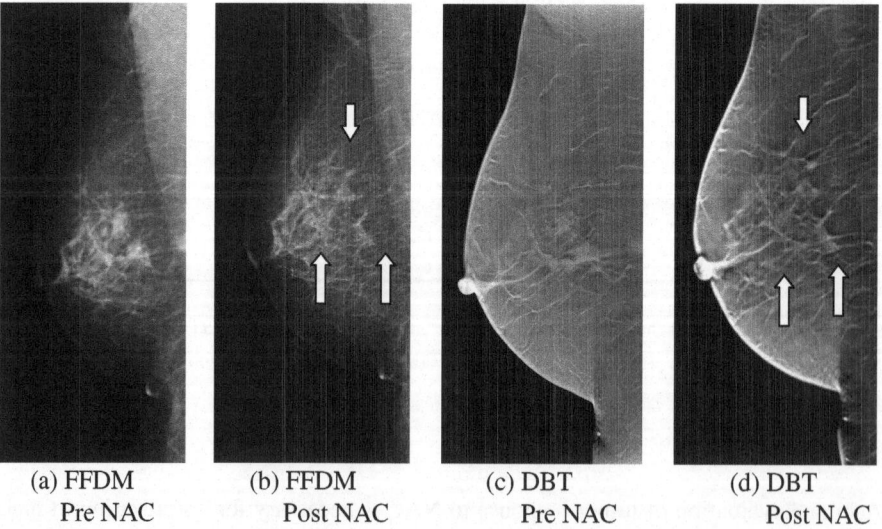

(a) FFDM	(b) FFDM	(c) DBT	(d) DBT
Pre NAC	Post NAC	Pre NAC	Post NAC

Fig. 1. (Grade 1 Case) FFDM (Fig.1a-b) showed reduced masses after NAC (white arrow). DBT (Fig.1c-d) showed reduced masses with scar with partial density inside of the corresponding lesion after NAC (white arrow).

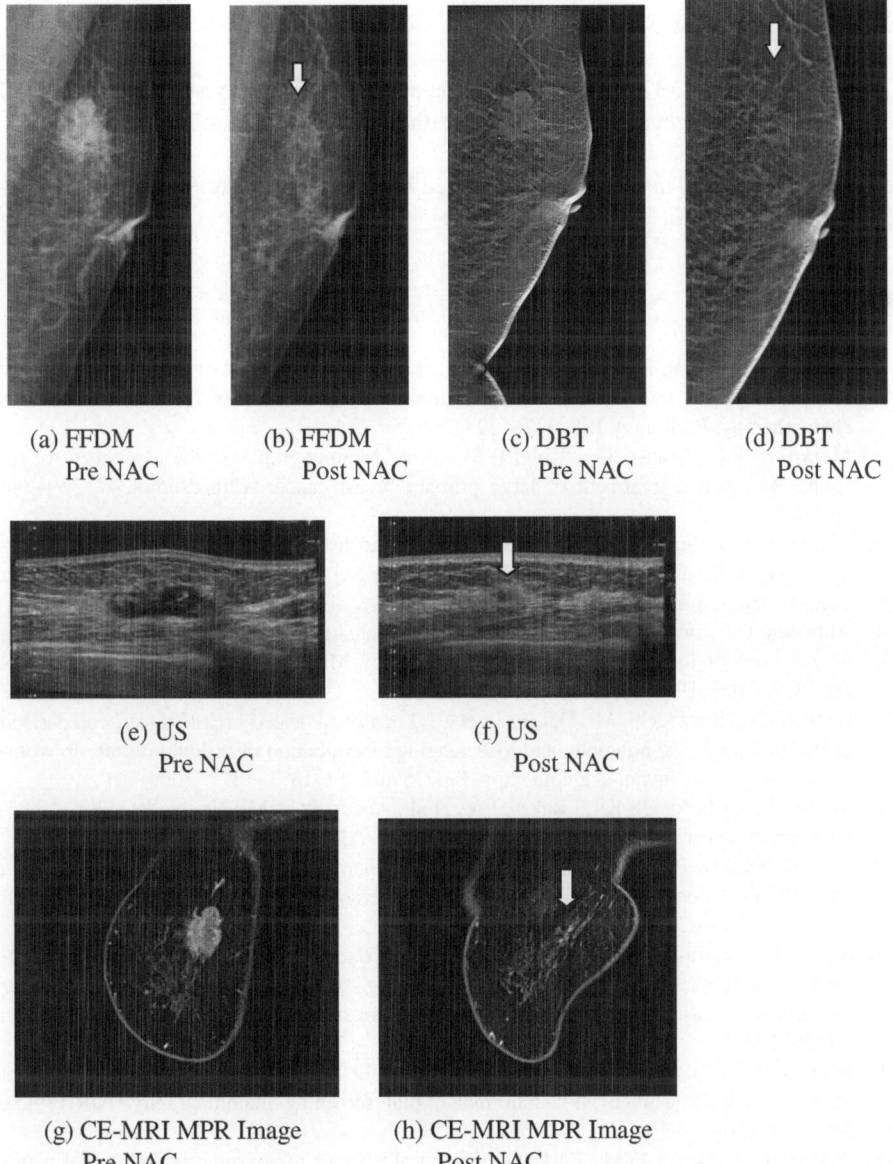

(a) FFDM   (b) FFDM   (c) DBT   (d) DBT
Pre NAC   Post NAC   Pre NAC   Post NAC

(e) US   (f) US
Pre NAC   Post NAC

(g) CE-MRI MPR Image   (h) CE-MRI MPR Image
Pre NAC   Post NAC

Fig. 2. (Pathological Grade 3 Case) FFDM (Fig.2a-b) demonstrated a reduced mass with microcalcifications after NAC (white arrow). DBT (Fig.2c-d) demonstrated microcalcifications with scar without core density inside of the corresponding lesion after NAC (white arrow). US (Fig.2e-f) demonstrated a reduced hypo-echoic mass as a suspicious residual lesion after NAC (white arrow). The coronal image of CE-MRI (Fig.2g-h) demonstrated small enhanced nodules as a suspicious residual lesion after NAC (white arrow). Pathological diagnosis demonstrated residual DCIS corresponding to the enhanced lesions by CE-MRI.

5   Conclusion

The adjunction of DBT to FFDM combined with other diagnostic modalities will contribute to more accurate assessment of pathological response to NAC.

Acknowledgment. This study was supported by Grant-in-Aid for Scientific Research (C) (No. 23591810) in Japan.

References

1. Helvie, M.A., Joynt, L.K., Cody, R.L., et al.: Locally advanced breast carcinoma: accuracy of mammography versus clinical examination in the prediction of residual disease after chemotherapy. Radiology 198, 327–332 (1996)
2. Moskovic, E.C., Mansi, J.L., King, D.M., et al.: Mammography in the assessment of response to medical treatment of large primary breast cancer. Clin. Radiol. 47, 339–344 (1993)
3. Keune, J.D., Jeffe, D.B., Schootman, M., et al.: Accuracy of Ultrasonography and Mammography in Predicting Pathologic Response after Neoadjuvant Chemotherapy for Breast Cancer. Am. J. Surg. 199(4), 477–484 (2010)
4. Abraham, D.C., Jones, R.C., Jones, S.E., et al.: Evaluation of neoadjuvant chemotherapeutic response of locally advanced breast cancer by Magnetic Resonance Imaging. Cancer 78, 91–100 (1996)
5. Londero, V., Bazzocchi, M., Del, F.C., et al.: Locally advanced breast cancer: comparison of mammography, sonography and MR imaging in evaluation of residual disease in women receiving neoadjuvant chemotherapy. Eur. Radiol. 14, 1371–1379 (2004)
6. Rosen, E.L., Blackwell, K.L., Baker, J.A., et al.: Accuracy of MRI in the detection of residual breast cancer after neoadjuvant chemotherapy. AJR 181, 1275–1282 (2003)
7. Yeh, E., Slanetz, P., Kopans, D.: Prospective Comparison of Mammography, Sonography, and MRI in Patients Undergoing Neoadjuvant Chemotherapy for Palpable Breast Cancer. A J R 184, 868–877 (2005)
8. Shien, T., Akashi-Tanaka, S., Yoshid, M., et al.: Usefulness of preoperative multidetector-row computed tomography in evaluating the extent of invasive lobular carcinoma in patients with or without neoadjuvant chemotherapy. Breast Cancer 16(1), 30–36 (2009)
9. Poplack, S.P., Tosteson, T.D., Koge, L.C.A., et al.: Digital breast tomosynthesis: initial experience in 98 women with abnormal digital screening mammography. AJR 189(3), 616–623 (2007)
10. Andersson, I., Ikeda, D.M., Zackrisson, S., et al.: Breast tomosynthesis and digital mammography: a comparison of breast cancer visibility and BIRADS classification in a population of cancers with subtle mammographic findings. Eur. Radiol. 18(12), 2817–2825 (2008)
11. Good, W.F., Abrams, G.S., Catullo, V.J., et al.: Digital breast tomosynthesis: a pilot observer study. AJR 190(4), 865–869 (2008)
12. Gennaro, G., Toledano, A., di Maggio, C., et al.: Digital breast tomosynthesis versus digital mammography: a clinical performance study. Eur. Radiol. 20(7), 1545–1553 (2010)

13. Uchiyama, N., Kinoshita, T., Akashi, S., et al.: Diagnostic Performance of Combined Full Field Digital Mammography (FFDM) and Digital Breast Tomosynthesis (DBT) in comparison with Full Field Digital Mammography (FFDM). In: CARS 2011, pp. 32–33. Springer (2011)

14. Förnvik, D., Zackrisson, S., Ljungberg, O., et al.: Breast tomosynthesis: Accuracy of tumor measurement compared with digital mammography and ultrasonography. Acta. Radiol. 51(3), 240–247 (2010)

15. Therasse, P., Arbuck, S.G., Eisenhauer, E.A., et al.: New Guidelines to evaluate the response to treatment in solid tumors. JNCI 92, 205–216 (2000)

The Morphology of Microcalcifications in 2D Digital Mammography and Breast Tomosynthesis: Is It Different?

Eman Shaheen[1,*], Chantal Van Ongeval[1], Federica Zanca[1], Lesley Cockmartin[1],
Nicholas Marshall[1], Frederik De Keyzer[1], Kenneth C. Young[2,3],
David R. Dance[2,3], and Hilde Bosmans[1]

[1] Department of Radiology, University Hospitals Leuven, Herestraat 49, 3000 Leuven, Belgium
{eman.shaheen,chantal.vanongeval,federica.zanca,
lesley.cockmartin,nicholas.marshall,frederik.dekeyzer,
hilde.bosmans}@uzleuven.be
[2] National Coordinating Centre for the Physics of Mammography,
Royal Surrey County Hospital, Guildford, GU2 7XX, United Kingdom
{ken.young,daviddance}@nhs.net
[3] Department of Physics, Faculty of Engineering and Physical Sciences, University of Surrey,
Guildford, GU2 7XH, UK

Abstract. The development of new 3D imaging systems in the mammographic field is raising questions on its superiority of performance over 2D digital mammography in all aspects. Researchers are currently investigating the performance of digital breast tomosynthesis (DBT) compared to 2D digital mammography in terms of detectability of lesions (masses and microcalcifications) and diagnostic accuracy. Since a morphological description of the shape of microcalcifications is a determining factor for recalling the patient or not, we have investigated the efficiency of DBT in describing the morphology of microcalcifications within clusters compared to digital mammography. Four radiologists participated in the study and have described the shapes of microcalcifications in 71 clusters in 2D images and DBT series that were read in separate blinded sessions. An agreement test based on the kappa statistic was applied to evaluate the consistency of each reader's evaluation in 2D and DBT. An inter-rater variability test was also applied for each modality. Results have shown that there is good agreement between the observers' evaluations in these two modalities. The inter-rater test also revealed good agreement between the observers performance of assessment. In conclusion, this preliminary study has shown that the morphology of microcalcification clusters does not differ substantially in 2D versus DBT.

Keywords: Digital mammography, breast tomosynthesis, microcalcifications, morphology of microcalcifications.

1 Introduction

Digital breast tomosynthesis (DBT) is a newly introduced 3D technology in the world of mammography. One major advantage of DBT systems is the possibility to

A.D.A. Maidment, P.R. Bakic, and S. Gavenonis (Eds.): IWDM 2012, LNCS 7361, pp. 362–368, 2012.
© Springer-Verlag Berlin Heidelberg 2012

overcome the problem of overlapping tissues, a known limitation of 2D planar mammography where normal breast structure could hide pathology of interest. Despite this extra 3D information, it is not yet clear whether DBT could be used in screening, or should be used for diagnostic evaluation only or in high risk women. Gennaro *et al.* [1] and Andersson *et al.* [2] have compared DBT to full-field digital mammography (FFDM) in terms of cancer detection and characterization. They have found that lesion conspicuity increases in DBT compared with FFDM and in [2] even concluded that DBT has a higher specificity for breast cancer detection. Moreover, Spangler *et al.* [3] have found that FFDM was more sensitive and specific than DBT for the detection of microcalcifications.

Microcalcifications are considered a characteristic sign for localization of malignancy [4]. Their morphology is one of the most important characteristics indicating malignancy or benignity [5]. Therefore, it is important for any mammographic system to allow not only detection but also correct categorization of breast microcalcifications since this impacts on the recall rate, an important indicator and performance measure for screening. Whereas most authors agree that DBT might have advantages in detecting and categorizing masses, its value for microcalcifications is not yet determined [2].

The aim of this study was to investigate characterization of microcalcifications, by comparing the morphological description of microcalcifications within clusters between DBT and 2D FFDM in an observer performance study. Whereas most observer studies comparing these two modalities apply a side by side reading, where the observer evaluates each case with the presence of both 2D and tomosynthesis, in our study, we opted to evaluate both techniques in separate, blinded sessions.

2   Materials and Methods

The observer study was performed with a total of 71 microcalcification clusters (cases). Thirty five cases were patients with real microcalcification clusters and 36 were clusters simulated into patient images [6]. Simulated clusters have been used to increase the number of cases. The 3D microcalcification clusters were previously validated for their realistic appearance against real clusters in an observer performance study and the results showed no statistically significant difference between real and simulated clusters of microcalcifications in both 2D FFDM and DBT [6]. The simulation framework ray traced 3D models of microcalcification clusters and adjusted the contrast for the x-ray spectrum that has been used in the patient image into which the calcifications were simulated. Each real microcalcification cluster present in a real breast was imaged in 2D and tomosynthesis using the same system (MAMMOMAT Inspiration TOMO, Siemens AG Healthcare, Erlangen, Germany). For the simulated clusters, the same patient background was also imaged using the same system and the cluster was simulated into the same position in 2D and DBT as described in [6]. All raw projection images were processed: the 2D images were processed using the default image processing software (OpView2, Siemens, Erlangen) and the projection tomosynthesis images were reconstructed using the Siemens software (TomoEngine,

Siemens, Erlangen, Germany) that is based on the Filtered Back-projection algorithm (FBP) [7]. The in-plane resolution of the reconstructed slices was 0.085 mm x 0.085 and the planes were reconstructed with 1 mm inter-slice distance. All patient doses in DBT are approximately double the dose of 2D FFDM, e.g. for a typical breast of thickness 45 mm the dose of one view 2D is 0.83 mGy and 1.79 mGy for one view DBT.

Four radiologists participated in the study. They evaluated the mediolateral (MLO) views of the patient cases using a user friendly software Sara[2] (Qaelum NV, Belgium) on a high resolution 5 megapixel monitor (Barco MDNG5121CB) in our mammography reading room. The radiologists were trained first to read tomosynthesis series containing microcalcifications along with the 2D images from the PACS environment. Afterwards, they had two training sessions one for 2D and one for DBT, to learn the use of the Sara[2] software. In the subsequent observer study, they evaluated the 2D images in separate sessions from the DBT sessions to guarantee an independent reading. As the goal of this study was to evaluate the morphology of the microcalcifications within the clusters and not detectability, each cluster was presented to the observers with a rectangle around it. The cases were presented to the radiologist one by one with the possibility to zoom in/out, change window level settings, toggle on/off the defining rectangle and scroll between planes in the case of DBT series. The radiologists were asked to describe the morphology of the microcalcifications in the cluster using one or more of the following four shapes: round, irregularly round, linear, and amorphous. Fig. 1 shows an example of the reading.

Comparison between the 2D and DBT setups was performed for each of the 4 shape categories (round, irregular round, linear and amorphous) separately using kappa statistics, and the observed agreement as well as the *p-value* were reported. No correction for multiple testing was performed in this preliminary study. Inter-rater agreement was assessed between each pair of the readers again using kappa statistics. A *p-value* of <0.05 was considered to indicate statistical significance.

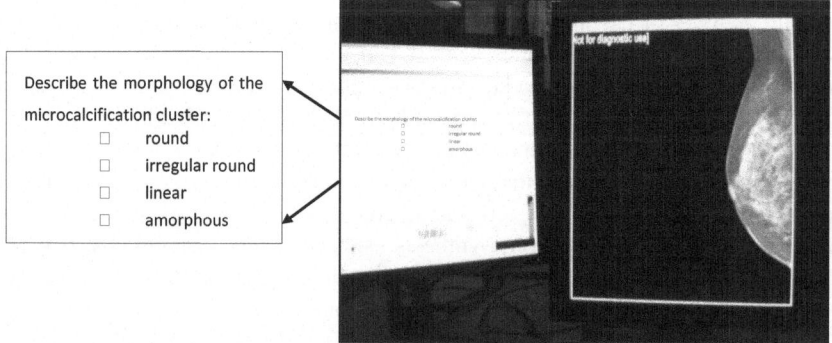

Fig. 1. Example of a reading session

3   Results

Table 1 shows the results of the agreement test based on kappa statistics with the corresponding p-value comparing 2D and DBT. The agreement was reported per shape category and observer. Agreements varied between 0.65 and 0.78 for the round shape, between 0.59 and 0.69 for the irregular round shape, between 0.75 and 0.83 for the linear shape, and between 0.76 and 1 for the amorphous shape. Generally, the agreement between the two modalities in the assessment of morphological description can be considered good, but only limited significance can be found in this limited population size.

Tables 2 and 3 show the results of inter-rater agreement between all observers for both 2D and DBT techniques, respectively. For 2D FFDM, the agreement varied from 0.73 to 0.78 indicating good agreement between readers in the evaluation of the morphological shapes of microcalcification clusters. For DBT, the agreement varied from 0.72 to 0.82 indicating good agreement as well.

Table 1. Agreement according to Kappa statistics and uncorrected *p-values* for comparison between 2D and DBT in terms of morphological description for the different shapes and observers

| Observer | Shape | | | |
| | Round | | irregular round | |
	Agreement	*p-value*	Agreement	*p-value*
1	0.65	0.028	0.61	0.099
2	0.79	0.070	0.62	0.094
3	0.78	0.478	0.59	0.315
4	0.78	0.025	0.69	0.018

| Observer | Shape | | | |
| | Linear | | Amorphous | |
	Agreement	*p-value*	Agreement	*p-value*
1	0.79	0.136	0.82	0.018
2	0.83	0.679	0.79	0.310
3	0.75	0.690	1	<0.0001
4	0.80	0.119	0.76	0.209

Table 2. Inter-rater observed agreement based on kappa statistics between the four observers for all evaluations in 2D

| | 2D FFDM | | | |
Observer	1	2	3	4
1	1	0.78	0.76	0.76
2	-	1	0.76	0.73
3	-	-	1	0.76
4	-	-	-	1

Table 3. Inter-rater observed agreement based on kappa statistics between the four observers for all evaluations in DBT

	DBT			
Observer	1	2	3	4
1	1	0.77	0.72	0.73
2	-	1	0.82	0.81
3	-	-	1	0.81
4	-	-	-	1

4 Discussion

The introduction of new technologies requires extensive research. Currently, a number of studies are investigating the role of DBT in the field of breast imaging. Some studies are interested in the physical development and optimization of the systems while other studies are evaluating the capabilities of DBT compared to 2D FFDM in clinical applications. Some studies show that DBT offers superior detectability for masses but is equal to 2D FFDM for microcalcifications. Other studies have focused on general detectability of microcalcifications and masses and found no significant difference between 2D and DBT [1, 2]. One major aspect that is not yet fully investigated is the characterization of microcalcifications. This study setup stems from the validation procedure of simulated microcalcification clusters when some differences were noticed between the appearance of clusters in 2D compared with the same clusters in DBT, as shown in Fig. 2. Fig. 2(a) is a microcalcification cluster in 2D and Fig. 2(b) is the same cluster in a DBT reconstructed plane (in focus plane). Table 4 shows the assessment of the cluster in Fig. 2 by all four observers in both 2D and DBT. It is clear that two observers have changed their interpretation from round to irregular round. The linear shape of calcifications was missed by all observers in DBT. When asked to provide feedback after having read all cases, the radiologists commented that generally the appearance of microcalcifications was slightly different in DBT when compared to 2D in terms of distribution over planes and reconstruction artifacts. But they didn't refuse the existence of reconstruction artifacts because they revealed the presence of irregularly shaped microcalcifications due to the peaks at the border of the microcalcification. The observers also commented that DBT images are noisier.

This study has focused on the morphological appearance of microcalcification clusters in 2D and DBT in highlighted regions. Although this was done intentionally, another approach would be to design the study as a search (detectability) and diagnostic task with a standardized descriptor such as Le Gal [8] or BIRADS [9]. Another limitation was the relatively low sample size, which was reflected in the non-significant correlation statistics (Table 1) where the *p-values* were reported for completeness. In future studies, a prospective setup in a larger patient population needs to be performed to further assess correlations between the 2D and DBT setups.

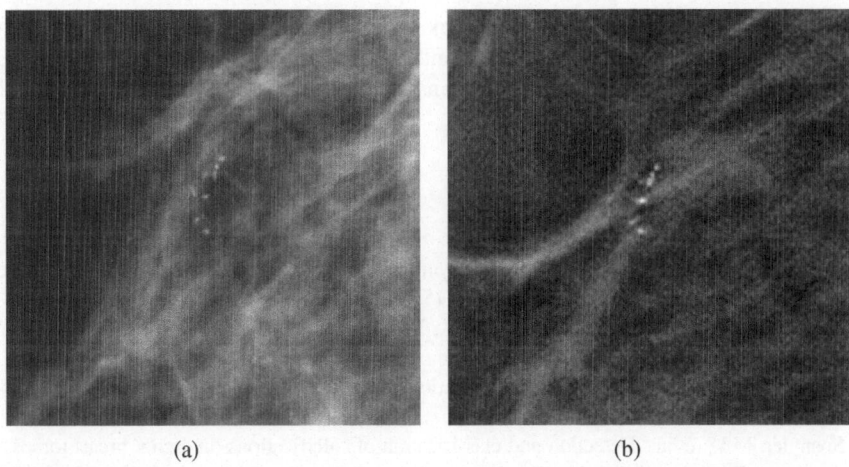

(a)   (b)

Fig. 2. An example of a microcalcification cluster in (a) 2D FFDM and in (b) DBT reconstructed plane (in focus plane)

Table 4. The assessment of the cluster in Fig. 2 by all four observers in both 2D and DBT

	Assessment in 2D FFDM	Assessment in DBT
Observer 1	round	irregular round
Observer 2	round, irregular round, linear	round, irregular round
Observer 3	round	irregular round
Observer 4	round, linear	Round

5   Conclusion

A comparison in terms of morphological description was applied between 2D FFDM and DBT. A total of 71 microcalcification clusters were evaluated by four radiologists who were asked to describe the shapes of the microcalcifications in the clusters in terms of round, irregular round, linear or amorphous. The observer study was implemented in blinded sessions, where the observers read the 2D images in separate sessions from the DBT series. An agreement test was calculated using kappa statistics between the two modalities (2D and DBT) and the results showed good agreement among readers per shaped category indicating that the morphology of microcalcification clusters does not substantially differ in 2D versus DBT.

Acknowledgements. This work is part of the OPTIMAM project which is funded by CR-UK & EPSRC Cancer Imaging Program in Surrey, in association with the MRC and Department of Health (England). The authors are grateful to the radiologists who participated in the study: Dr. Sandra Postema, Dr. Kirsten Joossens, and Dr. Riet

D'Hauwe. The authors would like to thank Jurgen Jacobs (Qaelum NV, Belgium) for providing the reading software "Sara[2]" and Thomas Mertelmeier from Siemens (Erlangen, Germany) for providing the reconstruction software "TomoEngine" and the reprocessing software "OpView2."

References

1. Gennaro, G., et al.: Digital breast tomosynthesis versus digital mammography: a clinical performance study. Eur. Radiol. 20, 1545–1553 (2010)
2. Andersson, I., Ikeda, D.M., Zackrisson, S., Ruschin, M., Svahn, T., Timberg, P., Tinberg, A.: Breast tomosynthesis and digital mammography: a comparison of breast cancer visibility and BIRADS classification in a population of cancers with subtle mammographic findings. Eur. Radiol. 18, 2817–2825 (2008)
3. Spangler, M.L., et al.: Detection and classification of calcifications on digital breast tomosynthesis and 2D digital mammography: a comparison. Am. J. Roentgenol. 196, 320–324 (2011)
4. Baker, R., Rogers, K.D., Shepherd, N., Stone, N.: New relationships between breast microcalcifications and cancer. Br. J. Cancer 103, 1034–1039 (2011)
5. Picca, D.A., De Paredes, E.S.: Calcifications in the breast: a radiologic perspective. Appl. Radiol., 29–37 (September 2003)
6. Shaheen, E., Van Ongeval, C., Zanca, F., Cockmartin, L., Marshall, N., et al.: The Simulation of 3D Microcalcification Clusters in 2D Digital Mammography and Breast Tomosynthesis. Med. Phys. 38, 6659–6671 (2011)
7. Mertelmeier, T., Orman, J., Haerer, W., Dudam, M.K.: Optimizing filtered backprojection reconstruction for a breast tomosynthesis prototype device. In: Proc. SPIE, vol. 6142, pp. 61420F1–61420F12 (2006)
8. Le Gal, M., Chavanne, G., Pellier, D.: Valeur diagnostique des microcalcifications groupees decouvertes par mammographies: a propos de 277 cas avec verification histologique et sans tumeur du sein palpable. Bull Cancer 71, 57–64 (1984)
9. American College of Radiology. Breast imaging reporting and data system (BIRADS). American College of Radiology, Reston (1993)

Comparison of 15° and 30° Angle Acquisition Digital Breast Tomosynthesis for Visualization and Characterization of Breast Abnormalities

Laurie L. Fajardo, Limin Yang, and Jeong Mi Park

Department of Radiology, University of Iowa, Iowa City, Iowa
L-Fajardo@uiowa.edu

Abstract. Investigations reporting digital breast tomosynthesis (DBT) describe better depiction of masses and architectural distortions and reduced recall for additional imaging. The purpose of this study was to evaluate the conspicuity and characterization of common findings (mass/distortion or calcifications) on DBT examinations performed by both 15° and 30° scan angles. Three readers independently reviewed 61 DBTs containing 78 findings, without knowledge which were 15° versus 30°acquisitions, and rated DBT lesion depiction using a 7-point Likert scale. An evaluation of image quality with respect to eliminating superimposed tissue and an overall DBT preference were also recorded. Our study showed no overall difference in readers' rating between 15^0 and 30^0 angle acquisition DBT exams for masses and distortions; for calcifications, there was a statistically significant preference favoring the narrow-angle scans. For overall image quality, a slight trend preferring narrow angle DBT was found, with readers' overall preference for narrow angle DBT being statistically significant.

Keywords: Digital Breast Tomosynthesis (DBT), acquisition angle, reader preference study.

1   Introduction

Breast cancer screening using x-ray projection mammography has contributed to reducing breast cancer mortality. Despite this success, lesion detectability in conventional digital mammography is limited by the anatomic background structure created by the projection of complex 3D parenchymal tissues onto a 2D image plane. To overcome this limitation, 3D breast imaging techniques are being developed, including digital breast tomosynthesis (DBT). Of interest is the variation in design of emerging DBT systems, particularly the angle of scanning used to acquire DBT image data.

In DBT, projection images acquired over a limited angular scan are reconstructed into a volume composed of thin slices (nominally 1 mm) oriented parallel to the detector plane and allowing the visualization of the breast at a specific depth while decreasing the obscuring effect of overlapping tissues. Minimizing the effect of overlapping tissue aids in the detection of masses, which is limited largely by breast tissue

A.D.A. Maidment, P.R. Bakic, and S. Gavenonis (Eds.): IWDM 2012, LNCS 7361, pp. 369–376, 2012.

structural noise. The detection of microcalcifications, however, is to a greater degree limited by quantum and detector noise. Preliminary clinical studies have shown that the removal of overlapping breast tissue reduces image clutter and increases detectability of large, low contrast lesions [1, 2]. However, other studies as well as anecdotal evidence, suggest decreased conspicuity of small, high contrast objects such as microcalcifications [3, 4].

The purpose of this study was to evaluate the conspicuity and characterization of common mammography findings on DBT examinations performed by both 15° and 30° scan angles in patients with BI-RADS® 0 (The American College of Radiology "Breast Imaging Reporting and Data System") assessment on screening digital mammography.

Table 1. DBT system scan Angles (α), no. of images acquired (n) and angular sampling distance ($\Delta\alpha$)

SYSTEM	SCAN ANGLE (α)	Number of images acquired (n)	Angular sampling distance ($\Delta\alpha$), degrees	Scan time (sec)
Hologic	15	15	1	4
Siemens	50	25	2	25
General Electric	25	9	2.8	10
Sectra	11	21	0.5	10

2   Methods

Rationale: DBT differs from conventional computed tomography in that it is a form of limited angle tomography. While DBT reduces overlap of parenchymal structures and potential breast lesions, the limited angle acquisition results in image slices that maintain some visibility of structures in the slices above and below the slice where an object of interest resides. This is similar to the characteristics of film-based linear tomography. As a general rule, wider angle tomosynthesis scans reduce the visibility of out-of-plane structures to a greater degree than narrow angle scans. Another general rule regarding in-plane resolution is that wider angle tomosynthesis scans produce images with poorer in-plane resolution while narrow angle scans have higher resolution. The degradation of resolution for wider angle scans results from several factors, including the oblique incidence of imaging photons on the detector and reconstruction artifacts. Though theoretical simulations and phantom studies have been reported [5,6], it is not immediately apparent what the optimal DBT scan angle for breast imaging should be. Wide angle scans will better reduce shadows from parenchymal breast tissue beyond a slice of interest; however, narrow angle scans will allow better visualization of microcalcification clusters due to the higher resolution and because more calcifications in a cluster will be imaged in a given slice. Similarly, a spiculated lesion might be better appreciated in a narrow angle DBT acquisition, because both the lesion's "mass" component and its out-of-plane spiculations can be seen sharply in a given slice. There are additional practical considerations in comparing narrow versus wider angle scans. For example, wide angle scans can result in smaller fields of view. They also require longer scan times that increase the potential for patient motion. Finally, wide angle scans result in x-rays travelling through a thicker effective breast, which may result in increased noise or increased patient dose.

Imaging System: For this trial, a Hologic Selenia Dimensions (Bedford, MA) DBT system was modified and used to acquire both 15° and 30° angle scans. The detector has 3328 X 4096 pixels with a 70 µm pitch. The target/filter combination of Tungsten (W)/Aluminum (Al) was used exclusively for DBT acquisition. For DBT acquisition in this study, the x-ray tube moved in a ± 7.5 degree or ±15 degree arc about a center of rotation located at the detector plane and acquiring 21 (15° angle acquisition) projection images or 30 (30° angle acquisition) projection views using 2x2 binned detector resolution of 140 microns (Figure 1). Image acquisition time was approximately 5 seconds for the 15 degree scan and 7.5 seconds for the 30

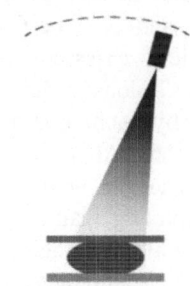

Fig. 1. X-ray tube rotates in an arc 15^0 or 30^0 above the breast

degree scan. The source to imager distance (SID) is 70 cm and the source to center of rotation distance is also 70 cm. Dose was controlled using auto AEC mode, and for any given subject, the same dose, equal to 1.5X standard screening digital mammography dose, was used for both 15° and 30° angle scans. The dose for a standard size (4.2 cm) and composition (50% fat, 50% glandular) breast was approximately 2.2 mGy.

Image Reconstruction: Tomosynthesis image reconstruction was performed using a modified filtered back projection algorithm and reconstructed into images with approximately 100 micron in-plane resolution and 1mm slice separation.

Subject Eligibility and Enrollment: Institutional Review Board Committee approval was obtained for this Health Insurance Portability and Accountability Act compliant protocol. Written informed consent was obtained. Females, at least 40 years of age, with a screening mammogram categorized as BI-RADS® 0 (The American College of Radiology "Breast Imaging Reporting and Data System" assessment category 0) because of suspected mass density, focal asymmetry, or calcifications were eligible for this study if they had both their screening and diagnostic mammograms performed on a Hologic 2D Selenia Mammography System. In addition to standard care diagnostic imaging, all participants underwent two experimental DBT acquisitions, in two projections (Cranio-Caudal and Mediolateral Oblique) on the breast of concern by both 15° and 30° acquisition angle, in a randomized order. A total of 110 subjects, including 3 African American and 107 Caucasian women (average age: 52 years; range: 40-74 years), were enrolled prospectively at a single institution and 106 subjects completed the experimental imaging. Four patients were excluded for the following reasons: 2 subjects did not have time to complete the imaging, 1 subject was discontinued for not meeting inclusion/exclusion criteria, and 1 subject could not be imaged because the technologist had not completed the DBT system QC testing. Of the 106 eligible subjects, 14 (13%) underwent biopsy of the lesion of concern; 4 (29%) subjects were confirmed pathologically to have cancer and the remaining 10 had benign lesions.

Reader Study: Of the 106 DBT scan pairs (15° and 30°) performed in this study, 61 "review" cases comprising a total of 78 different lesions, underwent independent evaluation by each of 3 readers from 3 separate locations. All readers were MQSA certified and had greater than 10 years of experience interpreting mammograms; 1 reader was an academic radiologist and 2 were community practice radiologists. Cases selected for this review were all cases proven to have a lesion of concern (mass density, architectural distortion, or calcifications) on diagnostic mammography work-up, including the 14 cases that went on to biopsy. Cases assessed at the originating institution as negative (summation artifact) were excluded from the reader study. Each reader evaluated and scored the 61 DBT "review cases" (78 lesions) at their own institution. The cases were viewed on a digital mammography workstation equipped with 2 high resolution 5 megapixel monitors using a specific DBT hanging protocol. The cranio-caudal (CC) narrow and wide angle DBT studies were displayed, followed by the medio-lateral oblique (MLO) narrow and wide angle DBT studies. Throughout the review, the narrow and wide angle tomo exams appeared randomly on the left or right screens, but for consistency, they were hung uniformly for a given case. For example, the wide angle CC and MLO exam were always shown on the same monitor for a given case, while the narrow angle exam will have hung on the opposite monitor. Readers were unaware which scans were 15° versus 30° DBT acquisitions. After viewing the CC and MLO DBT studies, the hanging protocol displayed the conventional 2-D screening mammogram and accompanying diagnostic work-up; however, these studies were available to the readers at any time by using the workstation's display "navigator". Each DBT study was evaluated for the presence of 2 common mammographic lesions: mass/distortion & calcifications. Readers were aware of what abnormality(ies) they were evaluating for each case because the 2D digital mammograms, including any diagnostic images for each case were available to them. For each case, readers compared the DBT scan on the left monitor to that on the right monitor. Specifically, for masses/architectural distortions readers recorded the conspicuity, margin sharpness and ability to characterize the lesion (by BI-RADS criteria) on a 7-point scale for each scan pair. For calcifications, similar comparisons, also using a 7-point scale, were made between the 2 DBT scans for conspicuity, sharpness/shape, ability to characterize and ability to assess distribution. Comparisons of which (if any) DBT scan best eliminated superimposed breast tissue, an overall scan preference, a BI-RADS lesion assessment for each scan and a rating of the breast

Table 2. Scoring Key

Wide Angle	
Diagnostically Better	-3
Moderately Better	-2
Slightly Better	-1
Equal	0
Narrow Angle	
Slightly Better	1
Moderately Better	2
Diagnostically Better	3

parenchymal density (based on standard BI-RADS criteria) were also collected. The data reporting form used for the reader study is given in Appendix A ("DBT Lesion Evaluation and Rating Form").

Table 3. Individual Readers' Assessments of 15^0 versus 30^0 DBT scans for Image Features and Quality

Mass/Distortion	Reader 1	Reader 2	Reader 3
Conspicuity	0.13	-0.09	0.07
Margin Sharpness	0.15	-0.05	0.09
Characterization	-0.04	-0.07	0.04
Calcium			
Conspicuity	0.85	0.29	0.43
Sharpness/Shape	0.80	0.33	0.50
Characterization	0.55	0.21	0.43
Distribution	0.20	0.00	0.56
Overall Image Quality			
Elimination of Superimposed Tissue	-0.01	0.05	0.18
Overall Preference	0.24	0.01	0.22

Data Analysis and Results
Each item evaluated by each reader on the wide (30° angle) versus the narrow (15° angle) scans was scored using the scale given in Table 2. Table 3 gives the results of individual readers' ratings for masses/ disotortions, calcifications and overall image quality when comparing narrow and wide angle DBT. Scores > 0 indicate a preference for narrow angles scans, scores < 0 a preference for wide angle. For masses and distortions, no one reader strongly preferred wide or narrow angle scans. For calcifications, readers more often preferred narrow angle DBT, except for Reader 2's evaluation of the distribution of calcifications, where there was no preference. Regarding overall scan angle preference, Readers1 and 3 strongly preferred the narrow angle scans and Reader 3 was neutral. Table 4 shows the distribution of pooled reader rating ratings, based on whether the wide or narrow angle DBT scan was rated as superior and gives the results of Wilcoxon Signed-Rank tests of statistical significance for pooled reader data comparing narrow (15^0) to wide (30^0) angle DBT scans. For cases with masses and/or architectural distortions, we found no difference between wide versus narrow angle scans with respect to readers' grouped ratings of lesion conspicuity, how well the mass margins were seen or ability to characterize the lesions as malignant or benign. The average reader ratings for all evaluations related to mass/architectural distortions were approximately 0 (Table 4), with variation in the responses for individual cases (some cases preferred in the narrow angle and others in the wide angle scans – Table 3). For microcalcifications, there were significant differences between the pooled reader ratings for the narrow vs. wide angle scans. Readers' rated narrow angle DBT scans significantly better for microcalcification conspicuity and sharpness, as well as the ability to evaluate shape and distribution and to characterize calcifications as benign or malignant. The pooled reader ratings of overall DBT

scan quality indicated a slight preference for the narrow angle scans. Finally, there was a statistically significant overall preference by readers for narrow angle DBT scans for evaluating commonly encountered breast abnormalities in this study.

Table 4. Pooled Results for All Readers and P-Values (*)

Ratings →	Wide angle superior			Narrow angle superior				Avg rating	P-value	Statistically significant?
	-3	-2	-1	0	1	2	3			
Mass/Distortion										
Conspicuity	2	4	15	114	27	4	0	0.04	0.45	No
Margin Sharpness	1	5	13	118	23	5	1	0.0.6	0.32	No
Characterization	1	7	10	128	17	3	0	0.02	0.60	No
Calcium										
Conspicuity	2	2	3	28	27	8	2	0.50	0.0001	Yes
Sharpness/Shape	2	2	3	27	25	13	0	0.53	<0.0001	Yes
Characterization	2	1	4	35	20	10	0	0.39	0.001	Yes
Distribution	2	0	4	44	15	4	2	0.27	0.011	Yes
Overall Image Quality										
Elimination of Superimposed Tissue	1	5	19	157	32	8	0	0.07	0.12	No
Overall Preference	2	8	14	140	46	12	0	0.15	0.007	Yes

(*) scores < 0 indicate preference for wide angle scans, scores > 0 indicate preference for narrow angle scans

3   Discussion

Our pilot study evaluated the effect of DBT image angle acquisition on readers' ratings of overall quality and how well common breast lesions (masses/distortions and calcifications) were depicted with respect to conspicuity, sharpness and ability to characterize lesion features. The study showed no overall difference between readers' ratings of narrow (15^0) angle acquisition and wide (30^0) angle acquisition DBT exams for masses and distortions, with a spread of responses indicating some cases were preferred in narrow angle and some with wide angle. Differences in readers' ratings of narrow vs. wide angle DBT scans for evaluating microcalcifications were statistically significant with respect to all metrics evaluated for microcalcifications, including conspicuity, sharpness, and readers' ability to evaluate shape, distribution and to characterize the calcifications as benign or malignant. Readers' ratings of overall DBT scan quality indicated a slight preference for the narrow angle scans. Finally, a statistically significant difference between readers' DBT scan preference ratings showed they more often preferred the narrow angle scans when evaluating commonly encountered breast abnormalities in the study. A limitation of our study is that it evaluated a single DBT system. The "standard" DBT acquisition commercially available on this system is the 15^0 angle acquisition and this DBT imaging mode may be best for screening and general evaluations. Because scan angles and scan times vary widely among different DBT systems, patient motion artifact might impact systems with longer scanning times. Even slight motion could affect the depiction and conspicuity of microcalcifications. Therefore, we recommend that further evaluation be performed to ascertain if and under what conditions, a 30^0 DBT scan might be valuable as an added diagnostic feature. This would provide the radiologist an option to further evaluate masses and architectural distortions differently from the standard 15-degree scan, if desired, for the isolated cases where a wider angle might offer an advantage.

References

1. Rafferty, E., Niklason, L., Halpern, E., et al.: Assessing radiologist performance using combined full-field digital mammography and breast tomosynthesis versus full-field digital mammography alone: results of a multi-center multi-reader trial. In: RSNA Annual Meeting, Chicago, IL (2007)
2. Skaane, P., Gullien, R., Eben, E.B., et al.: Reading time of FFDM and tomosynthesis in a population-based screening program. In: Radiological Society of North America Annual Meeting, Chicago, IL (2011)
3. Baker, J.A., Lo, J.Y.: Breast Tomosynthesis: state-of-the-art and review of the literature. Academic Radiology 18(10),1298–1310 (2011)
4. Poplack, S.P., Tosteson, T.D., Kogel, C.A., et al.: Digital breast tomosynthesis: initial experience in 98 women with abnormal digital screening mammography. Am. J. Roentgenol. 189, 616–623 (2007)
5. Sechopoulos, I., Ghetti, C.: Optimization of the acquisition geometry in digital tomosynthesis of the breast. Med. Phys. 36, 1199–1207 (2009)
6. Ren, B., Ruth, C., Zhang, Y., et al.: The CNR method in scan angle optimization of tomosynthesis and its limitations. In: Proc. SPIE, vol. 7258 (2009), doi:10.1117/12.813918

Appendix A. DBT Lesion Evaluation and Rating Form

DBT Study Score sheet

Case #				Radiologist Initials/Date:				
Lesion:								
Right Calcification 12:00 0mm								
Compare Left to Right Tomosynthesis Image								

Feature	Left Image				Right Image			
	Diagnostically Better	Moderately Better	Slightly Better	Equal	Slightly Better	Moderately Better	Diagnostically Better
Mass/Distortion								
Conspicuity								
Margin Sharpness								
Characterization								
Calcifications								
Conspicuity								
Sharpness/Shape								
Characterization								
Distribution								
Overall Image Quality								
Elimination of Superimposed Tissue								
Overall Preference								

BI-RADS Assessment Category (1-5) Normal – Highly Suggestive of Malignancy										
	Left Image						Right Image			
Assessment	1	2	3	4	5		1	2	3	4	5
Check Box										

BI-RADS Breast Composition (1-4) Fatty – Homogeneously Dense				
Density	1	2	3	4
Check Box				

Differences in Radiologists' Experiences and Performance in Breast Tomosynthesis

Tony Svahn[1], Kristina Lång[2], Ingvar Andersson[2], and Sophia Zackrisson[2]

[1] Medical Radiation Physics, Department of Clinical Sciences Malmö, Lund University,
Skåne University Hospital, Malmö, Sweden
[2] Medical Radiology, Department of Clinical Sciences Malmö, Lund University,
Skåne University Hospital, Malmö, Sweden
tony.svahn@med.lu.se

Abstract. The purpose was to study the ability of radiologists to detect breast cancers using 1-view breast tomosynthesis (BT) compared to 2-view digital mammography (DM) correlated with their experience in mammography. The patient population was enriched with difficult cases (89 abnormal and 96 normal/benign breasts). Eight breast radiologists with various experience levels in mammography interpreted the BT and DM image sets individually in a FROC study. Their performance was measured by the JAFROC figure-of-merit θ (non-parametric area under the AFROC curve) and analyzed as a function of experience level. The improvement was significant for the highly experienced radiologists, mean θ_{BT-DM} = 0.092; 95% CI: [0.023, 0.161] and for the experienced radiologists, mean θ_{BT-DM} = 0.094; 95% CI: [0.034, 0.149] while it was not for the less experienced radiologists, mean θ_{BT-DM} = 0.021: 95% CI: [-0.161, 0.202]. The results indicate that experience is necessary to achieve optimal performance in BT.

Keywords: Breast tomosynthesis, digital mammography, radiologist, experience, performance.

1 Background

Screening mammography plays a key role in the early detection of breast cancer, but reported sensitivities of 68-88% (as low as 48% for extremely dense breasts) and specificities of 82-98% indicate that the mammography performance can be improved further [1]. A problem with both screen-film mammography and digital mammography (DM) is that the anatomical noise (e.g. superimposed breast tissue onto the receptor plane) can hamper the detection of breast cancer. Breast tomosynthesis (BT) is a newly developed three-dimensional (3D) imaging modality with the potential to improve the performance of mammography by reducing the tissue overlap. To date this has been demonstrated in several clinical studies [1-5], but it needs to be confirmed in larger screening studies.

A.D.A. Maidment, P.R. Bakic, and S. Gavenonis (Eds.): IWDM 2012, LNCS 7361, pp. 377–385, 2012.

In general, reader variability in clinical studies is one of the largest source of variability and means that a larger number of readers need to be used in order to obtain a reliable average [6]. The choice of readers can affect the result significantly – experienced radiologists usually involve less intra-observer variations than inexperienced radiologists. While the use of highly experienced radiologists might require less numbers of readers, it is essential to realize that this might not reflect the clinical situation where various ranges of experience usually are involved. It can be hypothesized that the higher breast cancer visibility of BT [2, 3] would result in a larger performance improvement for inexperienced radiologists than for experienced radiologists; if the detection task is easier it should be less dependent on radiologist skill. Subtle signs of malignancy should on the other hand require more experience to detect. Smith et al [2] investigated the hypothesis and did not find any correlation between performance differences for BT and DM in relation to DM alone linked with radiologists' skill but found that all readers improved their performance with the BT modality. In a recent study that examined the diagnostic accuracy of 1-view BT and 2-view DM using an enriched population the authors demonstrated a statistically significant improvement using BT compared to DM [1]. The current work, based on the same patient population, was designed to investigate the performance using 1-view BT and 2-view DM related to various experience levels.

2   Methods

The study was approved by the Regional ethics comittee board at Lund University (Dnr 159/2006) and the local Radiation Safety Committee. The patients underwent informed consent and all examinations were voluntary. The BT system used and image acquisition for data collection has been described previously [1]. Each DM examination consisted of the mediolateral oblique (MLO) and craniocaudal (CC) views, while the MLO view was chosen for the BT examinations in 88% of the cases (the CC view was used in the remaining cases). The patient population was enriched with difficult cases by selecting cases with subtle signs of malignancy on DM and/or ultrasonography [1, 3]. Patients with suspicious lesions underwent surgery and histopathological examination of the specimens. Patients not undergoing surgery had a 1-year follow-up. Two experienced breast radiologists - non-participants in the studies - set the gold standard by determining the abnormal regions and their boundaries by aligning them using an electronic marker. This was done in the BT and DM images using all available information including BT, DM, ultrasonography, needle biopsy and pathology. Retrospectively, the study population comprised 89 abnormal cases (containing 95 abnormalities) and 96 normal/benign cases, which were entered into a reader study. The radiologists who participated in the reader study represent a range of clinical experience and were categorized into three experience levels: four were highly experienced (16, 23, 25 and 30 years of experience; mean 23.5 years), two were experienced (7 and 7 years of experience; mean 7 years) and two were less experienced (1 and 1 year of experience; mean 1 year). The readers were blinded to the true state (positive/negative) of the images. All radiologists were familiar with the DM interpretation, but none had any significant experience in reviewing BT images prior to a training session of 30 BT and the 30 corresponding DM cases before the study. BT had just been implemented at the institution and the study was performed before the readers had any clinical experience of BT. The intention with the training session was to familiarize the readers with the appearance of the normal tissue and the general appearance of various cancer types in BT. The readers did not receive any information of the case-mix of the study population (i.e. that it was enriched with difficult cases). The task was to mark and rate any finding suspicious for malignancy and any benign finding that they would normally report in the screening programme. The probability of malignancy was rated on a BIRADS-based scale with five levels (3, 4A, 4B, 4C and 5) of increasing probability for malignancy and no time limit was imposed on the readers' interpretations. A graphical user interface was used to display the images, and to collect and score the radiologist data. The radiologists' marks and ratings were recorded by the software at any given location in the DM and BT cases. The interpretations of the images were made on two 5 mega-pixel flat panel monitors (SMD21500, EIZO GmbH, Karlsruhe, Germany), calibrated according to DICOM part 14, using a Sun Microsystem Ultra 24 Workstation. The minimum luminance was 0.4 cd/m^2 and the maximum luminance was 355 cd/m^2. The ambient light level was lower than 3 lux. The cases were displayed one at a time using one 5 MP monitor per view. No limit was imposed on the interpretation time. The cases were presented in random order in eight reading batches of two blocks of 25 cases per modality: i.e., 25 1-view BT cases and 25 2-view DM cases. The modality presentation order was alternated and a period of 1-3 weeks separated consecutive viewings of the same case in the two modalities.

2.1   Statistical Analysis

If a mark with malignancy rating was located inside the aligned boundary of an abnormality it was scored as a lesion localization (LL), otherwise as a non-lesion localization (NL). The reader data was analyzed by the jackknife alternative free response receiver operating characteristic (JAFROC) method [6]. The JAFROC figure of merit (θ) is the probability that the rating of the highest rated and correctly localized lesion (LL) on an abnormal case exceeds the rating of the highest rated mark on a normal/benign case (NL); equivalent to the non-parametric area under the AFROC curve [6]; NLs on abnormal images were not used in the analysis. Significance testing was performed using the Dorfman-Berbaum-Metz multiple-reader multiple case (DBM-MRMC) mixed model analysis of variance (ANOVA) procedure applied to θ. The analysis was performed for random-readers random-cases, fixed-readers random-cases and random-readers fixed-cases.

Parametric reader-averaged AFROC curves fitted by search model are presented and the search-model parameters [6]. Parameter v is the probability that a breast cancer (signal-site) was considered for marking, while λ denotes the corresponding mean number of noise sites per image that were considered for marking in the preattentive stage. An inexperienced reader would be characterized by a smaller value of ν than an experienced reader. The parameter μ is the separation between these two distributions and represents lesion signal-to-noise ratio (SNR). It characterizes the ability of the reader to extract information from a signal site during cognitive evaluation and is influenced by external factors (e.g., complexity of the surround, lesion contrast, etc) and observer dependent factors (e.g., eyesight, expertise, etc).

A separate analysis was conducted to examine if the statistical dispersions of performance levels on BT was significantly different from that of DM. The dispersions were compared of computed reader-specific operating characteristics; the differences in spread were assessed of lesion-localization fractions (LLF), false positive fractions (FPF) and distances from reader-specific to reader-averaged operating points. The comparison of performance dispersion was performed on reader-specific subsets on BT and DM using Levene's equality test of variances [7].

3   Results

3.1   The JAFROC Figure-of-Merit (θ; Non-parametric Area under the AFROC Curve)

All radiologists increased their performance as measured by the JAFROC figure-of-merit (θ) using BT compared to DM (Table 1; the improvement was statistically

Table 1. The JAFROC figure-of-merit (θ; non-parametric area under the AFROC curve) for the highly experienced radiologists (reader 1-4), the experienced radiologists (reader 5 and 6) and the less experienced radiologists (reader 7 and 8). The 95-confidence intervals of differences (95-CI) are shown in the parenthesis in the final column for each category of experience.

Reader	Highly experienced			Experienced			Less experienced		
	BT θ	DM θ	θ$_{BT-DM}$ (95-CI)	BT θ	DM θ	θ$_{BT-DM}$ (95-CI)	BT θ	DM θ	θ$_{BT-DM}$ (95-CI)
1	0.759	0.641	0.118 (0.020, 0.217)						
2	0.838	0.704	0.134 (0.064, 0.204)						
3	0.813	0.736	0.077 (-0.003, 0.157)						
4	0.807	0.769	0.038 (-0.030, 0.106)						
5				0.828	0.681	0.147 (0.070, 0.224)			
6				0.774	0.733	0.041 (-0.033, 0.115)			
7							0.713	0.678	0.035 (-0.041, 0.110)
8							0.693	0.687	0.006 (-0.076, 0.088)
Average	0.804	0.712	+ 0.092 (0.023, 0.161)	0.801	0.707	+ 0.094 (0.034, 0.149)	0.703	0.683	+ 0.021 (-0.161, 0.202)

significant using all reader data: p = 0.0153, F-stat = 6.37; for random readers and random cases, p = 0.0041, F-stat = 8,47; for fixed readers and random cases and p = 0.0052, F-stat = 15.96; for random readers and fixed cases. The performance increase (mean θ_{BT-DM}) was statistically significant as indicated by the 95% confidence interval of differences (Table 1) for the highly experienced and experienced radiologists, but not for the less experienced radiologists. The performance was lower both on the BT and the DM modality for the less experienced radiologists, but substantially lower on the BT modality (0.804 and 0.801 vs. 0.703).

3.2   Parametric AFROC Curves and Search-Model Parameters

The average AFROC curves for each category of experience (Figure 1 a-c) illustrate that the highly experienced (a) and the experienced (b) radiologists operated further out on the y- and x-axis.

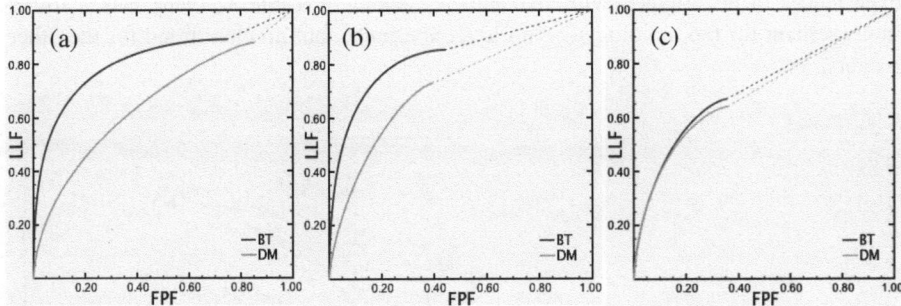

Fig. 1. The performance of breast tomosynthesis (BT) and digital mammography (DM) illustrated by AFROC curves for (a) highly experienced radiologists, (b) experienced radiologists and (c) less experienced radiologists.

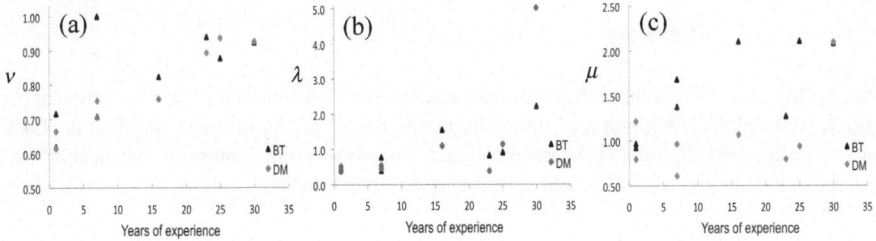

Fig. 2. The search-model parameters that constitutes the parametric AFROC curve as a function of reader experience: (a) ν - the probability that a breast cancer was considered for marking, (b) λ - the mean number of noise-sites considered for marking per image and (c) μ - the separation between the statistical distributions of ν and λ (e.g. the signal-noise-ratio).

The v parameter increased with years of experience in a linear fashion (Figure 2 a) (for BT $R^2 = 0.42$ and if the deviating point around 7 year is excluded $R^2 = 0.92$, and for DM $R^2 = 0.92$). The average v value for the radiologists on BT and DM was 0.668 and 0.640 (less experienced), 0.854 and 0.729 (experienced) and 0.892 and 0.879 (highly experienced), e.g. higher for BT for all experience categories. In general, the λ parameter increased with years of radiologist experience on BT and DM, but varied by modality (Figure 2 b): 0.436 and 0.445 (less experienced), 0.583 and 0.497 (experienced) and 1.373 and 1.909 (highly experienced). The characteristics of the slopes of the search model-fitted AFROC curves are determined by the μ parameter, which determines the sharpness of the transition from vertical slope at the origin to (λ, v), e.g. higher μ value is equivalent with a steeper transition to the plateau and usually higher performance. The difference in μ parameter between BT and DM was generally much larger for experienced readers (Figure 2 c).

Figure 3 shows the improvement in performance (θ) as a function of years of experience. In accordance with the data presented in Table 1, there was a lower improvement for the radiologists with less experience, but no clear trend for the other readers.

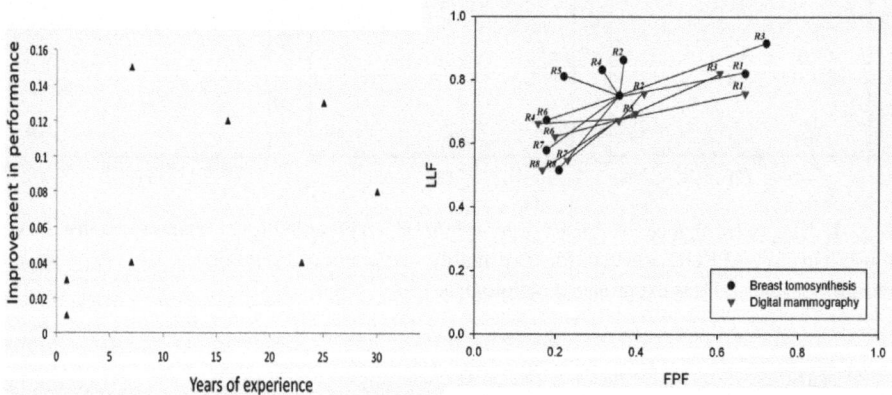

Fig. 3. (left plot). The improvement in performance (θ) as a function of years of experience.
Fig. 4. (right plot). Distribution of operating points for all the radiologists (R1-R8) for breast tomosynthesis and digital mammography (each operating point represents the accumulated lesion localization fraction, LLF, and false positive fraction, FPF).

The reader-averaged operating points (LLF, FPF) and standard deviations were 0.752 ± 0.144, 0.356 ± 0.219 and 0.672 ± 0.107, 0.354 ± 0.200 for BT and DM, respectively. There was no significant difference ($p = 0.622$) in the spreads of the operating points in BT versus those in DM on reader-specific sets (Figure 4). Two examples are shown (Figure 5) that were subject for different interpretation in BT in the experience categories.

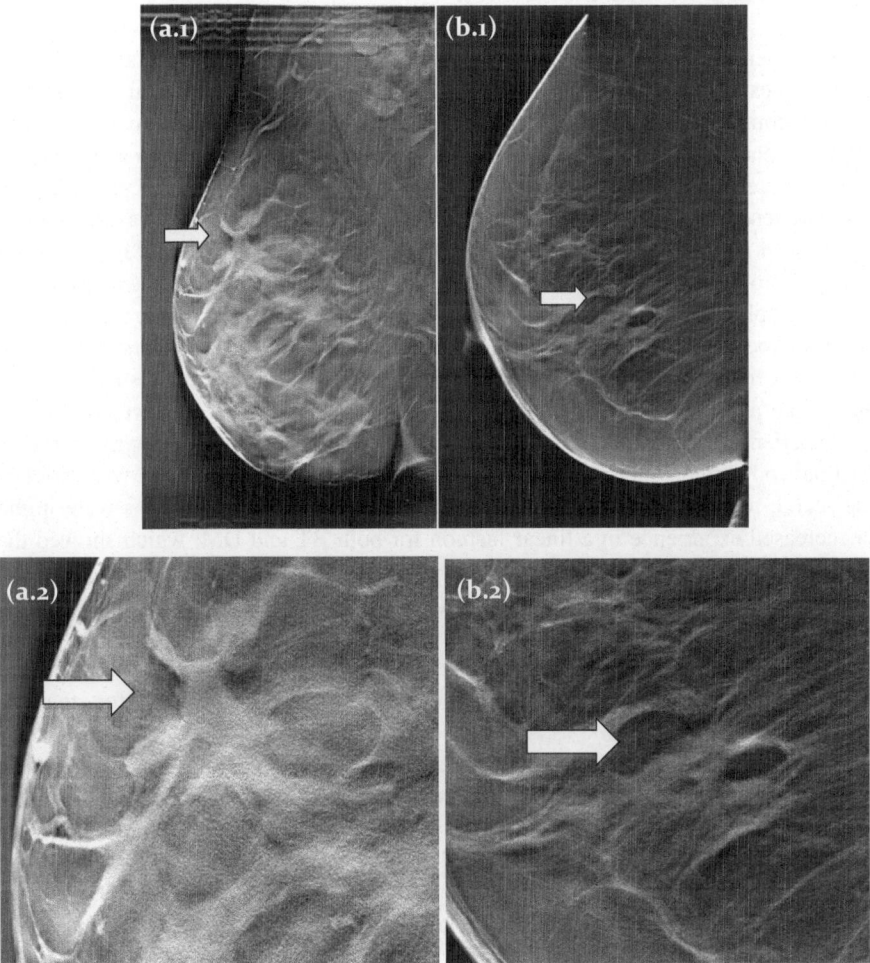

Fig. 5. Two BT cases that reflect differences in the experience categories, in medio lateral oblique views (a.1, b.1) and close-ups (a.2, b.2). (a.1): A 53-year old woman with a 20 mm, invasive ductal carcinoma grade 3. The tumor indicated by the arrow in (a.1-a.2) has a dense nucleus with somewhat irregular borders and quite coarse spiculations that in its caudal parts blend into the surrounding dense breast parenchyma. It was detected by the highly experienced and experienced radiologists but not by the less experienced radiologists. (b.1) A 64-year old woman with a 34 mm invasive ductal carcinoma grade 3. The tumor, indicated by the arrow in (b.1-b.2), was detected by all the highly experienced radiologists, none of the experienced, and one of the less experienced radiologists. It has fine spiculations in some slices causing a slight retraction in its cranial parts, but is located in an area with somewhat irregular breast parenchyma, which may have caused difficulties in the detection task.

4   Discussion and Conclusion

In this paper the performance of eight readers in BT and DM were analyzed with regards to experience in mammography. All radiologists improved their performance with BT compared to DM; the improvement was significant using all reader data for different generalizations of the populations of readers and cases. When analyzing the data separately in categories of reader experience, the performance improvement of less experienced radiologists was not statistically significant, while it was for both the experienced radiologists and the highly experienced radiologists. The AFROC curves averaged for each experience category illustrated that higher experience in mammography was related with both higher LLF and FPF. A probable reason is that the less experienced radiologists were not as good as the other readers at reporting breast cancer with subtler radiographic appearances. This may be a result of lack of knowledge and experience of the heterogeneity of breast cancer growth patterns in less experienced radiologists. Operating further out on the x-axis, allow the curves to level out and may have been particularly important since the population was enriched. The search-model parameters showed some interesting features; the v's were higher for increased experience in a linear fashion for both BT and DM, which showed that the probability that a breast cancer was considered for marking was higher in accordance with increased experience. The higher μ for BT characterizes the higher ability on BT of the radiologists to extract information from a signal site during cognitive evaluation. The difference in μ for BT in relation to DM was in general larger for increased experience, but not particularly pronounced for the less experienced radiologists.

There was a considerable spread among operating points (Figure 4) but it was not significantly different in between the modalities. Reader variability in operating points is attributable to the radiologists' variable thresholds for reporting disease. When this is accounted for in combined performance measures, the variability in diagnostic abilities of the radiologists is considerably smaller. Although, the results of this study were conclusive it should be noted that the numbers of readers were limited and the individual reader variation in performance within each experience category was rather large. Furthermore, an enriched study population was used, which may not reflect a true clinical or screening setting. Future work will involve increasing the reader data with more mid-level experience and less experienced readers, which is needed to confirm the initial findings of this work. This would help to determine how much experience with BT that is needed to reach the skill to identify more subtle lesions. Information about limitations in the BT interpretation is also desirable to devise targeted training strategies. In summary, although BT has the potential to provide 'clearer' images to the radiologist than DM the results indicate that there still will be detection and interpretation tasks that are highly experience-dependent.

Acknowledgements. The authors acknowledge the contribution from all the participating radiologists. The present study was supported by the Swedish Cancer Foundation, Cancer 450 Research Foundation at the Department of Oncology, Franke and Margareta Bergqvist Foundation.

References

1. Svahn, T., Chakraborty, D.P., Ikeda, D., Zackrisson, S., Do, Y., Mattsson, S., Andersson, I.: Breast tomosynthesis and digital mammography: A comparison of diagnostic accuracy. Accepted for publication in BJR (2012)
2. Smith, A.P., Rafferty, E.A., Niklason, L.: Clinical Performance of Breast Tomosynthesis as a Function of Radiologist Experience Level. In: Krupinski, E.A. (ed.) IWDM 2008. LNCS, vol. 5116, pp. 61–66. Springer, Heidelberg (2008)
3. Andersson, I., Ikeda, D.M., Zackrisson, S., Ruschin, M., Svahn, T., Timberg, P., et al.: Breast tomosynthesis and digital mammography: a comparison of breast cancer visibility and BIRADS classification in a population of cancers with subtle mammographic findings. Eur. Radiol. 18(12), 2817–2825 (2008)
4. Svahn, T., Andersson, I., Chakraborty, D., Svensson, S., Ikeda, D., Förnvik, D., et al.: The diagnostic accuracy of dual-view digital mammography, single-view breast tomosynthesis and a dual-view combination of breast tomosynthesis and digital mammography in a free-response observer performance study. Radiat. Prot. Dosim. 139(1-3), 113–117 (2010)
5. Michell, M.J., Wasan, R.K., Iqbal, A., Peacock, C., Evans, D.R., Morel, J.C.: Two-view 2D digital mammography versus one-view digital breast tomosynthesis. Breast Cancer Res. 12(suppl. 3) (2010)
6. Chakraborty, D.P.: New developments in observer performance methodology in medical imaging. Semin. Nucl. Med. 41(6), 401–418 (2011)
7. Levene, H.: Robust tests for equality of variances. In: Olkin, I. (ed.) Contributions to Probability and Statistics, pp. 278–292. Stanford University Press, Palo Alto (1960)

Proposing an Acquisition Geometry That Optimizes Super-Resolution in Digital Breast Tomosynthesis

Raymond J. Acciavatti and Andrew D.A. Maidment

University of Pennsylvania, Department of Radiology, Physics Section, 1 Silverstein Building,
3400 Spruce St., Philadelphia PA 19104-4206
racci@seas.upenn.edu, Andrew.Maidment@uphs.upenn.edu

Abstract. In digital breast tomosynthesis (DBT), oblique x-ray incidence shifts the image of an object in sub-pixel detector element increments with each projection angle. Our previous work has shown that DBT is capable of super-resolution as a result of this property. Although super-resolution is achievable over a broad range of positions for frequencies parallel to the chest wall side of the breast support, it is feasible at fewer positions for frequencies perpendicular to the chest wall. This finding arises because translational shifts in the image between projections are minimal in the chest wall-to-nipple direction. To optimize super-resolution, this work proposes an acquisition geometry in which the detector is translated in the chest wall-to-nipple direction between projections. At various increments of detector translation, we calculate the reconstruction of a sine input whose frequency is greater than the detector alias frequency. The model gives a proof-of-principle justification that detector translation promotes super-resolution.

Keywords: Digital breast tomosynthesis (DBT), aliasing, super-resolution, image reconstruction, Fourier Transform, spectral leakage, precision translation, optimization.

1   Introduction

In digital breast tomosynthesis (DBT), a 3D image of the breast is generated from a limited range of low-dose x-ray projections. Early clinical trials show that DBT has improved sensitivity and specificity for cancer detection relative to 2D digital mammography (DM), the current gold standard for breast cancer screening [1].

In DBT, the image of an object is translated in sub-pixel detector element increments with each increasing projection angle. Our previous work has demonstrated that DBT is capable of super-resolution (*i.e.*, sub-pixel resolution) as a result of this property [2]. The existence of super-resolution is dependent on the directionality of the input frequency and on position in the reconstruction. Although super-resolution is feasible over a broad range of positions for frequencies parallel to the chest wall side of the breast support, it is achievable at fewer positions for frequencies oriented along the posteroanterior (PA) direction. For example, super-resolution along the PA direction is not possible for input objects within the

A.D.A. Maidment, P.R. Bakic, and S. Gavenonis (Eds.): IWDM 2012, LNCS 7361, pp. 386–393, 2012.

mid-plane perpendicular to the chest wall and to the breast support. Since this mid-plane has extent in both the PA and source-to-support (SS) directions, it will be termed the mid PA/SS plane throughout the remainder of this work (Figure 1).

Super-resolution along the PA direction is not feasible in the mid PA/SS plane because translational shifts in the image between projections are minimal. To optimize super-resolution, this work proposes an acquisition geometry in which the detector is translated in the PA direction between projections. This design feature can be implemented through precision translation of the detector.

2   Methods

An analytical model of super-resolution is developed by calculating the reconstruction of a sine input whose frequency is greater than the alias frequency of the detector. Defining the xz plane as the chest wall (Figure 1), the input is taken to be a rectangular prism whose attenuation coefficient varies sinusoidally along the y direction. The input is positioned between the heights $z = z_0 \pm \varepsilon/2$ above the detector, where z_0 is the central height of the input and ε is its thickness (Figure 2). Denoting C as the amplitude of the waveform and f_0 as its frequency, the attenuation coefficient $\mu(x, y, z)$ can be written as $C \cdot \cos(2\pi f_0 y) \cdot \text{rect}[(z - z_0)/\varepsilon]$. The 1D Fourier transform of the input along the y direction is a sum of delta functions peaking at the frequencies $f_y = \pm f_0$. Since only the positive frequency is of interest in a physical measurement, this input is useful for modeling the reconstruction of a single input frequency.

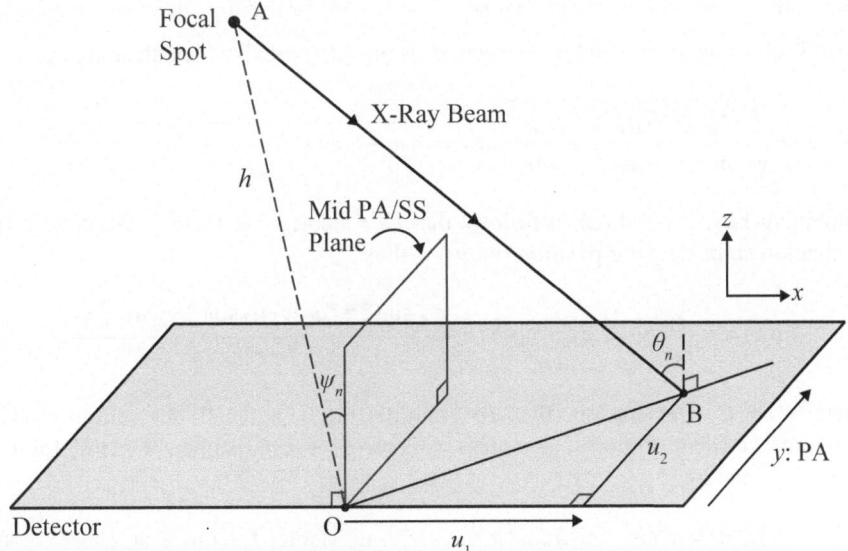

Fig. 1. In DBT, the nth x-ray projection is acquired within the plane of the chest wall (*i.e.*, the xz plane) at the angle ψ_n relative to the z axis.

In DBT, x-ray projections are acquired as the x-ray tube rotates in a circular arc within the plane of the chest wall. In many systems, the midpoint of the chest wall side of the detector serves as the center-of-rotation (COR) of the x-ray tube. Defining the origin O as the COR, the vector from O to any point A in the tube's arc is thus $\overline{OA} = (-h\sin\psi_n)\mathbf{i} + (h\cos\psi_n)\mathbf{k}$, where $\psi_n = n \cdot \Delta\psi$. In these expressions, h denotes the source-to-origin distance, ψ_n is the projection angle, n is the projection number, and $\Delta\psi$ is the angular spacing between projections. In a system with N total projections, the index n varies from $+(N-1)/2$ to $-(N-1)/2$ during the scan time.

The incident angle can now be calculated at any point B on the detector. Since $\overline{OB} = u_1\mathbf{i} + u_2\mathbf{j}$, it follows that $\overline{BA} = -\overline{OB} + \overline{OA} = -(u_1 + h\sin\psi_n)\mathbf{i} - u_2\mathbf{j} + (h\cos\psi_n)\mathbf{k}$, and hence the incident angle can be evaluated from the dot product

$$\cos\theta_n = \frac{\overline{BA}\cdot\mathbf{k}}{|\overline{BA}||\mathbf{k}|} \ , \ \theta_n = \arccos\left[\frac{h\cos\psi_n}{\sqrt{(u_1 + h\sin\psi_n)^2 + u_2^2 + (h\cos\psi_n)^2}}\right]. \tag{1}$$

Detector signal for each projection can now be determined by tracing the ray between points A and B. Defining w to be a free parameter, the equation of the ray can be written in terms of three parametric equations: $x = w(u_1 + h\sin\psi_n) - h\sin\psi_n$, $y = wu_2$, and $z = (1-w)h\cos\psi_n$. The focal spot at point A has been defined to correspond with $w = 0$, and the incident point at B has been defined to correspond with $w = 1$. The x-ray path length $\mathcal{L}_n$ through the input for the nth projection is determined from the intersection of the incident ray with the planes $z = z_0 \pm \varepsilon/2$. The values of w for these two points are $w_n^\pm = 1 - (z_0 \pm \varepsilon/2)h^{-1}\sec\psi_n$. For the nth projection, the total attenuation $\mathcal{A}\mu(n)$ is given by the integral $\int \mu ds$, where ds is the differential arc length along $\mathcal{L}_n$.

$$ds = \sqrt{\left(\frac{dx}{dw}\right)^2 + \left(\frac{dy}{dw}\right)^2 + \left(\frac{dz}{dw}\right)^2}\ dw = \sqrt{(u_1 + h\sin\psi_n)^2 + u_2^2 + (h\cos\psi_n)^2}\ dw \tag{2}$$

Combining Eqs. (1) and (2), it follows that $ds = h\cos(\psi_n)\sec(\theta_n)dw$. The total x-ray attenuation at the detector position (u_1, u_2) is thus

$$\mathcal{A}\mu(n) = \kappa_n \int_{w_n^+}^{w_n^-} \cos(2\pi f_0 u_2 w)dw = \frac{\kappa_n\left[\sin(2\pi f_0 u_2 w_n^-) - \sin(2\pi f_0 u_2 w_n^+)\right]}{2\pi f_0 u_2}, \tag{3}$$

where $\kappa_n = C \cdot h\cos(\psi_n)\sec(\theta_n)$. To simplify Eq. (3), recall the sum-to-product trigonometric identity $\sin(b_1) - \sin(b_2) = 2\cos[(b_1 + b_2)/2]\sin[(b_1 - b_2)/2]$ for real numbers b_1 and b_2.

$$\mathcal{A}\mu(n) = \kappa_n(w_n^- - w_n^+)\cos\left(\pi f_0 u_2\left[w_n^+ + w_n^-\right]\right)\text{sinc}\left(f_0 u_2\left[w_n^- - w_n^+\right]\right) \tag{4}$$

$$= \frac{\varepsilon\kappa_n \sec\psi_n}{h}\cos\left(2\pi f_0 u_2\left[1 - \frac{z_0 \sec\psi_n}{h}\right]\right)\text{sinc}\left(\frac{\varepsilon f_0 u_2 \sec\psi_n}{h}\right) \tag{5}$$

In Eq. (5), it is assumed that $\text{sinc}(u) \equiv \sin(\pi u)/(\pi u)$. This expression for total attenuation implicitly assumes that the detector possesses an x-ray converter with a modulation transfer function (MTF) of unity at all frequencies. An amorphous selenium (a-Se) photoconductor operated in drift mode is a good approximation for an x-ray converter with this property [3].

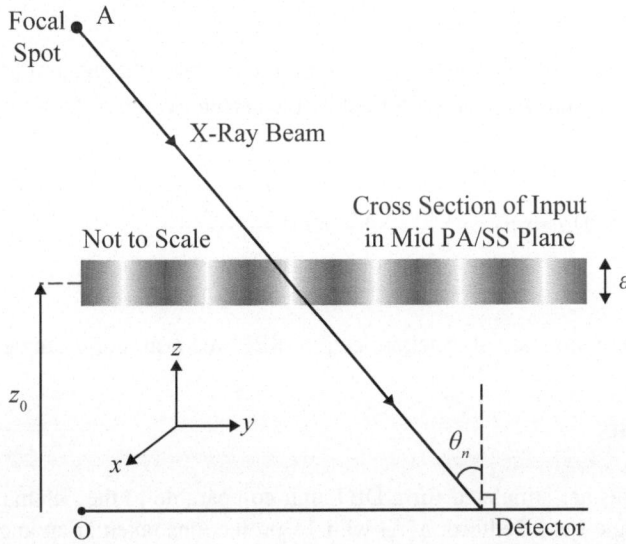

Fig. 2. In acquiring the central projection, a cross section of the input object in the mid PA/SS plane is shown. The attenuation coefficient varies sinusoidally along the PA direction (y).

In order to calculate the digitized detector signal, one must take into account the presence of a thin-film transistor (TFT) array which samples the total attenuation in pixels (*i.e.*, detector elements). The logarithmically-transformed signal for the nth projection is found by averaging the signal over the $\mathbf{m}^{\text{th}}$ detector element

$$\mathcal{D}\mu(\mathbf{m},n) = \int_{a(m_y - \delta[n-(N-1)/2])}^{a(m_y + 1 - \delta[n-(N-1)/2])} \int_{a(m_x - 1/2)}^{a(m_x + 1/2)} \frac{\mathcal{A}\mu(n)}{a^2} \cdot du_1 du_2 \quad , \quad m_x \in \mathbb{Z} \; , \; m_y \in \mathbb{Z}^* \; . \quad (6)$$

Detector elements are taken to be square with sides of length a. During the acquisition of the first projection for which $n = +(N-1)/2$, detector elements are centered on the coordinates $u_1 = m_x a$ and $u_2 = (m_y + 1/2)a$. In each subsequent projection, detector elements are translated in the PA direction ($+y$) by the amount δa, where δ is a parameter which expresses the translation between projections as a fraction of detector element length. Because θ_n should not vary considerably within each detector element, total attenuation can be approximated as

$$\tilde{\mathcal{A}}\mu(n) = \mathcal{A}\mu(n)\Big|_{\theta_n = \theta_{\mathbf{m}n}} \; , \; \theta_{\mathbf{m}n} \equiv \theta_n\Big|_{(u_1,u_2) = \left(m_x a, a\left[m_y + \frac{1}{2} - \delta\left(n - \frac{N-1}{2}\right)\right]\right)} \; , \quad (7)$$

where $\theta_{\mathbf{m}n}$ is the evaluation of the incident angle at the centroid of each detector element. Hence

$$\mathcal{D}\mu(\mathbf{m},n) \cong \int_{a\left(m_y-\delta[n-(N-1)/2]\right)}^{a\left(m_y+1-\delta[n-(N-1)/2]\right)} \frac{\tilde{\mathcal{A}}\mu(n)}{a} \cdot du_2 = \lim_{J_y \to \infty} \frac{1}{J_y} \sum_{j_y=1}^{J_y} \tilde{\mathcal{A}}\mu(j_y,n) \;, \qquad (8)$$

where

$$\tilde{\mathcal{A}}\mu(j_y,n) \equiv \tilde{\mathcal{A}}\mu(n)\Big|_{u_2=a\left(\frac{j_y-1/2}{J_y}+m_y-\delta\left[n-\frac{N-1}{2}\right]\right)} \cdot \qquad (9)$$

In Eq. (8), the midpoint formula has been used to evaluate the integral [4]. For the nth projection, the signal $\mathcal{S}\mu(u_1,u_2)$ recorded by the detector can now be written as

$$\mathcal{S}\mu(u_1,u_2) = \sum_{\mathbf{m}} \mathcal{D}\mu(\mathbf{m},n)\text{rect}\left(\frac{u_1-m_x a}{a}\right)\text{rect}\left(\frac{u_2-a\left(m_y+\frac{1}{2}-\delta\left[n-\frac{N-1}{2}\right]\right)}{a}\right). \qquad (10)$$

Using this expression, simple backprojection (SBP) reconstruction can be performed.

3   Results

Reconstructions are simulated for a DBT unit comparable to the Selenia Dimensions system (Hologic Inc., Bedford, MA) with 15 projections taken at an angular spacing ($\Delta\psi$) of 1.07°, assuming $z_0 = 50.0$ mm, $\varepsilon = 0.5$ mm, $h = 70.0$ cm, $C = 1/\varepsilon = 2.0$ mm^{-1}, and $a = 0.14$ mm. To illustrate the potential for super-resolution, an input frequency (f_0) of 5.0 lp/mm has been chosen, since this frequency is higher than the detector alias frequency $0.5a^{-1}$ (3.6 lp/mm).

In a conventional geometry in which the detector is not translated between projections ($\delta = 0$), Figure 3(a) shows SBP reconstruction versus position y measured perpendicular to the chest wall at the height $z = z_0 = 50.0$ mm within the mid PA/SS plane ($x = 0$). Super-resolution is not achievable since translational shifts in the image of the object are minimal between projections. SBP reconstruction resembles a single projection whose signal varies with position y in a step-like manner, with the width of each step matching the detector element length. The corresponding 1D Fourier transform of SBP reconstruction along the y direction has a major peak at 2.7 lp/mm as evidence of aliasing [Figure 3(b)]. Although Figure 3(a) is plotted over the region $y \in$ [29.4 mm, 30.6 mm], similar plots hold over a broad range of y values.

By translating the detector in the PA direction between projections, super-resolution in the mid PA/SS plane can be achieved. Figure 3(a) considers translations of 25% of detector element length between projections ($\delta = 0.25$). The major peak of the Fourier transform [Figure 3(c)] correctly occurs at the input frequency, 5.0 lp/mm.

Due to the PA detector translations, it would initially seem that the new geometry has the drawback of loss of x-ray coverage at the chest wall with each successive projection. However, it can be shown that the net translation of the detector during the scan time is minimal; in this example, the net translation is $(N-1)\delta a$ or 0.49 mm. For this reason, the loss of x-ray coverage at the chest wall is negligible.

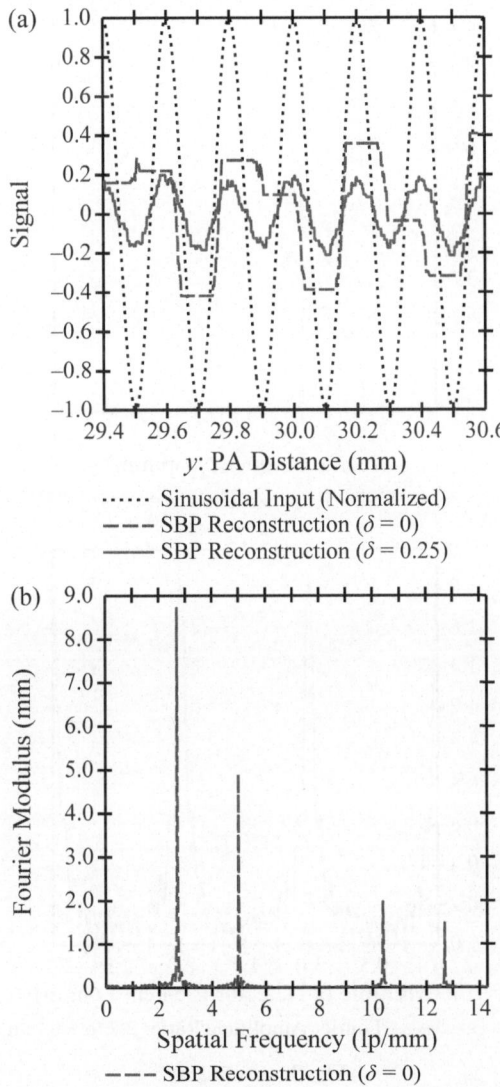

Fig. 3. Within the mid PA/SS plane, SBP reconstructions are plotted versus position y measured perpendicular to the chest wall for PA detector motions of 0% and 25% of detector element length between projections. The corresponding one-dimensional Fourier transforms along the y direction are also shown. The quality of super-resolution can be determined from the ratio (r) of the Fourier amplitudes at the aliased frequency (2.7 lp/mm) to the input frequency (5.0 lp/mm). By plotting this ratio versus δ, it is shown that super-resolution is not achievable at integer values of δ. That is, in order to maximize sub-pixel sampling gain between projections, the PA detector translation should occur in fractional multiples of detector element length.

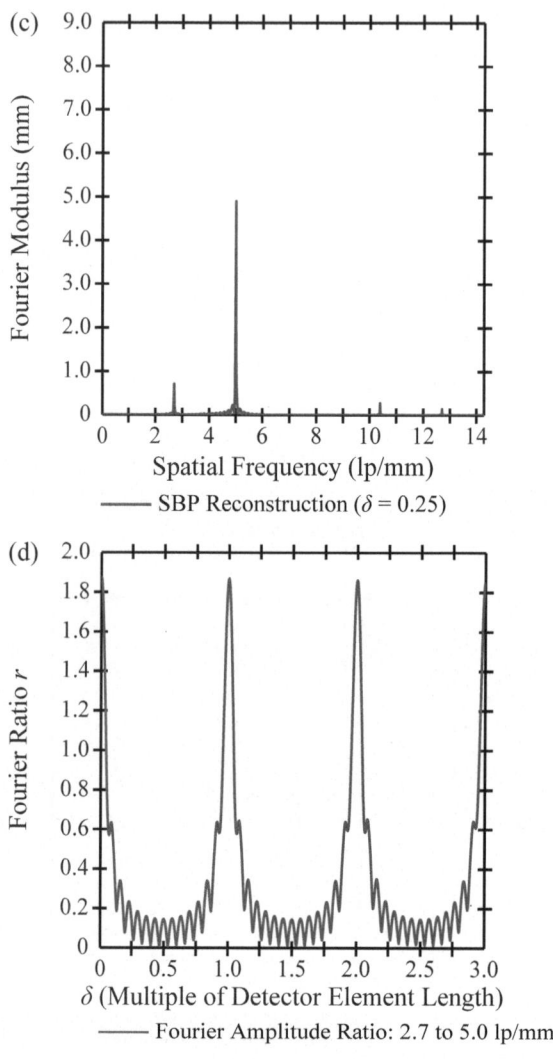

Fig. 3. (*continued*)

In order to assess the quality of super-resolution in the reconstruction, the ratio (r) of the amplitude of the Fourier peaks at 2.7 lp/mm to 5.0 lp/mm can be calculated. Super-resolution is present provided $r < 1$, and is absent provided $r \geq 1$. The dependency of r on δ is investigated in Figure 3(d). For measurements taken within the mid PA/SS plane, this plot illustrates that super-resolution along the PA direction is not feasible ($r > 1$) if detector translation between projections occurs in integer multiples of detector element length. To maximize sub-pixel sampling gain between projections, the PA translational shifts of the detector should occur in fractional multiples of detector element length. As shown in Figure 3(d), there is a relatively broad range of δ values over which r is sufficiently less than unity. For example, over the range $\delta \in [0.24, 0.76]$, the ratio of the amplitude of the Fourier peaks at 2.7 lp/mm to 5.0 lp/mm is less than 1:5 (*i.e.*, 0.20). Consequently, the existence of super-resolution in the mid PA/SS plane is relatively insensitive to the precise translational shifts between projections, provided that these shifts are not sufficiently close to integer multiples of detector element length.

A DBT detector may be designed with either discrete or continuous translations in the PA direction during the scan time. Although this work implicitly considers discrete translations, continuous translations should also show super-resolution in the mid PA/SS plane, since the detector translation during a typical exposure time for each projection should be significantly smaller than the detector element length.

4   Discussion

We have shown that translating the detector in the PA direction between projections broadens the positions over which super-resolution is achievable in DBT. Although SBP reconstructions are useful for illustrating this concept as proof-of-principle, future work should be directed at incorporating filters into the reconstruction [5]. In addition, other subtleties of the imaging system, such as noise [6] and focal spot blurring [5], can be modeled.

There are additional acquisition geometries which promote super-resolution in DBT. Future studies will investigate whether super-resolution can be optimized with x-ray tube motion having a component in the y direction in addition to the x and z directions.

Acknowledgments. The project described was supported by predoctoral training grant No. W81XWH-11-1-0100 through the Department of Defense Breast Cancer Research Program. The content is solely the responsibility of the authors and does not necessarily represent the official views of the funding agency.

References

1. Rafferty, E.: Tomosynthesis: New Weapon in Breast Cancer Fight. Imaging Economics 17(4) (2004)
2. Acciavatti, R.J., Maidment, A.D.A.: Investigating the potential for super-resolution in digital breast tomosynthesis. In: Pelc, N.J., Samei, E., Nishikawa, R.M. (eds.) Proc. of SPIE, Medical Imaging 2011: Physics of Medical Imaging, vol. 7961, pp. 79615K-1–79615K-12. SPIE, Bellingham (2011)
3. Lee, D.L., Cheung, L.K., Rodricks, B., Powell, G.F.: Improved imaging performance of a 14×17-inch Direct Radiography™ System using Se/TFT detector. In: Dobbins III, J.T., Boone, J.M. (eds.) Proc. of SPIE, Medical Imaging 1998: Physics of Medical Imaging, vol. 3336, pp. 14–23. SPIE, Bellingham (1998)
4. Stewart, J.: Calculus: Early Transcendentals, Belmont (2003)
5. Zhao, B., Zhao, W.: Three-dimensional linear system analysis for breast tomosynthesis. Med. Phys. 35(12), 5219–5232 (2008)
6. Barrett, H.H., Myers, K.J.: Foundations of Image Science. Bahaa E.A. Saleh, Hoboken (2004)

Converting One Set of Mammograms to Simulate a Range of Detector Imaging Characteristics for Observer Studies

Alistair Mackenzie[1], David R. Dance[1],
Oliver Diaz[2], Annabel Barnard[1], and Kenneth C. Young[1]

[1] National Coordinating Centre for the Physics of Mammography, Royal Surrey County Hospital, Guildford, GU2 7XX, UK and Department of Physics, University of Surrey, Guildford, GU2 7XH, UK
[2] Centre for Vision, Speech and Signal Processing, Faculty of Engineering and Physical Sciences, University of Surrey, Guildford, GU2 7XH, UK
alistairmackenzie@nhs.net

Abstract. A methodology for adjusting mammographic images taken on a given imaging system to simulate their appearance if taken on a different system for use in observer studies is presented. The process involves adjusting the image sharpness and noise, which takes into account the detector, breast thickness, and beam quality. The method has been tested by converting images acquired using an a-Se detector of a CDMAM test object and 'Rachel' anthropomorphic breast phantom. They were degraded to appear as if acquired using a computed radiography (CR) detector. Good agreement was achieved in the resulting threshold gold thickness for the simulated CR images with measured real values for CDMAM images. Power spectra comparisons of real and simulated images of the 'Rachel' phantom agree with an average difference of 4%. This tool in conjunction with observer studies can be used to understand the effects of the detector characteristics on cancer detection in mammography.

Keywords: simulation, noise power spectra, modulation transfer function.

1 Introduction

Clinical evaluation of image quality is expensive and time-consuming. Clinical trials to compare the effectiveness of different systems are rarely conducted as they would require large numbers of patients to achieve both sufficient numbers of detected cancers and statistical significance. In particular it would be desirable to repeat exposures on the same breast with the same positioning and compression to minimise confounding differences in the projection of the breast tissues, but this raises ethical issues. Alternative methods of evaluation involving some degree of image simulation have the potential to enable comparisons at reduced cost and time and without additional radiation exposure. For this purpose it is desirable to be able to acquire images on a given system and to simulate their appearance on a second system, so the

A.D.A. Maidment, P.R. Bakic, and S. Gavenonis (Eds.): IWDM 2012, LNCS 7361, pp. 394–401, 2012.

performance of the two systems can be compared. This may be possible when the performance of the second system is inferior to that of the first system. Such a method would enable the background tissue and compression to be matched in different arms of a study, either using real cancers or the insertion of simulated cancers.

The aim of this work is therefore to develop and test a methodology for adjusting mammographic images taken on a given imaging system to simulate their appearance if taken on a different system. The methodology presented extends previous work [1] with improved modelling of the noise power spectra, which takes into account the breast thickness and beam quality.

2   Method

2.1   Summary of Methodology for Changing Image Quality

The conversion methodology blurs the original image to match the blurring of a target system using measurements of the modulation transfer function. The difference in noise between the original system and the target system is then calculated and added in real space to the blurred image, ensuring that the magnitude and correlation of the noise matches the total noise in the target system. The method also accounts for the magnitude of the signal in the image. It has been validated using images of a contrast detail test object for situations where the noise characteristics were measured at the same beam quality as the image to be converted.

2.2   Linearisation of Images

The analysis below assumes that images have been linearised so that the pixel value is a measure of the energy absorbed per unit area of the detector. This can be achieved by a combination of measurements of the incident air kerma at the front face of the detector and Monte Carlo simulations. The Geant4 Monte Carlo code (http://geant4.cern.ch/) was used to calculate the absorbed energy per unit area for a reference beam quality, and to relate this to the incident air kerma at the front face of the image receptor. X-ray spectra from the work of Boone *et al* [2] filtered by the X-ray tube window, filter, compression paddle, object being imaged (test phantom or breast) and breast support were used for this purpose. The attenuation coefficients were obtained from Berger *et al* [3]. The signal transfer properties (STP) thus calculated for a given detector were assumed to apply to any beam quality for that detector so that the pixel value was a measure of the energy absorbed per unit area for all beam qualities.

2.3   Characterisation of Noise Power Spectra (NPS)

The noise was characterised by the NPS (W) which was split into components for electronic, quantum and structure noise at a reference beam quality. For this purpose, a series of collimated flat field images were acquired over a wide dose range using a

28 kV, Mo/Mo anode/filter combination and 4.5 cm polymethyl methacrylate (PMMA) at the tube head and the NPS was calculated for each dose. The three noise components for the reference condition were estimated by fitting a second order polynomial of NPS against absorbed energy for each spatial frequency.

2.4   Correction of Noise and Signal for Beam Quality

Clinical mammograms are acquired over a range of compressed breast thicknesses and radiographic factors and so the model needs to be able to take account of a range of beam qualities. When originally developed the methodology used measurements of the NPS appropriate to the beam quality used. In the present work we have improved the modelling of the NPS to take account of beam quality and breast thickness/composition. For this purpose, it was assumed that the three noise sources are affected by beam quality as follows:

- Electronic noise is independent of beam quality. No correction is required.
- The quantum noise is comprised of a number of different sources (primary quantum noise, excess noise, and secondary quantum noise) and is dependent on the number of photons detected and energy absorbed.
- Structure noise is proportional to the signal from the detector. No correction for beam quality is required.

The beam quality affects both the proportion of energy absorbed and the quantum noise. To estimate the effect of beam quality on the quantum noise, a series of flat field images were taken as described in section 2.3, but using a range of PMMA thicknesses, tube voltages and anode/filter combinations. These images were then linearised using the reference STP, so that the linearised pixel value equalled the absorbed energy per unit area irrespective of the beam quality.

Using the above flat field images, the NPS was calculated for each beam quality, and the results used to determine the parameters in a model of the NPS applicable to any beam quality (Eq. 1).

$$W(u,v) = \omega_e(u,v) + B(\lambda)\omega_q(u,v)\frac{E}{E_o} + \omega_s(u,v)\left(\frac{E}{E_o}\right)^2 \qquad (1)$$

In this equation ω_e, ω_q and ω_s (with units of mm^2) are 'noise coefficients' for electronic, quantum and structure noise respectively at absorbed energy per unit area at a reference beam quality E_o, E is the absorbed energy per unit area at the beam quality under consideration and u and v are spatial frequencies. In accordance with the assumptions in the bullet points above, the electronic and structure noise coefficients are independent of beam quality. The quantum noise coefficient, ω_q, is also independent of beam quality; the variation of the quantum noise with beam quality additional to the factor E in Eq. 1 is accounted for by the beam quality correction factor (B). The beam quality parameter λ is average photon energy of the beam incident on the detector and was calculated using the X-ray spectra model described in section 2.2. For breast images, λ can be calculated if an assumption about the breast composition is made [4].

2.5   Validation of the Conversion Using Images of CDMAM Test Object and Anthropomorphic Phantoms

The validation of the conversion from one detector to another was undertaken using the following two systems:

ASE: Hologic Selenia X-ray system, amorphous selenium (a-Se) detector. Pixel pitch 70 μm.

CR: Carestream CR900 reader with EHR-M2 CR plates. Pixel pitch 50 μm.

Sixteen images of the CDMAM contrast detail test object were acquired on both systems at two beam qualities. The CDMAM test object was imaged on the breast support on a base of 2 cm PMMA ('thin') using 26 kV, Mo/Mo and then with an additional 4 cm PMMA ('thick' – total of 6 cm PMMA) on top of the test object and imaged using 34 kV, Mo/Rh. The image conversion methodology was applied to the ASE CDMAM images to convert them to appear at the same image quality and dose as the CR images. The sets of target and simulated CDMAM images for CR were automatically read using CDCOM software version 1.5.2 (www.euref.org). Contrast detail curves were produced for both the simulated and target images, which were then compared [5].

The Rachel anthropomorphic breast phantom (Gammex RMI, WI, USA) was designed to mimic a 5 cm compressed breast. It was imaged five times using both detectors at 31 kV, Mo/Rh. The phantom was shifted slightly between images. The ASE images were converted to appear with the imaging characteristics of the CR detector and X-ray system used. The largest rectangular region of interest (ROI) away from the skin edge was extracted from the same location for the real CR and simulated CR images. Smaller overlapping sub-ROIs of size 256×256 were extracted from this ROI and the measured power spectra from all of the sub-ROIs were averaged for each system.

2.6   Clinical Images: Subjective Evaluation and Demonstration of Image Conversion

Mammography images have been collected for an image database. For the systems included in this study, images from 234 women (ASE) and 233 (CR) were collected. The ASE had 31 abnormal cases, while all of the CR images were as normal.

Firstly, a preliminary test of realism of the converted images was undertaken. A set of normal ASE and CR images were selected. A reasonable match between ASE and CR images in terms of compressed breast thickness, appearance of the breast and radiographic factors was made. The ASE images were converted to appear with the imaging characteristics of the CR system and its associated X-ray system. Both sets of images were processed using Agfa Musica 2. A simulated CR and a real CR image were shown to a set of 6 observers and they were asked to identify the real CR image. The observers were shown 10 pairs of images.

Secondly, a sub-set (six images) of the ASE images containing a confirmed cancer classified as being 'subtle' were selected. To demonstrate the conversion process, these images were changed to appear with the imaging characteristics of the CR detector using the same X-ray system and grid as the ASE system. Therefore no correction was made for differences in scatter and grid attenuation. The simulated images were visually examined for the effects of the conversion.

3   Results and Discussion

3.1   Conversion of CDMAM Test Object Images

The threshold gold thicknesses of simulated CR CDMAM images and the corresponding real CR images for two beam qualities and PMMA thicknesses show a close match (Fig. 1). The average differences between the results were 2.5% and 0.3% for the thin and thick phantoms respectively. This is an encouraging result because the CDMAM test object provides a good overall measure of the image quality in terms of noise, sharpness and contrast.

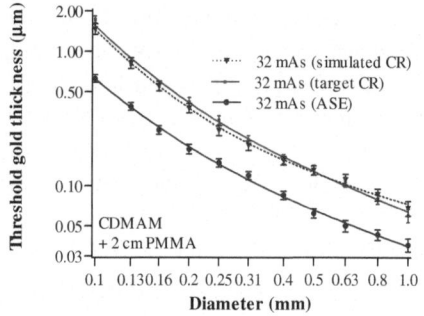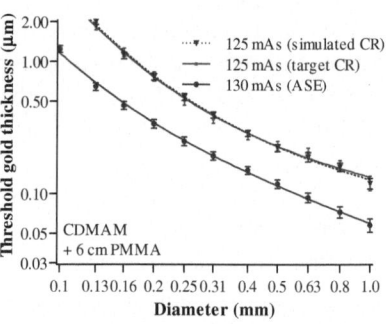

Fig. 1. Threshold gold thickness curves for CDMAM images acquired for the thin (2 cm PMMA) phantom (*left*), the thick (6 cm PMMA) phantom (*right*). Results are shown for simulated and target (real) images obtained with the CR detector and for the original ASE images from which the CR images were simulated.

3.2   Power Spectra of Conversion of Images of Rachel Anthropomorphic Phantom

No artefacts were seen in the simulated image of the Rachel phantom. The power spectra of real and simulated Rachel phantom images obtained with the CR system are shown in Fig. 2. The results show a good match between the images, with a maximum difference of 17% between the simulated and real images, the average difference was 2% over all spatial frequencies.

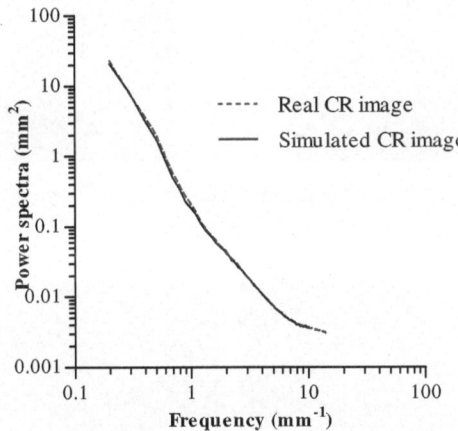

Fig. 2. Power spectra of 'Rachel' phantom of target CR and simulated CR

3.3   Subjective Evaluation of Realism of Converted Images

Using 6 observers and 10 image pairs of a real and simulated CR image, the real image was correctly identified 32 times out of 60 and the simulated CR image was incorrectly selected as the real CR image 28 times out of 60. There was a slight majority of the real image being correctly identified. While these number of results are very small, it does give an indication that the images produced do look realistic.

3.4   Examples of Conversion of Clinical Images Suitable for an Observer Study

Figs. 3 & 4 show on the left a high quality image of a lesion acquired on a ASE system. The image on the right shows the image after it has been degraded to have the image quality of a CR system. There are noticeable differences between the ASE and simulated CR images in terms of sharpness and noise. The cancers are still visible in the CR images but the interest of this work is whether the detector used affects the detection and diagnosis of cancer in breast imaging. An observer study has been undertaken using this image modification process. The study showed a difference in the detection of subtle calcifications between ASE detector and a generic CR detector [6]. The advantage of this method is that the only difference between the two sets of images is the detector, and that differences due to breasts, compression, anti-scatter grid, X-ray tube have been removed.

This methodology can be applied to simulate images from different detectors or even theoretical detectors. A range of observer studies can be undertaken on the effect of the receptor performance and dose on the detection of different signs of breast cancer (e.g. masses, calcifications).

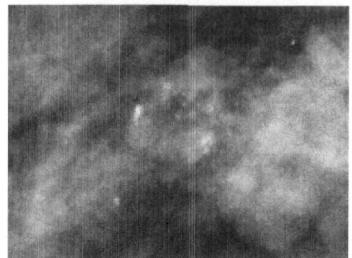 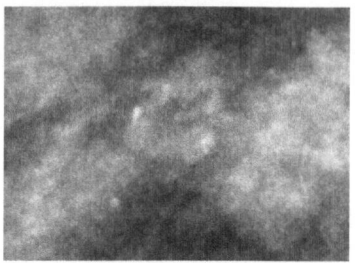

Fig. 3. Example images of micro-calcification cluster for the original ASE system (*left*) and simulated CR (*right*)

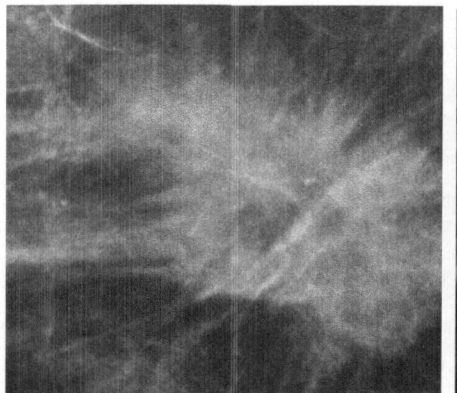 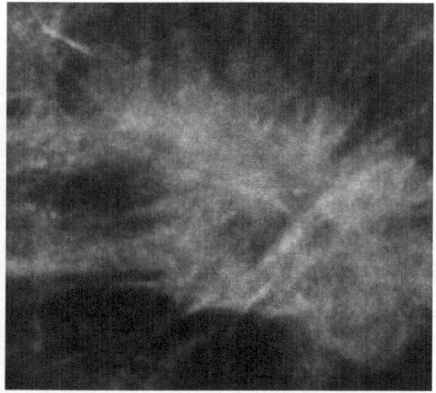

Fig. 4. Example images of mass for the original ASE system (*left*) and simulated CR (*right*)

4   Conclusions

We have developed a conversion methodology to change an image to appear as if acquired on a different imaging system which accounts for the change in detector, X-ray system and beam quality. The methodology has been successfully applied to contrast detail measurements. Images with the appearance of a realistic clinical CR mammogram can be produced without artefacts. The use of this tool in conjunction with observer studies can be used to understand the effects of detector characteristics on cancer detection.

Acknowledgements. This work is part of the OPTIMAM project and is supported by Cancer Research-UK & EPSRC Cancer Imaging Programme in Surrey, in association with the MRC and Department of Health (England).

The authors are grateful for the help and support of staff from St George's Hospital, London, and Jarvis Breast Screening Unit, Guildford. The authors acknowledge Hologic Inc., MIS Healthcare, and Carestream Healthcare for their help in accessing images and Agfa Healthcare for the use of their image processing package. We thank our NCCPM colleagues Lucy Warren and Faith Green who have helped with the collection of images, and all of our colleagues who took part in the observer study. We thank our colleagues at Katholieke Universiteit Leuven for helpful discussion of this work.

References

1. Mackenzie, A., Dance, D.R., Workman, A., Yip, M., Wells, K., Young, K.C.: Development and validation of a method for converting images to appear with noise and sharpness characteristics of a different detector and X-ray system. Med. Phys. 39, 2721–2734 (2012)
2. Boone, J.M., Fewell, T.R., Jennings, R.J.: Molybdenum, rhodium, and tungsten anode spectral models using interpolating polynomials with application to mammography. Med. Phys. 24, 1863–1874 (1997)
3. Berger, M.J., Hubbell, J.H., Seltzer, S.M., Chang, J., Coursey, J.S., et al.: XCOM: Photon cross sections database. NIST Standard Reference Database 8, 87-3597 (1998)
4. Dance, D.R., Skinner, C.L., Young, K.C., Beckett, J.R., Kotre, C.J.: Additional factors for the estimation of mean glandular breast dose using the UK mammography dosimetry protocol. Phys. Med. Biol. 45, 3225–3240 (2000)
5. Young, K.C., Alsager, A., Oduko, J.M., Bosmans, H., Verbrugge, B., et al.: Evaluation of software for reading images of the CDMAM test object to assess digital mammography systems. In: Proc. SPIE, vol. 6913, pp. 69131C-1–69131C-11 (2008)
6. Warren, L.M., Mackenzie, A., Cooke, J., Given-Wilson, R., Wallis, M.G., et al.: Mammographic calcification cluster detection and threshold gold thickness measurements. In: Proc. SPIE, vol. 8313, p. 83130J (2012)

Quantification of Tc-99m Sestamibi Distribution in Normal Breast Tissue Using Dedicated Breast SPECT-CT

Steve D. Mann[1], Kristy L. Perez[2], Emily K.E. McCracken[3], Jainil P. Shah[2], Kingshuk R. Choudhury[2], Terence Z. Wong[2], and Martin P. Tornai[1,2,4]

[1] Medical Physics Graduate Program, Duke University, Durham, NC, USA
[2] Department of Radiology, Duke University Medical Center, Durham, NC, USA
[3] Duke University Medical School, Durham, NC, USA
[4] Department of Biomedical Engineering, Duke University, Durham, NC, USA
{steve.mann,kristy.perez,emily.mccracken,jainil.shah,
kingshuk.roy.choudhury,terence.wong,martin.tornai}@duke.edu

Abstract. The use of Tc-99m-Sestamibi in molecular breast imaging is common due to its preferential uptake in malignant tissue. However, quantification of the baseline uptake in normal, healthy breast tissue is not possible using planar-imaging devices. Using our dedicated breast SPECT-CT system, an IRB approved pilot study is underway to quantify mean activity in normal breast tissue, and to differentiate uptake between adipose and glandular tissues. A cohort of patients at normal breast cancer risk undergoing another diagnostic Sestamibi study was imaged using the breast SPECT-CT system. SPECT images were corrected and quantitatively reconstructed using previously developed methods, and registered with the CT images. The CT images were segmented, and the average activity concentration was measured for glandular, adipose, and total breast tissue. Results indicate no preferential uptake between tissues and low average uptake, which may be used to determine a universal threshold for cancer detection.

Keywords: breast cancer, breast imaging, quantification, SPECT, CT, Sestamibi.

1 Introduction

The utilization of nuclear medicine imaging devices in the diagnosis and staging of breast cancer is on the rise. Nuclear medicine offers unique functional information different from other imaging modalities. The use of Tc-99m-Sestamibi (MIBI) as a tracer for breast cancer has been well established, and serves as the primary tracer for a number of commercially available 2D molecular breast imaging (MBI) or breast specific gamma imaging (BSGI) systems [1]. The tracer has shown preferential uptake in malignant breast tissue, potentially offering a useful tool for diagnosis or staging of breast cancer [2], especially with the use of high performance dedicated breast

A.D.A. Maidment, P.R. Bakic, and S. Gavenonis (Eds.): IWDM 2012, LNCS 7361, pp. 402–409, 2012.

imaging devices. However, absolute quantification of tracer uptake is not possible with current commercially available planar (2D) MBI/BSGI imaging devices [3]. Several commercially available systems use planar detectors with mild/moderate compression, similar to mammography, which are only capable of relative measures of tracer uptake [4, 5]. Furthermore, studies have shown standard whole body clinical gamma cameras for breast scintigraphy are similarly unsuited for quantitative breast imaging: limitations in energy and spatial resolution lead to partial volume averaging, and bulkiness prevents proximal access to the breast. We have developed a compact, hybrid high-performance SPECT-CT system for dedicated breast imaging, which allows for fully 3D breast imaging and accurate quantification of tracer uptake [6].

While MIBI has a 6:1 tumor-to-background uptake in breast tissue, the baseline quantitative uptake values for normal healthy tissue have not been established per se [7]. Such data could be useful for establishing a lower threshold for distinguishing cancerous regions from regions of healthy tissue. This study aims to image a small cohort of patients to quantitatively determine the average activity concentration of MIBI in normal risk, cancer-free women for use in establishing this threshold. Furthermore, the ability to differentiate between fatty and glandular tissue with the dedicated breast CT sub-system offers the possibility to determine the (non)uniformity of the non-specific uptake of the tracer as quantitatively determined by dedicated breast SPECT.

2   Materials and Methods

A dedicated breast SPECT-CT system has been developed [8] with the potential to diagnose and/or stage cancer in patients, with minimal discomfort to the patient. The system is designed such that the patient lies prone on a bed with a hole in the center, allowing one of the patient's breasts to be positioned pendant through the opening. Below the bed, a CT and SPECT system are mounted orthogonally to each other on a common gantry, and rotate around the uncompressed breast while acquiring data, and yield 3D image volumes.

The CT system uses a RAD94 (*Varian Medical Systems, Inc.*) and a 20x25cm^2 digital flat-panel detector (Paxscan 2520, *Varian Medical Systems, Inc.*) which rotate in a simple circle azimuthally around the uncompressed, pendant breast in a step-and-shoot fashion. All CT images are scatter corrected with measurements using a beam stop array (BSA), and iteratively reconstructed using an OSC algorithm [9]. Additionally, the quasi-monochromatic cone beam source imparts an overall CT dose <5mGy [10] and minimal beam hardening, yielding little cupping artifact in CT [11].

The SPECT system consists of a LumaGEM 3200S gamma camera (*Gamma Medica, Inc.*) with a hexagonal close-packed parallel hole collimator. The high-Z compound, near room-temperature CZT semi-conductor detector has 2.5mm pixilation and 6.7% energy resolution at 140keV. The gamma camera system has been described in detail elsewhere [12]. In brief summary, it has three degrees of freedom (azimuthal, polar tilt, radius of rotation) that allow for customized, contoured non-traditional trajectories to be acquired; specifically, the projected sinusoidal

(PROJSINE) trajectory, illustrated in Figure 1, has been shown to yield optimal reconstructions with accurate quantification. Due to the implementation of non-traditional 3D trajectories, resultant data are reconstructed using an iterative OSEM algorithm.

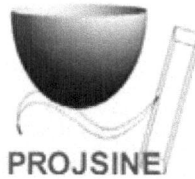

PROJSINE

Fig. 1. Image illustrating the projected sine-wave (PROJSINE) 3D trajectory used in acquisitions. The PROJSINE orbit allows for nearly-complete sampling of the breast volume while providing useful data from the chest wall that may otherwise not be collected.

Women undergoing diagnostic parathyroid SPECT studies are consented and scanned using the dedicated breast SPECT-CT system as part of this ongoing IRB-approved study. Subject volunteers are excluded if they have a positive breast cancer history, current pregnancy, or weight >160kg. Subjects are injected with 25mCi MIBI for their parathyroid study and imaged with breast SPECT-CT between their routine scintigraphy (10 minutes post injection) and diagnostic SPECT scan (2 hours post injection). The left or right breast is randomly selected for dedicated imaging, and dual-modality fiducial markers are attached to the breast to allow for accurate image registration of the reconstructed images.

The procedure for data collection and quantification is outlined in Figure 2. For SPECT, a flood and point source acquisition are used for quality assurance purposes. ListMode data is processed to generate projections at the lower, scatter energy window for scatter correcting the SPECT data using the well-established dual-energy window method [13]. SPECT data are first reconstructed to 2 iterations (8 subsets); the images are then used to define a mask for attenuation correction using the NIST value for water of $0.1545cm^{-1}$ at 140keV. The SPECT data are then reconstructed with attenuation and scatter corrections to 20 iterations (8 subsets) and decay corrected to the injection time point. For CT, 240 projections are acquired azimuthally about 360 degrees. Additionally, 6 BSA projections (at 60 degree increments) are acquired. The BSA projections are spline fit across 60 degrees for the full 360 degree acquisition, and used to estimate and subtract scatter from the CT projections. Scatter-corrected images are iteratively reconstructed using OSC to 5 iterations (16 subsets). Resultant SPECT and CT images are registered using the fiducial markers and AMIDE visualization software.

In CT datasets, the skin boundary, which would normally be visible in the glandular-only data sets, was manually removed so that it would not contribute to the distribution measurements. After skin removal, all breast tissue below the lower threshold of $0.26cm^{-1}$ was assumed to be fatty, while all tissue above the upper threshold

0.28cm^{-1} was assumed to be glandular (Figure 3); attenuation coefficient thresholds were chosen based on one patient who exhibited easily distinguishable distributions of glandular and fatty tissue in the histogram. The crossover point (minimum) was estimated for the two distributions, and the thresholds of $\pm0.01\text{cm}^{-1}$ where chosen in an attempt to minimize overlap between tissue regions. Corresponding VOIs for each tissue volume were superimposed on the registered SPECT data, and the average activity concentration of adipose, glandular, and the total breast were determined for each patient.

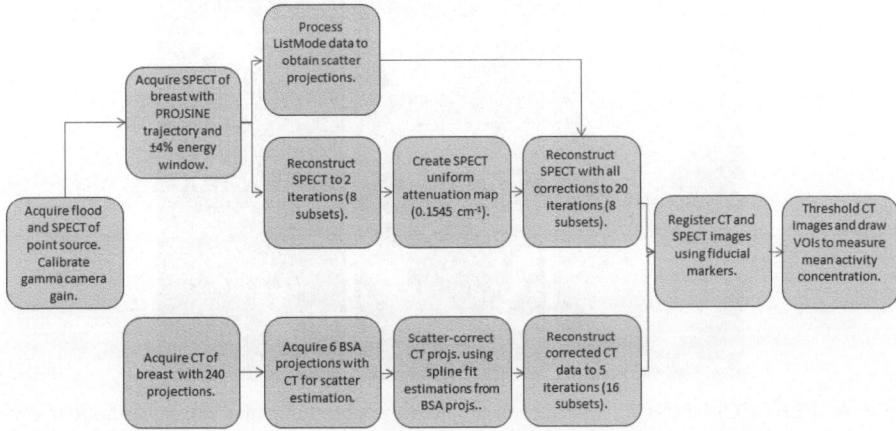

Fig. 2. The flowchart above outlines the protocol for acquiring data and quantifying SPECT images and registering SPECT and CT image volumes

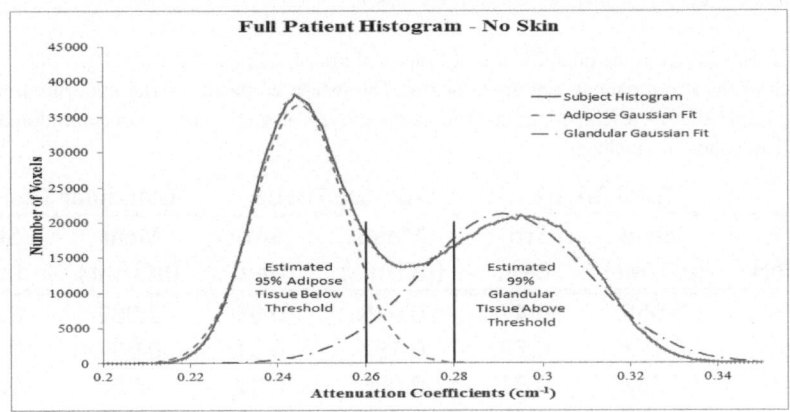

Fig. 3. A representative histogram from a subject data set. Two peaks are easily discernible, representing the different tissue types within the breast. Vertical bars indicate the lower and upper threshold values used to segment the breast into fatty and glandular tissue.

3   Results

To date, seven women undergoing diagnostic parathyroid studies were consented and
scanned for this study. Four subject data sets were of sufficient quality to allow the

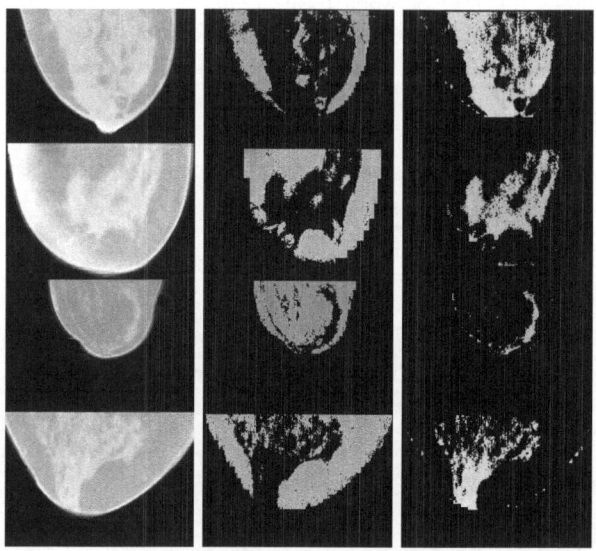

Fig. 4. (LEFT COLUMN) CT sagittal image slices through the medial breast of the four seg-
mentable subjects. Images reveal the glandular, skin and adipose tissue within the breast. The
CT images were segmented into adipose (CENTER COLUMN) and glandular (RIGHT
COLUMN) tissue types using the described dual-threshold procedure. Segmented images were
used for VOI quantification of SPECT images after registration. Note that segmented edges
appear blocky due to the manual removal of the skin.

Table 1. Results from the quantification of the total breast, adipose tissue, and glandular tissue
for each of the seven patients are given below. The measured mean activity concentration and
standard deviation for each patient, as well as the overall average activity concentration across
the patient cohort are included.

	Total Breast		Adipose Tissue		Glandular Tissue	
Subject	Mean (μCi/mL)	Std. Dev.	Mean (μCi/mL)	Std. Dev.	Mean (μCi/mL)	Std. Dev.
1	0.055	0.47	0.045	0.35	0.082	0.49
2	0.152	0.58	0.152	0.51	0.097	0.41
3	0.052	0.31	0.056	0.31	0.06	0.29
4	0.148	0.61	0.125	0.49	0.165	0.68
5	0.061	0.42	-	-	-	-
6	0.036	0.24	-	-	-	-
7	0.11	0.62	-	-	-	-
Total:	0.09	0.18	0.09	0.21	0.10	0.23

CT images to be segmented using the dual threshold method described; unusable subject CT images had severe motion artifacts (major patient shift) or truncation due to a breast size larger than the CT and/or SPECT system FOVs. Figure 4 illustrates the CT images for which tissue segmentation was performed, and Figure 5 shows an example of a fused SPECT-CT patient data set. Note that the skin boundary was manually removed prior to the segmentation. The results of the quantification of the seven patients are given in Table 1.

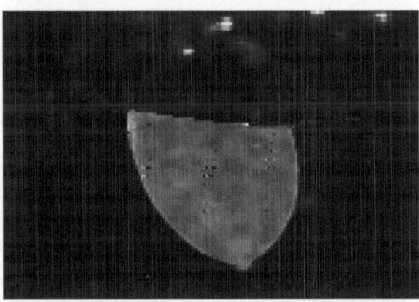

Fig. 5. Representative fused SPECT-CT image of a patient's breast. SPECT activity (hot color scale) seen above the breast is due to allowing views into and beyond the chest wall allowed by the 3D PROJSINE trajectory.

4   Discussion

The results given in Table 1 indicate an average tracer activity concentration of $0.09\mu Ci/mL$ in normal breast tissue, with no preferential uptake of MIBI by either glandular or adipose tissue. The lack of preferential uptake between tissue types is different from results seen with FDG PET imaging, but is not necessarily surprising since the metabolic mechanisms of FDG and MIBI uptake and utilization are different [14]. The standard deviation of these initial results is large due to some potential factors: the low overall radioactivity within the breast; the acquired projections having few counts, leading to noisy reconstructed images; a majority of the voxels within the breast having zero or near zero values. These zero valued voxels, as well as a few unrealistically high (noisy) voxels, are included within the measurements and yield a large standard deviation. Such trends in the data indicate that assuming a Gaussian distribution of tracer uptake values may not be appropriate. More patients are also needed to increase the precision and confidence of the measurements, especially with the limited tissue-segmentation group. The current results indicate that approximately 30 subjects must be quantified to have 95% confidence that the mean tracer uptake in normal breast tissue has been established. We are actively recruiting more subjects. Further study on subjects with known breast cancer would also be beneficial to determine average measured values of non-malignant background regions and how similar they are to the normal tissue uptake measured here. Additionally, imaging those cancer patients' foci of uptake will establish the typical differences in absolute activity concentration seen between suspected lesions and the non-specific uptake in otherwise normal, background volumes.

5   Conclusions

No preferential uptake or distribution of MIBI was observed in fatty or glandular breast tissue with dedicated breast SPECT-CT. This is different from results seen with FDG PET imaging, but is not necessarily surprising. No preferential uptake may indicate that breast composition would not interfere with a global threshold-based method for determining malignancy. While the overall noise seen in the SPECT images is high, the trends for values within the seven patients suggest that it may be possible to designate a low, normal-tissue threshold for characterizing regions of interest within breast tissue. However, more patients are needed to increase the precision and confidence of our measurements.

Acknowledgements. This work has been funded by the National Cancer Institute of the National Institutes of Health (R01-CA096821 and T32-EB007185). MPT is the inventor of this SPECT-CT technology and is named as an inventor on the patent for this technology awarded to Duke (#7,609,808). If this technology becomes commercially successful, MPT and Duke could benefit financially. The IRB protocol for this study is Pro000026702.

References

1. O'Connor, M., Rhodes, D., Hruska, C.: Molecular breast imaging. Expert Rev. Anticancer Ther. 9, 1073–1080 (2009)
2. Khalkhali, I., et al.: Technetium-99m-Sestamibi Scintimammography of Breast Lesions: Clinical and Pathological Follow-up. J. Nucl. Med. 36, 1784–1789 (1994)
3. Rosenthal, M.S., et al.: Quantitative SPECT imaging: a review and recommendations by the Focus Committee of the Society of Nuclear Medicine Computer and Instrumentation Council. J. Nucl. Med. 36, 1489–1513 (1995)
4. Hruska, C.B., O'Conner, M.K.: Quantification of Lesion Size, Depth and Uptake Using a Dual-Head Molecular Breast Imaging System. Med. Phys. 35, 1365–1376 (2008)
5. Brem, R.F., et al.: Breast-specific gamma imaging as an adjunct imaging modality for the diagnosis of breast cancer. Radiology 247, 651–657 (2008)
6. Perez, K.L., Cutler, S.J., Madhav, P., Tornai, M.P.: Towards Quantification of Dedicated Breast SPECT Using Non-Traditional Acquisition Trajectories. IEEE Trans. Nucl. Sci. 58, 2219–2225 (2011)
7. Maublant, J., et al.: Technetium-99m-Sestamibi Uptake in Breast Tumor and Associated Lymph Nodes. J. Nucl. Med. 37(6), 922–925 (1996)
8. Madhav, P., Crotty, D.J., McKinley, R.L., Tornai, M.P.: Evaluation of Tilted Cone-Beam CT Orbits in the Development of a Dedicated Hybrid Mammotomograph. Phys. Med. Biol. 54, 3659–3676 (2009)
9. Madhav, P., et al. In: vivo characterization of breast tissues through absolute attenuation coefficients using dedicated cone-beam CT. In: Proc. SPIE 7622, 762209 (2010)

10. Crotty, D.J., et al.: Evaluation of the Absorbed Dose to the Breast Using Radiochromic Film in a Dedicated CT Mammotomography System Employing a Quasi-Monchromatic Beam. Med. Phys. 38(6), 3232–3245 (2011)
11. McKinley, R.L., et al.: Initial Study of a Quasi-Monochromatic Beam Performance for X-ray Computed Mammotomography. IEEE Trans. Nucl. Sci. NS-52(5), 1243–1250 (2005)
12. Brzymialkiewicz, C.N., et al.: Evaluation of Fully 3D Emission Mammotomography with a Compact Cadmium Zinc Telluride Detector. IEEE Trans. Med. Imag. MI-24(7), 868–877 (2005)
13. Jaszczak, R.J., et al.: Improved SPECT Quantification Using Compensation for Scattered Photons. J. Nucl. Med. 25, 893–900 (1984)
14. Vranjesevic, D., et al.: Relationship Between 18F-FDG Uptake and Breast Density in Women with Normal Breast Tissue. J. Nucl. Med. 44, 1238–1242 (2003)

Impact of Digitalization of Mammographic Units on Average Glandular Doses in the Flemish Breast Cancer Screening Program

An De Hauwere and Hubert Thierens

Ghent University, Department of Medical Physics, Proeftuinstraat 86, B-9000 Gent, Belgium
an.dehauwere@UGent.be

Abstract. The impact of digitalization on the average glandular doses in 49 mammographic units participating in the Flemish Breast Cancer Screening Program was studied. Screen-film was changed to direct digital radiography and computed radiography in 25 and 24 departments respectively. Average glandular doses were calculated before and after digitalization for different PMMA-phantom thicknesses and for groups of 50 successive patients. For the transition from screen-film to computed radiography both phantom and patient dose data show a significant increase of dose with digitalization. For the transition from screen-film to direct digital radiography the evolution of the average glandular dose depends on the phantom thickness. For 20mm PMMA a significant increase in dose was found, for 45mm and 70mm PMMA there was a significant decrease in dose. The median average glandular dose of the patient dosimetry showed a smaller but significant decrease.

Keywords: mammography, screening, breast cancer, digitalization, average glandular dose, screen-film, computed radiography, direct digital radiography.

1   Introduction

After a typetesting procedure [1-2] the first digital mammographic units were accepted within the Flemish Breast Cancer Screening Program in 2007. It is often claimed by manufacturers and in the media that "digitalization" in mammography leads to a dose reduction. However over the past 5 years, medical physicists in Flanders encountered that for individual mammographic centers the dose is sometimes higher after digitalization than before. Since asymptomatic woman between age 50 and 69 are systematically screened for breast cancer every two years in Flanders, it is necessary to assure the balance between benefit and the risk of the screening program. Therefore it is important to check the impact of the changes in average glandular dose caused by digitalization of the screening units on the radiation-induced breast cancer risk of the Flemish Breast Cancer Screening Program.

2   Method

The impact of digitalization on the average glandular doses was studied in 49 mammographic units participating in the Flemish Breast Cancer Screening Program.

A.D.A. Maidment, P.R. Bakic, and S. Gavenonis (Eds.): IWDM 2012, LNCS 7361, pp. 410–417, 2012.

Screen-film (SF) was changed to direct digital radiography (DR) and computed radiography (CR) in 25 and 24 departments respectively.

For all centers data regarding the yearly and half yearly physical-technical quality assurance test are available, in accordance with the European Guidelines [3-4]. On one hand average glandular doses (AGDs) before and after digitalization could be calculated for PMMA-phantom thicknesses between 20mm and 70mm applying the method of Dance et al. [5] based on automatic exposure control data, combined with output and half value layer measurements.

On the other hand a real patient dose study was performed in all centers after digitalization. Average glandular doses were calculated for a group of at least 50 successive patients. A large fraction of the centers conducted also a patient dose study prior to digitalization. Periodic patient dose studies are required by Belgian legislation [6]. A first registration period ended in the beginning of 2010. At that time some mammographic centers were already working digital, others were still working conventional. For each center that digitalized later on, a second patient dose study was requested.

For each patient dose study, the median of the average glandular doses was plotted against the average glandular dose corresponding with the 45mm PMMA-phantom at the time. These data could be represented satisfactory by a linear fit (y=1.066x ± 0.235, r^2=0.738, Fig. 1). For centers who did not perform patient dosimetry of a patient population prior to digitalization, the linear fit was used to deduce the median of the average glandular doses for a group of patients from the phantom dose data obtained prior to digitalization.

AGDs before and after digitalization were compared for each mammographic unit individually and significance of difference was evaluated by Wilcoxon signed rank test (p<0.05). Mean AGDs were calculated over the different units.

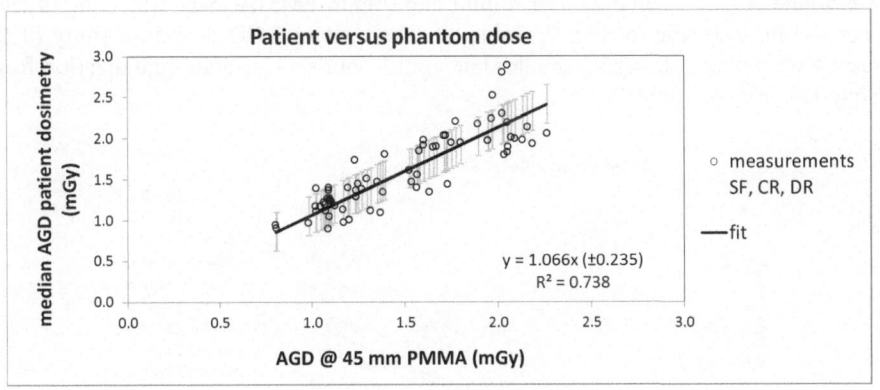

Fig. 1. Correlation between the median of the AGDs of a group of 50 patients and the AGD of a 45mm PMMA phantom

3   Results

Before digitalization there was a large variation in average glandular dose as a function of phantom-thickness between the 49 mammography units (Fig. 2). The dose differences were mainly due to the brand and type of the screen-film combination. For larger compressed breast thicknesses the observed dose differences are also linked to the brand and type of the corresponding x-ray units. Older x-ray units operate at Mo/Mo for all thicknesses. However the automatic exposure control of newer x-ray units changes at larger compressed breast thicknesses automatically to other target/filter combinations and/or higher kilovoltages, which reduces the AGD in such a way that the image quality remains acceptable.

For all CR-systems phantom-doses are quite high and there is a smaller variation in doses between the different brands of CR-cassettes (Fig. 3). This because the automatic exposure controls had to be calibrated close to the acceptable dose limit stated in the European Quality Control Protocol in order to reach acceptable image quality for small details.

For DR-systems phantom-doses are generally lower than for CR-systems (Fig. 4) and comparable to the lower dose SF-systems. Only one DR-system operated at a dose level lower than the lowest SF-system, this was a mammography unit with a photon counting detector instead of an amorphous silicon or amorphous selenium detector.

These trends were also seen in the patient dosimetry, though differences in individual breast composition and in the executed compression force have an influence on the correlation between phantom en patient dosimetry.

For the transition from SF to CR (25 screening units) phantom AGD increased significantly for 20mm, 45mm and 70mm PMMA in nearly all mammographic units (Fig. 5, Fig. 6, Fig. 7, Table 1). The median AGD of a dose study of 50 successive patients was also significantly higher after digitalization from SF to CR (Fig. 8, Table 1).

For the transition from SF to DR (24 screening units) the evolution of the AGD depends on the phantom thickness. For 20mm PMMA a significant increase in dose was found (Fig. 5, Table 2). For 45mm and 70mm PMMA there was a significant decrease in dose (Fig. 6, Fig. 7, Table 2). The median AGD of a dose study of 50 successive patients showed a smaller but significant decrease after digitalization from SF to DR (Fig. 8, Table 2).

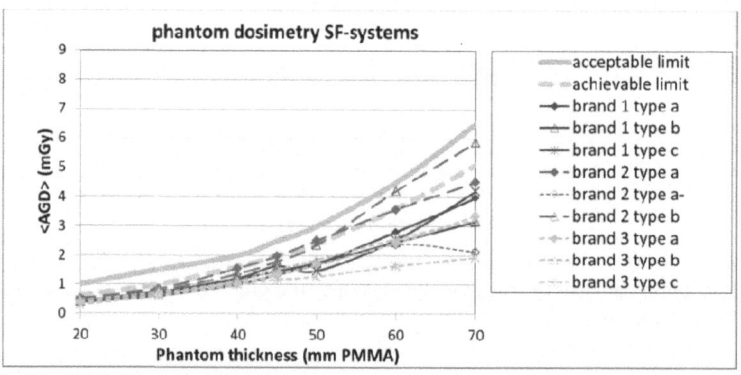

Fig. 2. Screen-film phantom dosimetry: AGD versus phantom thickness averaged over different brands and different screen-film combination types

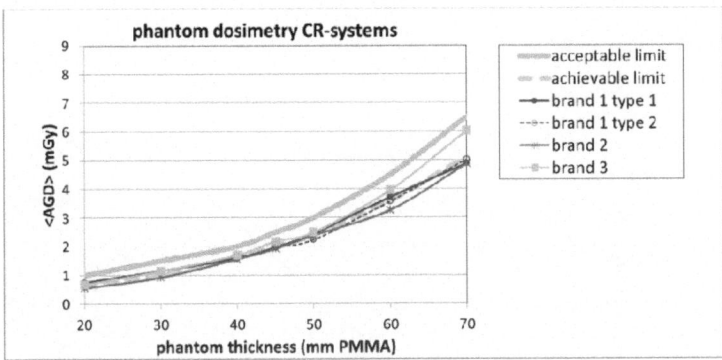

Fig. 3. Computed radiography phantom dosimetry: AGD versus phantom thickness averaged over different brands and different imaging plate types

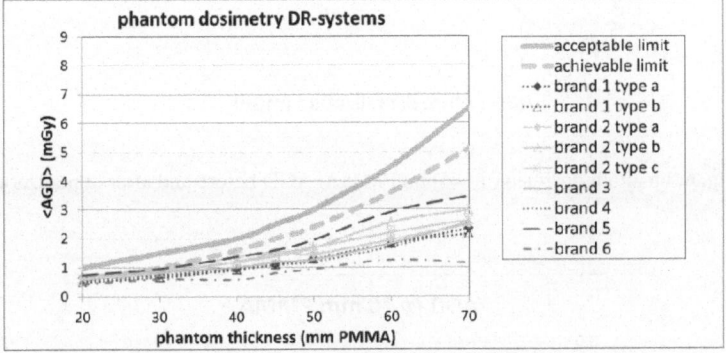

Fig. 4. Direct digital radiography phantom dosimetry: AGD versus phantom thickness averaged over different brands and different models of mammography equipment

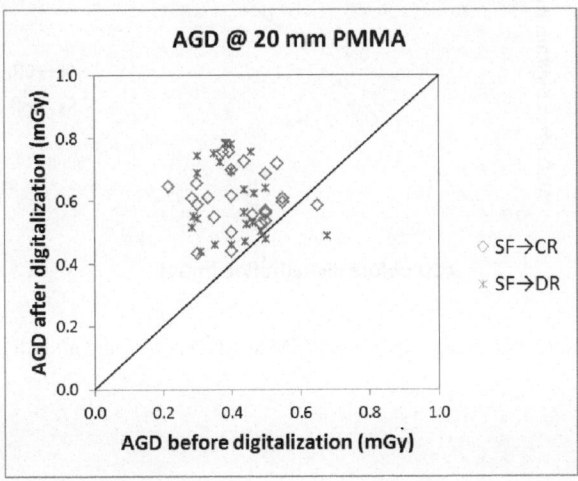

Fig. 5. Phantom dosimetry at 20mm PMMA: AGD before and after digitalization

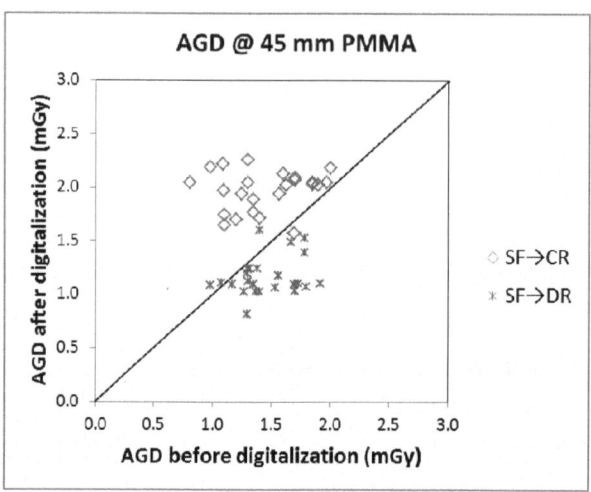

Fig. 6. Phantom dosimetry at 45mm PMMA: AGD before and after digitalization

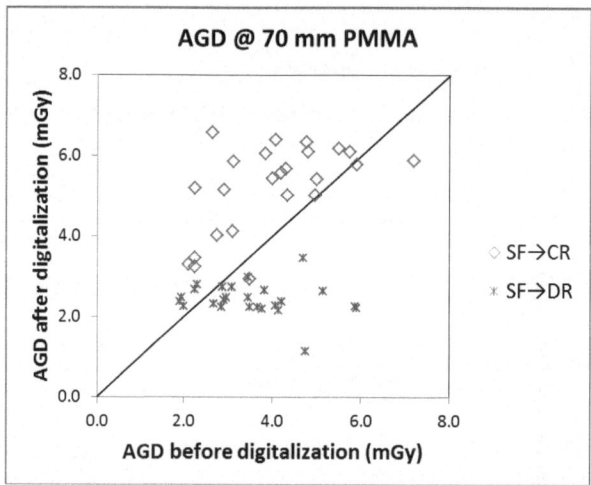

Fig. 7. Phantom dosimetry at 70mm PMMA: AGD before and after digitalization

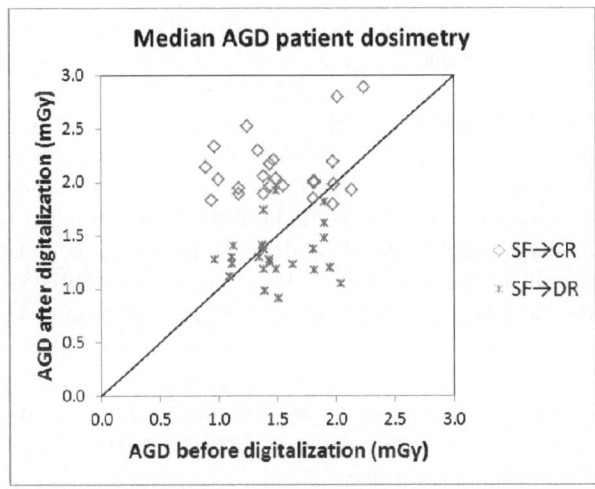

Fig. 8. Median AGD of a patient dose study of 50 successive patients before and after digitalization

Table 1. Statistical analysis of the transition from SF to CR

	SF mean	CR mean	normalized dose difference	p*
AGD @20 mm PMMA (mGy)	0.42	0.60	43%	0.000
AGD @45 mm PMMA (mGy)	1.45	1.97	36%	0.000
AGD @70 mm PMMA (mGy)	3.98	5.21	31%	0.000
median AGD patient dosimetry (mGy)	1.53	2.11	38%	0.000

* Wilcoxon Signed Ranks Test

Table 2. Statistical analysis of the transition from SF to DR

	SF mean	DR mean	normalized dose difference	p*
AGD @20 mm PMMA (mGy)	0.41	0.61	49%	0.000
AGD @45 mm PMMA (mGy)	1.45	1.16	-20%	0.000
AGD @70 mm PMMA (mGy)	3.53	2.43	-31%	0.001
median AGD patient dosimetry (mGy)	1.50	1.32	-12%	0.032

* Wilcoxon Signed Ranks Test

4   Discussion

It is a misconception that digitalization in mammography always leads to a dose reduction. Our results demonstrate that the transition from screen-film mammography to computed radiography on average in fact leads to a 38% higher AGD for an average patient. This higher dose is necessary to reach an acceptable image quality level for small details. In contrast a reduction of 12% in AGD was achieved on average for an average patient with a transition from screen-film mammography to direct digital radiography. We believe a stronger dose reduction for the transition from SF to DR can be accomplished by optimizing the automatic exposure control of the DR systems. This because for 20mm PMMA phantom doses are higher for DR than for SF. From our yearly and half yearly test results, we know that image quality in terms of contrast-to-noise ratio is much higher at 20mm PMMA than at larger thicknesses. As the European Quality Control Protocol [4] demands a constant contrast-to-noise ratio for all thicknesses, there is a potential of dose reduction for DR-systems at smaller thicknesses. Care must be taken that the overall contrast-to-noise level stays high enough to see small low-contrast details even in dense and thick breasts.

Whether and to what extent the patient dose decreases or increases in an individual mammographic unit after digitalization therefore largely depends on the choice for CR or for DR and is also determined by the brand and type of the formerly used screen-film combination and x-ray unit.

An increase of 38% in average glandular dose for the transition from SF to CR could change the detection over induction ratio (DIR) of the Flemish breast cancer program from 50 to 35 provided that the cancer detection rate stays the same. Therefore we plan to investigate for the same 49 mammography units, the impact of digitalization on the breast cancer screening performance parameters such as recall rate, cancer detection rate, fraction of invasive cancers, fraction of invasive cancers smaller than 1cm, fraction of ductal carcinoma in situ (DCIS) and the positive predictive value. This in order to calculate the DIR for digital mammography screening in Flanders and to ensure the overall quality of the digitalized Flemish breast screening program.

5   Conclusion

In present study it was shown that transition from screen-film to digital mammography will not necessarily result in a dose reduction. In fact the use of computed radiography leads to an important increase in average glandular dose (38%). On the other hand direct digital mammography contributed to a small but significant decrease in average glandular dose (12%). Direct digital mammography can be further optimized for smaller compressed breast thicknesses without compromising image quality.

From patient dose point of view, direct digital mammography has to be preferred over computed radiography in digitalization of mammography screening. A close collaboration between radiographers and medical physicists is indicated.

Manufacturers of direct digital mammography systems are advised to investigate how the automatic exposure control can be further optimized for smaller thicknesses: care should be taken that clinical as well as physical image quality parameters meet all requirements in lowering the dose setting.

Results obtained in present study are clearly in favor of direct digital radiography in digitalization of the screening program.

References

1. Thierens, H., Bosmans, H., Buls, N., Bacher, K., De Hauwere, A., Jacobs, J., Clerinx, P.: Typetesting of physical characteristics of digital mammography systems: first experiences within the Flemish Breast Cancer Screening Programme. JBR–BTR 90, 159–162 (2007)
2. Thierens, H., Bosmans, H., Buls, N., De Hauwere, A., Bacher, K., Jacobs, J., Clerinx, P.: Typetesting of physical characteristics of digital mammography systems for screening within the Flemish breast cancer screening programme. EJR 70, 539–548 (2009)
3. Van Engen, R., van Woudenberg, S., Bosmans, H., Young, K., Thijssen, M.: The European protocol for the quality control of the physical and technical aspects of mammography screening: Screen-film mammography. In: Perry, N., Broeders, M., de Wolf, C., Törnberg, S., Holland, R., von Karsa, L., Puthaar, E. (eds.) European Guidelines for Quality Assurance in Breast Cancer Screening and Diagnosis, 4th edn., Part 2a, pp. 61–104. Office for Official Publications of the European Communities, Luxembourg (2006)
4. Van Engen, R., Young, K., Bosmans, H., Thijssen, M.: The European protocol for the quality control of the physical and technical aspects of mammography screening: Digital mammography. In: Perry, N., Broeders, M., de Wolf, C., Törnberg, S., Holland, R., von Karsa, L., Puthaar, E. (eds.) European Guidelines for Quality Assurance in Breast Cancer Screening and Diagnosis, 4th edn., Part 2b, pp. 105–165. Office for Official Publications of the European Communities, Luxembourg (2006)
5. Dance, D.R., Skinner, C.L., Young, K.C., Beckett, J.R., Kotre, C.J.: Additional factors for the estimation of mean glandular dose using the UK mammography protocol. Phys. Med. Biol. 45, 3225–3240 (2000)
6. Royal Decree of 20 July 2001 laying down the general rules and regulation for the protection of the general public, of the workers and the environment against the danger arising from ionising radiation. Chapter VI: Medical Applications of ionising radiation. Belgian Law Gazette, 171(245), 28982–28996 (2001)

An Examination of Silver as a Radiographic Contrast Agent in Dual-Energy Breast X-ray Imaging

Roshan Karunamuni[1], Ajlan Al Zaki[2], Anatoliy V. Popov[1], E. James Delikatny[1],
Sara Gavenonis[1], Andrew Tsourkas[2], and Andrew D.A. Maidment[1]

[1] University of Pennsylvania, Department of Radiology, Philadelphia USA
[2] University of Pennsylvania, Department of Bioengineering, Philadelphia, USA
aros@seas.upenn.edu, andrew.maidment@uphs.upenn.edu

Abstract. Silver nanoaprticles have been investigated as an alternative to iodine in dual-energy breast x-ray imaging. Dual-energy imaging involves acquiring images at two distinct energy windows (low and high). Weighting factors are then applied to create an image where the contrast between background tissues has been suppressed. Silver (Ag) represents an attractive contrast material due to its favorable x-ray attenuation properties (k-edge of 25.5 keV). Theoretical analysis using polychromatic spectra shows that silver can provide similar, if not better, contrast to iodine. Spherical Ag nanoparticles with an average diameter of 4 ±2 nm were synthesized using the Brust method in water. The particles were surface stabilized with polyethylene glycol and showed little cellular toxicity in T6-17 fibroblast cells. These results have encouraged further investigation into validation and testing in living system models. Silver nanoparticles represent an exciting avenue for the development of a novel dual-energy, x-ray breast imaging agent.

1 Introduction

Contrast-enhanced dual-energy (DE) x-ray imaging provides a technique to increase the contrast of radiographic imaging agents by suppressing the variation in signal between various tissue types. In the breast, this involves the suppression of the signal variation between admixtures of glandular and adipose tissue. By reducing the effect of this "anatomical noise", it is then possible to more accurately segment and quantify the signal from the contrast agent. Dual-energy imaging utilizes two distinct energy windows (low- and high-) to quantify the variation in attenuation with energy. To achieve a suitable contrast between imaging agent and tissue, it is therefore necessary that their respective attenuation profiles do not follow the same general trend from low- to high- energy. This can be done by using a contrast material whose k-edge lies between the two energy windows. The discrete jump in attenuation due to the photoelectric effect of the extra k-shell electrons means that the contrast material exhibits a markedly different attenuation profile to the surrounding tissue.

Currently, the majority of research that is performed in dual-energy x-ray imaging involves iodinated contrast agents. Silver (Ag) represents an attractive alternative due

A.D.A. Maidment, P.R. Bakic, and S. Gavenonis (Eds.): IWDM 2012, LNCS 7361, pp. 418–425, 2012.
© Springer-Verlag Berlin Heidelberg 2012

to the location of its k-edge (25.5 keV) within the range of clinically-used mammographic energies. Silver filtration is also common in the clinical setting, which could provide additional benefit with a silver imaging agent. The aim of this study is to provide an experimental argument for Ag in breast DE x-ray imaging, and to develop a prototype Ag nanoagent for testing in living systems.

2   Results (Theoretical Simulations)

Monoenergetic Analysis: A monoenergetic analysis was first performed to identify candidate combinations of low (LE) and high (HE) energies. Linear attenuation coefficients (LAC) were calculated for various admixtures of glandular and adipose tissues ranging from 0 to 100% glandular. Separately, the LAC were calculated for a 50% glandular, 50% adipose composite with increasing concentrations of contrast material.   Mass attenuation coefficients needed for this calculation were obtained from the NIST XCOM online physics database [1]. Energy pairs ranging from 15 to 45 keV (in 1 keV intervals) were studied.   For each energy-pair, two-dimensional maps of linear attenuation coefficients for tissue were calculated in terms of glandularity and concentration of silver (see Figure 1). Linear relationships were observed for both variables. The metric R was defined as the angular separation between these two linear fits.

An energy pair of (20, 30) keV was identified to maximize R (44°) using a silver contrast agent. A similar calculation for iodine showed that R was maximum at an energy pair of (30, 40) keV with a value of 39°. These energy pairs were further studied with polychromatic spectral analysis.

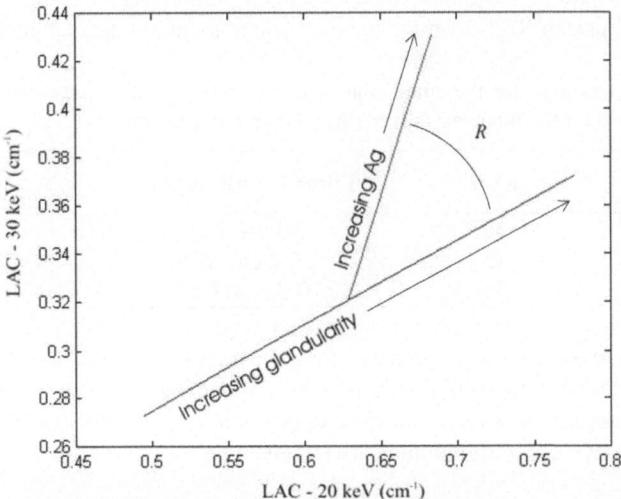

Fig. 1. Two dimensional map of LAC for variations of glandularity and concentration of silver, the metric R was defined as the angle between the two linear fits

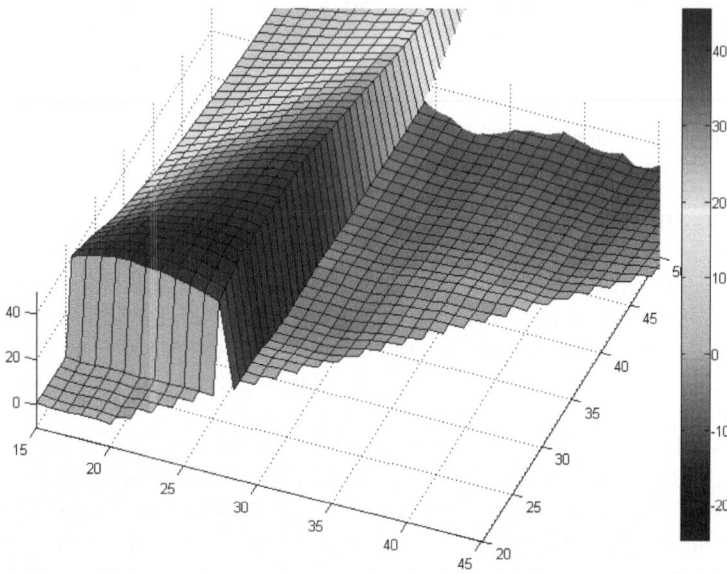

Fig. 2. Surface plot of R for various combinations of low- and high- energy pairs. A maximum occurs at (20, 30) keV providing an R of 44°.

Polychromatic Spectra: Tungsten polychromatic spectra were designed using the interpolating method of Boone et al [2]. Hundreds of combinations of kVp and filter materials were tested until three spectra with mean energies of roughly 20 (S1), 30 (S2) and 40 keV (S3) were chosen, as shown in Table 1. It is expected that a spectral pair of S1, S2 would be more beneficial to a silver contrast agent compared to iodine while a spectral pair of S2, S3 would be better suited to an iodinated contrast agent.

Table 1. Parameters used for the simulation of the 3 spectra with various average energies. Abbreviations used for the filter: Ag (silver), Al (aluminum), Cu (copper).

	kVp	Filter Combination	Average Energy (keV)
S1	32	80 µm Ag	21.6
S2	45	0.2 cm Al	30.0
S3	49	0.03 cm Cu	38.0

Weighting Factors: For each spectrum, the transmission through 1 cm of tissue of varying breast tissue composition (0% to 100 % glandular) was calculated. A thickness of 1 cm was chosen as an initial starting point for our calculations. The transmission was then converted to signal intensity (S) given by:

$$S = ln\left(\sum_{E=0}^{kVp} E \times I_E \times e^{-\mu_E t} \right) \tag{1}$$

Where E is the energy in keV, I_E is the incident photon fluence (photons/mm^2) at that energy, μ_E is the linear attenuation coefficient of the breast tissue composition at that energy E, and t is the thickness of tissue.   This formulation assumes that an ideal energy-integrating detector is used. The dual-energy signal (S_D) was defined as the weighted subtraction of the low- and high-energy SI:

$$S_D = S_{HE} - w \times S_{LE} \tag{2}$$

For a given pair of tissue glandularities (see Figure 3, G1 and G2), a weighting factor was determined such that the DE signal from G1 was equal to that of G2.

$$S_D(G1) = S_D(G2) \rightarrow w = \frac{H1 - H2}{L1 - L2} \tag{3}$$

Thus, in a DE image no contrast would be observed between these two tissue types using this calculated weighting factor.

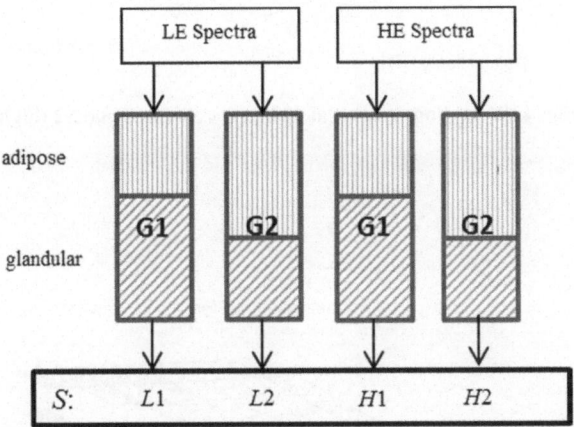

Fig. 3. Schematic setup for determining the weighting factor for a given pair of tissue glandularities (G1, G2). A weighting factor is chosen so as to equate the S_D of the two materials. S_D is given by a weighted subtraction of the high and low signal intensities.

The weighting factor needed to suppress various combinations of tissue glandularities are shown for a high/low spectral combination of S0, S1 (Figure 4) and S1, S2 (Figure 5). The weighting factor is relatively invariant with tissue composition. This would imply that for a given spectral pair of low- and high-energy beams, it should be possible to effectively null the contrast between the underlying tissue structures in the breast.

Contrast Calculation: The calculated values of w were used to determine DE signals for background tissue (50% adipose, 50 % glandular) and contrast enhanced tissue (50% adipose, 50% glandular + 1mg/mL of contrast material). The contrast (C) was calculated as the difference in S_D of tissue with and without contrast material. Values of C using silver, iodine and various low/high spectral pairs are tabulated in Table 2. The data correlates well with those predicted by monoenergetic calculations.

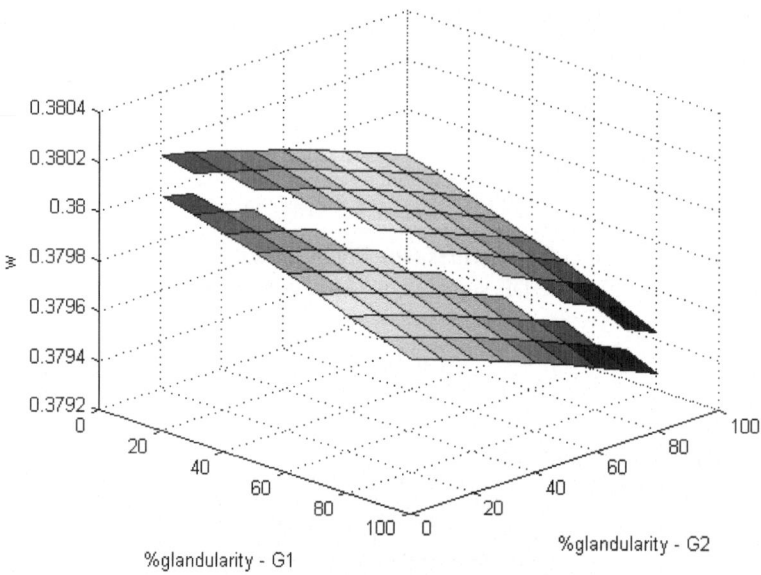

Fig. 4. Weighting factors calculated for S1 (low) and S2 (high)

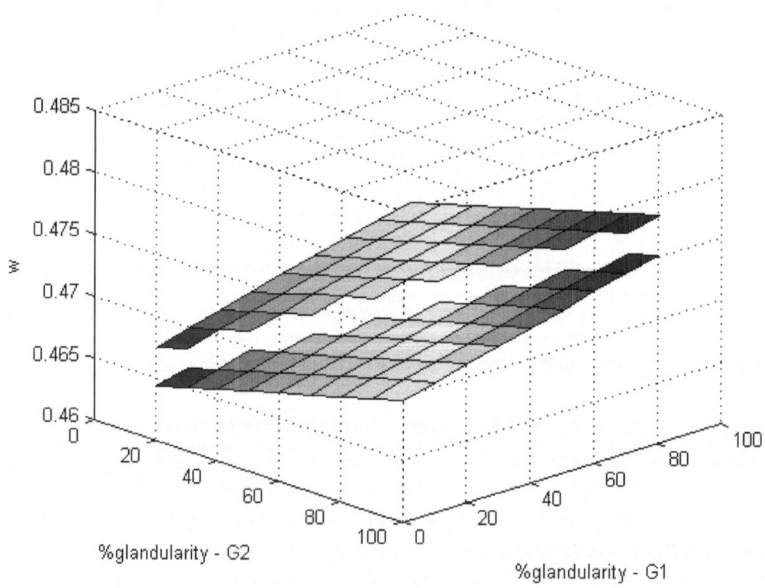

Fig. 5. Weighting factors calculated for S2 (low) and S3 (high)

1. The contrast observed for each contrast material is greater when using the spectral pair that brackets the k-edge of that material. The contrast observed for silver is greater when using the (S1,S2) spectral pair. Conversely, the contrast observed for iodine is greater when using the (S2,S3) spectral pair.

2. The maximum contrast observed for silver is greater than that of iodine. By comparing the spectral pairs that best suited each material, it was found that the contrast observed for silver was roughly twice that of iodine.

Although these results are not conclusive, they do support our initial hypothesis that silver demonstrates significant potential as a contrast material for dual-energy breast x-ray imaging.

Table 2. Signal Differences tabulated for silver and iodine using various low- and high – energy spectral combinations

| C (Digital Units) | Spectral Combinations | |
	Low E: S_1 High E: S_2	Low E: S_2 High E: S_3
Silver	20.8 ± 0.003	7.44 ± 0.08
Iodine	9.88 ± 0.004	11.70 ± 0.05

3   Results (Nanoparticle Development)

Silver nanoparticles (AgNP) have been synthesized using the Brust [3] method in water. This is preferred over the Turkevich method as it provided a more reliable size distribution of particles from batch to batch. Figure 6 shows a transmission electron micrograph (TEM) of the synthesized particles. Analysis of the size distribution yielded a mean diameter of 4 ±2 nm. Initial analysis showed two populations of nanoparticles present which accounts for the high standard deviation in mean diameter. The AgNP were surface stabilized using polyethylene glycol (PEG, M_w = 5000) to improve solubility in cell media and phosphate buffered solutions. A molar ratio of 1.5:1 was used between the PEG stabilizing ligand and silver.

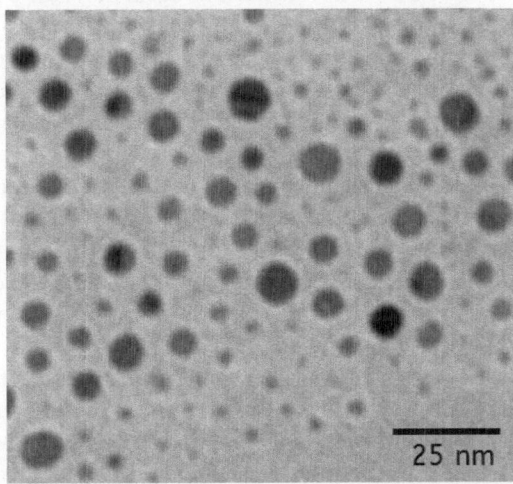

25 nm

Fig. 6. TEM of the colloidal silver nanoparticles synthesized using the Brust method in water. The particles have been stabilized using a polyethylene glycol surface chain.

The cellular toxicity of the stabilized AgNP was measured in T6-17 fibroblast cells using the MTT assay. Figure 7 shows the relationship between concentration of Ag in AgNP and percent cell viability after 24 hour incubation. Compared to a sham treated control, total cell viability of 50% was maintained at an Ag concentration of 10 mM (roughly 1 mg Ag/mL). These results show marked improvement over cell viability studies using AgNP in the literature [4-5] and have encouraged us to begin analysis of the particles in living systems.

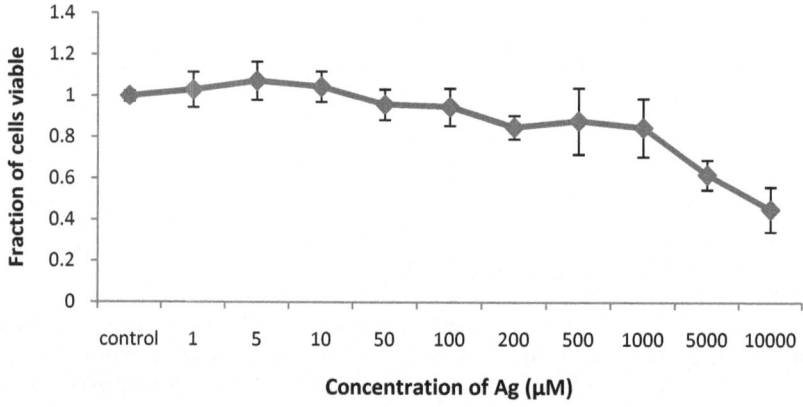

Fig. 7. Cellular toxicity of AgNP in T6-17 cells after 24-hour incubation

4   Discussion

Silver is being investigated as a novel imaging agent for dual-energy breast x-ray imaging. Monoenergetic analysis of linear attenuation coefficients showed that compared to iodine it is possible to achieve a greater separation between tissue with and without contrast when silver is used. These results were corroborated by polyenergetic spectra simulation where silver showed up to twice the radiographic contrast of iodine.

It should be noted that only a small subset of the possible spectral pairs were tested in the polyenergetic simulations. The results should therefore not be considered as conclusive as the true optimal contrast values for each material may differ slightly if a more extensive search was performed. However, both the monoenergetic and polyenergetic simulations demonstrate that there exists enormous potential for the use of silver in DE breast x-ray imaging.

Initial work has been completed on the synthesis and testing of AgNP. Spherical AgNP (d = 4 ±2 nm) were synthesized using the Brust method, and stabilized with PEG surface ligands. Little cellular toxicity was observed in cells for silver concentrations up to 1mg/mL. The testing of these particles in living systems is currently underway.

Silver nanoparticles represent an exciting avenue for the development of a novel DE breast x-ray imaging agent. Simulations have demonstrated that within the mammographic energy range, silver is able to offer comparable, if not greater DE contrast to iodine. This work provides the initial groundwork for a rich, new direction in contrast-enhanced DE breast imaging.

Acknowledgements. The project described was supported by grants W81XWH-09-1-0055 and W81XWH-11-1-0246 through the Department of Defense Breast Cancer Research Program. The content is solely the responsibility of the authors and does not necessarily represent the official views of the funding agency.

References

1. National Institute of Standards and Technology (NIST) Physical Measurement Laboratory. XCOM: Photon Cross Sections Database (retrieved December 10, 2011)
2. Boone, J.M., Fewell, T.R., Jennings, R.J.: Molybdenum, rhodium, and tungsten anode spectral models using interpolating polynomials with application to mammography. Med. Phys. 24(12), 1863–1874 (1997)
3. Brust, M., Walker, M., Bethell, D., Schiffrin, D.J., Whyman, R.: Synthesis of thiol derivatized gold nanoparticles in a 2-phase liquid-liquid system. J. Chem. Soc. Chem. Commun., 801–802 (1994)
4. Hussain, S., Hess, K.L., Gearhart, J.M., Geiss, K.T., Schlager, J.J.: In Vitro Toxicity of nanoparticles in BRL 3A rat liver cells. Toxiciology in Vitro, 975–983 (2005)
5. Navarro, E., Piccapietra, F., Wagner, B., Marconi, F., Kaegi, R., Odzak, N., Sigg, L., Behra, R.: Toxicity of Silver Nanoparticles to Chlamydomonas reinhardtii. Environmental Science and Technology, 8959–8964 (2008)

Initial Evaluation of a Newly Developed High Resolution CT Imager for Dedicated Breast CT

Jainil P. Shah[1], Steve D. Mann[1,2], Andrew M. Polemi[2],
Martin P. Tornai[1,2], Randolph L. McKinley[3], George Zentai[4],
Michelle Richmond[4], and Larry Partain[4]

[1] Department of Radiology, Duke University Medical Center, Durham, NC 27710
[2] Medical Physics Graduate Program, Duke University Medical Center, Durham, NC 27705
{jainil.shah,steve.mann,andrew.polemi,martin.tornai}@duke.edu
[3] Zumatek, Inc., Research Triangle Park, NC 27709
randolph.mckinley@zumatek.com
[4] Ginzton Technology Center, Varian Medical Systems, Mountain View, CA 94043
{george.zentai,michelle.richmond,larry.partain}@varian.com

Abstract. A new, high resolution 40x30cm^2 area CsI-TFT based CT imager having 127μm pixel pitch was developed for fully-3D breast CT imaging as part of a SPECT-CT system. The imager has two narrow edges suited for pendant breast CT imaging close to the chest wall. The scintillator thickness of 600 microns provides >90% absorption for the 36keV mean x-ray energy of the cone beam source. The 2D MTF is ~7.5% at the 3.9 lp/mm Nyquist frequency. The imager has excellent linearity over the full dynamic range. The imager is mounted on the CT device and initial tomographic imaging of geometric and breast phantoms demonstrate the reliable and robust imaging capabilities of this device for breast CT.

Keywords: Imaging, X-ray imaging, breast CT, mammography, mammotomography, tomosynthesis, flat panel imaging arrays.

1 Introduction

We have developed a dual modality SPECT-CT system for dedicated breast imaging [1-2]. The CT subsystem of the scanner uses an ultra-thick K-edge filtered, quasi-monochromatic x-ray cone beam and a 20x25cm^2 active sensor area for 3D imaging of a pendant, uncompressed breast. For developing the advanced version of the dedicated SPECT-CT mammotomography device that will enable fully-3D CT imaging including near chest-wall access in an improved system design, a new, high resolution detector with smaller pixels than currently available in commercial units of this size has been developed. Importantly, the imager has very narrow bezels at two edges, rendering it well suited for pendant breast CT imaging close to the chest wall. This paper evaluates the high resolution, large area digital imager for inclusion in the breast CT portion of the hybrid imaging device, or as a stand-alone breast CT system.

A.D.A. Maidment, P.R. Bakic, and S. Gavenonis (Eds.): IWDM 2012, LNCS 7361, pp. 426–433, 2012.

2   Methods

2.1   4030 Flat Panel Imager

Varian Medical Systems (Mountian View, CA) developed a new imager having a 127μm pixel size (identical in pixel size and configuration to the *Varian Paxscan* 2520) for an active 40x30cm^2 area with 3200×2304 total pixels. The readout and driver ASIC TAB bonding pads were arranged only on two sides of the imager plate, to facilitate the extra space requirements by having two narrow edges (the contra-lateral side with wider edge is now more densely packed with electronics). A special housing was necessarily developed to accommodate this imaging plate providing very narrow 8mm edges (bezels) on two orthogonal sides (Fig. 1), where there are no TAB bonding pads. The TFT array imager was coated with 600μm thick micro-columnar CsI layer, which provides >90% absorption in the breast CT (65kVp and 36keV mean, quasi-monochromatic) x-ray energy range. Our system operates at 60kVp and with the Ce-filtration yields a 36keV mean, quasi-monochromatic x-ray spectrum [2]. It provides better than 70% absorption for RQA5 (70kVp 21mm Al filter) x-ray radiation [3]. The readout ASICs are connected to 14 bit A/D converters and special *Varian* readout ASICs with dynamic gain switching capability provide an additional 4 bit virtual (2-3 effective) bits of resolution [4]. The data are transmitted via a Gigabit Ethernet interface at a maximum rate of 7fps in 2x2 pixel binned mode, and 3fps in full resolution mode, and has a simple high voltage (HV) supply line for power. In the current configuration, this would allow for a 34sec full 360° CT acquisition on our system, given 240 projections that we have collected with the earlier *Paxscan 2520*.

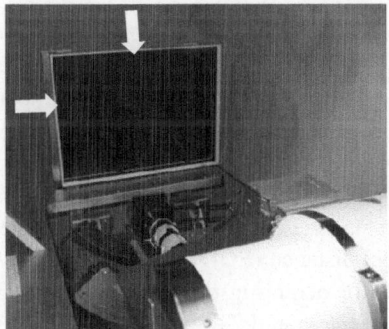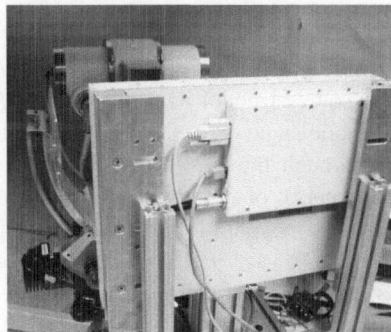

Fig. 1. Photographs of the 4030 flat panel imager mounted on the current system: (LEFT) front view with detector in background and source in foreground, and (RIGHT) back view with detector in foreground. White arrows indicate narrow bezel edges.

2.2   2D MTF Measurements

The 2D MTF of the imager was evaluated based on edge techniques [5-6]. Measure-ments were made with a 117cm source-to-image distance (SID), a *Varian* G-1092 x-ray source (rotating anode, metal insert type) at 70kVp and 100mA. Aluminum filtration (21mm) was added to meet RQA5 requirements [3]. The image acquisition was with 1x1 binning at 2 fps. 32 calibrations frames are used to apply corrections for offset, gain and defective pixels prior to object imaging. An MTF edge is arranged on the imager with its measurement edge producing a 2-3 degree angle relative to the panel. Two sets of data are taken, one with the MTF pattern in portrait vertical as shown below (Fig. 2) and one with the pattern landscape horizontal. An offset calibration is performed prior to each data set. Gain and defect calibrations are performed only once. For each arrangement of the MTF pattern, a sequence of 32 exposed frames is gathered and averaged to produce a single image.

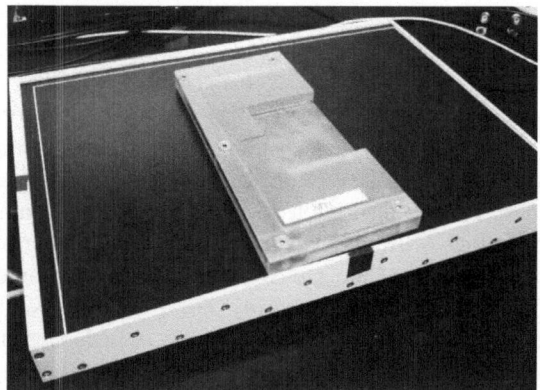

Fig. 2. Photo of the 2D MTF edge arranged on detector for 2D MTF characterization

2.3   CT Data Acquisition

The CT sub-system of our hybrid imaging device uses a rotating tungsten target x-ray source (model Rad 94, *Varian Medical Systems)* with a 0.4mm focal spot and 14° anode angle (Fig. 1). The tube potential was set to 60kVp with a 1.25 mAs exposure through the 0.7cm Ce filter rendering the beam quasi-monochromatic, with a mean energy of 36keV and FWHM of 15%. The new 4030 flat panel imager was externally mounted to the azimuthal rotation stage (Fig. 1). The source-to-image distance (SID) was 79.6cm, and source-to-object distance (SOD) was 47.8cm. *Varian*'s image acquisition software, *VIVA* was used for acquiring the data. Phantoms were positioned near the iso-center of the imaging system and 240 projection images were acquired over a 360 degree azimuthal acquisiton. Images were acquired in 2x2 pixel binned "Fluoro" mode at 0.33 fps leading to a slower, 12 min scan on the current system configuration. The projections were reconstructed using a ray driven, iterative ordered subsets algorithm (OSC). Reconstruction parameters were set to 5 iterations, 16 subsets and a reconstruction grid size up to 1000x1000x1000, with a reconstructed voxel size of 254µm on a side. Reconstructions took approximately 6 min on the *Intel* Core i7 2nd Generation (Extreme Edition) CPU.

2.4   Phantoms

An acrylic mini-rod phantom (rods with diameters from 1.1mm to 4.6mm spaced on twice their diameter, and with 2cm axial extent, *Data Spectrum*, Hillsborough, NC) was initially used to measure directional offsets as well as the center of rotation offset for the newly mounted detector. The cylinder was 8.2cm in diameter with a 3.25mm thick wall. Once determined, these offsets were used as input parameters for the OSC reconstruction algorithm.

A novel 3D MTF phantom was imaged based on our previous work [7]. The phantom consists of three nearly-orthogonally positioned tungsten wires, each of a uniform 50.8 μm diameter and ~11cm length, tightly suspended in an acrylic box frame [7].

The imager was also assessed using two geometric phantoms (cylinder and cone) and one anthropomorphic breast phantom (~800 mL) (*Radiology Support Devices*, Newport Beach, CA). Diameters of these phantoms varied from 8-15cm and were filled with water.

3   Results

3.1   2D MTF Measurements

The horizontal and vertical MTF was calculated from the measured projection images. A 2D MTF of ~7.5% was measured at the 3.9 lp/mm Nyquist frequency in both horizontal and vertical dimensions (Fig. 3).

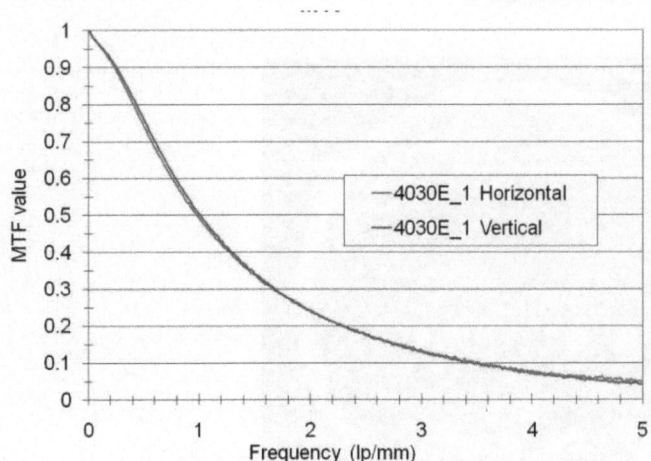

Fig. 3. Horizontally and vertically measured MTFs

3.2   Cold Rod Phantom

Projection images of the rod phantom were obtained and reconstructed with different directional and rotation offsets due to centering of the detector. Some shimming and

J.P. Shah et al.

leveling of the detector relative to the source and rotation axis was implemented in an effort to minimize blurring in the reconstructions. Line profiles were drawn across the reconstructed rods to determine offset values due to detector offsets and reconstruction that resulted in the narrowest line profiles. The resultant images demonstrate both the clear separation of the rods as well as some scatter between them (Fig. 4 and 5) seen by the non-zero values between rods in the profiles.

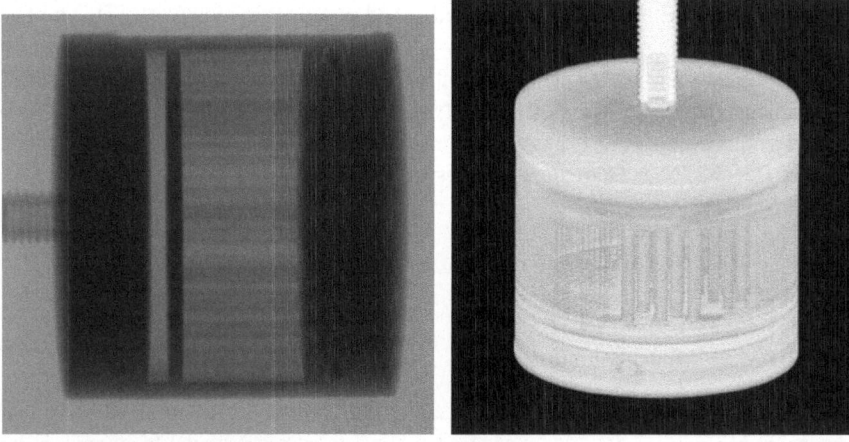

Fig. 4. (LEFT) Projection image of the cold rod phantom, and (RIGHT) 3D volume rendering of the reconstructed object image

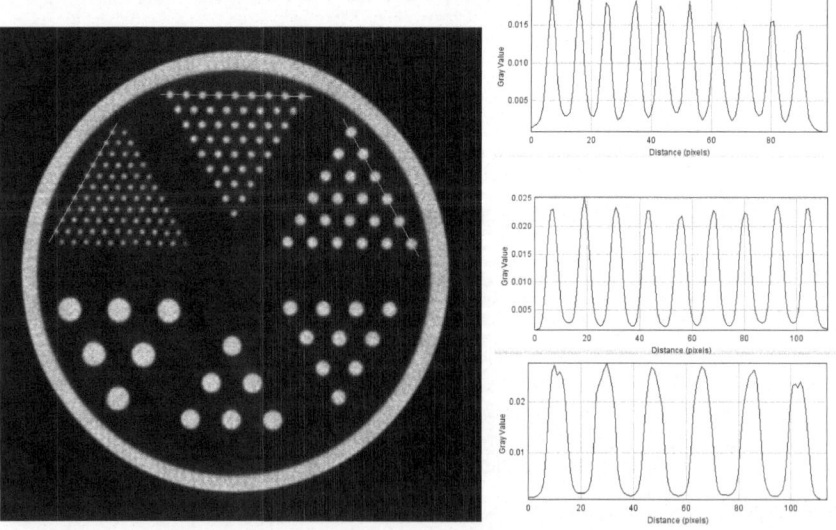

Fig. 5. (LEFT) Reconstructed image of the cold rod phantom having 254micron isotropic voxels, and (RIGHT) plotted profiles at the illustrated (blue) lines at LEFT

The offset correction values initially used to correct the reconstructed cold rod phantom are sufficient for larger objects and lower frequencies. However, use of those same values resulted in some artifacts in the reconstructed images of the very high frequency 3D MTF phantom. Thus, the reconstructed 3D MTF phantom data is initially presented qualitatively; as we believe even better system alignment can be achieved prior to fully-3D MTF analysis. Notably, the tungsten wires are all visible throughout their entire expanse in the projections (Fig. 6). The reconstructed image, however, still yielded non-converged line sources shaped like tubes and split lines, indicating that the detector positioning shifts, rotations, etc. have not been completely accurately determined at this point. Therefore, 3D MTF measurements could not be made on this data. Nonetheless, an initial surface rendered volumetric image of the 3D MTF phantom is shown alongside the projection images (Fig. 6).

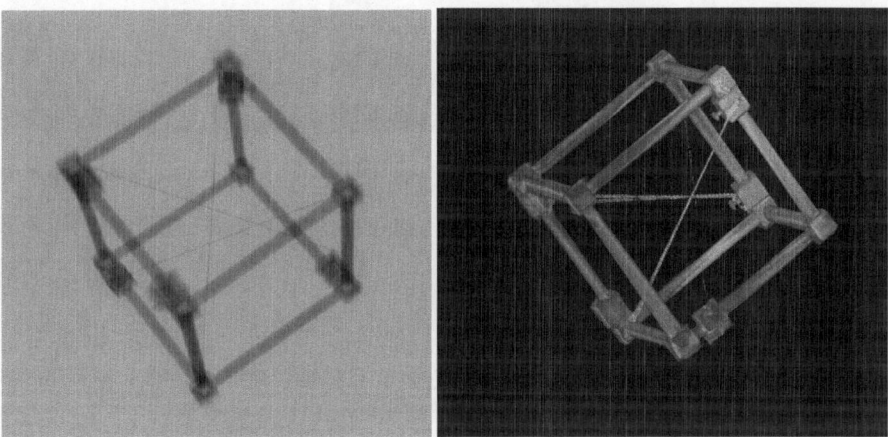

Fig. 6. (LEFT) Projection image of the 3D MTF phantom with three orthogonal tungsten wires, and (RIGHT) 3D Volume rendering of the reconstructed MTF phantom

3.3   Geometric and Anthropomorphic Breast Phantoms

The water-filled cylinder, cone and anthropomorphic breast phantoms were also scanned using the same techniques as for the geometric phantoms. Initial reconstructions show artifacts similar to the cold rod and 3D MTF phantoms, where the edges of the phantoms are slightly blurred (Fig. 7). Additionally, some ring artifacts are also visible on these uniform phantoms, with no egregious circular artifacts that would indicate pixel or line errors in projection space. The observed large centrally located cylinder has consistently appeared in images of uniformly filled phantoms with our 2520 detector, and is a visual artifact with slightly lower noise characteristics in the center. Based on our previous experience, we do not expect it to be as obvious in non-uniformly filled or structurally noise containing phantoms.

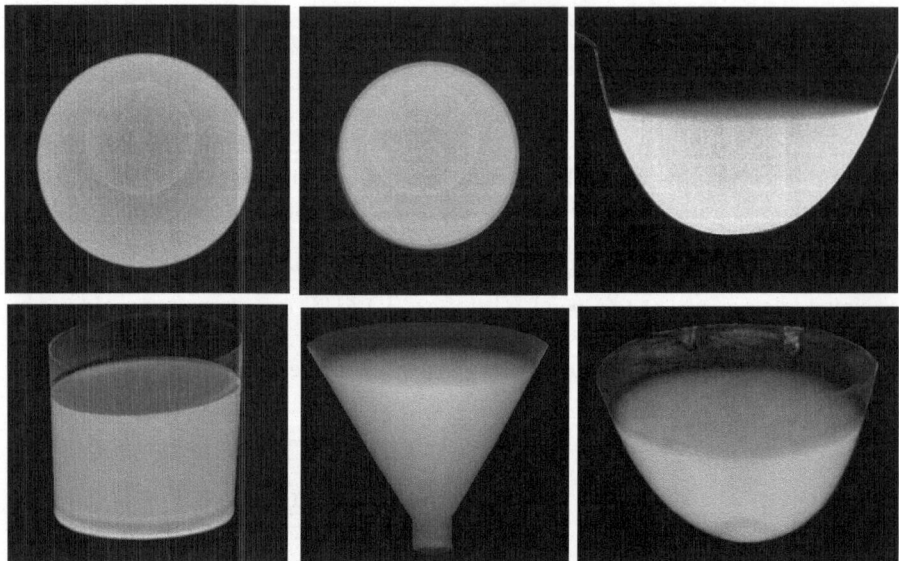

Fig. 7. (TOP LEFT & MIDDLE) Coronal slices and (TOP RIGHT) one sagittal slice along with (BOTTOM) volume renderings of reconstructed images of (LEFT) cylinder, (MIDDLE) cone and (RIGHT) anthropomorphic breast phantoms

4   Discussion

This newly developed imager will contribute to the new SPECT-CT system under development to obtain very high resolution, fully-3D sampled breast CT images without truncation. That system under development has fully-3D motion incorporated into the data acquisition sequence, and with this very narrow edge (at chest wall) imager will allow for routine chest wall and whole breast imaging. With an SID of 60cm, the current *Paxscan 2520* provides an untruncated FOV of 15.4cm diameter. For the increased SID of 79cm and near-identical magnification, the new 4030 considerably improves the untruncated FOV to 24.4cm. The increased imaging area along with high intrinsic resolution and wide dynamic range, should lead to improved imaging capabilities for a very large number of breast sizes.

Acknowledgements. This work has been funded by the National Cancer Institute of the National Institutes of Health (R01-CA096821 and R44-CA125924) and partly by internal funds at *Varian*. MPT is the inventor of this SPECT-CT technology and is named as an inventor on the patent for this technology awarded to Duke (#7,609,808). If this breast CT technology becomes commercially successful, MPT and Duke could benefit financially. In addition, MPT and RLM are founders and Board Members of *Zumatek*. MPT is also a consultant to *Zumatek*.

References

1. Madhav, P., Crotty, D.J., McKinley, R.L., Tornai, M.P.: Initial Development of a Dual-Modality SPECT-CT System for Dedicated Mammotomography. In: IEEE Nuclear Science Symposium & Medical Imaging Conference Record, vol. 4, pp. 2382–2386 (2006)
2. Tornai, M.P., McKinley, R.L., Brzymialkiewicz, C.N., et al.: Design and development of a fully-3D dedicated xray computed mammotomography system. In: Proc. SPIE: Phys. of Med. Imag., vol. 5745(1), pp. 189–197 (2005)
3. International Standard, IEC 62220-1 (2003)
4. Roos, P.G., Colbeth, R.E., Mollov, I., Munro, P., Pavkovich, J., Seppi, E.J., Shapiro, E.G., Tognina, C.A., Virshup, G.F., Yu, J.M., Zentai, G.: Multiple-gain-ranging readout method to extend the dynamic range of amorphous silicon flat-panel imagers. In: Proc. SPIE: Phys. of Med. Imag., vol. 5368, p. 139 (2004)
5. Samei, E., Flynn, M.J.: A method for measuring the presampled MTF of digital radiographic systems using an edge test device. Med. Phys. 25(1), 102–113 (1998)
6. Greer, P.B., van Doom, T.: Evaluation of an algorithm for the assessment of the MTF using an edge method. Med. Phys. 27(9), 2048–2059 (2000)
7. Madhav, P., McKinley, R.L., Samei, E., Bowsher, J.E., Tornai, M.P.: A novel method to characterize the MTF in 3D for computed mammotomography. In: Proc. SPIE: Phys. of Med. Imag., vol. 6142 (2006)

Comparison of Lesion Extent and Contrast-Agent Uptake in Breast Tomosynthesis versus Cone-Beam Breast CT

Pablo M. de Carvalho[1,2], Ann-Katherine Carton[2], Răzvan Iordache[2],
Sylvie Saab-Puong[2], and Serge Muller[2]

[1] Université Paris Sud XI, Orsay, France
[2] GE Healthcare, 283 rue de la Minière, 78533 Buc, France
pablo.milionidecarvalho@ge.com

Abstract. This study compares the quantitative potential of cone-beam dedicated breast CT (bCT) and digital breast tomosynthesis (DBT) for contrast-enhanced (CE) imaging in the assessment of 3D lesion extent and iodinated contrast-agent uptake. bCT and DBT topologies were modeled assuming perfect energy-integrating detectors. Projection images were simulated using optimized spectra for iodine imaging and primary photons only. Lesion extent and lesion-to-background-contrast were measured in reconstructed images of breast tissue equivalent phantoms containing iodinated lesions. Lesion extent was estimated using an automatic estimator. A full factorial experiment was used to evaluate the effect of 3D lesion dimension, position and iodine concentration on measurement precision. Preliminary results show that for CE-DBT and CE-bCT, precision is similar in the in-plane direction, while CE-bCT is superior in the depth direction. Lesion-to-background-contrast greatly depends on lesion diameter in CE-DBT and is almost independent of lesion diameter for CE-bCT.

Keywords: quantitative imaging, breast, computed tomography, digital breast tomosynthesis, contrast-enhanced imaging, dual energy.

1   Background

In a breast cancer therapy setting, quantitative imaging methods for the characterization of tumors play an important role for improved clinical decision making and disease outcome. Today, CE-MRI, CE full-body CT, PET and PET/CT are used for quantitative assessment of breast tumors before, during and after therapy. These techniques have shown to correlate strongly with pathology. CE-MRI is however very costly and not widely available, while two key disadvantages of CE full-body CT and PET/CT are their high radiation dose and limited spatial resolution.

An alternative less expensive imaging technique dedicated for the breast providing accurate quantitative information on breast lesions' location, morphology, and functional information is of high clinical and economical interest. CE-DBT and CE-bCT are two potential candidates. It is anticipated that the quantitative potential of CE-DBT is however limited, due to the inherent low depth-resolution of reconstructed CE-DBT images. CE-bCT with quasi-isotropic spatial resolution and voxel signal

A.D.A. Maidment, P.R. Bakic, and S. Gavenonis (Eds.): IWDM 2012, LNCS 7361, pp. 434–441, 2012.

intensity proportional to the linear attenuation coefficient is believed to offer more accurate quantitative information.

This paper investigates the quantitative potential of CE-DBT and CE-bCT in the assessment of 3D lesion extent and iodinated contrast-agent uptake through theoretical modeling. As a first step, previously described cone-beam topologies and acquisition techniques were compared. For CE-DBT, a topology similar to that of a prototype GE Senographe DS-based CE-DBT system (GE Healthcare, Chalfont St Giles, UK) using a dual-energy (DE) subtraction technique was investigated [1]. For CE-bCT, a cone-beam topology similar to that published by Boone *et al.* [2] scanning the breast before and after contrast agent injection was simulated.

2   Method

2.1   Image System Simulations

Fig. 1 demonstrates the investigated CE-DBT and CE-bCT topologies and phantoms. Table 1 summarizes the model parameters to simulate the CE-DBT and CE bCT implementations. Two 50% fibro-glandular equivalent mathematical phantoms were simulated (Fig. 1 and Table 1). For CE-DBT, a 5 cm thick half-cylinder was used to mimic the breast under compression, while for CE-bCT a 14 cm diameter cylinder was used to mimic the same breast without applying compression and with the patient in prone position [3]. Spherical lesions with 2 to 20 mm diameters and 0.5, 1.0, 2.5 and 5.0 mg/cm^3 iodine concentrations were embedded in the phantoms. They were positioned at three distances from the chest wall side of the detector, in order to to assess the effect of the cone-beam artifact.

For CE-DBT and CE bCT, perfect energy-integrating detectors that do not generate any kind of noise or blurring were assumed. X-ray projections were simulated using mono-energetic and poly-energetic spectra [4–6] assuming primary x-rays only. The simulations were repeated without quantum noise and with quantum noise corresponding to a total average glandular dose (AGD) equal to 3 mGy. AGD was computed using previously described methods [7, 8]. For CE-DBT, a DE subtraction technique was used [9]. For CE-bCT two breast scans, one before and one after contrast-agent injection were simulated [10]. For CE-DBT, x-ray spectra and AGD allocations between the low-energy (LE) and high-energy (HE) images delivering optimal iodine enhanced images were used [11, 12]. For CE-bCT, an x-ray spectrum was used that has previously been shown to deliver optimally enhanced iodine images [13]. The AGD was the same for the pre- and post-contrast images.

For CE-DBT, LE and HE projection images were recombined into iodine projections using the algorithm of Puong *et al.* [9]. Tomographic reconstruction of the iodine projections was then performed using a filtered-back-projection (FBP), with a filter designed following the methodology described in [14], to obtain reconstructed iodine images parallel to the detector array with 1 mm spacing and an in-plane voxel pitch of 0.1 mm. CE-bCT pre- and post-projection images were also reconstructed by FBP, using a ramp filter and a 0.410 mm isotropic voxel size, to obtain pre- and post-contrast reconstructed breast volumes.

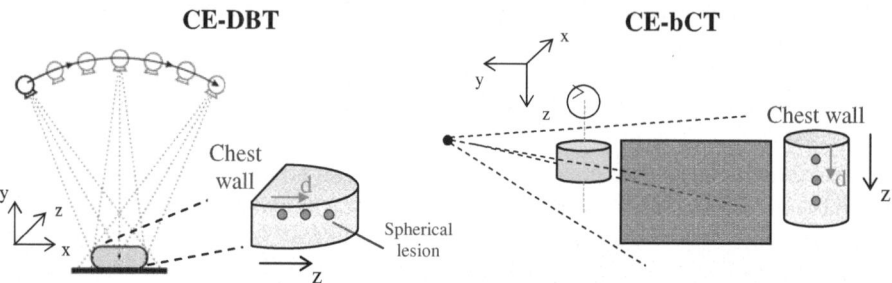

Fig. 1. CE-bCT and CE-DBT topologies and phantom configurations. Iodine-enhanced lesions were positioned along the rotation axis, at distance d from the chest wall side of the detector.

Table 1. Parameters used to simulate the CE-bCT and CE-DBT implementations

Model parameters		CE-DBT	CE-bCT
Spectrum	Mono-energetic	20 & 34 keV	34 keV
	Poly-energetic	Rh/Rh 27kV & Mo/Cu 49kV	W/Cu 47kV
Geometry	Magnification (SDD/SID)	660mm / 620mm	880mm / 460mm
	no. of projections	15 & 40° range	300 & 360° range
Phantom		Thickness: 5 cm	Diameter: 14 cm
	Composition	50 % fibro-glandular equivalent	
	Lesions	Diameter: 2, 5, 10, 15, 20 mm	
		Iodine concentration: 0.5, 1.0, 2.5,5.0 mg/cm³	
		Distance from chest wall: 20, 45, 70 mm	
Flat detector	Pixel size	0.100 mm	0.394 mm
Reconstruction		FBP	FBP
	Voxel size	0.1x0.1x1.0 mm	0.410x0.410x0.410 mm

SDD: source-to-detector distance / SID: source-to-isocenter distance

All simulations were performed using CatSim, a software package previously developed and validated at GE Healthcare [15].

2.2   Quantitative Analysis

Lesion extent was evaluated independently in the x, y, z directions (Fig. 1), using the reconstructed iodine images for CE-DBT and the post-contrast reconstructed volume for CE-bCT. Lesion extent, $\tilde{D}$, was estimated using an automatic estimator, A. $\tilde{D}$ was computed as the maximum of the convolution of a 1D profile through the lesion's center of mass (COM), f, with a sliding rectangle function, h, with varying width D_W. For example, $\tilde{D}$ in the x-direction was computed as:

$$\tilde{D} = \arg max_{D_W}\{f(x) * h(x)\}, \text{ with } h(x) = \begin{cases} 1/D_W, |x| \leq D_W/2 \\ -1/(N - D_W), elsewhere \end{cases} \quad (1)$$

where N is the length of $h(x)$. A calibration was performed to exclude any bias in lesion extent estimation due to the inherent imaging characteristics of CE-DBT and CE-bCT; the difference between $\tilde{D}$ and D_{true}, the true lesion dimension, was minimized through linear regression:

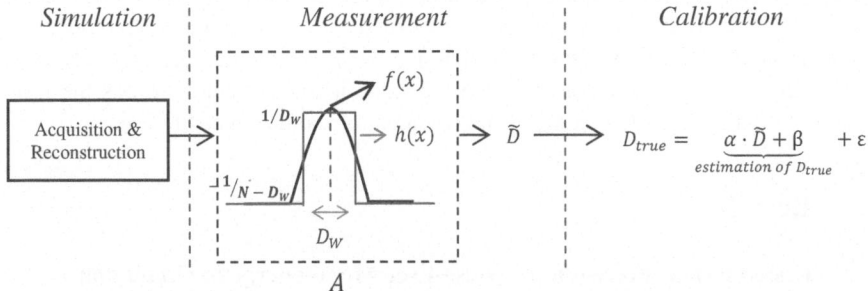

Fig. 2. Method for automatic lesion extent assessment; A represents the automatic estimator, $f(x)$ and $h(x)$ a 1D lesion profile and the rectangle window function in the x direction

$$D_{true} = \underbrace{\alpha \cdot \tilde{D} + \beta}_{estimation\ of\ D_{true}} + \varepsilon \tag{2}$$

where α and β are calibration parameters and ε is the residual error. The regression was repeated for each axis direction separately and included all lesion diameters, positions and iodine concentrations.

Since digital detectors are not shift invariant, the imaged lesion size depends on its alignment with respect to the sampling grid. Therefore, the simulations were repeated by shifting the lesions' COM by sub-voxel values in all three directions. The large obtained dataset (>1000 simulated lesions) allowed to calculate the residual error's mean, $\bar{\varepsilon}$, and standard deviation, σ_ε. Since $\bar{\varepsilon}$ tends towards zero (Equation 2), lesion size estimation precision is only characterized by σ_ε.

Finally, a full factorial experiment was designed to understand the impact of iodine concentration, lesion diameter and position (the independent variables) on the measurement precision, described by σ_ε (the observations). A general linear equation with crossed terms describes the interactions within the model:

$$\sigma_\varepsilon = a_0 + a_s X_s + a_p X_p + a_c X_c \dots + a_{sp} X_s X_p + \dots + a_{spc} X_s X_p X_c \tag{3}$$

where X_s, X_p and X_c represent lesion size, position and iodine concentration values, respectively. Statistical hypothesis tests were applied to verify the statistical significance of each factor in the model. The significance level for the p-values was set at 0.05. The data analysis was performed using software package MINITAB®.

Relative lesion-contrast-to-background contrast, C_{rel}, was computed in the reconstructed slices centered at the lesion's COM as:

$$C_{rel} = \frac{SI_{iodine} - SI_{bg}}{SI_{iodine}^{10\ mm} - SI_{bg}} \tag{4}$$

where SI_{iodine} and SI_{bg} are the mean per-pixel signal intensity in a ROI inside the iodine enhanced lesion and a background region. In DE CE-DBT, SI_{bg} is measured in a ROI surrounding the lesions, while in CE-bCT SI_{bg} is measured in a ROI of lesions in the pre-contrast image. To account for the different signal intensity scaling of the

CE-DBT and CE-bCT reconstruction algorithms, the absolute lesion-contrast-to-background (numerator in Equation 4) was normalized to the absolute lesion-contrast-to-background of a 10 mm diameter reference lesion, positioned at 20 mm from the chest wall side of the detector and with the same iodine concentration as the lesion under consideration. Note that C_{rel} is independent of iodine concentration.

3   Results

3.1   Lesion Extent Precision for Noise-Free Mono-energetic Simulation

Our results indicate that the linear regression fit is adequate to estimate D_{true}; R^2 values were found to be larger than 0.999 (t-test, p<0.001) for all axes and both topologies, except for the y-direction in CE-DBT (R^2=0.79). Due to CE-DBT's limited depth resolution in the y-direction, lesions appear ~3 times larger in that direction. Assuming that the reconstructed volume is limited to the 5 cm phantom thickness, the automatic estimator is unable to differentiate lesions >15 mm in diameter positioned at mid-depth in the phantom. To assess the precision to estimate lesion dimension in the y-direction, we repeated the analysis with 10 cm thick phantoms and lesions positioned at mid-depth. This resulted in an improved fit in the y-direction (R^2>0.995, t-test, p<0.001) without affecting the original calibration parameters in the x- and z-direction.

Fig. 3a summarizes the overall precision in lesion diameter estimation; for both topologies σ_ε is shown for the x-, y- and z-directions. For CE-DBT, the precision to estimate lesion diameter in the in-plane direction is about twice the in-plane voxel dimension (0.1 mm), while the precision in the y-axis direction is about half the spacing between reconstructed slices. For CE-bCT the precision to estimate lesion dimension is similar in all three axes directions; the precision is approximately half the voxel dimension (0.410 mm).

Fig. 3b summarizes the factorial analysis experiment; for both topologies σ_ε is shown as a function of each independent variable and for the x-, y- and z-direction. In CE-DBT, measurement precision is affected by the true lesion diameter in the three directions (t-test, p-values, 0.001, 0.064, and 0.001 for the x-, y- and z-direction respectively) and by the lesion's iodine concentration (t-test, p=0.029). The magnitude of these effects is however smaller than the voxel dimensions, in all three directions. In CE-bCT, measurement precision is only affected by the true lesion diameter (t-test, p<0.001). Again, the magnitude of this effect is smaller than the voxel dimension. In CE-DBT and CE-bCT, measurement precision is not affected by lesion position in the phantom.

3.2   Contrast Uptake for Noise-Free Mono-energetic Simulation

Fig. 4 shows average C_{rel} values as a function of lesion diameter and position in the phantom for quantum noise-free mono-energetic simulations. For CE-DBT, C_{rel} is greatly affected by lesion diameter. For CE-bCT, C_{rel} is almost constant as a function of lesion diameter, except for the 2 mm diameter lesion which has a slightly lower

a)   b)

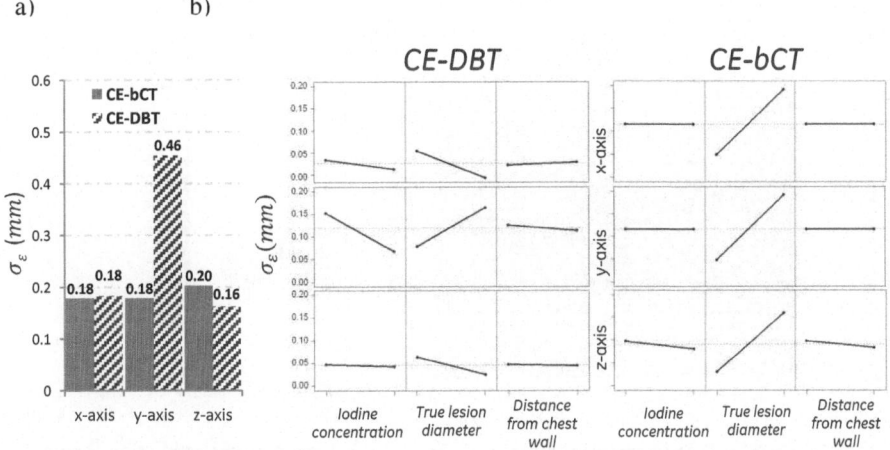

Fig. 3. a) Overall precision to estimate lesion diameter with CE-DBT and CE-bCT by evaluating the standard deviation, σ_ε, of the residual errors, ε, in the three axis directions; b) Main effect of independent variables on lesion extent estimation precision.

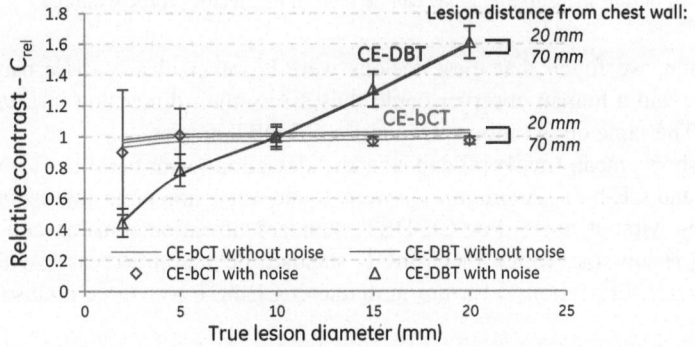

Fig. 4. C_{rel} as a function of lesion diameter, for lesions positioned at different distances from the chest wall. For CE-DBT, C_{rel} is 60% higher for 20 mm diameter lesions than for 10 mm lesion, while for CE b-CT C_{rel} is almost independent of lesion diameter.

C_{rel}. In this case, measurement accuracy is affected by the voxel dimension. For CE-DBT and CE-bCT the cone-beam artifact has only a small effect on C_{rel}; for lesions positioned further away from the chest-wall side C_{rel} decreases up to 1% and 5% for CE-DBT and CE-bCT respectively.

3.3   Lesion Extent Estimation and Contrast Uptake for Poly-energetic Simulation, Including Quantum Noise

Fig. 5a illustrates ROIs in CE-bCT slices through the lesions' COM, for simulations using poly-energetic spectra and quantum noise corresponding to a total AGD equal to 3 mGy. As illustrated in Fig 5b, it was found that the automatic estimator was not reliable for lesions with low inherent contrast-to-noise ratio's (CNR). After some

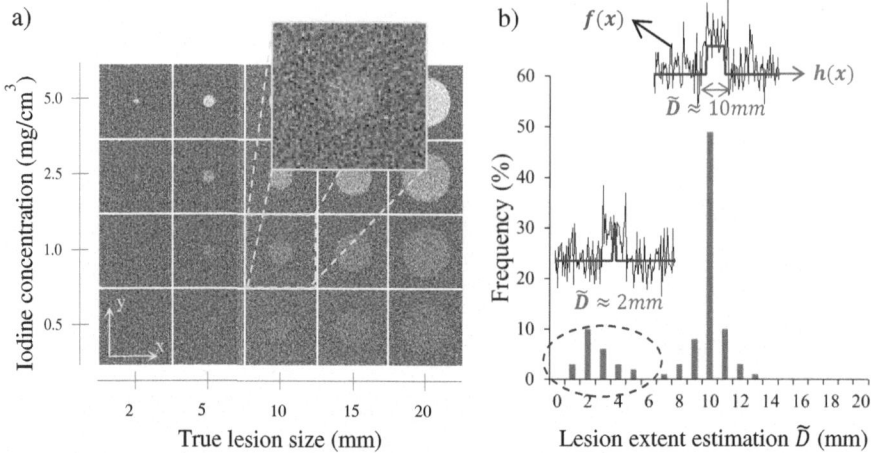

Fig. 5. a) Set of ROIs from different reconstructed CE-bCT slices passing through the lesions' COM; b) histogram from a hundred automatic measurements in one axis direction for a 10 mm diameter lesion containing 1.0 mg/cm³ of iodine. The left band in the histogram highlights the percentage of outlier measurements, as can be seen in the nearer profile example.

investigation, we found that these lesions were however clearly discernable by the human eye and a human observer could thus assess their dimension in a more accurate way. The same observation was made in CE-DBT images.

Fig. 4 shows mean (markers) and standard deviation (error bars) in C_{rel} values for CE-DBT and CE-bCT. Average C_{rel} were found very similar to those obtained for simulations without noise. For CE-DBT, standard deviation remains constant with increasing lesion size, while for CE-bCT, standard deviation decreases with increasing lesion size. For lesions >10 mm in diameter CE-bCT was more precise than CE-DBT.

4   Discussion

This paper compares the quantitative potential of a cone-beam CE-bCT and a cone-beam CE-DBT topology in the assessment of lesion extent and iodinated contrast-agent uptake. To assess lesion extent in the reconstructed slices, a calibrated automatic estimator was proposed. Without quantum noise, this estimator was shown to be robust to all simulated lesions and a factorial experiment demonstrated the effect of lesion size, position and iodine concentration on estimation precision. With quantum noise, the automatic estimator was shown to be inefficient for lesions with low CNR. In addition, the efficiency of the estimator with respect to the human observer (*i.e.* the radiologist) is not understood. Further studies, including human observers, are necessary to properly assess the accuracy and precision of lesion extent estimation in the presence of noise.

To assess iodine concentration, relative image contrast between iodine enhanced lesions and background breast tissue was used as figure of merit. As suggested previously, relative image contrast can be used to estimate the iodine area density when the appropriate transformation is known. Since contrast in CE-DBT depends on lesion size (Fig. 4), the accuracy of iodine concentration estimation could be improved by including the estimated lesion extent as *a priori* information. Relative image contrast showed very good agreement in simulations with and without quantum noise.

Our results are a first step in the comparison of CE-DBT and CE-bCT for their quantitative performance. Inclusion of more realistic physics phenomena in the image simulation chain and a comparison of dual-energy CE-DBT and bCT are underway.

Acknowledgements. This study was funded by the ANRT, under the PhD CIFRE convention 2010/756.

References

1. Carton, A.-K., et al.: Effects of image lag and scatter for dual-energy contrast-enhanced digital breast tomosynthesis using a CsI flat-panel based system. In: Proceedings of SPIE, pp. 79611D–79611D-5 (2011)
2. Lindfors, K.K., Boone, J.M., et al.: Dedicated Breast CT: Initial Clinical Experience. Radiology 246, 725 (2008)
3. Boone, J.M., Kwan, A.L.C., et al.: Technique factors and their relationship to radiation dose in pendant geometry breast CT. Radiology, 3767–3776 (2005)
4. Birch, R., et al.: Computation of bremsstrahlung Xray spectra and comparison with spectra measured with a Ge(Li) detector. Physics in Medicine and Biology 24, 505–517 (1979)
5. Cranley, K., et al.: Catalogue of Diagnostic X-Ray Spectra and Other Data (1997)
6. Boone, J.M., Seibert, J.A.: An accurate method for computer-generating tungsten anode x-ray spectra from 30 to 140 kV. Medical Physics 24, 1661–1670 (1997)
7. Boone, J.M.: Normalized glandular dose (DgN) coefficients for arbitrary x-ray spectra in mammography: Computer-fit values of Monte Carlo derived data. Medical Physics 29, 869 (2002)
8. Boone, J.M., et al.: A comprehensive analysis of DgN_{CT} coefficients for pendant-geometry cone-beam breast computed tomography. Medical Physics 31, 226 (2004)
9. Puong, S., et al.: Dual-energy contrast enhanced digital mammography using a new approach for breast tissue canceling. In: Proceedings of SPIE, vol. 6510, pp. 65102H–65102H-12 (2007)
10. Prionas, N., Lindfors, K., Ray, S., Huang, S.: Contrast-enhanced Dedicated Breast CT: Initial Clinical Experience. Radiology 256 (2010)
11. Puong, S., et al.: Dual-energy contrast enhanced digital mammography: theoretical and experimental study of optimal monoenergetic beam parameters using synchrotron radiation. In: Proceedings of SPIE, vol. 7258, pp. 72583U–72583U-10 (2009)
12. Puong, S., et al.: Optimization of beam parameters and iodine quantification in dual-energy contrast enhanced digital breast tomosynthesis. In: Proceedings of SPIE, vol. 6913, pp. 69130Z–69130Z-11 (2008)
13. Weigel, M., Vollmar, S.V., Kalender, W.A.: Spectral optimization for dedicated breast CT. Medical Physics 38, 114 (2011)
14. Kunze, H., Haerer, W., et al.: Filter determination for tomosynthesis aided by iterative reconstruction techniques. In: 9th International Meeting on Fully Three-Dimensional Image Reconstruction in Radiology and Nuclear Medicine, pp. 309–312 (2007)
15. Man, B.D., Basu, S., et al.: CatSim: a new computer assisted tomography simulation environment. In: Proceedings of SPIE, vol. 6510, pp. 1–8 (2007)

Development and Initial Demonstration of a Low-Dose Dedicated Fully 3D Breast CT System

Randolph L. McKinley[1], Martin P. Tornai[2,3], Laura A. Tuttle[4], Doreen Steed[4], and Cherie M. Kuzmiak[4]

[1] *Zumatek, Inc.*, Research Triangle Park, NC 27709
rmckinley@zumatek.com
[2] Department of Radiology, Duke University Medical Center, Durham, NC 27710
[3] Medical Physics Graduate Program, Duke University Medical Center, Durham, NC 27705
[4] Department of Radiology, University of North Carolina, Chapel Hill, NC 27599

Abstract. Based on earlier work demonstrating more complete, 3D cone beam sampling acquisition approaches that additionally facilitate chest wall imaging posterior to an uncompressed breast, a new, clinic-ready, low-dose breast CT system was developed and is undergoing initial clinical validation. The system includes a small focal spot pulsed x-ray source and 30x30cm^2 flat panel detector having 3 degrees of freedom of motion, and a radiopaque patient support that facilitates whole-breast and universal anterior chest-wall imaging. Data is acquired with fully-3D trajectories and iteratively reconstructed within minutes of acquisition. Performance characteristics include: sub-200 micron isotropic reconstructed resolution, low-dose (<4.5 mGy) fully-3D scans acquired in ~1.5 min, clinic throughput of 1patient/11min, and DICOM compatible images. To date, 25 subjects have been successfully scanned. Characterization results and volumetric clinical images are presented including demonstration of routine anterior chest wall imaging and comparison with digital mammography.

Keywords: Breast imaging, computed tomography, mammography, breast CT, breast cancer, screening, diagnostic imaging.

1   Introduction

We have developed a clinic-ready 3D breast CT system for dedicated breast imaging. The system was based on an earlier, fully-3D prototype with which more complete cone-beam sampling and anterior chest wall imaging was demonstrated, through the use of polar titling trajectories[1,2,3,4]. The unique orbiting capability[3,4] together with a custom formed patient support allow for full breast and chest wall access while maximizing patient comfort and consequently minimizing patient motion. A custom user interface has been developed whereby scans can be operated independently by a (mammography) technologist, raw image results are packaged in DICOM format, and reconstructions are performed automatically and rapidly. This paper presents the first imaging results of the system including a pilot clinical study.

A.D.A. Maidment, P.R. Bakic, and S. Gavenonis (Eds.): IWDM 2012, LNCS 7361, pp. 442–449, 2012.
© Springer-Verlag Berlin Heidelberg 2012

2   Methods

2.1   Breast CT System

The clinic ready breast CT system development is built upon earlier work on prototypes developed at Duke University [2,3]. The development of a commercially realizable system took place with the following goals in mind: (1) increase scan speed to reduce scan time from ~10 min down to ~1.5 min/breast; (2) increase patient comfort; (3) achieve a total procedure time faster than current mammography; (4) increase the number of degrees of freedom of motion from 2 to 3; (5) achieve full breast and chest wall access; (6) develop a custom user interface to allow a imaging technologist to perform the scans independently; (7) develop a DICOM compatible flow through from acquisition through reconstruction, with final 3D results viewable in 3rd party DICOM viewers; and (8) reduce the reconstruction time from hours to minutes.

The basic system components used to build the cone-beam CT system include: a $30x30cm^2$ CsI flat panel detector with 197 micron pixels and 8mm narrow dead-edge; a single pole 0.3mm focal spot x-ray tube capable of output to 49 kVp; an x-ray generator capable of fast pulsed x-ray generation up to 30 fps; direct drive motors for 3 degrees of freedom of motion in step-and-shoot mode up to 10 fps. This system is capable of being moved around the pendant, uncompressed breast of a prone patient in any arbitrary trajectory. The elements were arranged on a custom developed and machined chassis. Multi-threaded software was written in C# to sychronize all components and perform a step and shoot acquisition. The completed system is shown in Figure 1. The device has a METLab certification indicating conformance with UL electrical safety standards and is considered a non-significant risk device.

2.2   Geometric and Anthropomorphic Phantoms

A large variety of geometric and anthropomorphic phantoms (in addition to supermarket produce) were scanned with the system prior to any human scanning. These phantoms include resolution (acrylic rod and tube) and materials phantoms in various media having different target to background ratios to simulate breasts of different densities containing known objects. Additionally, a cadaver breast was imaged under various conditions, with and without addition of a silicone implant above the suspended biological tissue. Then, radiation dose measurements were performed using a calibrated ionization chamber (*Radcal* model 10X5-6M) located at the system isocenter, and read-out by a *Radcal Accu-Pro* monitor.

2.3   Healthy Volunteers

The first cohort of 7 subjects were healthy volunteers who have been through the "mammography experience", but with no history of breast cancer and at otherwise normal risk for the disease. The left breast was scanned first in all cases. Each subject placed their breast through the visible hole in the patient support (Figure 1). The technologist verified that their breast was centered in the FOV through open shielded doors on the side of the system, both visually and with the assistance of a laser sight, then began the scan. After one breast was scanned, the procedure was repeated for the opposite breast without the subject leaving the support structure. After the scan, the subject stepped off the system and got dressed. Then she was asked to fill in a brief questionnaire about her experience.

2.4   BIRADS 4/5 Subjects

Scans of 20 BIRADS 4 and 5 patients have been completed at the time of this paper submission. The ultimate goal of this pilot study is to perform a reader study comparison of both screening and diagnostic mammograms (where available) with that of breast CT for a total of 20 BIRADS 4/5 subjects with suspicious masses. Two cases are qualitatively presented in this paper comparing mammograms to breast CT for cases of: (1) a cyst, and (2) suspicious non-spiculated mass.

3   Results

3.1   Completed Breast CT System

A complete clinic-ready system is shown in its current configuration in Figure 1. The custom contoured patient support allows for comfortable uncompressed patient imaging procedures to image both breasts in 11 min ± 47sec, with a repositioning time between breasts of less than 1 min. Not shown in the figure is a set of stairs for the patient to ease the effort in climbing on to the system. In addition, the system has been designed with an open geometry allowing for the future addition of interventional devices. To date, with a total of 27 subjects scanned (mean age: 56, range: 41-75, breast cup size range: A-DD), all patients have rated the system in a post scan questionnaire as 4/5 or 5/5, where 5 is Easy for getting on and off the system. It is recognized that there may be patients who may have some difficulty in getting on and off the system. However, with proper assistance from clinic staff, our initial experience is that the vast majority of patients will be able to get on and off the system and sustain a scan without discomfort.

With scans operated by a clinical mammography technologist, raw data sets are automatically forwarded to a reconstruction server. The CPU-based reconstruction server performs ordered subsets convex (OSC) reconstructions with 5 iterations, 15 subsets in under 15 minutes, where these reconstructions would previously have taken several hours.

Figure 2 illustrates the existing technologist interface for operating the breast CT system. Training time for the operation of the system is approximately 1 hour. This includes going through the user interface as well as the procedure for positing the patient, centering the breast, and conducting scout images to ensure proper positioning prior to starting the scan.

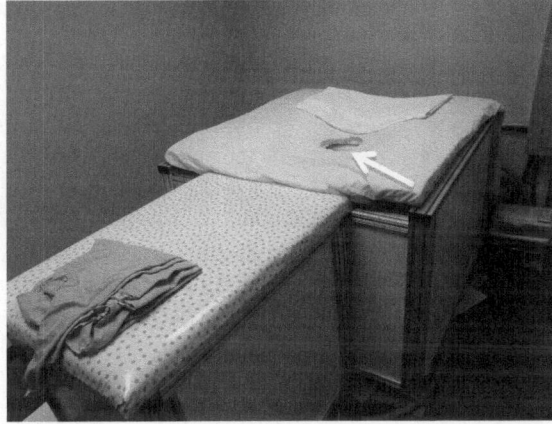

Fig. 1. Completely shielded breast CT system enclosure used for imaging. Upper right section covered in a yellow sheet is where the patient lies prone and extends her breast through the opening (white arrow). Lower left section covered in pink polka-dots is for hip and leg support. The inside of this section is also used for housing various motion control components.

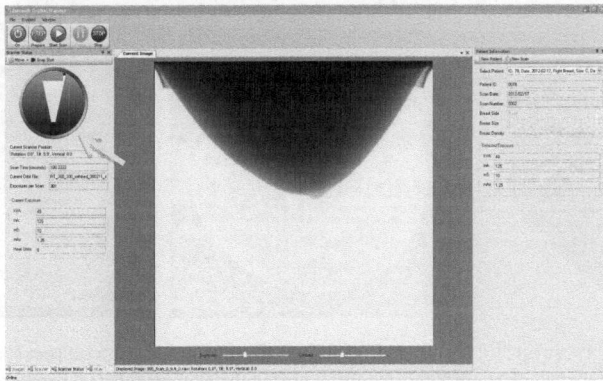

Fig. 2. Screen shot of the user interface used by the technologist to control the breast CT scan and post-scan data publishing. The technologist has access to an animation (upper left – yellow arrow) that shows the actual system position in real time. The large central area also comprises a real time projection by projection view of the actual individual projections being taken by the scanner. The right column contains patient data and technique information.

3.2   Geometric and Anthropomorphic Phantom Results

Initial results from geometric and anthropomorphic phantom scans, as well as a cadaver breast scan, were completed prior to any human scanning (Figure 3).

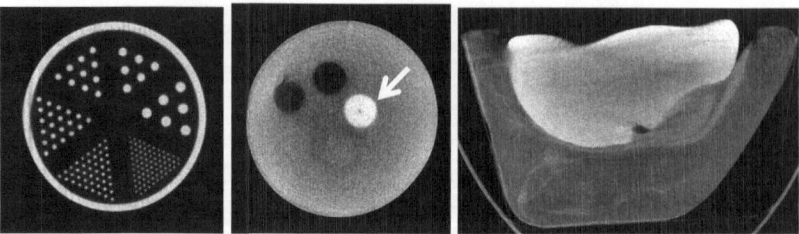

Fig. 3. (Left) Resolution phantom scan completed as early test scan on the newly constructed system. Acrylic rod sizes are from 1.1mm to 4.6mm in diameter, with spacing on twice their diameters throughout. (Middle) Materials phantom scan results with the following materials (clockwise from white arrow): delrin, acrylic, glandular-equivalent, fat, and polyethylene equivalent bathed in water. (Right) Sagittal cadaver breast image slice from 58y.o. donor with posterior breast implant placed by researchers to observe contrast differences between breast tissue and implant as well as performance of new system on human tissue prior to human volunteers. Black region between implant and breast is an air space; darker grey region near air pocket is portion of chest muscle.

3.3   Healthy Volunteer Results

Initial human results are shown in Figure 4. Figure 5 illustrates the capability of the system to easily access the chest wall. A close look at the sagittal view shows significant access to the chest wall as indicated by viewable pectoralis muscle and several ribs (at arrows).

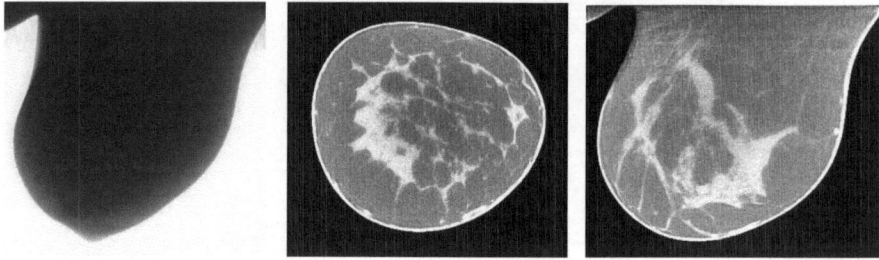

Fig. 4. (Left) Raw projection image obtained of the suspended uncompressed breast from a patient lying prone on the support. (Middle) Coronal slice of fully-3D reconstructed images which can be sliced in any orientation. (Right) Sagittal view of the same breast.

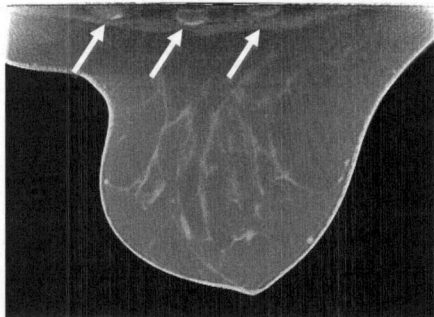

Fig. 5. Sagittal view of a subject whose anterior ribs and pectoralis muscle are clearly visible at arrows, in addition to the full volume of her breast

3.4   BIRADS 4/5 Subjects Breast CT versus Mammography

Two cases are presented illustrating breast CT results versus diagnostic and screening mammography for BIRADS 4/5 volunteers. Note that our reader study has not yet begun so the following are for illustrative purposes only and do not represent quantitative reader results.

Case 1: 51y.o. white female presenting with palpable subareolar lump in right heterogenously dense breast. Mammogram findings indicate obscured mass in 6 o'clock position without associated architectural distortion or microcalcifications. Ultrasound indicated 0.7x0.6x0.6 cm irregular hypoechoic mass with microlobulations. Breast CT clearly indicates an oval circumscribed cystic mass approximately 4.1cm in diameter (Figure 6). Breast CT finding confirmed by follow-up diagnostic work-up and aspiration.

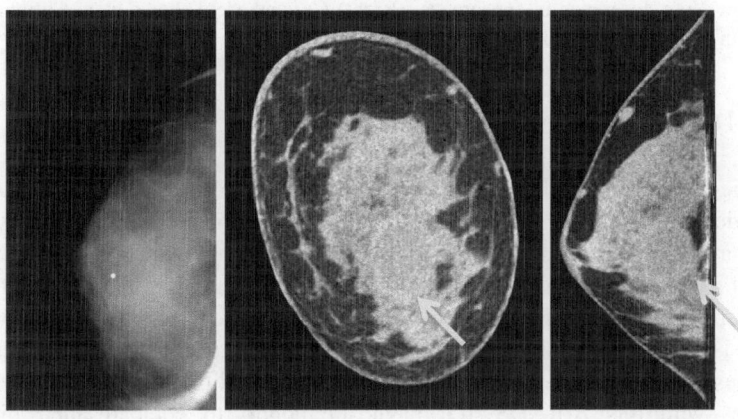

Fig. 6. (Left) Diagnostic mammogram right MLO mag-view. Patient presents with palpable subareolar lump in position indicated by BB marker. (Middle) Single sagittal slice from breast CT through cyst indicated by arrow. (Right) Coronal view shows different perspective of cyst in a different plane of the 3D reconstruction.

Case 2: 48y.o. African-American female with screening mammogram finding of 8mm lobular mass at 4 o'clock position in left breast with additional 7mm asymmetry identified in MLO view only. Diagnostic mammogram indicates 7mm asymmetry as normal tissue and identifies 1.0cm mass in 6 o'clock position. This correlates with 0.8x0.5x0.6cm hypoechoic lobular mass seen in ultrasound. Breast CT indicates 3 distinct lobular masses in right breast (Figure 7).

Based on the exposure measurements and comparisons with our earlier work [5], the dose delivered to the subjects ranged between 4.1 and 4.8 mGy with an average dose of approximately 4.5 mGy.

448   R.L. McKinley et al.

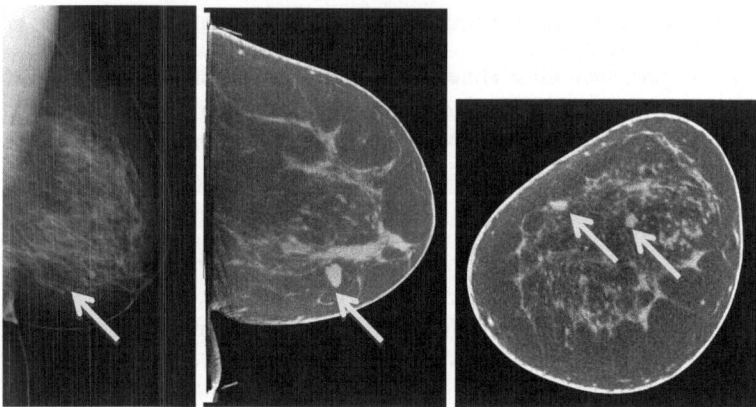

Fig. 7. (Left) Diagnostic mammogram MLO view left breast. Radiology report indicates suspicious mass at arrow. (Middle) Single sagittal slice from breast CT through same mass indicated by arrow. Note difference in appearance. (Right) Coronal view shows two additional lobular masses in a different plane of the 3D reconstruction.

4   Discussion and Conclusion

A clinic-ready dedicated breast CT system has been developed that achieves the initial design goals. The scans are performed by an imaging technologist with total procedure times faster than conventional mammography. Surveys indicate a high level of patient comfort and satisfaction with a scan, yielding minimal patient motion. Reconstructions are achieved within minutes of the scan and are ready while the patient is still present. Initial patient scans have shown access to the complete breast and chest wall across the variety of 27 subjects. Additional patient studies are in progress with this BIRADS 4/5 diagnostic cohort to compare their diagnostic mammograms with 3D breast CT. Initial results comparing breast CT to digital mammography are promising. The breast CT system will initially be used for diagnostic purposes, but with technological improvements, isotropic image resolution, patient comfort, low dose, and speed, we ultimately foresee the device as having the potential to replace screening mammography.

Acknowledgements. This work has been funded by the National Cancer Institute of the National Institutes of Health (R44-CA125924). The UNC IRB protocol for this study is # 10-1383. RLM and MPT are founders and Board Members of *Zumatek*. MPT is also a consultant to *Zumatek*.

References

1. McKinley, R.L., Tornai, M.P., Samei, E., Bradshaw, M.L.: Simulation study of a quasi-monochromatic beam for X-ray computed mammotomography. Med. Phys. 31(4), 800–813 (2004)

2. Tornai, M.P., McKinley, R.L., Brzymialkiewicz, C.N., Madhav, P., Cutler, S.J., Crotty, D.J., Bowsher, J.E., Samei, E., Floyd, C.E.: Design and Development of a Fully-3D Dedicated X-ray Computed Mammotomography System. In: 2005 Proc. SPIE: Physics of Medical Imaging, vol. 5745(1), pp. 189–197 (2005)

3. McKinley, R.L., Tornai, M.P., Brzymialkiewicz, C.N., Samei, E., Bowsher, J.E.: Analysis of a novel offset cone-beam computed mammotomography imaging system for attenuation correction of SPECT in a proposed dual modality dedicated breast mammotomography system. Physica Medica XXI(supplement 1), 48–55 (2006)

4. Madhav, P., Crotty, D.J., McKinley, R.L., Tornai, M.P.: Evaluation of Tilted Cone-Beam CT Orbits in the Development of a Dedicated Hybrid Mammotomograph. Phys. Med. Biol. 54, 3659–3676 (2009)

5. Crotty, D.J., Brady, S.L., Jackson, D.C., Toncheva, G.I., Anderson, C.E., Yoshizumi, T.T., Tornai, M.P.: Evaluation of the Absorbed Dose to the Breast Using Radiochromic Film in a Dedicated CT Mammotomography System Employing a Quasi-Monchromatic Beam. Med. Phys. 38(6), 3232–3245 (2011)

Correspondence among Subjective and Objective Similarities and Pathologic Types of Breast Masses on Digital Mammography

Chisako Muramatsu[1], Kohei Nishimura[1], Mikinao Oiwa[2], Misaki Shiraiwa[2], Tokiko Endo[2], Kunio Doi[3,4], and Hiroshi Fujita[1]

[1] Department of Intelligent Image Information, Graduate School of Medicine, Gifu University, 1-1 Yanagido, Gifu 501-1194, Japan
chisa@fjt.info.gifu-u.ac.jp
[2] Department of Radiology, National Hospital Organization, Nagoya Medical Center, 4-1-1 Nakaku Sannomaru, Nagoya, Aichi 460-0001, Japan
[3] Gunma Prefectural Collage of Health Sciences, 328-1 Kamiokimachi, Maebashi, Gunma 371-0051, Japan
[4] Department of Radiology, The University of Chicago, 5841 South Maryland Avenue, Chicago, Illinois 60637

Abstract. In multi-modality, multi-information breast cancer diagnosis framework, radiologists take into account all the information available in making diagnosis, one of which can be the information from reference cases. The purpose of this study is to investigate the relationship between pathological concordance and image similarity of breast masses for exploring the utility of similar images and determining the effective similarity index for image retrieval. Twenty-seven images of masses, three from each of 9 pathologic types, were used in this study. Subjective similarity ratings for all possible pairs (351 pairs) were provided by 8 expert readers. Thirteen image features were determined, and their usefulness as a similarity index was examined. Generally, masses with the same pathologic types were considered more similar (0.75) than those with different types (0.43) by the experts, although cysts and fibroadenomas appeared very similar on mammograms. Perimeter, ellipticity, radial gradient index, and full-width at half maximum of radial gradient histogram were considered potentially useful (correlation, r>0.4) for estimating subjective similarity among image features. Similar images together with their clinical data may serve as a useful reference for diagnosis of breast lesions.

Keywords: subjective similarity, objective similarity, breast masses, reference images, image retrieval, pathological classification.

1 Introduction

Mammography is considered a very effective examination for screening breast cancer in women with normal risk [1-3]. When a suspicious lesion is found on mammograms, usually it would be evaluated with other imaging modalities. Even in such

A.D.A. Maidment, P.R. Bakic, and S. Gavenonis (Eds.): IWDM 2012, LNCS 7361, pp. 450–457, 2012.
© Springer-Verlag Berlin Heidelberg 2012

multimodality diagnostic framework, it is important to independently assess findings on mammograms and to anticipate results from other examinations before a final decision is made on the basis of the combined information. It can be, however, difficult to diagnose and classify lesions on mammograms. In order to assist radiologists in differentiating lesions between benign and malignant, computer-aided diagnosis systems that provide the likelihood of malignancy of lesions have been suggested and found potentially useful in observer performance studies [4-6]. Although the probability is straightforward and easy to interpret, the reasons for the computed probability are blinded to radiologists. For providing more descriptive and evidential data, researchers have suggested to present reference cases with known diagnoses in the field of breast lesions on mammograms and lung nodules in CT [7-12].

Conventionally, image retrieval methods were often based on the difference in image feature values or the distance in feature space [7-11]. However, to select reference images that may be helpful in the diagnosis, it is important to quantify and evaluate image similarity in the radiologists' point of view. There have been a small number of studies that investigated the subjective similarity of lesions by radiologists [12-13]. To select visually similar images, we have been investigating a similarity measure that correlates with radiologists' visual impression [14-16]. In the previous study, radiologists' subjective similarity ratings for pairs of masses on digitized mammograms were obtained to be used for determination and evaluation of similarity measures. In that study, we found that presentation of similar images may be useful to radiologists in the distinction between benign and malignant masses; however, it was also found that some atypical cases, i.e., benign masses that are very similar to malignant masses, as well as malignant masses that are very similar to benign masses, can cause detrimental effects [17]. In our previous studies, masses are largely categorized to benign and malignant types, although it is known that masses with different pathologic types are expected to have different characteristics. In this study, to analyze the similarity of masses in more detail, we investigated subjective similarities of masses within and between different pathologic types, and also the usefulness of image features in classifying subtypes and determining objective similarity.

2   Material and Methods

2.1   Database

Digital mammograms used in this study were acquired at Nagoya Medical Center, Nagoya, Japan from December 2006 to April 2010. They were obtained with use of phase contrast mammography (PCM) system (Mermaid or Pureview, Konica Minolta Holdings, Inc.), Fuji digital mammography (DM) system (Amulet, Fujifilm Corporation), or computed radiography (CR) systems (MAMMOMAT 3000, Siemens, with C-Plate, Konica, or Profect, Fujifilm). The pixel size of the original images is 25, 43.75, or 50 μm, and the pixel values are stored in gray levels of 10, 12, or 14 bits depending on the systems used. To facilitate image comparison and computation, the pixel size was adjusted to 50 μm by the linear interpolation, and the gray level was down-sampled to 10 bits.

On the basis of the radiologic and pathologic reports, two radiologists placed square regions of interest (ROIs) in confining masses on both craniocaudal and mediolateral oblique views if a lesion was visible. The size of the ROIs varied from 168 x 168 to 1888 x 1888. As a result, the mass database consisted of 552 ROIs extracted from 272 cases. The numbers of lesions and ROIs with different pathologic types are listed in Table 1. All of the malignant cases were confirmed by biopsy and/or surgery, and benign cases were confirmed by biopsy or follow-up by mammography and ultrasonography.

In this study, 9 pathologic types with at least 5 lesions, except invasive ductal carcinoma (IDC) without other specification (unknown subcategories), were considered. The 9 types included ductal carcinomas in situ (DCIS), invasive lobular carcinomas (ILC), mucinous carcinomas (MC), papillo-tubular carcinomas (PTC), scirrhous carcinomas (SC), solid-tubular carcinomas (STC), cysts, fibroadenomas (FA), and benign phyllodes tumor (PT). Note that PTC, SC, and STC are the 3 subcategories of IDC. From each of the 9 groups, 3 ROIs with representative characteristics of the subtype were selected and included in this study. No ROIs from the same patients were selected. The effective diameters of these 27 masses ranged from 8 to 34 mm with mean of 15.5 mm. Subjective and objective similarities were determined for all possible 351 pairs.

Table 1. Numbers of lesions and ROIs obtained

	Number of lesions	Number of ROIs
Ductal carcinoma in situ	10	17
Invasive lobular carcinoma	9	17
Mucinous carcinoma	7	12
Papillotubular carcinoma	21	41
Scirrhous carcinoma	50	91
Solid-tubular carcinoma	24	44
Other malignant types	37	74
Cyst	68	112
Fibroadenoma	71	118
Benign phyllodes tumor	6	10
Other benign types	9	16

2.2   Subjective Similarity Data

Subjective similarity ratings for the 351 pairs were obtained from 8 physicians who are certified for breast image reading by the Central Committee on Quality Control of Mammographic Screening in Japan. The mean years of experience in reading mammograms was 12 years with the range of 4 to 25 years. Each expert reader individually provided the subjective similarity for the pairs of masses on a continuous rating scale between dissimilar to similar based on the overall impression for diagnosis including shape, density, and margin with consideration of predicted pathologic types. The observers were told that the masses include 9 pathologic types.

They were asked not to consider the size of lesions and the surrounding normal tissue. During the reading session, a pair of ROIs was placed side by side on a 17 inch (1280 x 1024 pixel resolution) liquid crystal display (LCD) monitor (Eizo Nanao Co.), and thier corresponding mammograms (entire views) were provided on a 27 inch (2560 x 1440 pixel resolution) LCD monitor (Dell Inc.). The observers could adjust the contrast and density levels of the ROIs, if desired. In the begining of the session, 5 training cases including pairs with the same and different pathologic types were provided for readers to become familier with appearances of similar and dissimilar pairs. The order of the pairs was randomized for each observer.

2.3   Image Features

Thirteen image features were determined: shape features included the area, effective diameter, perimeter, circularity, irregularity, ellipticity, elliptical irregularity, and ratio of minor-to-major axis of the fitted ellipse; density features included the contrast and standard deviation of pixel values; and edge features included the average edge strength, radial gradient index (RGI), and full-width at half-maximum (FWHM) of radial gradient histogram. The definitions of these features are described elsewhere [14]. The shape features were based on mass outlines determined manually by a co-author (CM), although they should be replaced by the automatic contours in the future. The edge features which can characterize smoothness or spiculation were determined in the margin area around the outline.

3   Results

Interreader agreement on subjective similarity ratings between observers in terms of Pearson's correlation coefficient ranged from 0.43 to 0.71, with the mean of 0.58. The observers strongly agreed on those of the cyst pairs and the sirrhous carcinoma pairs, inferred by the small standard deviations of 0.09 for both. These two types of lesions have characteristic features in the opposite extreme. On the other hand, the observers tended to disagree on pairs including mucinous carcinomas, although such results may be due to specific cases included in this study rather than the pathologic trend.

In general, the observers considered pairs with the same pathologic types more similar than those with the different types, indicated by the average ratings of 0.75 and 0.43, respectively. Figure 1 shows the average subjective ratings for pairs within and between different pathologic types. Only the highest 3 types for each are shown in the figure. Note that for each type, the result for pairs within group is the average of 3 ratings, while that for pairs between groups is the average of 9 ratings. It can be seen that although the masses with the same pathologic types are often rated high, except for the mucinous carcinomas, masses with other pathologic types could be considered similar. Especially, cysts and FAs were considered very similar to each other, while they were considered dissimilar to those of malignant types. SCs were considered very similar to ILCs and somewhat similar to STCs; however, they were

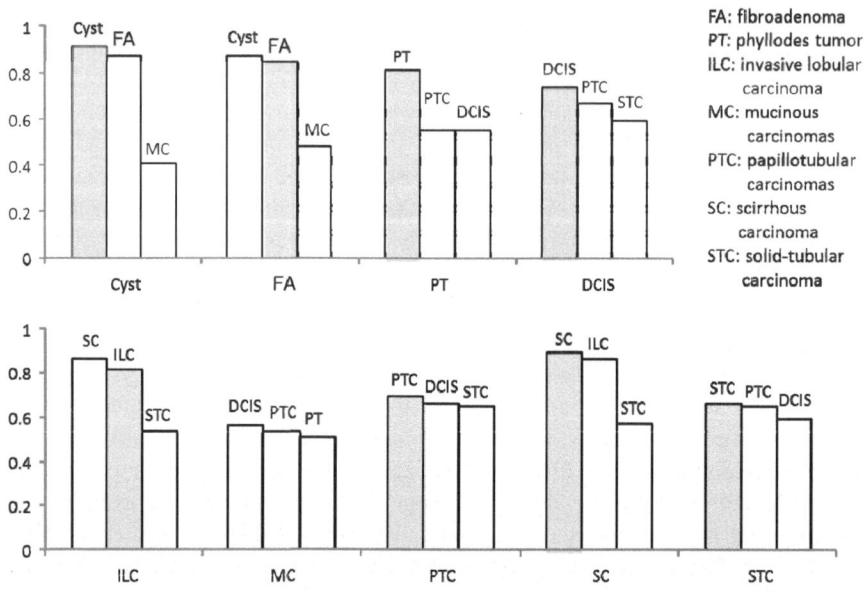

FA: fibroadenoma
PT: phyllodes tumor
ILC: invasive lobular
    carcinoma
MC: mucinous
    carcinomas
PTC: papillotubular
    carcinomas
SC: scirrhous
    carcinoma
STC: solid-tubular
    carcinoma

Fig. 1. Average similarity ratings for masses with same and different pathologic types

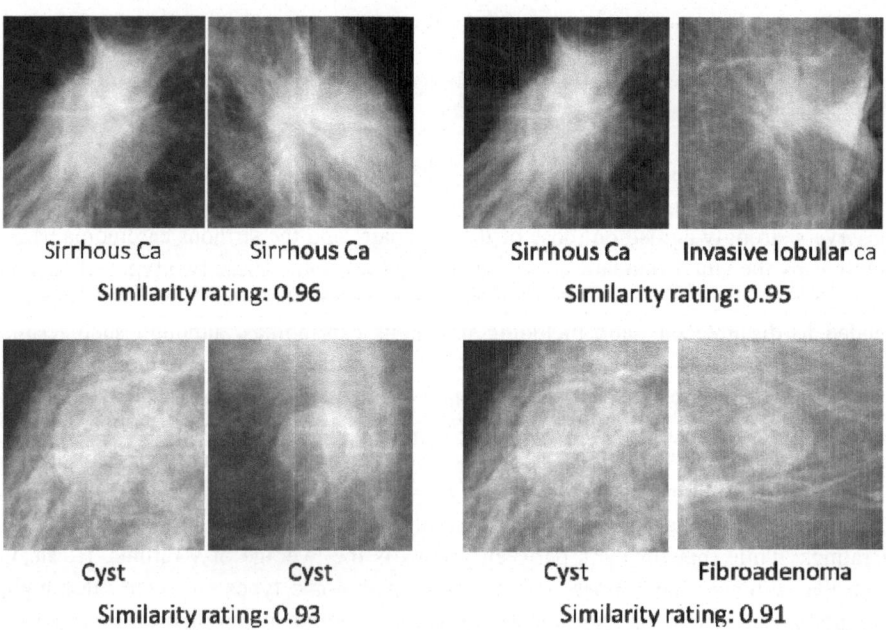

Fig. 2. Pairs with the high average subjective similarity ratings for masses of the same and different pathologic types

dissimilar to other types (similarities < 0.41). DCIS, PTC, and STC are considered to have similar apparence. The pairs with the high average ratings for masses of the same and difference pathologic types are shown in Fig. 2. The difficulty of distinguishing these masses with the different pathologic types is apparent.

When the differences in feature values were compared with the average subjective similarity ratings, the perimeter of the lesion, degree of ellipticity, RGI, and FWHM could be considered potentially useful for determining objective similarity measures, indicated by the moderate correlation above 0.40. The correlation coefficients between the subjective ratings and the differences in the feature values are listed in Table 2. The highest correlation was obtained with the FWHM for the 351 pairs. Three cysts used in this study had comparable values in shape and edge features. SCs and ILCs, which often appears spiculated, had smaller RGI values and larger FWHM values than the other types of lesions as expected. However, the ranges of the values are larger than that of the cysts. This fact indicates that the differences in feature values may not be simply and linearly related to the subjective similarity.

Table 2. Correlation coefficients between the average subjective ratings and the differences in feature values for 351 pairs

Image features	Pearson's correlation coefficient
FWHM of radial gradient histogram	-0.63
Degree of ellipticity	-0.54
Perimeter of a mass	-0.50
Radial gradient Index (RGI)	-0.46
Circularity	-0.28
Contrast	-0.23
Degree of elliptical irregularity	-0.23
Effective diameter	-0.21
Area of a mass	-0.12
Minor-to-major axis ratio	-0.07
Standard deviation in pixel values	-0.06
Average edge gradient	-0.01

4   Discussion and Conclusion

In general, masses with the same pathologic type were considered very similar to each other by the experts, indicating a potential utility of presenting similar cases as a diagnostic reference. It must be noted, however, that masses with some pathologic types could appear very similar, such as cysts and fibroadenomas, which may be differentiated by ultrasonography. Some mucinous carcinoma lesions could appear similar to fibroadenomas, while others may look similar to malignant lesions. Therefore, when reference images would be presented, the pathologic information, not only the benignity and malignancy, should be provided along with similar images preferably with the prevalence of such lesions.

For the 351 pairs used in this study, some shape and edge features were found potentially useful for determining the objective similarity measures. On the other hand, the correlation coefficients for the contrast and stadard deviation of pixel values were not very high. Since the density of masses are also considered an important feature for diagnosing masses by the experts, better definition of density features must be explored. Although edge features were considered useful, the ranges of the values for circumscribed lesions could be much smaller than those for spiculated lesions, causing non-linearity between the difference in feature values and subjective similarity. The relationship between subjective similarity and image features must be investigated further.

Acknowlededement. This study was partly supported by Grants-in-Aid for Scientific Research by Ministry of Education, Culture, Sports, Science and Technology, Japan. Authors are grateful to the following physicias for their contribution in this study; T. Horiba, MD, M. Kato, MD, N. Kobayashi, MD, T. Morita MD, M. Nishikawa, MD, T. Niwa MD, and M. Sassa MD.

References

1. Tabar, L., Fagerberg, G., Duffy, S.W., Day, N.E., Gad, A., Grontoft, O.: Update of the Swedish two-county program of mammographic screening for breast cancer. Radiol. Clin. North Am. 30, 187–210 (1992)
2. Shapiro, S., Venet, W., Strax, P., Venet, L., Roeser, R.: Selection, follow-up, and analysis in the health insurance plan study: A randomized trial with breast cancer screening. J. Natl. Cancer Inst. Monogr. 67, 65–74 (1985)
3. Humphrey, L.L., Helfand, M., Chan, B.K.S., Woolf, S.H.: Breast cancer screening: A summary of the evidence for the U.S. preventive services task force. Annals. of Internal Medecine 137, E-347-3-367 (2002)
4. Chan, H.P., Sahiner, B., Roubidoux, M.A., Wilson, T.E., Adler, D.D., Paramagul, C., Newman, J.S., Sanjay-Gopal, S.: Improvement of radiologists' characterization of mammographic masses by using computer-aided diagnosis: An ROC study. Radiology 212, 817–827 (1999)
5. Huo, Z., Giger, M.L., Vyborny, C.J., Metz, C.E.: Breast cancer: Effectiveness of computer-aided diagnosis - observer study with independent database of mammograms. Radiology 224, 560–568 (2002)
6. Jiang, Y., Nishikawa, R.M., Schmidt, R.A., Metz, C.E., Giger, M.L., Doi, K.: Improving breast cancer diagnosis with computer-aided diagnosis. Acad. Radiol. 6, 22–33 (1999)
7. Swett, H.A., Fisher, P.R., Cohn, A.I., Miller, P.L., Mutalik, P.G.: Expert system-controlled image display. Radiology 172, 487–493 (1989)
8. Qi, H., Snyder, W.E.: Cotent-based image retrieval in picture archiving and communications systems. J. Digit. Imaging 12, 81–83 (1999)
9. Sklansky, J., Tao, E.Y., Bazargan, M., Ornes, C.J., Murchison, R.C., Teklehaimanot, S.: Computer-aided, case-based diagnosis of mammographic regions of interest containing microcalcifications. Acad. Radiol. 7, 395–405 (2000)

10. Giger, M.L., Huo, Z., Vyborny, C.J., Lan, L., Bonta, I., Horsch, K., Nishikawa, R.M., Rosenbourgh, I.: Interlligent CAD workstation for breast imaging using similarity to known lesions and multiple visual prompt aids. In: Proc. SPIE Medical Imaging, vol. 4684, pp. 768–773 (2002)

11. Aisen, A.M., Broderick, L.S., Winer-Muram, H., Brodley, C.E., Kak, A.C., Pavlopoulou, C., Dy, J., Shyu, C.R., Marchiori, A.: Automated storage and retrieval of thin-section CT images to assist diagnosis: System description and prekliminary assessment. Radiology 228, 265–270 (2003)

12. Li, Q., Li, F., Shiraishi, J., Katsuragawa, S., Sone, S., Doi, K.: Investigation of new psychophysical measures for evaluaation of similar images on thoracic CT for distinction between benign and malignant nodules. Med. Phys. 30, 2584–2593 (2003)

13. Nishikawa, R.M., Yang, Y., Huo, D., Wernick, M., Sennett, C.A., Papioannou, J., Wei, L.: Observers' ability to judge the similarity of clustered calcifications on mammograms. In: Proc. SPIE Medical Imaging, vol. 5371, pp. 192–198 (2004)

14. Muramatsu, C., Li, Q., Suzuki, K., Schmidt, R.A., Shiraishi, J., Newstead, G.M., Doi, K.: Investigation of psychophysical measure for evaluation of similar images for mammographic masses: Preliminary results. Med. Phys. 32, 2295–2304 (2005)

15. Muramatsu, C., Li, Q., Schmidt, R.A., Shiraishi, J., Doi, K.: Investigation of psychophysical similarity measures for selection of similar images in the diagnosis of clustered microcalcifications on mammograms. Med. Phys. 35, 5695–5702 (2008)

16. Muramatsu, C., Li, Q., Schmidt, R.A., Shiraishi, J., Doi, K.: Determination of similarity measures for pairs of mass lesions on mammograms by use of BI-RADS lesion descriptors and image features. Acad. Radiol. 16, 443–449 (2009)

17. Muramatsu, C., Schmidt, R.A., Shiraishi, J., Li, Q., Doi, K.: Presentation of similar images as a reference for distinction between benign and malignant masses on mammograms: Analysis of initial observer study. J. Digit. Imaging 23, 592–602 (2010)

A Hypothesis-Test Framework for Quantitative Lesion Detection and Diagnosis

Christopher Tromans[1], Guido van Schie[2],
Nico Karssemeijer[2], and Sir Michael Brady[3]

[1] Wolfson Medical Vision Laboratory, Department of Engineering Science,
University of Oxford, Parks Road, Oxford, United Kingdom, OX1 3PJ
[2] Radboud University Nijmegen Medical Centre, Department of Radiology,
Geert Grooteplein Zuid 18, 6525 GA Nijmegen, The Netherlands
[3] Department of Oncology, Old Road Campus Research Building,
Oxford, United Kingdom, OX3 7DQ
cet@robots.ox.ac.uk

Abstract. A method is presented which quantifies the radiodensity of lesions in projection images, providing a diagnostic indicator to better inform the decisions of both human readers and computer algorithms. The models of image formation underlying the Standard Attenuation Rate (SAR) are used to facilitate the forward simulation of the appearance of a lesion in a breast. By forming hypotheses, informed from measurements on the acquired image, virtual 3D scenes are constructed which predict the size, position and radiodensity of a suspect lesion and the surrounding breast tissue. Comparisons between simulations of this scene, and the acquired image enable both the refinement of the hypothesis, and the assessment of the likelihood of the hypothesis being correct. In the event of a high likelihood of correctness, the hypothesised lesion informs diagnosis. The application of the method to a patient image containing a cyst shows it has an attenuation corresponding to water (SAR 1.246), and an invasive carcinoma which is considerably denser at SAR 2.27. Thus the technique yields a quantitative radiodensity measure for discrimination in diagnostic decision making.

Keywords: Quantitative mammography, mass, cyst, computer-aided diagnosis.

1 Introduction

An enormous number of mammograms are acquired annually, each of which has to be read expertly, primarily to avoid false-negatives. Unfortunately, false-positive results are also too frequent, which result in a stressful and unpleasant patient experience. For example, Román et al found the cumulative false-positive risk for women who started screening at age 50-51 was 20.39%, ranging from 51.43% to 7.47% in the highest and lowest risk profiles, respectively [1]. In order to improve the sensitivity and specificity of mammography double reading is employed, as well as the use of

A.D.A. Maidment, P.R. Bakic, and S. Gavenonis (Eds.): IWDM 2012, LNCS 7361, pp. 458–465, 2012.

computer aided detection/diagnosis (CAD) algorithms. In this paper we propose a technique which supplements the information available to human readers and current CAD systems, beyond that which may be gleaned solely from visual image features, by providing quantitative measurements of the radiodensity of suspect lesions and calcifications. By applying the technique in reverse, a method is developed to predict the appearance of a lesion, for use as a search template in computer aided detection. This extra information has the potential to improve sensitivity, and perhaps more importantly, specificity rates.

The Standard Attenuation Rate (SAR) [2-4] has been developed for tissue quantification and incorporates a complete model of the imaging process, including photon production in the x-ray tube, explicit consideration of both absorption and scattering phenomena within the breast, and detector signal formation. This is used to quantify relative attenuation against a reference material on a continuous scale (analogous to the Hounsfield unit). The SAR image thus depends only on the attenuation of the underlying anatomy (decoupled from the x-ray characteristics used for imaging). The underlying models of primary and scattered photons used in SAR, as well as the normalised radiodensity measure, are adopted as the foundation of the technique presented here.

The appearance of a lesion, be it a mass, or a microcalcification, in a raw x-ray depends upon a multiplicity of factors regarding the image acquisition settings (tube voltage, exposure, anode and filter materials and the detector response characteristics) and the anatomical surroundings. The computation of the SAR image addresses the effect of the acquisition settings. Here, we propose a method to remove the dependency of the rest, which relate to the anatomical surroundings of the lesion, i.e. it normalises the lesion within an image with respect to both breast thickness and density of the surrounding tissue.

The results presented here relate to a pilot study we have undertaken to establish the efficacy of the proposed technique in order to establish if it is worth the investment in undertaking a more complete study. The technique is applied to a single case selected at random from the clinic, which whilst allowing the potential of the technique to be assessed, lacks the statistical power to draw definitive conclusions regarding the population at large.

2 Materials and Methods

To illustrate the image formation process consider the case of solely the primary photon fluence and a monoenergetic beam. This is a reasonable simplification given the use of the SAR image which depends solely on the underlying tissue radiodensity, and is thus normalised with respect to the beam quality selected and the effects of scatter. If one were to consider a ray passing through a compressed breast, of thickness, H, comprising of a homogenous tissue background, $\mu_{background}$, and containing a lesion of attenuation μ_{lesion}, and thickness t_{lesion}, and for which the incident photon fluence is I_0, then the resulting image signal, I, at any given pixel would be given by:

$$I = e^{-(\mu_{background}(H-t_{lesion})+\mu_{lesion}t_{lesion})}I_0$$

Note that the appearance of the lesion depends not only on its size and attenuation, but also on the thickness of the compressed breast and the attenuation of the tissues in its background surroundings. Fig. 1 illustrates the effects of the thickness and tissue composition of the surrounding anatomy, using pixel plots along the minor axis, through an ellipsoidal lesion with major and minor axes of length 8mm and 5mm respectively, and of 80/20 fibroglandular/adipose composition. Despite the x-ray acquisition parameters being held constant, notable differences in both contrast across the lesion, and the absolute pixel values may be observed for both varying breast thickness (between 40 and 80mm) and background composition (from pure adipose to 60/40). Our approach to normalising these effects, and thereby quantifying the radiodensity of the lesion, which itself is a direct function of its underlying chemical composition, adopts a classic hypothesis-test methodology, and may be summarised by the following steps:

1. Compute the SAR image for the raw x-ray image, to remove the effects of beam quality and scatter, yielding the radiodensity encountered by the primary ray [4].
2. Segment the suspect lesion of interest within the SAR image.
3. Build a "virtual" three dimensional scene comprising of the compressed breast containing the suspect lesion (the hypothesis). These scenes may be of vastly varying complexity. For example, they may be as simple as assuming that a calcification or cyst is an ellipsoid; measuring the dimensions of the major and minor axes from the segmentation, and assuming the length of the axis in the "unknown" projection image plane perpendicular to the image receptor surface is the average of the measured major and minor axial lengths; using the average of the SAR values around the boundary of the segmentation as the radiodensity of the background tissue; and the measured compressed breast thickness from the DICOM header. Conversely, a highly complex scene describing an invasive mass may require the use of a voxelised volume in which SAR values are set for each individual voxel, allowing stellate shapes and spicules to be included.
4. The three dimensional virtual scene is passed as the input to the forward simulator using the primary photon model underlying the SAR calculation. The normalised SAR image is then calculated for this simulated image.
5. Direct comparison between the simulation and actual observed SAR images (the test) using a suitable similarity metric (for example root mean squared difference over the area of the lesion) yields a value quantifying the likelihood the hypothesis as to the lesions attenuation in the virtual scene is valid.
6. Steps 3 to 5 may be repeated to iterate the hypothesis in light of the similarity observed in step 5.

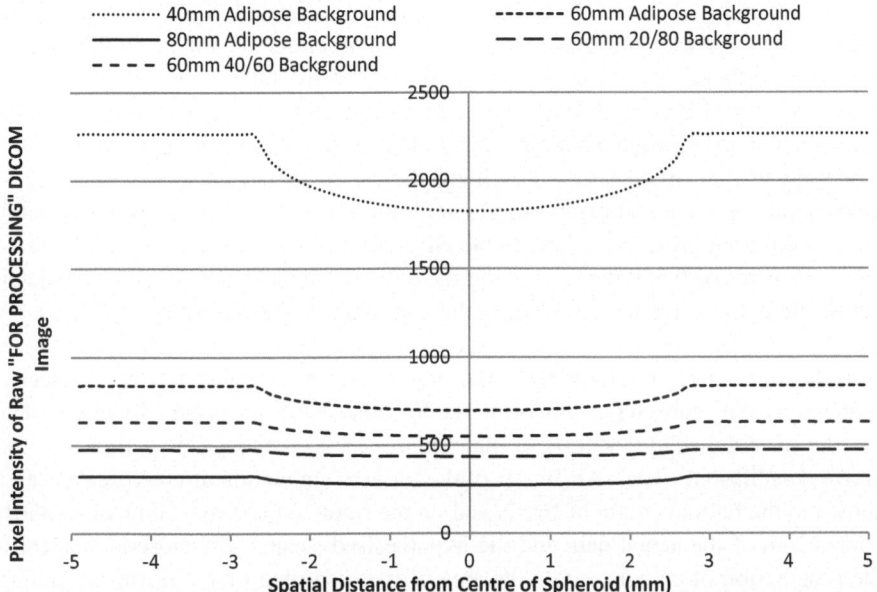

Fig. 1. Simulations of a spheroid lesion in a homogenous background of a range of thicknesses and compositions using the SAR models at 29kVp Mo-Rh 71mAs on a GE Essential

The measurements taken from the segmentations in step (2) and which are subsequently used to build the virtual 3D scene in step (3) in effect set values for $\mu_{background}$ and t_{lesion}, and the degree of freedom to be resolved is the hypothesis of the lesion radiodensity, μ_{lesion}. The image signal is computed at each pixel by forward situation of the image in step (4). Quantification of the differences between the acquired and simulated image measures the likelihood of the validity of the hypothesis in step (5), hence the likely validity of μ_{lesion} in the virtual scene.

3 Results and Discussion

To illustrate the method, the technique is applied here to images of a 64 year old women, exhibiting multiple lesions, imaged on a GE 2000D. The original radiologists report concluded with a BIRADS 4 (suspicious abnormality - biopsy should be considered) verdict. Two features of note included in the report are: "a circumscribed hyperdense spherical structure in upper lateral quadrant right, probably a cyst", and "directly behind nipple, dense area badly differentiated with spicules and microcalcs". The case went on to needle biopsy and mastectomy, where the pathology report confirmed the cyst and declared the "dense area" to be an invasive ductal carcinoma.

The left of fig. 2 shows the normalised, scatter accounted, SAR radiodensity image of the "circumscribed hyperdense spherical structure" identified by the radiologist as a probable cyst. The major/minor axes of the ellipse measure 9.2/7.5mm respectively, and it is assumed to consist of water (SAR value 1.246, compared to Hammerstein [5] Fibroglandular at 1.207). This may be seen in blue in the 3D visual rendering of the virtual scene describing the breast in the upper centre of fig. 2. What would appear to be feature noise, in all likelihood a Cooper's ligament running along a different projection plane to the ellipsoid, can be seen crossing its centre. It has a diameter of 0.539mm, and using the area of "quiet" background immediately below the bottom right corner of the sphere an iterative search using hypothesis-test cycles, finds the SAR radiodensity of the structure to be 3.5. This radiodensity being considerably higher than fibroglandular tissue, suggests a dense fibrous connective tissue, providing substantial support to the hypothesis it is a Cooper's ligament. This may be seen in the 3D rendering of the virtual scene as the long fine yellow structure above the ellipsoid. The SAR image of the forward simulation of the virtual scene is shown in the bottom centre of fig. 2, and on the right colour maps allow quantitative comparison of the actual data and the hypothesised scene. The close agreement of the progression of colours across the area of the suspected cyst confirm the validity of the prediction the lesion comprises of primarily water, and the change in colour of the linear structure as it leaves the lower right of the suspected cyst confirms the hypothesis of a superimposed linear structure, as opposed to a spicule emanating from within it. Fig. 3 allows more accurate quantification of the agreement between the simulation of the hypothesised breast and lesion structure, by presenting horizontal pixel intensity plots through the centre of the lesion. The high level of agreement shown shows this lesion is largely water, and hence provides substantial evidence it is a cyst.

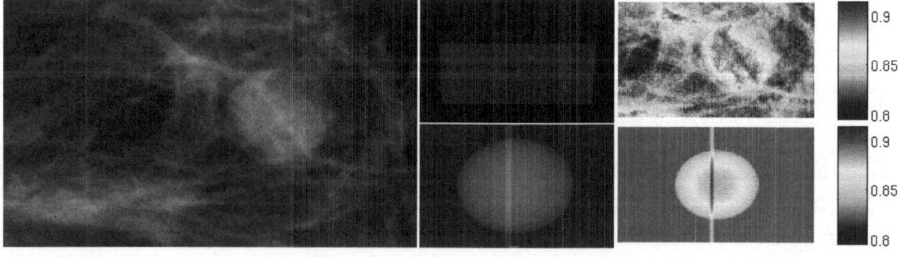

Fig. 2. The region in the SAR image identified by the radiologist as hyperdense and being suspicious of a cyst (left); a visual rendering of the 3D virtual scene built to describe the lesion, comprising of a spheroid containing water with a linear structure passing over it (upper centre); the SAR image of the simulated x-ray of the 3D virtual scene (lower centre); and the observed SAR image of the cyst and the simulated hypothesised scene plotted using identical colour maps (right).

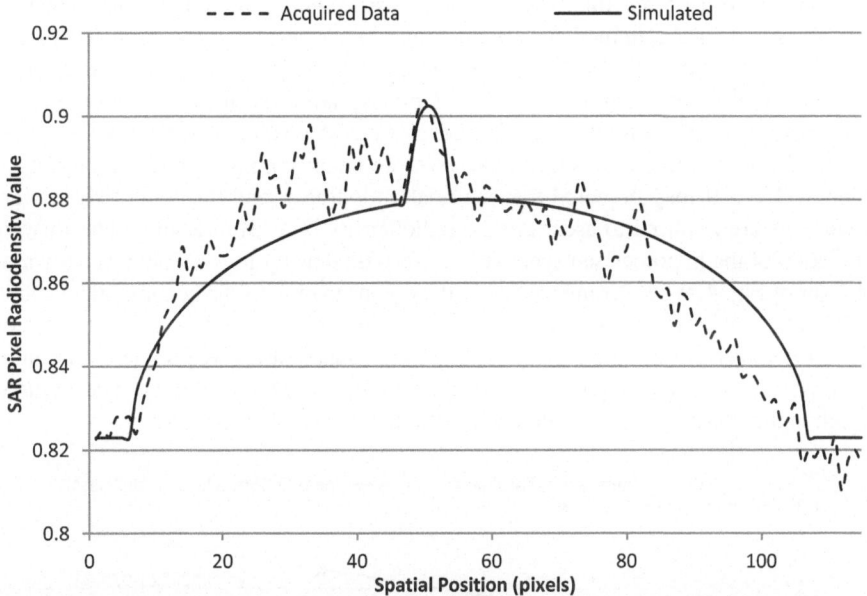

Fig. 3. Horizontal pixel intensity plots through the actual and simulated SAR images

Turning attention now to the region identified by the radiologist as "dense area badly differentiated with spicules and microcalcs". The left of **Fig. 4** shows the area in question of the SAR image. Whilst the mass in the greyscale image does appear to be badly differentiated, as noted by the radiologist, once the region is plotted on a colour map, the extent of the mass becomes clear, and it can be seen to have the characteristics of a spheroid in shape.

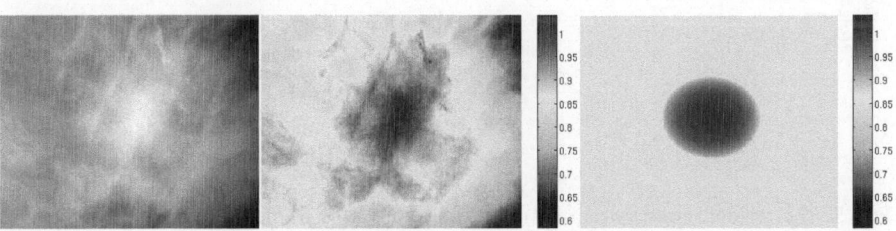

Fig. 4. The region in the SAR image identified by the radiologist as "a dense area badly differentiated with spicules and microcalcs" and latter confirmed as being an invasive ductal carcinoma (left); the region plotted on a colour map (centre); and the simulated SAR image of the hypothesised ellipsoid of SAR 2.27 plotted on an identical colour map (right).

Measuring the major and minor axes of the projected ellipse give sizes of 8.7mm and 7.2mm respectively. Taking the "thickness" of the spheroid in the z-direction to be the average of these two lengths, gives 7.95mm. Fig. 5 shows a plot relating the radiodensity observed in the SAR processed projection image of a 7.95mm thick ellipsoid within a 65mm thickness of breast tissue with a SAR attenuation of 0.85 (that measured in the immediate surroundings of the lesion in the acquired patient image), to the SAR radiodensity at the centre of the lesion. Measuring the average radiodensity of a small circle of pixels (13 pixels diameter) in the centre of the suspected lesion in the acquired patient image, gives a SAR value of 1.019 for the case in Fig. 4. Using the relation in Fig. 5, this gives an underlying SAR radiodensity of the lesion as 2.27. It may be noted that the relation is linear, and thus only two forward simulations are required to ascertain the radiodensity of a given lesion. The forward simulation of the hypothesised scene using this radiodensity for the lesion is shown on the right of Fig. 4, where comparison via the colour map with the acquired data shows good agreement across the entire area of the lesion. Unfortunately the current version of our ray tracer doesn't yet support orientating a shape at a given angle, so aligning the simulation with the acquired data is not possible, and hence it is not yet possible, though highly desirable, to calculate a quantitative measure of agreement.

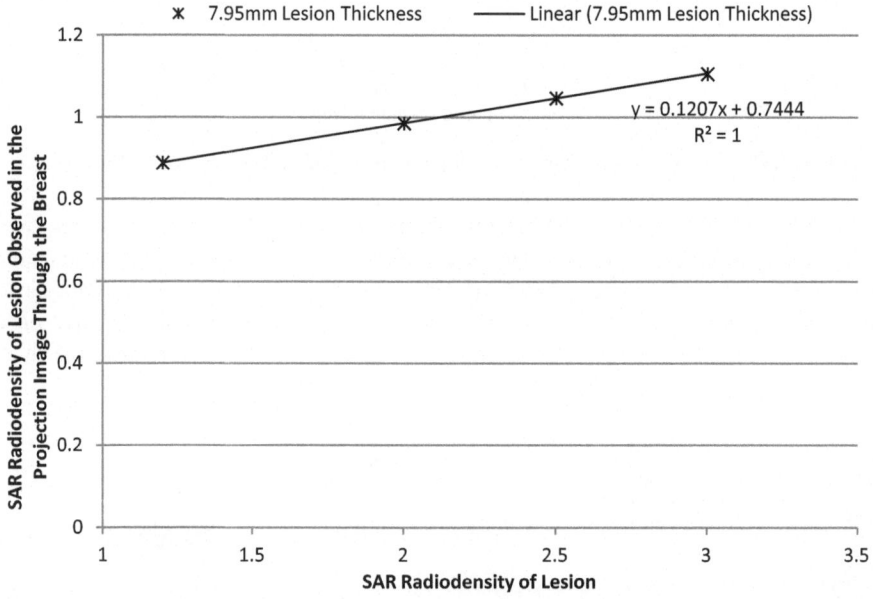

Fig. 5. The relationship between the radiodensity observed in the SAR processed projection image of a 7.95mm thick ellipsoid within a 65mm thickness of breast tissue with a SAR attenuation of 0.85, and that of the underlying SAR radiodensity of which said lesion comprises

In order to assess the sensitivity of measuring the lesion radiodensity using the method described, the linear relation plotted in Fig. 5 were calculated for lesion ellipsoid thicknesses equal to both the sizes measured for the major and minor axes from the acquired patient data. The resulting lesion SAR radiodensities for 7.2mm and 8.7mm thick were 2.41 (5.3% above the value resulting from averaging the lengths of the major and minor axes to glean the thickness) and 2.15 (6.2% below) respectively.

Comparing the SAR radiodensity for this pathology proven infiltrating ductal carcinoma at 2.27, to the SAR radiodensity of water at 1.246, which was observed to match that of the cyst in this patient, the potential to discriminate between the benign cyst, and the malignant lesion, on the basis of in-vivo measurements of their radiodensity using this technique clearly exists.

An area we wish to pursue in our further work is the comparison of in-vivo measurements of lesion radiodensity, with radiodensity values measured from "pure" in-vitro samples, such as slices prepared for histological analysis by the pathology laboratory, or fluid aspirated from cysts.

4   Conclusion

A technique for quantifying the radiodensity of a suspect lesion is presented using hypothesis-test cycles comparing the observed acquired images and simulated images of the hypothesis (as it is iteratively refined) computed using the image formation models within SAR. The potential shown in the results to discriminate between an invasive carcinoma (seen to exhibit a radiodensity of 2.27) and a cyst (seen to exhibit the radiodensity of water at 1.246) based on the radiodensity measured by the presented technique, in a study for which the radiologist concluded BIRADS 4 "suspicious abnormality - biopsy should be considered", illustrates the positive effect the technique offers on improving the specificity of the screening programme. The promise shown by these results suggest merit lies in fuller investigation on a larger dataset to establish robustness across the population.

References

[1] Roman, M., Fau-Sala, R., et al.: Effect of protocol-related variables and women's characteristics on the cumulative false-positive risk in breast cancer screening, 20111222
[2] Tromans, C.: DPhil Thesis: Measuring Breast Density from X-Ray Mammograms. DPhil Thesis, Engineering Science. Oxford University (October 2006)
[3] Tromans, C., Brady, M.: An Alternative Approach to Measuring Volumetric Mammographic Breast Density. In: Astley, S.M., Brady, M., Rose, C., Zwiggelaar, R. (eds.) IWDM 2006. LNCS, vol. 4046, pp. 26–33. Springer, Heidelberg (2006)
[4] Tromans, C.E., Brady, S.M.: The Standard Attenuation Rate for Quantitative Mammography. In: Martí, J., Oliver, A., Freixenet, J., Martí, R. (eds.) IWDM 2010. LNCS, vol. 6136, pp. 561–568. Springer, Heidelberg (2010)
[5] Hammerstein, G.R., et al.: Absorbed radiation dose in mammography. Radiology 130, 485–491 (1979)

Breast Density into Clinical Practice

Ralph Highnam[1], Natascha Sauber[1], Stamatia Destounis[2],
Jennifer Harvey[3], and Dennis McDonald[4]

[1] Matakina Technology, 86 Victoria Street, Wellington, New Zealand
Ralph.Highnam@matakina.com
[2] Elizabeth Wende Breast Care, LLC, Rochester, New York, USA
sdestounis@ewbc.com
[3] University of Virginia, Charlottesville, Virginia, USA
JAH7W@hscmail.mcc.virginia.edu
[4] Sutter Health North Bay Women's Health, Santa Rosa, USA
mcdonadn@sutterhealth.org

Abstract. It is well established that breast density is related to breast cancer risk; making that connection precise, and understanding how to use it in clinical practice, has been a major academic focus since the 1970's. However, it transpires that the first clinical uses of breast density have not been for risk prediction, rather they are for judging when to recommend further imaging. In this paper, we show how scientific research has had to be adapted in order to create the automated volumetric breast density assessment tool, Volpara®, to make it ready for actual clinical use and how it is impacting patient management.

Keywords: Breast density, BI-RADS®.

1   Introduction

Since the mid-1970's, breast density has been a major area of epidemiological research because of its increasingly established connection to breast cancer risk. However, clinical application of such research has been hampered by a lack of ability to automatically and objectively measure breast density, the lack of a risk model including breast density and the lack of options once a woman is recognized as being of high risk of developing breast cancer due to breast density.

However, the need for breast density assessment in clinical practice is now accelerating in the US, and elsewhere, due to a wider understanding of how the sensitivity of mammography becomes worse with denser breasts [1,2] and that supplementary imaging techniques such as whole-breast ultrasound or MRI can pick up extra cancers in those breasts. For example, from reports it appears that whole-breast ultrasound has the ability to detect almost twice the number of cancers in women with denser breasts, albeit at the cost of more false positives [3,4]. Thus, the major question now for clinical application of density is how best to measure it in order to convey sensitivity of mammography and how to use that measurement to ensure the correct women are selected for supplemental imaging.

A.D.A. Maidment, P.R. Bakic, and S. Gavenonis (Eds.): IWDM 2012, LNCS 7361, pp. 466–473, 2012.

The judgment of what is a "dense" breast that is commonly used today is based on the radiologist's own density assessment which is generally based on visually assessed area-based categories as outlined in the 4th Edition of BI-RADS® :

Category 1: The breast is almost entirely fat (<25% glandular).
Category 2: There are scattered fibroglandular densities (approximately 25-50% glandular).
Category 3: The breast tissue is heterogeneously dense, which could obscure detection of small masses (approximately 51% – 75% glandular).
Category 4 : The breast tissue is extremely dense. This may lower the sensitivity of mammography (>76% glandular).

Though at first sight these definitions appear to be quantitative and thus objective, in reality BI-RADS breast density assessments are highly subjective. As the American College of Radiology's own submissions to the FDA have stated: "There is significant observer variability in the assignment of a breast density category" and "The assessment of breast density is not reliably reproducible". The published literature [3-10] shows that readers only agree moderately in their assessments of density.

It is because of the subjectivity and time requirements of BI-RADS breast density, that automated and objective volumetric techniques of determining breast density have been developed as demanded by some physicians [11]. With such techniques, models of the physics of mammogram formation are used to find x-ray attenuation. From the attenuation, the actual physical breast composition in terms of the volume of fibroglandular tissue cm^3, the volume of breast tissue cm^3, and the ratio of the two, which is equated to the volumetric breast density can be estimated [10, 12-14].

However, there have been further more technical issues with getting volumetric breast density measurements into clinic practice, including:

1. Current clinical information systems (in the USA) are all built around a BI-RADS breast density category. They store a number, from 1 to 4, not volumetric measures, and many such systems incorporate automated reporting mechanisms based upon that number. In particular, certain terms from the BI-RADS definitions are inserted into the letters sent to the individual woman automatically based upon the 1-4 categories.

2. The volumetric densities are in the range 0-35% [12, 13], whereas area-based visual assessment of density is 0-100%. Further, it has been seen that area-based estimates can change dramatically according to the vendor specific post-processing applied to the mammogram prior to presentation and the subjective assessment of the reader. This mis-match of actual (volumetric) density versus area-based, visual density needs to be addressed to ensure confidence in the volumetric results.

3. Many imaging centres have mammography machines from multiple vendors in regular usage, which implies that to be useful and used in practice, the volumetric technique has to produce comparable numbers across vendors else there is lack of confidence and confusion for the radiologist.
4. Volumetric techniques need reliable calibration data, and in clinical practice it should be expected that some errors in the calibration data are inevitable compared to a more research based setting.

In this paper, we described how we modified our original work on volumetric density estimation [15, 16] into software in a form ready for clinical use, namely Volpara® [12,13]. Questions 3 & 4 were addressed in [12,13] for Volpara and we cover more of Q3 in this paper, but the focus is on questions 1 & 2 - how do we get breast density measurements into the clinical systems used today and in a way which the radiologists trust? The answer is to translate the volumetric numbers into the BI-RADS scale. We start the paper by addressing that before we detail one clinical use of volumetric breast density as assessed by Volpara in which accuracy is important, but patient workflow and convenience turn out to be the critical factors.

2 Translating Volumetric Density for Clinical Use

In order to facilitate a comparison to the radiologist's assessment of BI-RADS, we had to map the volumetric breast density measures to a BI-RADS density category; we did this using data reported from DMIST [1,12,13] and we optimized the matching to maximize the agreement between the radiologist and what we termed the Volpara Density Grade (VDG®). That latter term was specifically chosen so that the radiologist would recognize that it is a volumetric driven grade, rather than a BI-RADS category per se which also has a non-quantitative element, as is evident from the BI-RADS definitions provided above. The following thresholds were used for version 1.5 of Volpara Imaging Software to partition the volumetric densities into VDG: 0-4.5%, 4.5-7.5%, 7.5-15.5%, and over 15.5%.

Table 1 show confusion matrices for Volpara versus radiologist(s) at two major breast imaging clinics (UVA = University of Virginia, EWBC = Elizabeth Wende Breast Clinic) and with different mammography systems (HX stands for Hologic, GE for GE). EWBC-2 represents a second set of data from EWBC but with images from mixed machines and the BI-RADS assessed in a more clinical than research fashion.

From the data in Table 1 we generated Table 2 where we show the overall agreement percentage between the radiologist(s) and Volpara. More importantly, we show the percentage of times that Volpara agreed with the radiologist's assessment that a woman should be classified as BI-RADS 3 or 4, which is generally the criterion that is used in the United States to determine whether or not a woman has an abnormally dense breast.

Table 1. Volpara versus radiologists at different sites and on different x-ray machines

UVA

		GE X-ray BI-RADS				
		1	2	3	4	
	1	60	22	1	0	83
Volpara	2	16	34	28	0	78
	3	0	5	52	14	71
	4	0	0	13	51	64
		76	61	94	65	296

EWBC-1

		GE X-ray BI-RADS				
		1	2	3	4	
	1	12	6	0	0	18
Volpara	2	4	15	6	0	25
	3	0	7	18	7	32
	4	0	1	4	17	22
		16	29	28	24	97

EWBC-1

		HX X-ray BI-RADS				
		1	2	3	4	
	1	15	2	1	0	18
Volpara	2	7	16	5	0	28
	3	0	4	22	5	31
	4	1	1	3	15	20
		23	23	31	20	97

EWBC-2

		HX & GE BI-RADS				
		1	2	3	4	
	1	49	41	2	0	92
Volpara	2	6	94	28	0	128
	3	0	26	99	3	128
	4	0	0	11	25	36
		55	161	140	28	384

Table 2. % Agreement between Volpara and radiologist at various sites across the US

Site	%Overall Agreement	%Agreement on 3 & 4
UVA - GE	66.6	81.8
EWBC 1 - GE	63.9	88.5
EWBC 1 - HX	70.1	88.2
EWBC 2 - Mix	69.5	85.4

We note that these results show strong and repeatable consistency across sites and across the machines from different vendors. We should not expect perfect agreement due to reader subjectivity and the inherent differences between volumetric and area based assessment of density. We also note that such results also highlight a number of trends that are found in clinical practice, as compared to academic research; for example, many radiologists tend to avoid using BI-RADS categories 1 & 4 in clinical practice and that is demonstrated in the EWBC-2 data.

As further evidence in support of our claim of consistency across sites, we compare our BI-RADS assessments to those of Kopans [17]. First, collaborators took 15,000 mammography studies from Toronto and applied Volpara Imaging Software 1.4. The top graph in Figure 1 shows as a function of age the percentage of mammograms for which Volpara recommended a BI-RADS score of 3&4 versus 1&2. The lower graph compares this to the equivalent percentages reported by Kopans [17] from a study of 3,000 film-screen mammograms.

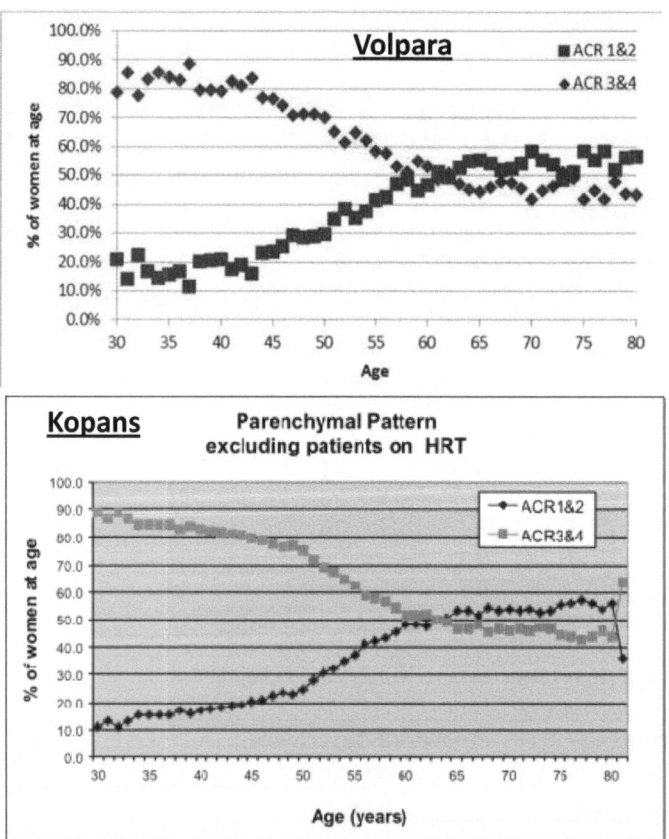

Fig. 1. % of women at each age with BIRADS 1&2 v 3 as judged by Kopans and Volpara

3   Density in Clinical Use - Recommending Ultrasound

We next focus on a specific breast imaging clinic, namely Sutter Health North Bay Women's Health, in Santa Rosa, California which has an automated whole breast ultrasound available.

This site was reporting that few of the women when told of their visually assessed breast density by letter were scheduling a breast ultrasound despite having dense breasts. The site implemented Volpara which allowed them to assess and talk about breast density whilst the woman was still in the clinic; that increased the take up rate by a factor of 3. The take-up rate was further increased by a factor of 5 when the ultrasound was performed straight after the mammograms were performed. Full studies still need to be conducted about the effect of cost, convenience and fear of false positives, but clearly convenience plays a major factor not opting for ultrasound.

The need for accuracy of density assessment becomes very clear when considering the numbers of women being screened each year in the USA. Currently, 30M women are screened each year in the USA alone.   A whole breast ultrasound image costs approximately US$100-US$250.   There are thus huge cost and false-positive implications if, for example, a radiologist were to over-read BI-RADS density and send too many women for ultrasound. Taking the Toronto data-set as our model population, as shown in Figure 2, we can compute the numbers of women, as well as the extra cost involved, for various cut-off percentages. Table 3 shows the implications of different density cut-offs across the US.

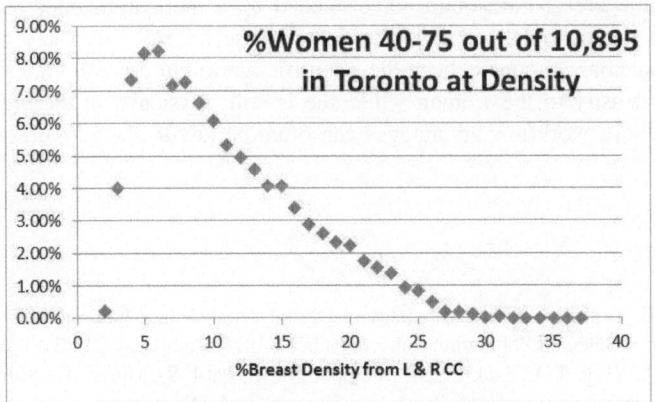

Fig. 2. % of women with a certain density

Table 3. Ultrasound cut-offs versus cost

Cut-Off For Ultrasound	# Women	Extra Cost
8%	49%, 14.7M	$1.5-3.7Bn
12.5%	27%, 8.1M	$0.8-2.0Bn
15%	18%, 5.4M	$0.6-1.4Bn

Clearly, these numbers are very high and they show how critical it is going to be to have objective, reliable density scoring across the US. Note that these cost numbers are highly conservative: they do not for example take account of reduced surgery or adjuvant therapy costs from cancers being found early and do not include false-positive related costs.

4   Discussion

The translation of scientific findings into routine clinical use inevitably takes time: clinicians need to be confident that any new science will improve their performance and that it will do so within practical constraints.   Such translation can take a frustratingly long time, especially when clinical practice and systems are already established. In the case of measuring volumetric breast density, the BI-RADS breast density categories have existed for many years and are incorporated in the mammography information systems which dominate breast screening, especially in the USA. Working out how volumetric breast density relates to BI-RADS categories and ensuring that we get consistent results across sites and x-ray machines has been critical to gain acceptance into clinical use.

Further, whereas our initial essentially academic focus concerned breast cancer risk, there remains uncertainty in clinical breast screening what such epidemiological research implies for an individual woman deemed to be at high risk. However, the women's advocacy groups in the US concerned about breast density, coupled with the trials of whole breast ultrasound, have opened up a more immediate use for breast density assessment tools. Judging what is a "dense breast" and a key factor in our success to date has, of course, been the scientific work; but critically it is the ability to give breast density to the woman while she is still physically at the breast imaging center. In short, workflow advantages can often be key to the adoption of scientific ideals.

References

1. Pisano, E., et al.: Diagnostic Accuracy of Digital versus Film Mammography: Exploratory Analysis of Selected Population Subgroups in DMIST. Radiology 246(2), 376 (2008)
2. Arora, N., King, T.A., Jacks, L.M., Stempel, M.M., Patil, S., Morris, E., Morrow, M.: Impact of Breast Density on the Presenting Features of Malignancy. Ann. Surg. Oncolol. 17, S211–S218 (2010)
3. Berg, W.A., et al.: Combined Screening with Ultrasound and Mammography vs Mammography Alone in Women at Elevated Risk of Breast Cancer. JAMA 303(15), 1482 (2008)
4. Steenbergen, S., Weigert, J.: The Connecticut Experiment: The Role of Ultrasound in the Screening of Dense Breasts. RSNA (2011)
5. Berg, W.A., Campassi, C., Langenberq, P., Sexton, M.J.: BIRADS: Inter-and Intra-Observer Variability in Feature Analysis and Final Assessment. AJR 174(6), 1769–1777 (2000)
6. Harvey, J.A., Bovbjerg, V.E.: Quantitative Assessment of Mammographic Density: Relationship with Breast Cancer Risk. Radiology 230, 29–41 (2004)

7. Nicholson, B.T., LoRusso, A.P., Smolkin, M., Bovbjerg, V.E., Petroni, G.R., Harvey, J.A.: Accuracy of Assigned BI-RADS Breast Density Category Definitions. Acad. Radiology 13(9), 1143–1149 (2006)
8. Ciatto, S., Visioli, C., Paci, E., Zappa, M.: Breast Density As a Determinant of Interval Cancer At Mammographic Screening. Breast Journal of Cancer 90, 393–396 (2004)
9. Martin, K.E., Helvie, M.A., Zhou, C., Roubidoux, M.A., Bailey, J.E., Paramaqul, C., Blane, C.E., Klein, K.A., Sonnad, S.S., Chan, H.P.: Mammographic Density Measured with Quantitative Computer-Aided Method: Comparison to Radiologists' Estimates and BI-RADS categories. Radiology 240(3), 656–665 (2006)
10. Ren, B., Smith, A.P., Marshall, J.: Investigation of Practical Scoring Methods for Breast Density. In: Martí, J., Oliver, A., Freixenet, J., Martí, R. (eds.) IWDM 2010. LNCS, vol. 6136, pp. 651–658. Springer, Heidelberg (2010)
11. Ng, K.-H., Yip, C.-H., Taib, N.A.M.: Standardization of Clinical Breast Density Measurement. Lancet Oncology 13, 334 (2012)
12. Highnam, R., Brady, S.M., Yaffe, M.J., Karssemeijer, N., Harvey, J.: Robust Breast Composition Measurement - Volpara^{TM}. In: Martí, J., Oliver, A., Freixenet, J., Martí, R. (eds.) IWDM 2010. LNCS, vol. 6136, pp. 342–349. Springer, Heidelberg (2010)
13. Jeffreys, M., Harvey, J., Highnam, R.: Comparing a new volumetric breast density method (Volpara^{TM}) to cumulus. In: Martí, J., Oliver, A., Freixenet, J., Martí, R. (eds.) IWDM 2010. LNCS, vol. 6136, pp. 408–413. Springer, Heidelberg (2010)
14. Shepherd, J.A., Herve, L., Landau, J., Fan, B., Kerlikowske, K., Cummings, S.R.: Novel Use of Single X-ray Absorptiometry for Measuring Breast Density. Technol. Cancer Res. Treat. 4(2), 173–182 (2005)
15. Highnam, R., Brady, M.: Mammographic Image Analysis. Kluwer Academic Press (1999)
16. Van Engeland, S., Snoeren, P.R., Huisman, H., Boetes, C., Karssemeijer, N.: Volumetric Breast Density Estimation From Full-Field Digital Mammograms. IEEE Medical Imaging 25(3) (2006)
17. Kopans, D.: Breast Imaging. Lippincott Williams & Wilkins (2003)

Intensity Independent Texture Analysis in Screening Mammograms

Xi-Zhao Li, Simon Williams, and Murk J. Bottema

Flinders University, Bedford Park 5042, SA, Australia
{li0691,s.williams,murk.bottema}@flinders.edu.au

Abstract. Image texture features for detecting malignant masses in screening mammograms are proposed that are independent of background intensity mean and variation. Subtracting local means and dividing by local standard deviation reveals linear structures of approximately 0.7 mm width in screening mammograms. A simple texture feature calculated from on this derived image is used to demonstrate that texture information associated with the location of cancer is retained in the mean and standard deviation normalized image. Such texture features have the potential to provide evidence of malignancy that better complements intensity based features for detecting breast cancer in screening mammograms.

Keywords: computer-aided mammography, breast cancer, texture, mass detection.

1 Introduction

Changes in tissue texture patterns have been associated with increased risk of breast cancer [13],[6],[14]. In addition, measures of texture have been used along with other computed image features to distinguish between benign and malignant masses in computer-aided mammography schemes [2], [3], [9], [7], [1]. Some texture measures are motivated by the experience of radiologists. For example, the quantification of the spiculated pattern associated with malignant masses is such a texture measure [10] as is the quantification of patterns of fibrous structure associated with architectural distortions [4], [8]. Other measures of texture, particularly measures based on textons, are not linked directly to known biology of cancer [11], [1]. Studies of this nature are motivated by the conjecture that cancer tissue may differ from normal tissue in ways that manifest in mammograms at levels of contrast and scale that are not be visible to human readers and thus do not form part of the experience of radiologists. Evidence exists that this is indeed the case [12], but accurate characterization of such texture differences is the subject of ongoing research.

One problem in searching for texture measures that are not motivated directly by biological understanding of breast tissue and cancer is the difficulty of evaluating if proposed texture measures are indeed associated with cancer and if so, that information provided by the texture measure is independent of existing image

A.D.A. Maidment, P.R. Bakic, and S. Gavenonis (Eds.): IWDM 2012, LNCS 7361, pp. 474–481, 2012.

features. This problem is exacerbated by the nonlinear relation between tissue density (actually X-ray attenuation) and image intensity in screening mammograms. For example, in texture analysis based on textons, a filterbank is used to establish a high-dimensional texture signature for every pixel in the image [5]. These responses are clustered to form textons and classification of a region within the image is based on the distribution of textons associated with the region. The difficulty is that regions of high image intensity result in high filter responses. Since malignant masses are high intensity features, classification based on textons may result in high sensitivity (albeit with poor specificity) if the textures are, in fact, surrogates for intensity. Correcting for background intensity does not solve this problem (Section 2) because of the nonlinear response of the imaging system.

Here texture features are proposed based on images corrected so that local mean intensities are zero and local standard deviations are one. Texture patterns in these normalized images are thus independent of mean intensity and variation and thus have the potential to provide information regarding the disease state independent of intensity based features. Section 2 demonstrates problems that result from basing texton analysis on images that are not normalized and Section 3 demonstrates that texture patterns in normalized image have the potential to contribute distinguishing cancer from normal tissue.

2   Texton Analysis without Normalization

Several studies were conducted to ascertain the value of texton based texture features for detecting malignant masses in screening mammograms. These studies differed mainly in terms of the choice of filterbank and number of textons chosen in the clustering step. Only one of these studies is reported here in detail but the results are representative.

2.1   Materials and Methods

For this initial study, 89 cases were chosen from the Digital Database for Screening Mammography (DDSM). In all cases, a confirmed malignant mass was present in one breast. Annotation information from the DDSM data base was used to extract regions of interest (ROI) containing the malignant mass from each MLO and each CC view in the set, resulting in a collection of 178 ROI with malignancies present. For each such ROI (referred to here as a malignant ROI) a corresponding normal ROI was extracted from the breast image without the cancer from the same woman at the corresponding location of the malignant ROI. The site of the normal ROI was determined manually based on the left-right symmetry between breasts. Of the original 89 cases, 49 were randomly selected for training and 40 were reserved for testing. The images were subsampled to 250 μm resolution.

For each pixel, the intensities at the eight neighboring pixels were recorded to form an eight-dimensional feature space. This is tantamount to applying a

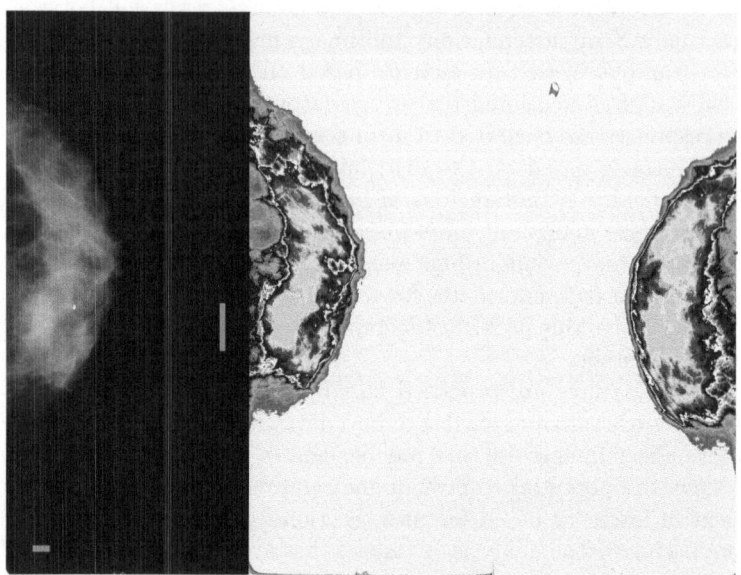

Fig. 1. On the left is the original mammogram X. The bars show the horizontal and vertical extent of a malignant mass. The middle panel shows the "backpmap" image obtained by replacing each pixel in X by the classification label. The result shown is for the case of $K = 16$ textons. The right panel shows the backmap image for the right breast. The backmap images indicate that the texture features are identified with high intensity regions and not specifically with cancer.

filterbank of size eight where filter i comprises a 3×3 array with zeros in every position except at position i where the value is one. K-means clustering was used with values $K = 8, 16, 20, 25, 30, 34, 40$ to produce seven different texton dictionaries. All the pixels in an ROI were mapped to a texton using nearest the neighbor criterion and each ROI was then represented by the distribution of textons to which its pixels were mapped. The Fisher criterion was used for classification.

2.2   Results and Consequences

One complication in texton analysis is deciding on the number of textons, or in other words, the value of K in the clustering step. The larger the number of textons, the larger the feature space for classification. Hence, several values of K were tested. As expected, the A_z score for classification performance on the training data increased with K (Table 1) with a top A_z score of 0.812 for $K = 40$ textons. Also as expected, A_z scores for testing data was consistently lower and with no obvious relation to K. A top score of $A_z = 0.644$ was found for $K = 8$. These numerical performance results do not indicate if these texture measures are indeed useful for distinguishing between normal and cancer tissue because

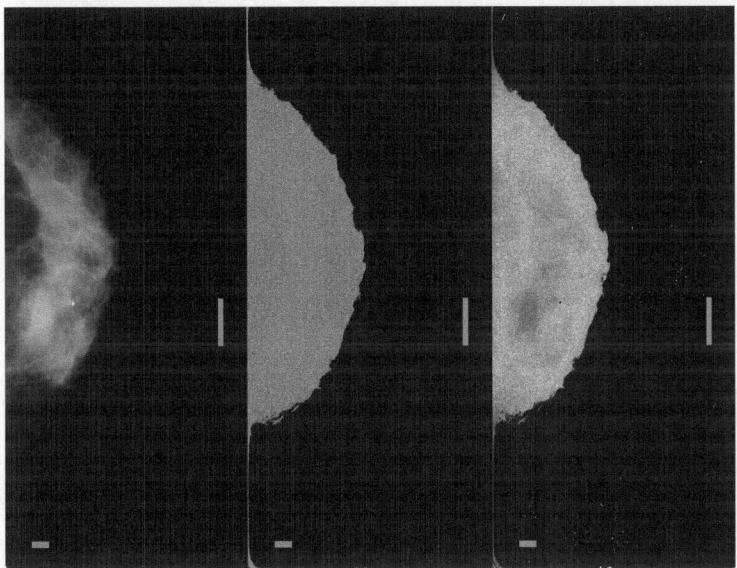

Fig. 2. On the left is the original mammogram X. The bars show the horizontal and vertical extent of a malignant mass. The middle panel is the local mean subtracted image D_r (in this panel, the background has been set to the minimum value of the image to facilitate the display) and the right panel is the local standard deviation image S_r. Due to the nonlinearity of the imaging process, bright regions in X appear as a relatively dark regions in S_r. For this example $r = 5$ pixels.

Table 1. Classification scores for seven texton dictionaries

K	8	16	20	25	30	34	40
A_z Training	0.691	0.710	0.735	0.747	0.758	0.780	0.812
A_z Testing	0.644	0.629	0.571	0.594	0.586	0.614	0.563

inflated performance scores are expected when high-dimensional features spaces are used for classification.

To explore the connection between the texture features and cancer, texton combinations allegedly associated with cancer were mapped back to the original full images (Fig. 1). The results indicate that these texton combinations were associated with high intensity regions generally and not specifically with cancer. Accordingly, these texture measures provide little if any additional value to detection of cancer, despite some reasonable performance scores.

3   Texture in Normalized Images

One method for testing if texture features can provide information about the presence of breast cancer independent of background intensity is to compute

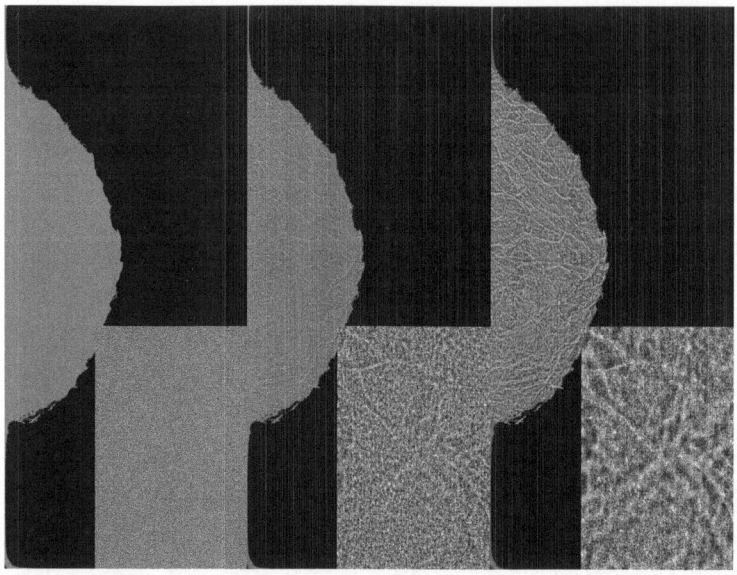

Fig. 3. Normalized mammograms. Each panel shows the normalized image N_r obtained from the image in Fig. 2 for values of $r = 1, 10, 22$ respectively (left to right). The insets in the lower right of each panel show the region of the known malignant mass indicated by the bars in Fig. 2. The left panel shows essentially no structure for $r = 1$, not even the breast outline, but structure emerges with increasing r. In each panel, the background has been set to the minimum image value to facilitate display.

texture features on "flattened" images. An example of a flattened image is D_r defined by

$$D_r(p) = X(p) - \text{mean}(X(B(p, r))),$$

where X is the original image and $B(p, r)$ is the disk of radius r centered at pixel p. However, due to the nonlinearity of the imaging process, the local variation is also a function of background intensity (Fig. 2). Thus texture measures extracted from D_r will still reflect local background intensity.

In order to remove dependence on local variation, the normalized image N_r is defined by

$$N_r(p) = \frac{D_r(p)}{S_r(p)}, \qquad \text{where } S_r(p) = \text{std}(X(B(p, r))).$$

To explore textures based on these normalized images, N_r was computed using radii $r = 3n + 1$ for $n = 0, 1, \ldots, 7$ (pixels) on full resolution ($\approx 50\mu$m per pixel) mammograms. No structure could be seen for low values of r, but significant linear structure appeared for larger values of r (Fig. 3).

To see if the linear structures found in the normalized images N_r could be used as a feature to distinguish normal and cancer tissue, an experiment was conducted to check if the distributions of orientations of the linear structures

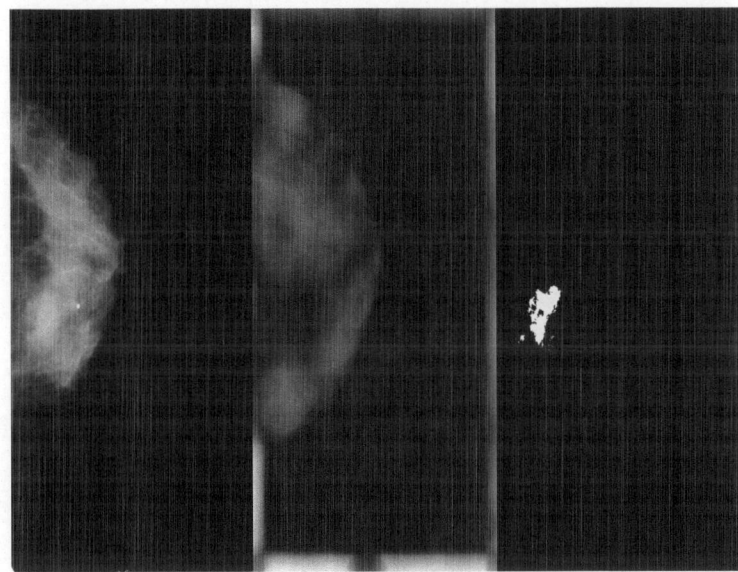

Fig. 4. On the left is the original image. The middle panel shows the variation of the oriented filterbank responses at each pixel. The combination of high intensity (above a fixed threshold T_1) and low variation (below a fixed threshold T_2) identifies the region shown in the far right panel.

is different. A filterbank comprising ten oriented filters was applied to N_r with $r = 22$ (the image in the far right panel of Fig. 3). Filter j consisted of a rounded rectangular filter of width 15 pixels (≈ 0.7 mm) and length 60 pixels (≈ 3.0 mm) oriented at an angle $(j - 1)\pi/10$, $j = 1, 2, \ldots, 10$. Thus for every pixel, a feature vector comprising oriented filter responses at ten angles was constructed. The variation of these filter responses was recorded as a single texture feature (middle panel of Fig. 4). Using the image intensity (original image) and this single texture feature the mass region of the image was correctly delineated in the example image with no false positive regions within the image (right panel of Fig. 4) simply by setting an empirically defined thresholds for each of the two features (Fig. 5).

4 Discussion

The image in the right panel of Fig. 3 is flat in the sense that the bright regions in the original image (left panel in Fig. 3) do not appear in this image. The texture feature computed from this image (variation of oriented filter outputs) is therefore independent of background intensity. This texture feature shows a clear response in the region of the mass (middle panel in Fig. 4). Thus this response is viewed as associated with the texture properties of the mass but independent of background intensity. Neither this texture feature alone nor image intensity

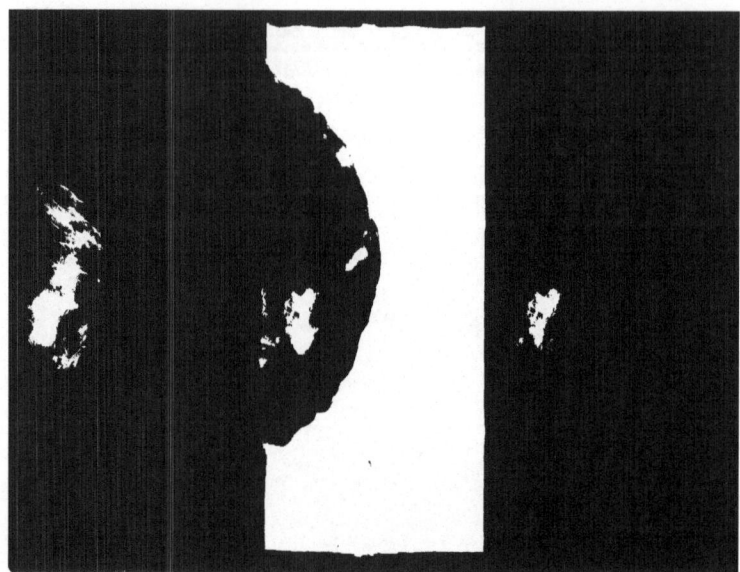

Fig. 5. The panel on the left shows the regions of the original image with intensity above threshold T_1. The middle panel shows the image of variation to oriented filter response (the middle panel of Fig. 4) below threshold T_2. The right panel shows the intersection of the previous two panels.

alone suffice to classify tissue as cancerous (Fig. 5). However, when the texture feature is combined with image intensity, the result is that the region of the mass is identified but other bright regions in the original image are not identified.

The purpose of this paper is to establish that texture features exist that contribute to the identification of breast cancer independently of image intensity. The purpose is not to quantify this contribution and so no effort was made to test the observation on a large data set. A more complete analysis of texture on flattened images is currently underway.

References

1. Grim, J., Somol, P., Haindl, M., Daneš, J.: Computer-aided evaluation of screening mammograms based on local texture models. IEEE Transaction on Image Processing 18(4), 765–773 (2009)
2. Gupta, R., Undrill, P.E.: The use of texture analysis to delineate suspicious masses in mammography. Phys. Med. Biol. 40, 835–855 (1995)
3. Karssemeijer, N.: Automated classification of parenchymal patterns in mammograms. Physics and Medicine in Biology 43, 365–378 (1998)
4. Karssemeijer, N., te Brake, G.M., et al.: Detection of stellate distortions in mammograms. IEEE Transactions on Medical Imaging 15(5), 611–619 (1996)
5. Malik, J., Belongie, S., Shi, J., Leung, T.: Textons, contours and regions; Cue integration in image segmentation. In: IEEE Int. Conf. on Comp. Vision, Corfu, Greece. IEEE (1999)

6. McCormack, V.A., dos Santos Silva, I.: Breast density and parenchymal patterns as markers of breast cancer risk: A meta-analysis. Cancer Epidemiology, Biomarkers and Prevention 15(6), 1159–1169 (2006)

7. Mudigonda, N.R., Rangayyan, R.M., Desautels, J.E.L.: Detection of breast masses in mammograms by density slicing and texture flow-field analysis. IEEE Transactions on Medical Imaging 20(12), 1215–1227 (2001)

8. Palma, G., Bloch, I., Muller, S.: Spiculated Lesions and Architectural Distortions Detection in Digital Breast Tomosynthesis Datasets. In: Martí, J., Oliver, A., Freixenet, J., Martí, R. (eds.) IWDM 2010. LNCS, vol. 6136, pp. 712–719. Springer, Heidelberg (2010)

9. Sahiner, B., Chan, H.-P., Petrick, N., Halvie, M.A., Goodsitt, M.M.: Computerized characterization of masses on mammograms: The rubber band straightening transform and texture analysis. Medical Physics 25(4), 516–526 (1998)

10. Sahiner, B., Chan, H.-P., Petrick, N., Helvie, M.A., Hadjiiski, L.M.: Improvement of mammographic mass characterization using spiculation measures and morphological features. Medical Physics 28(7), 1455–1465 (2001)

11. Tourassi, G.D., Delong, D.M., Floyd Jr., C.E.: A study on the computerized fractal analysis of architectural distortions in screening mammograms. Phys. Med. Biol. 51, 1299–1312 (2006)

12. Wessel, C., Schnabel, J.A., Brady, S.M.: Towards More Realistic Biomechanical Modelling of Tumours under Mammographic Compressions. In: Martí, J., Oliver, A., Freixenet, J., Martí, R. (eds.) IWDM 2010. LNCS, vol. 6136, pp. 481–489. Springer, Heidelberg (2010)

13. Wolfe, J.N.: Risk for breast cancer development determined by mammographic parenchymal pattern. Cancer 37(5), 2486–2492 (1976)

14. Zwiggelaar, R.: Local Greylevel Appearance Histogram Based Texture Segmentation. In: Martí, J., Oliver, A., Freixenet, J., Martí, R. (eds.) IWDM 2010. LNCS, vol. 6136, pp. 175–182. Springer, Heidelberg (2010)

Inter- and Intra-Observer Variability of Radiologists Evaluating CBIR Systems

Lubomir Hadjiiski[1], Hyun-chong Cho[1], Heang-Ping Chan[1], Berkman Sahiner[2], Mark A. Helvie[1], Chintana Paramagul[1], and Alexis V. Nees[1]

[1] University of Michigan, Department of Radiology, Ann Arbor, MI 48109
lhadjisk@umich.edu
[2] Center for Devices and Radiological Health, US Food and Drug Administration, Silver Spring, MD 20993

Abstract. The purpose of the study is to evaluate the inter- and intra-observer variability of the radiologists in evaluation of the similarity between the query and retrieved ulatasound images containing breast masses by the Content-Based Image Retrieval (CBIR) CADx system. Three radiologists rated the similarity between the query masses and the computer-retrieved (ED-CBIR) masses. Three CBIR systems based on each radiologist's subjective similarity ratings (R-CBIRs) were formed and compared with the ED-CBIR. The intra-observer variability was smaller than the inter-observer variability for all three radiologists. The radiologists' performance with the R-CBIRs produced similarity ratings results close to the radiologists' performance with the ED-CBIR. The average difference in classification accuracy (Az) between the ED-CBIR and the R-CBIRs was slightly lower than the average difference in Az between the R-CBIRs. The relatively large intra- and inter-observer variability may make more difficult to evaluate the effect of the CBIR CADx systems on radiologists' performance.

Keywords: computer-aided diagnosis, content-based image retrieval, inter-observer variability, intra-observer variability, breast masses, breast ultrasonography.

1 Background

We are developing a Content-Based Image Retrieval (CBIR) CADx system to assist radiologists in characterizing masses on ultrasound (US) images [1-3]. We have designed and studied the performance of CBIR CADx systems that incorporated input-feature-based similarity measures such as Euclidean distance measure (ED) and cosine distance measure [1], output-score-based similarity measures such as linear discriminant analysis and Bayesian neural network [1], as well as decision tree based similarity measures [2]. A relevance feedback was also used in the design of our ED-based CBIR CADx (ED-CBIR) system [3]. In order to compare the performance of the different retrieval methods, we performed a number of observer studies with

A.D.A. Maidment, P.R. Bakic, and S. Gavenonis (Eds.): IWDM 2012, LNCS 7361, pp. 482–489, 2012.

radiologists. An important factor influencing the effect of CBIR CADx on radiologists' performance is the radiologists' variability in perceiving the similarity between the query case and the retrieved cases. In this study, we evaluated the inter- and intra-observer variability of the radiologists in evaluation of the similarity between the query and retrieved US images containing breast masses by the CBIR CADx system based on radiologists' visual similarity assessment.

2   Methods

Two observer studies were performed to evaluate the radiologists' inter- and intra-observer variability in visual similarity assessment of pairs of masses in US images.

In Study 1, for a query mass, 3 most similar masses were retrieved with ED-CBIR [1] and were presented to the radiologists in random order. Three Mammography Quality Standards Act (MQSA) approved radiologists (R1, R2, R3) rated the similarity between the query mass and the computer-retrieved masses using a 9-point similarity scale (1=very dissimilar, 9=very similar). The data set included 100 query masses on 100 (49 malignant and 51 benign) images and 121 reference library masses on 230 (79 malignant and 151 benign) images collected with IRB approval. All masses were biopsy-proven. Therefore, 300 image pairs (query mass - retrieved mass) ((100query) X (top 3 retrieved)=300) were evaluated by the radiologists R1, R2 and R3 (defined as Reading 1). Approximately a year later the same 300 image pairs were evaluated again by the same radiologists R1, R2 and R3 (defined as Reading 2).

In Study 2 a second data set consisting of 62 (31 malignant and 31 benign) masses was used. All masses were biopsy-proven. The similarities of 1891 image pairs from the 62 masses (full combination set, 62X61/2=1891) were also rated by the 3 radiologists R1, R2 and R3 using the 9-point similarity scale.

By using the radiologists' similarity ratings from Study 1 (Reading 1 and Reading 2), we estimated the intra- and inter-observer variability of radiologists in evaluation of the similarity between pairs of the retrieved mass and query mass. By using the radiologists' similarity ratings from Study 2 we were able to estimate the inter-observer variability of radiologists in evaluation of all possible 1891 image pairs obtained from 62 masses.

Using the similarity ratings of the three radiologists from Study 2, we formed three CBIR systems (R1-CBIR, R2-CBIR, R3-CBIR), each of which used one of the radiologists' similarity ratings for image retrieval. We estimated the inter-observer variability of the radiologists by simulation experiments as follows. For each R-CBIR system, a leave-one-out method was used for image retrieval, 10 most similar masses to each query mass (the left out-mass) were retrieved from the reference library (the remaining 61 masses). The retrieved images were evaluated by using the R1, R2 or R3 similarity ratings, allowing the estimation of the inter-observer variability. In addition, a similar experiment using the computerized ED-CBIR was performed with the same 62 masses and the retrieved images were also evaluated by using the R1, R2 and R3 similarity ratings. The performance of the computerized ED-CBIR was compared with that of the R-CBIR systems in terms of classification accuracy. The ratio of the number of retrieved malignant masses to the total number of retrieved masses (10) was used as a decision variable for every query mass.

The intra-observer variability was estimated as the average difference and the average absolute difference between the radiologist's ratings from Reading 1 and Reading 2. The inter-observer variability was estimated as the average difference and the average absolute difference between the radiologists' ratings (R1-R2, R1-R3, and R2-R3). For example, the inter-observer variability (IOV) for R1 was IOV(R1) = (|R1-R2|+|R1-R3|)/2.

3   Results

3.1   Intra-observer Variability

The estimated intra-observer variability for R1, R2 and R3 are presented in Table 1 and Figure 1. For all 3 radiologists the difference in similarity ratings between Reading 1 and Reading 2 was statistically significant. R1 had the smallest average absolute difference and R2 had the largest average absolute difference. From Figure 1 it can be observed that R1 has the largest number of ratings with difference of 0, 1 or -1 compared to the other two radiologists.

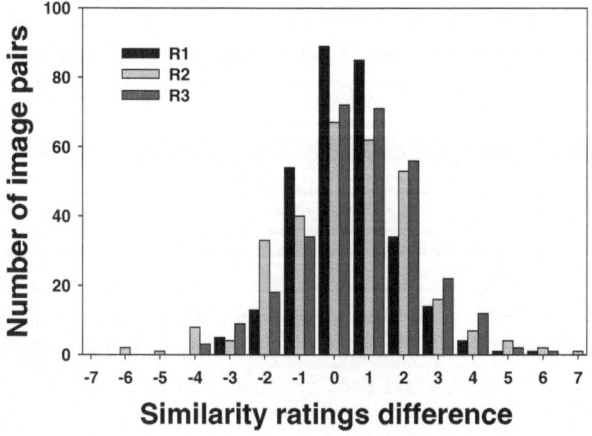

Fig. 1. Distribution of the difference between Reading 1 and Reading 2 similarity ratings for radiologists R1, R2 and R3

Table 1. Average similarity ratings of radiologists R1, R2 and R3 performing Reading1 and Reading 2 one year apart for 300 image pairs

	Evaluated by		
	R1	R2	R3
Reading 1	5.71	4.63	5.61
Reading 2	6.13	5.02	6.29
Difference	0.42±1.38	0.39±1.95	0.68±1.70
AbsoluteDifference	1.06±0.98	1.50±1.30	1.41±1.17
p (paired t-test)	<0.001	<0.001	<0.001

3.2   Inter-observer Variability

The trends of the average absolute differences and corresponding standard deviations between similarity ratings of radiologists R1, R2 and R3 in Study 2 are similar to those observed in Study 1 (both for Reading 1 and Reading 2). The results are presented in Tables 2 and 3 and Figures 2, 3 and 5.

Table 2. Average difference and average absolute difference between similarity ratings of radiologists R1, R2 and R3 based on the evaluation of 300 pairs of mass US images

	R1-R2	|R1-R2|	R1-R3	|R1-R3|	R2-R3	|R2-R3|
Reading 1	1.08±2.02	1.76±1.46	0.10±1.85	1.46±1.13	-0.98±2.23	1.89±1.53
Reading 2	1.11±1.74	1.66±1.23	-0.16±1.74	1.37±1.08	-1.27±2.16	1.99±1.52

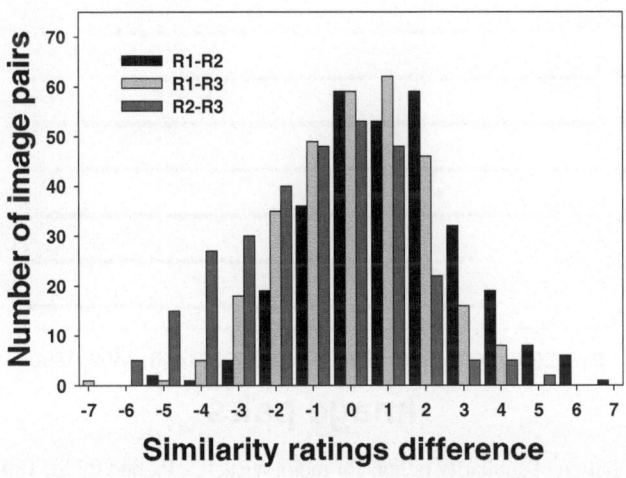

Fig. 2. Distribution of the differences in similarity ratings for Reading 1

Table 3. Average difference and average absolute difference between similarity ratings of radiologists R1, R2 and R3 based on the evaluation of 1891 pairs

	R1-R2	|R1-R2|	R1-R3	|R1-R3|	R2-R3	|R2-R3|
Study 2	0.59±1.78	1.45±1.20	-0.01±1.71	1.30±1.11	-0.60±1.95	1.52±1.37

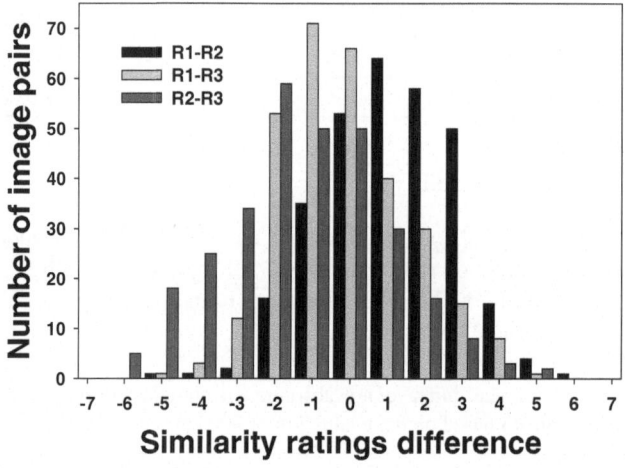

Fig. 3. Distribution of the differences in similarity ratings for Reading 2

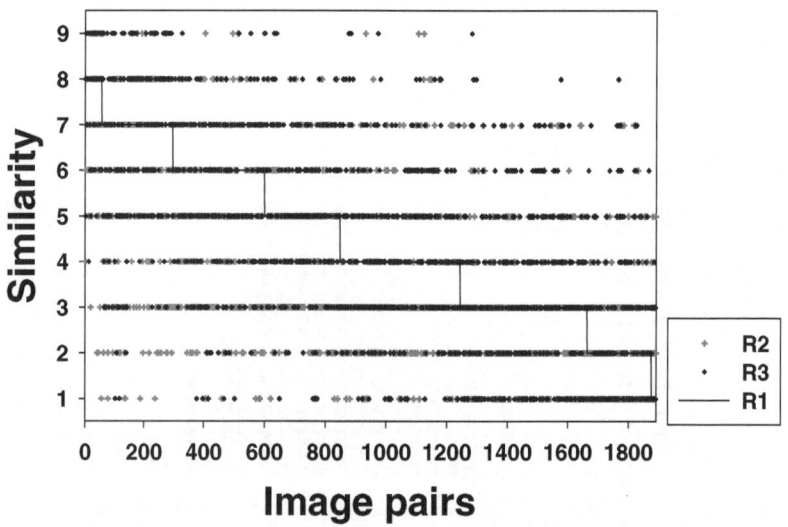

Fig. 4. Distribution of similarity ratings for radiologists R1, R2 and R3 for 1891 image pairs

The smallest average absolute difference and standard deviation were between R1 and R3. The largest average absolute difference and standard deviation were between R2 and R3. The inter-observer variability for Reading 1 was IOV(R1)= 1.61±1.31, IOV(R2)= 1.83±1.50, IOV(R3)= 1.68±1.34; for Reading 2 was IOV(R1)= 1.52 ±1.16, IOV(R2)= 1.83±1.38, IOV(R3)= 1.68±1.32; and for Study 2 was IOV(R1)= 1.38±1.16, IOV(R2)= 1.49±1.29, IOV(R3)= 1.41±1.25.

The inter-observer variability was the smallest for R1, followed by R3, and the largest for R2. The similarity ratings for radiologists R1, R2 and R3 for 1891 image pairs are plotted in Figure 4, using R1's ratings in descending values to order the 1891 pairs.

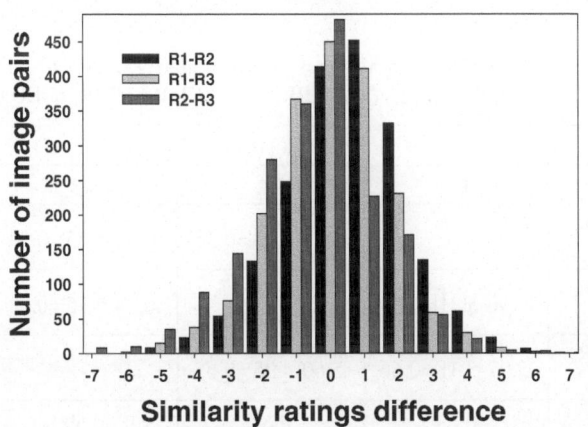

Fig. 5. Distribution of the difference in similarity ratings in Study 2

3.3   Comparison of the Accuracy of the Automated ED-CBIR System to the R-CBIR Systems and Inter-observer Variability of the Radiologists When Evaluating the CBIR Systems

For the comparison of the accuracy of the ED-CBIR system to the R-CBIR systems, the similarities of 1891 image pairs were used. For all 62 query masses, the Az values of R1-CBIR, R2-CBIR, R3-CBIR, and ED-CBIR at k=10 were 0.93±0.03, 0.85±0.05, 0.92±0.04, and 0.89±0.03, respectively. The average absolute difference in Az among the R-CBIRs was 0.05±0.04. The average absolute difference in Az between the ED-CBIR and the R-CBIRs was 0.04±0.03.

Table 4. Average similarity ratings of R1, R2 and R3 for retrievals from different CBIR systems (R1-CBIR, R2-CBIR, R3-CBIR, or ED CBIR) for k=10

	Evaluated by					
Retrieved by	R1	R2	R3	IR1-R2I	IR1-R3I	IR2-R3I
R1-CBIR	**6.85**	5.53	6.29			0.76
R2-CBIR	5.90	**7.14**	6.38		0.48	
R3-CBIR	5.97	5.60	**7.57**	0.37		
ED CBIR	5.31	4.95	5.75			

The average similarity ratings for the different CBIR systems are presented in Table 4. The absolute difference of the average similarity ratings for evaluation of R1-CBIR by the other two radiologists (i.e. the absolute difference between the average similarity ratings of R2 evaluating R1-CBIR retrievals and that of R3 evaluating the same retrievals) was 0.76 (Table 4). The absolute difference for evaluation of R2-CBIR by R1 and R3, and R3-CBIR by R1 and R2 were 0.48 and 0.37, respectively (Table 4). The average absolute difference in similarity ratings in test mode (averaged over the 3 CBIRs retrievals) was 0.54. These estimations reveal the inter-observer variability of the three radiologists evaluating the three R-CBIR systems.

Table 5. Absolute difference between averages of the similarity ratings of R1, R2 and R3 for retrievals from different CBIR systems (R1-CBIR, R2-CBIR, R3-CBIR, or ED CBIR) for $k=10$

	Evaluated by			
Difference	R1	R2	R3	**Average**
Diff(R1-CBIR, ED CBIR)	-	|5.53-4.95|=0.58	|6.29-5.75|=0.54	
Diff(R2-CBIR, ED CBIR)	|5.90-5.31|=0.59	-	|6.38-5.75|=0.63	
Diff(R3-CBIR, ED CBIR)	|5.97-5.31|=0.66	|5.60-4.95|=0.65	-	
Average	0.63	0.62	0.59	**0.61**

The average absolute differences in the similarity ratings for R1 when evaluating the ED-CBIR system and CBIR systems based on the other two radiologists (i.e., absolute differences in similarity ratings between R1 evaluating ED-CBIR retrievals, R1 evaluating R2-CBIR retrievals and R1 evaluating R3-CBIR retrievals) was 0.63 (Table 5). These absolute differences for R2 and R3 were 0.62 and 0.59, respectively (Table 5). The average absolute difference in similarity ratings was 0.61. The above estimations show the variability of every individual radiologist evaluating the ED-CBIR and the R-CBIR systems. For the three radiologists these variabilities were relatively consistent. The average variability of 0.61 was slightly higher than the inter-observer variability of the three radiologists evaluating the three R-CBIR systems (0.54).

4   Discussion

The intra-observer variability was smaller than the inter-observer variability for all three radiologists. The inter-observer variability was consistent for the three radiologists in the repeat experiments Reading 1 and Reading 2, and slightly smaller when evaluating Study 2. The rank order of the radiologists, based on the magnitude of their intra- and inter-observer variability, was consistent in both observer studies. The radiologists' performance with the R-CBIR systems in the simulated evaluation experiments produced results close to the radiologists' performance with the ED-CBIR system. The average difference in classification accuracy between the ED-CBIR and the R-CBIRs was slightly lower than the average difference in accuracy among the R-CBIRs. The ED-CBIR may be useful for classification of US breast masses as malignant and benign. However, the relatively large intra- and inter-observer variability may make more difficult to evaluate the effect of the CBIR systems on radiologists' performance.

Acknowledgements. This work is supported by USPHS grant CA 118305.

References

1. Cho, H.C., Hadjiiski, L., Sahiner, B., Chan, H.P., Helvie, M., Paramagul, C., Nees, A.V.: Similarity Evaluation in a Content-Based Image Retrieval (CBIR) CADx System for Characterization of Breast Masses on Ultrasound Images. Medical Physics 38, 1820–1831 (2011)
2. Cho, H.C., Hadjiiski, L., Chan, H.P., Sahiner, B., Helvie, M., Paramagul, C., Nees, A.V.: A similarity study between the query mass and retrieved masses using decision tree content-based image retrieval (DTCBIR) CADx system for characterization of ultrasound breast mass images. In: Proc. SPIE Medical Imaging, vol. 8315, pp. 831528-1–831528-7 (2012)
3. Cho, H.C., Hadjiiski, L., Sahiner, B., Chan, H.P., Paramagul, C., Helvie, M., Nees, A.V.: Interactive content-based image retrieval (CBIR) computer-aided diagnosis (CADx) system for ultrasound breast masses using relevance feedback. In: Proc. SPIE Medical Imaging, vol. 8315, 831509-1–831509-7 (2012)

Quantification of Detection Probability of Microcalcifications at Increased Display Luminance Levels

Tom R.L. Kimpe[1] and Albert Xthona[2]

[1] Barco Healthcare, President Kennedypark 35, 8500 Kortrijk, Belgium
[2] Barco Healthcare, 15425 SW Beaverton Creek Court, 97006 Beaverton, OR, USA
`{tom.kimpe,albert.xthona}@barco.com`

Abstract. Only 70-80% of breast cancer is detected in the screening environment. Detection of microcalcifications is generally incomplete and limits effectiveness of controlling breast cancer through early detection. Any advantage in detection of microcalcifications would be highly welcome. Anecdotal comments from practicing radiologists suggest that increased luminance provides one way to increase the detection of relevant microcalcifications. This paper aims to study the effect of increased display luminance on the detection probability of microcalcifications.

1   Background

The ACRIN DMIST trial found significantly better diagnostic accuracy of digital mammography, as compared with screen-film mammography, in women with dense breasts; Studying the cancers, this was most likely attributable to differences in *image contrast*, attributable primarily to differences in the display and acquisition characteristics [1]. Small calcifications provide evidence of breast cancer. The specific size, shape, and clustering of these microcalcifications can be used to categorize breast images following examples in an atlas [2]. The microcalcifications of interest are on the order of 0.5mm. Determination of the shape of such objects is possible with digital mammography detectors having a range of 50-100 microns. Categorization of microcalcifications per atlas is well correlated with breast cancer [3].

Breast-screening images are typically presented to radiologists for interpretation on multiple medical-grade displays with a resolution of 5 mega pixels (5MP). These displays have a typical luminance of 500 cd/m² (AAPM TG18 and FDA require a minimum luminance of 450 cd/m² for primary reading of mammography images). When seated at such a display system, 500 – 600 mm is a typical viewing distance. 0.125 mm – 1mm (in the breast) calcifications are the size of interest. The spatial frequency is thus between 3.1 and 29.8 cycles/degree, when using the whole 5MP screen to view each image.

Contrast and luminance affect our ability to see details in mammography and other medical images. Consider the typical image below in figure 1. On the left it is presented with nominal luminance, on the right with twice that luminance (The exact ratio being subject to the limitations of print and digital media).

A.D.A. Maidment, P.R. Bakic, and S. Gavenonis (Eds.): IWDM 2012, LNCS 7361, pp. 490–497, 2012.
© Springer-Verlag Berlin Heidelberg 2012

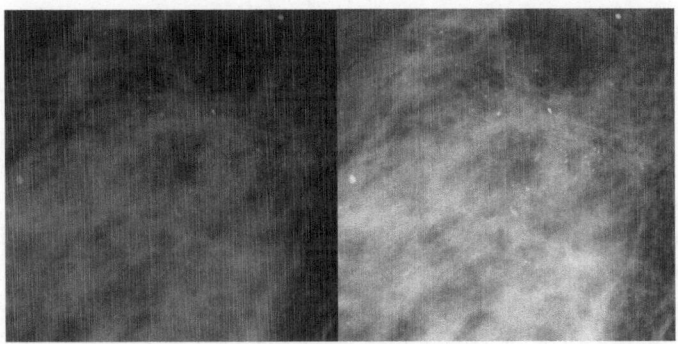

Fig. 1. Example of how luminance affects visibility of image details

The luminance of softcopy displays has evolved over the past 10 years. When the FDA first approved Full Field Digital Mammography for breast screening as an alternative to film-screen mammography, softcopy displays were based primarily on CRT technology. There was a trade-off between focus and electron beam current that limited the practical luminance. With the advent of LCD displays, its luminance has evolved upwards.

Table 1. Overview of display luminance evolution

Year display was introduced	Technology	Luminance in candela per square meter
1997	CRT	300
2002	CRT	450
2004	LCD	600
2011	LCD	1000

Contrast and luminance are both strongly correlated with conspicuity of mammographic targets. Using FDA-trained inspectors to score phantoms, it was found that the mass and speck scores were significantly higher both with higher luminance and with greater contrast [4].

Anecdotal comments from practicing radiologists about superiority of higher luminance need to be tested before the importance of this observation can be determined. Failure to perceive mammographic details is an important category of error in missed breast cancer [5]. Breast cancer, when present, is detected in screening 70-80% of the time. When cancer is detected in subsequent screenings, visible evidence can often be found in the prior screening images. Based on data collected in the Dutch screening program based in Nijmegen, half of undetected cancers have minimal signs present [6]. From this we can assume a detection probability in the original screening to be on the order of 85% - accounting for half of the 30% missed in the screening.

This paper aims to quantify the clinical value of increasing the luminance of medical displays by determining the advantage in microcalcification detection.

2   Method

In order to determine the clinical value of higher display luminance, detection probability of typical microcalcifications will be calculated as a function of display luminance. These calculations will be based on generally accepted models of the human visual system. The calculations will be performed for a 21.3 inch 5 Mega Pixel medical display with contrast ratio of approximately 900:1. Many medical displays used for mammography have a typical calibrated luminance value of 500 cd/m². This means that over the entire lifetime of the display, the white-point will be at 500 cd/m². We will use 500 cd/m² as a reference point and we will compare higher calibrated luminance values of 1000 cd/m² and 2300 cd/m² with the reference point.

As a first step, the simple DICOM GSDF (Grayscale Standard Display function) model [7] will be used. The GSDF forms the basis of current medical display calibration technology. The GSDF curve (see figure 2) defines the luminance (cd/m²) in function of JNDs (Just Noticeable Differences). A JND is the difference in luminance that is necessary such that a typical observer will be able to see the target in luminance in 50% of the cases. The GSDF curve allows computing the total number of just noticeable differences that a display system can generate, as well as the JNDs per step that reflect the perceived contrast of a medical display system.

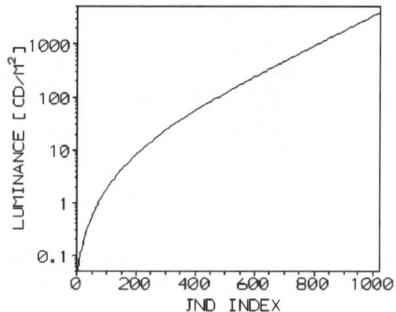

Fig. 2. DICOM Grayscale Standard Display Function

The Grayscale Standard Display function is based on Barten's model [8] of the Contrast Sensitivity Curve (CSF). The CSF represents the amount of minimum contrast at each spatial frequency that is necessary for a visual system to distinguish sinusoidal gratings or Gabor patterns over a range of spatial frequencies surrounded by a uniform field. Barten's CSF model has been heavily validated by means of multiple psycho visual studies and as of today is considered to be one of the most accurate contrast sensitivity models of the human visual system. In this paper we will make use of the general CSF model of Barten of which the main formula is shown in figure 3.

$$CSF(u) = \frac{1}{m_t(u)} = \frac{M_{opt}(u)}{k} \cdot \frac{1}{\sqrt{\dfrac{2}{T}\left(\dfrac{1}{X_0^2}+\dfrac{1}{X_{max}^2}+\dfrac{u^2}{N_{max}^2}\right)\left(\dfrac{1}{\eta pE}+\dfrac{\Phi_o}{1-e^{-(u/u_0)^2}}\right)}}$$

X_0: the angular size of the object
X_{max}: the maximum aungular size of the integration area
N_{max}: the maximum number of cycles over which the eye can integrate the
information
η: the quantum efficiency of the eye
p: the photon conversion factor for the conversion of light units in units for the flux
density of the photons
E: retinal illuminance

k	= 3.0	T	= 0.1 sec	η	= 0.03
σ_0	= 0.5 arc min	X_{max}	= 12°	Φ_0	= 3×10^{-8} sec deg^2
C_{ab}	= 0.08 arc min/mm	N_{max}	= 15 cycles	u_0	= 7 cycles/deg

Fig. 3. Barten's model of Contrast Sensitvity Function

When DICOM/NEMA generated the GSDF curve, Barten's CSF model was used where the target is assumed to have a 4 cycles degree spatial frequency and a angular size of 2 degrees and for a 'typical' medical display. Therefore, a more accurate result can be obtained by using the CSF model with specific parameters corresponding to the correct spatial frequency and size of microcalcifications, correct display size and luminance, etc.

Finally, the link will be made between sensitivity of the eye and actual detection probability of microcalcifications. This relationship is described by the psychometric function [9] that can be approximated with a Weibull function.

3   Results

3.1   GSDF Model Calculations

As a first result, the total number of available JNDs (Just Noticeable Differences) is calculated based on the GSDF curve and this for the three calibrated luminance levels.

The medical display running at 500 cd/m² has a black point of 0.556 cd/m² (and of course a white-point of 500 cd/m²). Note that this corresponds to a contrast ratio of +/- 900:1. As can be derived from the GSDF curve, 500 cd/m² corresponds to JND value 706 and 0.556 cd/m² corresponds to JND value 50. This means that this display has 657 available JNDs (706-50+1) or 2.566 JNDs per step if images of 256 grey levels are shown.

The medical display running at 2300 cd/m² has a black point of 2.556 cd/m² (and of course a white-point of 2300 cd/m²), again corresponding to a contrast ratio of +/- 900:1. As can be derived from the GSDF curve, 2300 cd/m² corresponds to JND value 938 and 2.556 cd/m² corresponds to JND value 138. This means that this display has 801 available JNDs or 3.129 JNDs per step if images of 256 grey levels are shown.

This means that increasing the calibrated luminance of a medical display from 500 cd/m² to 1000 cd/m² results into a 12% increase in perceived contrast (even though the physical contrast ratio remains unchanged). A further increase to 2300 cd/m² results into a 22% increase in perceived contrast compared to the 500 cd/m² reference. These results have been summarized in the table below.

Table 2. Influence of display luminance on #JNDs and perceived contrast

	Black point		White point		Contrast Ratio	Available JNDs	JNDs/step	Increase in
	Luminance	JND number	Luminance	JND number				perceived contrast
500 cd/m²	0,556	50	500 cd/m²	706	900	657	2,566	
1000 cd/m²	1,111	76	1000 cd/m²	811	900	736	2,875	12,02%
2300 cd/m²	2,556	138	2300 cd/m²	938	900	801	3,129	21,92%

As has been explained before, the GSDF model is based on Barten's more general model of the Contrast Sensitivity Function where the target is assumed to have a 4 cycles per degree spatial frequency and a angular size of 2 degrees and for a 'typical' medical display. The next section will calculate more accurate results of the CSF for the specific medical display used in this paper and micro calcifications as targets to be detected.

3.2   Refined CSF Model Calculations

Based on Barten's CSF model and the formula shown in figure 3, calculations have been made for the same 21.3 inch 5 Mega Pixel medical displays, viewing distance 50 cm, three calibrated luminance levels (500 cd/m², 1000 cd/m² and 2300 cd/m²) and target size corresponding to typical microcalcifications. Microcalcifications of interest (that are often missed) are in the order of 0.5 mm. The relevant spatial frequencies are around 15 cycles/degree, when using the whole 5MP screen to view each image. The resulting CSF curves are shown in the left side of figure 4 (please note the logarithmic scale of this figure).

In line with the expectations, there is mostly improvement for higher spatial frequencies. This also perfectly corresponds with previously received feedback from radiologists that higher luminance mostly helps for detecting subtle, small microcalcifications (that correspond to higher spatial frequencies).

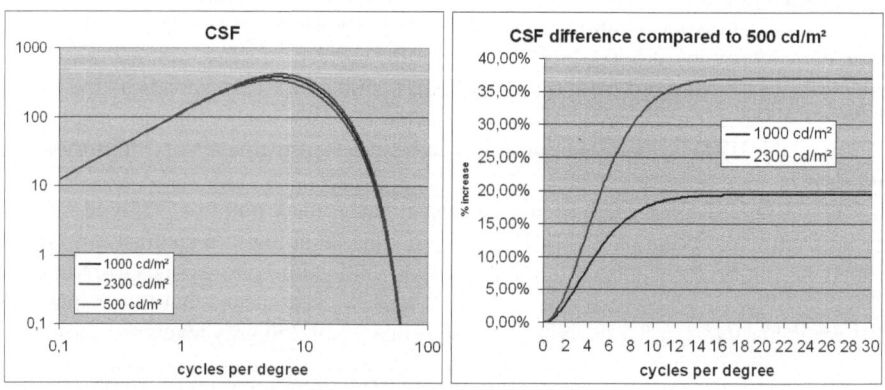

Fig. 4. (left) Contrast Sensitivity curves, (right) Improvement in sensitivity

Figure 4 (right side) shows the increase in contrast sensitivity for calibrated luminance levels 1000 cd/m² and 2300 cd/m² compared to the reference 500 cd/m². It is confirmed that the higher luminance mostly makes a difference for higher spatial frequencies (>4 cycles per degree) with maximum benefit for spatial frequencies of 10 cycles per degree and higher. In that range of spatial frequencies, increasing the luminance from 500 cd/m² to 1000 cd/m² results into a 19.4% higher sensitivity, while increasing from 500 cd/m² to 2300 cd/m² even results into a 37.0 % higher sensitivity. Simple GSDF model only predicted an increase of 12.0% (1000 cd/m² versus 500 cd/m²) and 21.9% (2300 cd/m² versus 500 cd/m²).

3.3   Detection Probability of Microcalcifications

To finally estimate the clinical value of higher luminance of medical displays we need to know the increase in detection probability for microcalcifications. The JND values and CSF results need to be related back to detection probability of microcalcifications. The psychometric function [10] is used to convert signal strength/sensitivity into detection probability. For this paper we use a Weibull function [9] to estimate the psychometric function. The Weibull function has one parameter 'k'. For details about this parameter 'k' we refer to [9; 10] and [8] pp. 11-15. Generally accepted values for 'k' are in the range 2-3. Figure 5 shows detection probability as a function of signal strength.

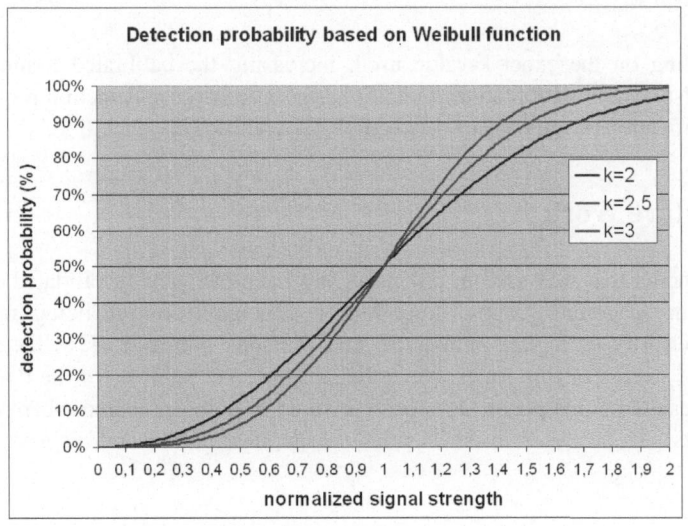

Fig. 5. Weibull function for k-values 2; 2.5 and 3

In order to calculate what the effect of increased luminance is on detection probability we need to have one calibration point on the psychometric curve. We choose a detection probability for microcalcifications on a display with calibrated luminance 1000 cd/m² of 85%, based on the Netherlands data [6] that was collected with very bright analog displays. By means of this calibration point we can now calculate the detection probability for 500 cd/m² and 2300 cd/m².

Sensitivity has shown to be 37% higher at 2300 cd/m² and 19% higher at 1000 cd/m² compared to 500 cd/m². Similarly, but now putting the reference point at 1000 cd/m²: sensitivity is 15.1% higher at 2300 cd/m² compared to 1000 cd/m², and sensitivity is 16.0% lower at 500 cd/m² compared to 1000 cd/m².

By inspecting the psychometric function, we observe that 85% detection (for k-value 2.5) corresponds to normalized signal strength 1.42. Increasing luminance from 1000 cd/m² to 2300 cd/m² corresponds to increasing the sensitivity and normalized signal strength with 15.1%. Therefore detection probability at 2300 cd/m² can now be read from the psychometric function (k-value 2.5) at normalized signal strength 1.42 x 1.151 = 1.635 and equals 94.1% probability of detection. Detection probability at 500 cd/m² can also be read from the psychometric function (k-value 2.5) at 1.42x0.840= 1.193 and equals 68.3% probability of detection. The table below also shows this calculation but now for all three k-values (2; 2.5; 3).

Table 3. Detection probability in function of display luminance

		Normalized signal strength			Detection probability		
		500 cd/m²	1000 cd/m²	2300 cd/m²	500 cd/m²	1000 cd/m	2300 cd/m²
k-value	2	1,303	1,55	1,784	71,8%	85,0%	92,6%
	2.5	1,193	1,42	1,635	68,3%	85,0%	94,1%
	3	1,126	1,34	1,543	65,0%	85,0%	95,3%

Depending on the exact k-value used, increasing the calibrated luminance of a medical display from 1000 cd/m² to 2300 cd/m² will increase detection probability of microcalcifications from 85% to between 92.6% and 95.3%.

4   Future Work

Barten's model that was used in this paper has been extensively validated by several independent academic groups. Anecdotal comments from practicing radiologists about superiority of higher luminance, and previous publications in literature also support the results of this paper. Nevertheless, observer studies will be done to confirm the results of this paper. An observer study is being prepared where practicing radiologists will be asked to detect microcalcifications at several display luminance settings.

5   Conclusions

Detection of microcalcifications is generally incomplete and limits effectiveness of controlling breast cancer through early detection. As shown in the Nijmegen study [6], as many as 50% of prior exams had unrecognized evidence of malignancy. Any advantage in detection would be welcome.

Two models of the human visual system have been used to estimate the increase in detection when luminance is increased from 500 cd/m² to 1000 cd/m² and even 2300 cd/m². Increasing the calibrated luminance of a medical display from 1000 cd/m² to 2300 cd/m² increases detection probability of microcalcifications from 85% to 92.6%-95.3%.

Therefore, recent technological advances of medical display systems that offer luminance levels up to 2300 cd/m² hold a lot of promise for increased clinical performance of breast cancer screening.

References

1. Pisano, E., Acharyya, S., Cole, E., Marques, H., Yaffe, M., Blevins, M., Conant, E., Hendrick, R., Baum, J., Fajardo, L.: Cancer Cases from ACRIN Digital Mammographic Imaging Screening Trial: Radiologist Analysis with Use of a Logistic Regression Model. Radiology 252, 348 (2009)
2. D'Orsi, C.: Breast imaging reporting and data system, breast imaging atlas, 4th edn. American College of Radiology (2003)
3. Liberman, L., Abramson, A., Squires, F., Glassman, J., Morris, E., Dershaw, D.: The breast imaging reporting and data system: positive predictive value of mammographic features and final assessment categories. American Journal of Roentgenology 171, 35–40 (1998)
4. Pisano, E., Britt, G., Lin, Y., Schell, M., Burns, C., Brown, M.: Factors affecting phantom scores at annual mammography facility inspections by the US Food and Drug Administration. Academic Radiology 8, 864–870 (2001)
5. Martin, J., Moskowitz, M.: Breast cancer missed by mammography. American Journal of Roentgenology 132, 737–739 (1979)
6. Van Dijck, J., Verbeek, A., Hendriks, J., Holland, R.: The current detectability of breast cancer in a mammographic screening program. A review of the previous mammograms of interval and screening detected cancers. Cancer 72, 1933–1938 (1993)
7. NEMA, Digital Imaging and Communications in Medicine (DICOM), Supplement 28: Grayscale standard display function (GSDF) (1998)
8. Barten, P.G.J.: PhD thesis Technical University of Eindhoven. Contrast sensitivity of the human eye and its effects on image quality (1999)
9. Nachmias, J.: On the psychometric function for contrast detection. Vision Research 21(2), 215–223 (1981)
10. Wichmann, F.A., Hill, N.J.: The psychometric function: I. Fitting, sampling, and goodness of fit. Attention Perception and Psychophysics 63(8), 1293–1313 (2001)
11. Krupinski, E.A., Roehrig, H., Furukawa, T.: Influence of film and monitor display luminance on observer performance and visual search. Acad. Radiol. 6, 411–418 (1999)

Development of Computer Techniques Designed to Aid Tests of Digital Mammography Systems Quality Evaluation with the Phantom CDMAM 3.4

Maria A.Z. Sousa[1], Homero Schiabel[1], and Regina B. Medeiros[2]

[1] Dept. Electrical Engineering – EESC/USP, S.Carlos/SP
[2] Dept. Imaging Diagnosis – UNIFESP, S.Paulo/SP – Brasil
angelicazucareli@usp.br

Abstract. Image quality in digital mammography can be achieved by conducting periodic tests. It is recommended that some quality parameters be measured from images acquired by exposing specific phantoms, as CDMAM 3.4, in such systems. Whereas this task is hard-working and time consuming, this study has attempted to develop and compare two computational methods in order to assist the technical professional in performing the tests with such phantom images, reducing the subjectivity due to the observers. Tests used 27 phantom images obtained from six different digital mammography systems – five CR-type and one DR-type. Both methods proved to be effective in detecting structures. However, the first one allowed the complete image processing and not just a region of interest, which makes it quite advantageous.

Keywords: digital mammography, quality assurance in mammography, phantom CDMAM, computer-assisted detection.

1 Introduction

Mammography image quality can be assured by performing periodic tests to check for instance high contrast details and the low contrast threshold. These parameters can be evaluated by phantom images, which can determine the distinction between the signal of interest and the background.

With the growing development of digital mammography systems, as CR and DR units, new procedures have been developed to evaluate the image quality produced by such equipment. Phantom CDMAM 3.4 [1] was developed specially for performing high and low contrast tests. It is consisted by an aluminum plate inside acrylic, composing a matrix. Four other acrylic plates simulate the breast thickness. In each matrix cell two identical gold discs are randomly disposed. They are between $0.03\mu m$ and $2.0\mu m$ thick and their diameters diverge from 0.06mm up to 2.0mm. The matrix is rotated $45°$ so that to eliminate structures which are easily detectable and those which will surely not be detected. Figure 1 illustrates an image from phantom CDMAM 3.4.

A.D.A. Maidment, P.R. Bakic, and S. Gavenonis (Eds.): IWDM 2012, LNCS 7361, pp. 498–505, 2012.

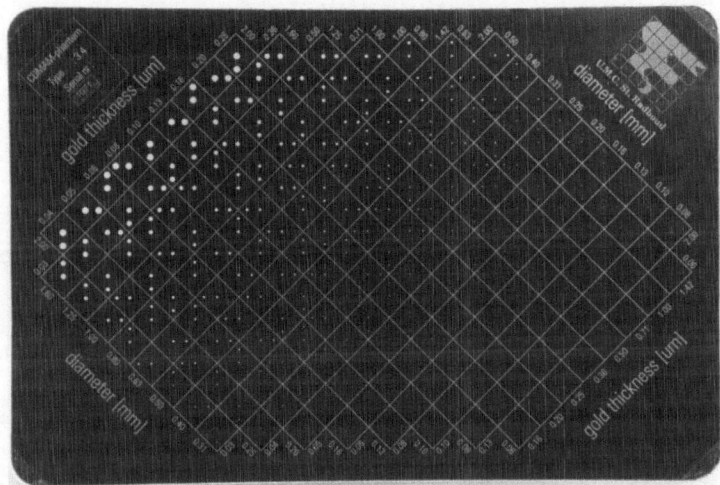

Fig. 1. Frontal view of phantom CDMAM 3.4 – Artinis Contrast-Detail Phantom

As stated by the European Protocol [2], the test should be done annually by 3 observers who read two images verifying the discs location by means of a template in order to determine the contrast threshold. However the phantom image reading is considered tiresome and time consuming. In addition, this reading is quite dependent on the reader subjectivity, which can cause errors, mainly among different observers. In order to minimize this subjectivity, a software named CDCOM was proposed by Karssemeijer [3]. CDCOM searches for finding the accurate discs positioning in DICOM images. Nevertheless, an optimal method to interpret data is not defined, which impairs the search for contrast threshold, and a data correction or validation is necessary [4,5].

Thus, this work proposes the development of computer techniques to detect the discs in these phantom images, working as an aid tool to the digital mammography systems quality control, allowing to reduce the subjectivity due to the human observer. Furthermore, we attempted to correlate these techniques to the human vision, which can discard the need of correcting the measured threshold values.

2   Methods

Two methodologies were developed and compared relatively to the detection accuracy and computational cost. The first is based on the correlation matching technique, consisted by developing circular filters. The filters external ring matches with the image background and the internal ring matches with the structure (disc) to be detected. In the second methodology, the discs were found from their contrasts, calculated by means of circular filters providing the average of pixels values as those corresponding to the image background as well as to the discs.

To correlate these measures with the human vision, we are studying the experiment proposed by Tseng [6], in which the human vision threshold is obtained by the Weber ratio modified by parameters defining the structure visibility as its contrast relative to the background.

2.1   Techniques for Computer Detection

CDMAM 3.4 images from five CR units and one DR system were obtained. Parameters as kVp and mAs were set according to the European Protocol. Twelve images were acquired from a Selenia® Hologic/Lorad DR mammography system; other 15 images were obtained from the following CR units (3 from each one): Agfa 75, Agfa 85, Fuji 50, Fuji 100 and Kodak 975.

The first methodology was developed by using Java and plugins from the software ImageJ®. This eliminated the need of developing a new interface.

In the procedure the first step is determining the initial scanning point. A Sobel borders detector was used allowing to apply the Hough Transform in order to determine the coordinates corresponding to the vertices of the matrix cells in the (x,y) plane. The correlation matching [7] technique was used to detect the discs. It was applied with concentric circular filters composed by two peripheral regions (one external and other internal, according to the illustration in Fig. 2). The internal region is a circle which comprises the structure and attempts to match its interior, while the external one is a ring which attempts to match the background. Filters were made by varying their diameters according to the diameters of the discs existent in the phantom image used as template.

The procedure of locating the structures returns a list of structures marked for each detection. The image is 45° rotated to allow the scanning to be made for each line of the image. The decision on the detection or not of a single structure of interest is based on the contrast between the structure and the background as well as on the background gray scale.

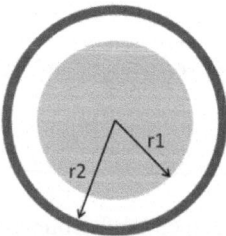

Fig. 2. Filter model used for discs detection

In the second methodology, also concentric circular filters (Fig. 2) are used. The internal filter comprises the structure and the average of pixel values inside the circle is calculated. The external filter is a ring which provides the calculation of the average of pixel values in a region embracing the image background. The number of pixels of the circle and the ring is the same. The contrast is calculated by the difference between the averages of pixel values corresponding to the background and the structure of interest. The center of a singular disc and the vertices of the searching region should be selected, according to Fig. 3.

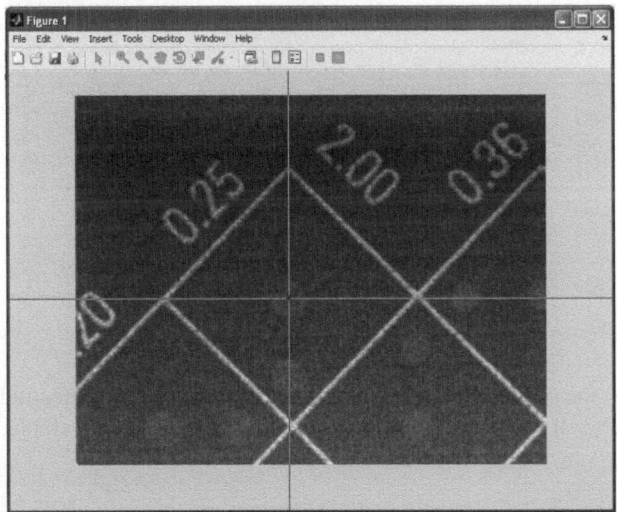

Fig. 3. Selecting the center of the structure to be located

2.2   Correlation with the Human Vision

In order to correlate the image reading made by the computer and the human vision reading, the technical report was used to select the threshold disc which predominates in 50% or more of images [6]. By using ImageJ®, for each image the average of pixel values of image background (B) as well as of 12 chosen threshold discs (B_0) was obtained. Then, the Weber ratio was calculated from the relation $\Delta B/B$, were $\Delta B = B_0 - B$.

This ratio describes the human vision behavior in discriminating the contrast in images analysis [8]. The Weber ratio is close to a constant, β, on a significant range of gray intensities, which can be obtained from the information on the graph ($\Delta B/B$ x B), as well as the maximum value of $|\Delta B/B|$. From these data, the graph corresponding to $\log(\Delta B)$ x $\log(B)$ can be determined [6].

3   Results

3.1   Correlation Matching Technique

In the correlation matching method, when a structure of interest is detected, the software marks the location corresponding to the found disc, illustrated by Fig. 4. In the thumbnail, there is an example of two found discs located in one of the matrix cells.

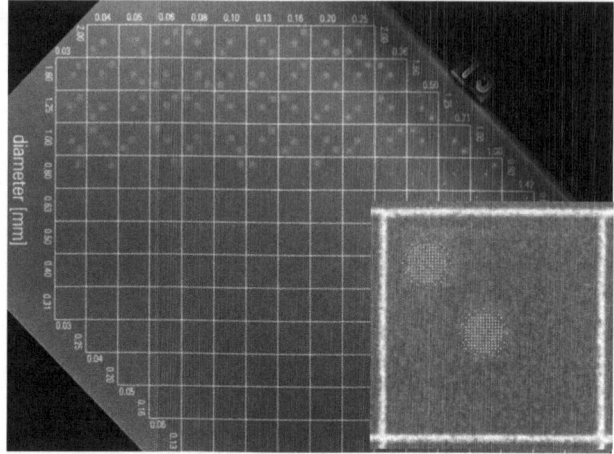

Fig. 4. Result from the discs detection with the method of correlation matching

In this case, the purpose was only detecting the discs in the center and in one of the vertices of each cell. This allowed to detect indeed all the discs in all phantom images, including those not visible to the human eye.

3.2   Average of Pixel Values

After the first test above, the average of filters pixel values were determined comprising only the diameters considered visible according to the technical report. The purpose was reducing the execution time and the computational cost, since the searching is performed cell by cell. The diameters were defined according to a reference image. As a result, in the region of interest comprising one cell, both the discs were located and marked. The center of each mark was stored as a variable.

However, each disc was marked more than once. And, in some cases, the software yielded a wrong result, detecting one of the matrix borders as a structure of interest. This is due to the fact that the border gray level is very close to that corresponding to the disc in such phantom region. As this problem is inherent to the region selected by the user, we could observe that the detection still can be influenced by the user.

As the searching was being done in regions with thinner but larger diameter discs, the detection hardness was increasing, considering that the disc fills big part of the searching region. This limits the region belonging to the background, where the contrast is smaller. Thus, the number of discs detections increased significantly. This error can be minimized by enlarging the searching step.

We could verify that this improvement is valid only for discs with larger diameters. Applying a 3 pixels step for discs smaller than 0.5mm in diameter, the error happens again. So, the results were obtained by using only a 1 pixel step as searching interval, since knowing the exact discs positioning was not necessary in this case. Therefore, we have considered correctly detected the marked structures, even when indicated more than once.

For most of the cases of threshold structures selected by the technical report, only one disc was detected inside the cell. The considered accuracy rate involved all the right detections indicating both discs inside a cell in each image. Results regarding only one disc detected in a single cell were considered erroneous, as well as when the matrix border was detected. Table 1 shows the discs detection rate for the second methodology, for the 27 images used, considering those obtained by CR systems, as well as those acquired from a DR Selenia® Hologic/Lorad unit.

Table 1. Accuracy detection rate corresponding to the method of pixel values average

	Detection Rate
Accuracy rate	83%
Matrix borders detection	6%
Detection of only one disc in the cell	11%
Total of errors	17%

Such errors sometimes can be corrected by changing the searching step or decreasing the region of interest, which however makes the technique relatively dependent on the user.

When analyzed separately, the results obtained for images acquired by the DR Selenia® were verified superior relatively to those obtained for CR systems – reaching an accuracy rate of 86%, while for the CR systems, this rate was 81%. In addition, a decrease of 5% in border detections was also observed. In 9% of cases, only one disc was detected in the cell for the DR images.

Even so, in a general comparison, results for all equipment were similar, with differences no larger than 10% among them.

We should stress that such analysis allow us to compare our software sensitivity, considering the different equipment under study. This means that all the performed investigations compare the single units and not necessarily the different technologies of digital mammography images acquisition.

3.3   Parameters for Correlation with the Human Vision

Contrast for each threshold disc as well as the Weber ratio were calculated in order to determine the parameter β needed for the final equations (Table 2).

Graph in Fig.5 shows the curve obtained from experimental data. Approximation by parts was performed by the minimum squares method, resulting in parameters $B_1=10960$, $B_2=13000$ e $B_3=19000$ required to complete the equations to establish the human vision threshold.

With all the parameters, the human vision threshold can be estimated for each disc to be located in the image in order to allow that the software only determines the limit discs perceptible by human vision.

Table 2. Result from contrast calculation for each selected threshold disc (respective parameter β obtained equal to 0.07)

Threshold	Background (B)	Contrast
1	27543	0.15
2	26962	0.08
3	25690	0.10
4	24185	0.11
5	23592	0.06
6	21974	0.05
7	21447	0.08
8	21790	0.06
9	21347	0.04
10	20309	0.04
11	20443	0.03
12	21218	0.03
Average	23042	0.07
Stand. Dev.	2521	0.04

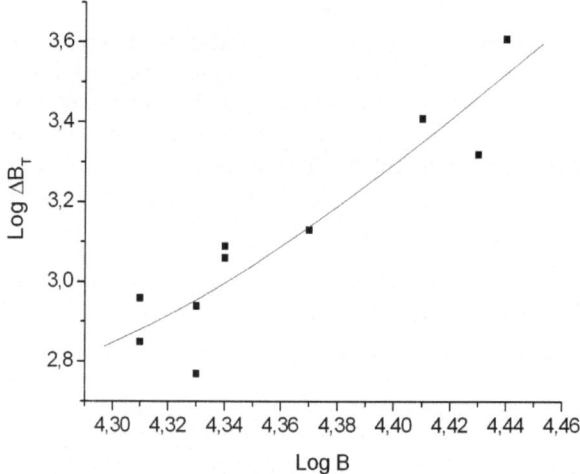

Fig. 5. Graph referent to log(ΔB) x log(B)

4   Conclusions

The first methodology was verified efficient in discs detection, performing the scanning in the entire image, being not time consuming and of low computational cost. Besides, the interface associated to the ImageJ® software made the method totally automatic and simple to be performed. All the discs could be detected, which characterizes the method as a random process, since it does not allow to classify detections between right or wrong. This leads to the need of applying also procedures such as the correlation with the human vision, presented in the test stage, in order to achieve the adequate classification.

The second procedure, although also with a simple interface, has been quite dependent on the user, which causes variation in the results. The double detection of some structures was not a problem, since the purpose was only to check the presence of discs in the cell center and in one of its corners. The scanning by regions of interest instead of the entire image implied a long time expended in the software execution, being also tiresome to the user. However the technique also could be considered efficient, since it was able to detect discs in 83% of all the tests.

Thus, comparatively, the first methodology could be considered more adequate to the procedure of automatic detection of contrast threshold from the CDMAM 3.4 phantom image analysis.

New tasks could be incorporated to the software in the future by using the ImageJ® interface. Our estimative is that this work is an initial process to optimize the quality evaluation of digital mammography systems in determining the image quality parameter describe by the detail-contrast curve.

Acknowledgment. To FAPESP and CAPES due to the financial support and to the team from Laboratório de Qualificação de Imagens Médicas (QualIM) – UNIFESP, by acquiring and providing the images used in our tests.

References

1. Bijker, K.R., Thijssen, M.A.O., Arnoldussen, T.J.M.: Manual of CDMAM-phantom type 3.4. University Medical Centre Nijmegen, St. Radboud (2002)
2. Perry, N., Broeders, M., Wolf, C., Törnberg, S., Holland, R., Von Karsa, L.: European Guidelines for Quality Assurance in Mammography Screening and Diagnosis, 4th edn. European Communities, Luxembourg (2006)
3. Karssemeijer, N., Thijssen, M.A.O.: Determination of contrast-detail curves of mammography systems by automated image analysis. In: Proceedings of the 3rd International Workshop on Digital Mammography, pp. 155–160. Elsevier, Amsterdam (1996)
4. Hummel, et al.: Factors for conversion between human and automatic read-outs of CDMAM images. In: SPIE Medical Imaging 2011: Physics of Medical Imaging (2011)
5. Monnin, et al.: Image quality assessment in digital mammography: part II. NPWE as a validated alternative for contrast detail analysis. Phys. Med. Biol. 56, 4221–4238 (2011)
6. Tseng, Huang: Automatic thresholding based on human visual perception. Image and Vision Computing 11(9) (1993)
7. Gonzalez, R.C., Woods, R.E.: Digital Image Processing, 2nd edn. Prentice Hall, New Jersey (2002)
8. Buchsbaum, G.: An analytical derivation of visual nonlinearity. IEEE Trans. Biomed. Engrg. 27, 237–242 (1980)

Towards Breast Anatomy Simulation Using GPUs

Joseph H. Chui[1], David D. Pokrajac[2],
Andrew D.A. Maidment[3], and Predrag R. Bakic[4]

[1] Department of Radiology, University of Pennsylvania, Philadelphia PA 19104
{Joseph.Chui,Andrew.Maidment,Predrag.Bakic}@uphs.upenn.edu
[2] Applied Mathematics Research Center, Delaware State University, Dover, DE 19901
dpokrajac@desu.edu

Abstract. We have developed a method for massively parallelized breast anatomy simulation and a corresponding GPU implementation using OpenCL. The simulation method utilizes an octree data structure for recursively splitting the simulated tissue volume. Several strategies to optimize the GPU utilization were proposed and evaluated, including the use of synchronization constructs in the language and minimization of buffer allocations. The task of tissue classification was separated from the voxelization to further improve the balance of the control flow. The proposed anatomy simulation method provides for fast generation of high-resolution anthropomorphic breast phantoms. Currently, it is possible to generate an octree representation of 450 ml breasts with 50 μm voxel size on a AMD Radeon 6950 GPU with 2GB of memory at a rate of 7 phantoms per minute, 32 times faster than a multithreaded C++ implementation.

Keywords: Digital mammography, anthropomorphic breast phantom, Parallelization, GPU.

1   Introduction

Breast tissue simulation is of great importance for pre-clinical testing and optimization of imaging systems or image analysis methods. Currently, the standard for imaging systems validation includes pre-clinical evaluation performed with simple geometric phantoms, followed up by clinical imaging trials involving large numbers of patients and repeated imaging using different acquisition conditions. Such an approach frequently causes delays in technology dissemination, due to the duration and cost of these trials. In addition, there are many factors which place strict limitations on the number of test conditions, such as the use of radiation in x-ray imaging trials.

Use of software anthropomorphic phantoms for pre-clinical evaluations offers a valuable alternative approach which can reduce the burden of clinical trials. In this paper, we present a GPU (Graphical Processing Unit) implementation of a method for generating software anthropomorphic breast phantoms. The breast anatomy simulation method is based upon recursive partitioning of the simulated volume utilizing octrees. The octree-based algorithm allows generation and processing of octree nodes at the same tree level independently (i.e., in any arbitrary order), which makes the

A.D.A. Maidment, P.R. Bakic, and S. Gavenonis (Eds.): IWDM 2012, LNCS 7361, pp. 506–513, 2012.

algorithm a good candidate for parallelization. Using profiler analysis we have identified the bottleneck steps in the CPU implementation of the algorithm and developed a corresponding GPU implementation using OpenCL. The performances of the GPU and CPU implementations were compared in terms of the time needed for generating phantoms of various voxel sizes. The effects of several implementation parameters are discussed.

2   Methods

Our proposed method of breast anatomy simulation using GPUs is based on the algorithm originally proposed by Pokrajac et al [1]. The paper proposed a method of using octrees to represent simulated volumes of various tissue types. We recently proposed a roadmap [2] to migrate its implementation to a platform that directly utilizes massively parallel processors such as GPUs. Specific milestones were defined to allow incremental migration in implementations and regression testing. A multiple threaded, concurrent version targeting multiple-core CPUs had been implemented along the roadmap. Figure 1 shows the flowchart of this version of algorithm.

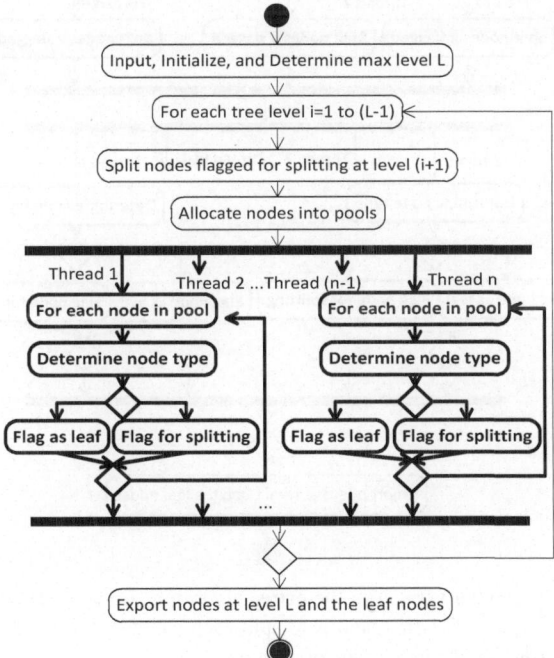

Fig. 1. Flowchart of the concurrent version of the octree-based algorithm, where nodes are processed concurrently to determine their tissue types

We chose OpenCL [3] as our software platform to implement a massively parallel version of the algorithm. Each individual octree node is identified as the finest granularity in the parallelization. To map it to OpenCL, each OpenCL work item is indexed to a unique node at each tree level. The concurrent part of the algorithm is ported into OpenCL kernels which are functions invoked and executed by the GPUs.

Profiling was performed on the initial OpenCL implementation to identify its potential bottlenecks using AMD APP SDK v2.6 [4]. The data transfer between the host memory and the device memory was identified as the major bottleneck in the pipeline. To reduce the amount of data transferred between the host and the devices, the process of splitting the nodes into child nodes was ported as an OpenCL kernel, so that the uploading of octree data to the devices was no longer needed. Figure 2 shows a float chart where the node splitting is parallelized on the GPU.

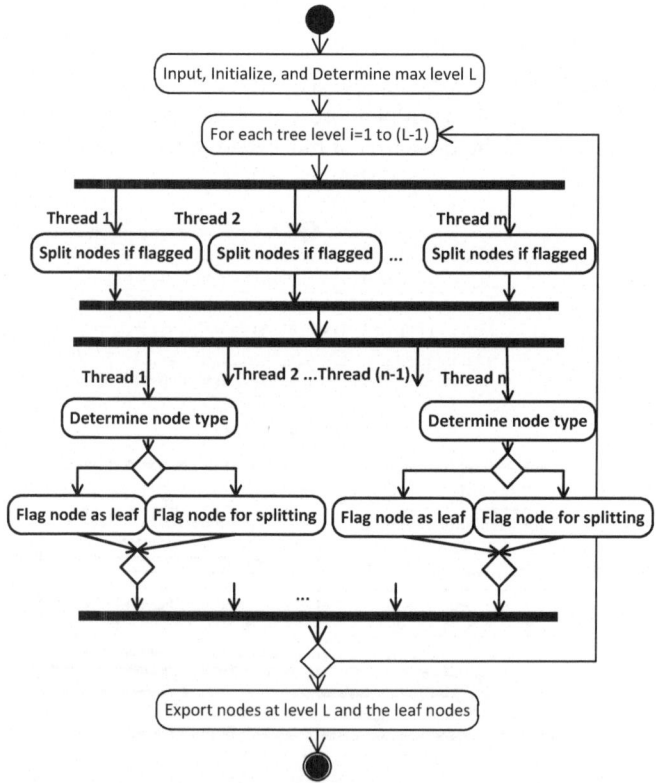

Fig. 2. A massively parallel version of the octree algorithm. At each octree level, two parallelized steps are performed. The first step is to split each splitable node into 8 child nodes. The second step is determining the tissue type of each node.

Because OpenCL does not allow allocation of memory by its kernels, buffers of sufficient sizes have to be allocated by the host in advance. Therefore, the GPU implementation has to determine, in advance, the number of octree nodes requiring for splitting. A technique similar to reduction [5] is used to accelerate the counting process. The implementation first counts the number of nodes which require splitting in each work group using a counter in local memory. Next, the counts of each workgroup are accumulated so that the accumulation result multiplied by 8 would be the index where each workgroup starts splitting its nodes in parallel. Figure 3 shows an example of the parallelized splitting process.

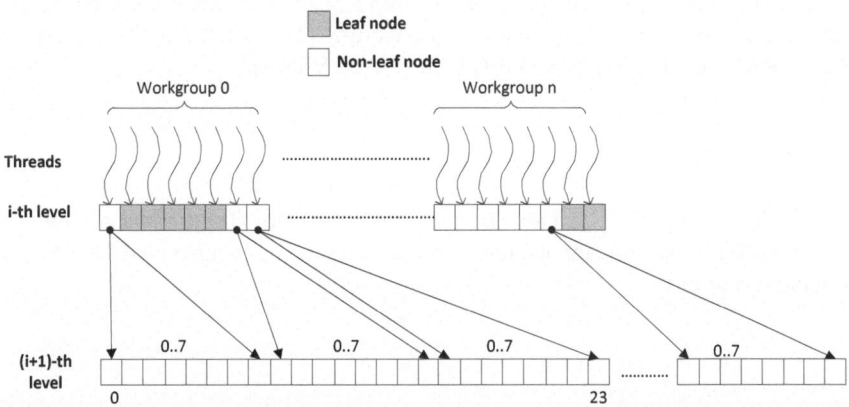

Fig. 3. Illustration of GPU threads splitting its each node into eight nodes in parallel. In this example, workgroup 0 has 3 nodes (0, 6, and 7) requiring splitting. Indexes 0 to 23 (= 3 x 8 - 1) are reserved for workgroup 0, while the next workgroup splits the nodes into child nodes starting from index 24.

Built-in OpenCL atomic functions `atom_inc()` and `atom_add()` were utilized to increment and add the counters on multiple threads to guard against a race condition.

During software profiling, several other GPU-specific bottlenecks were also identified. First, buffer allocations on GPUs require significant time. Secondly, excessive use of flow control in the kernels running on the GPUs slows down the execution of work groups.

To address the buffer allocation problem, instead of re-allocating new buffers for every level of octrees, buffers were retained on the devices until the current ones were no longer big enough for the next tree level. This was especially effective for phantoms of high resolution, where the buffers created for an octree section could often be reused for subsequent sections.

To tackle the issue of excessive use of flow control, the OpenCL kernels implemented in this study were refactored manually. Programming methods using branching that are designed for sequential computation are often unsuitable for parallel computation [6]. Instead, costly functions called on different control paths can be consolidated into a single call on the main path.

Our concurrent, non-parallel version of the algorithm conditionally voxelizes volumes on some of its control paths based on each node's tissue types. The whole workgroup is blocked when there is a work item in this group requires voxelization of its octree node. To improve the utilization of the GPU, the voxelization was separated from the kernel that determines each node's tissue type.

We validated the implementation by comparing the generated octrees with the ones generated by previous implementations using the same set of parameters. In order to assess the performances of various implementations, the simulation times at different target resolutions were compared. We also measured the effects of workgroup sizes on the performance. Performances of the implementations were assessed by their duration times on a desktop PC with Intel® Core™ i7-2600K CPU @ 3.40GHz and 16GB of RAM and Radeon 6950 GPU with 2GB of VRAM.

3   Results

Figure 4 shows the orthogonal sections of a phantom with 400 µm and 50 µm voxel resolutions. With the same inputs, the identical octrees were constructed by the different implementations.

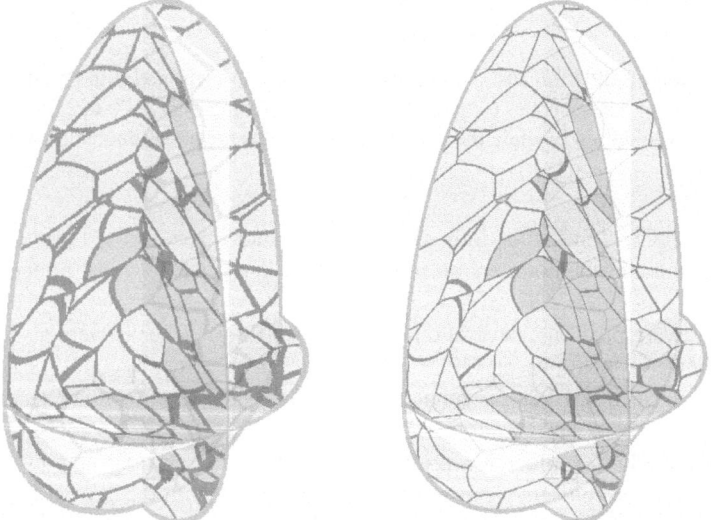

Fig. 4. Orthogonal sections of a simulated breast phantom of (a) 400µm and (b) 50µm resolutions

The performance of the OpenCL implementation was assessed by comparing the duration times to generate phantoms of various voxel sizes. The duration time of each configuration was measured by averaging the duration times of 5 independent phantoms; each phantom was generated from a different set of ellipsoids modeled randomly inside the simulated breast. Figure 5 is a graph showing the duration times of 2 implementations at different voxel resolutions. Figure 6 shows the duration times measured for 25µm resolution using different OpenCL workgroup sizes.

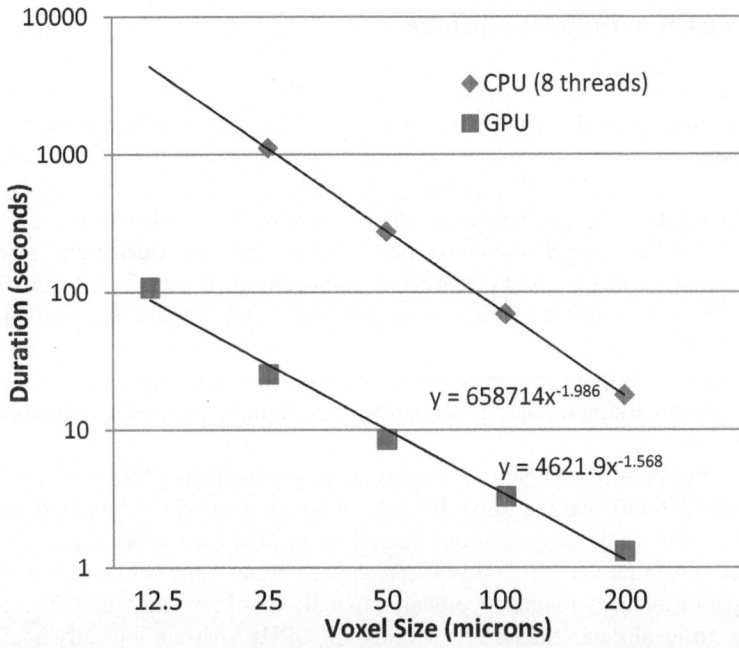

Fig. 5. Average duration times of different implementations of the octree-based algorithm for various voxel sizes (12.5, 25, 50, 100 and 200 μm)

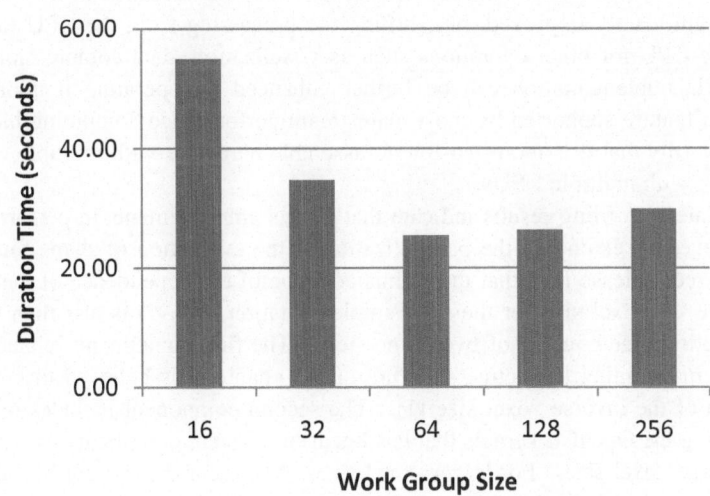

Fig. 6. The duration times using different OpenCL workgroup sizes (16, 32, 64, 128, and 256)

4   Discussion and Conclusions

We have successfully implemented an efficient parallelized version of an algorithm to simulate the breast anatomy for anthropomorphic phantoms by utilizing some of the strategies targeted for GPUs such as reuse of buffers and reduction of flow control. We measured, on average, a 32-fold improvement for the GPU implementation over the multi-threaded CPU implementation when simulating 50 μm phantoms.

Based on the measured duration times using different workgroup sizes, a workgroup of 64 yielded the best performance. Since the GPU used in this study has a wavefront size of 64 work items, any work group size less than 64 may underutilize the GPUs. On the other hand, a workgroup of more than 64 items would increase the memory contention among the units. Since the optimal workgroup size is hardware dependent, benchmarking on individual hardware is required to determine the optimal work group size.

The performance of the implementation is sufficient to create phantoms of reasonably high resolution in near real time. By generating and storing the data on the GPU, it becomes feasible to develop real time visualization software that interoperates with the same set of data on the GPU. This arises, in part, because the octree data structure offers a superior memory footprint compared to a 3D voxel representation. Therefore, an octree is an ideal data structure for storage on GPUs (that are typically available with limited memory). For simulations requiring higher resolution, the simulated phantom can be subdivided into sub-volumes small enough for the individual GPUs.

We observed a CPU usage of 2% by the application when the octrees are generated on the GPU. Thus, porting the code to the GPU not only resulted in the performance being significantly improved, but shifting the processing from the CPU to the GPU frees the CPU for other operations such as voxelization, data compression and I/O. Our GPU implementation can be further enhanced by operating it upon multiple GPUs; a feature supported by most mainstream performance computing hardware. It is noteworthy that it is more feasible to assemble hardware with multiple GPUs than hardware with multiple CPUs.

Our latest profiling results indicate that further improvements in performance can be achieved by extending the parallelization to the evaluation of shape functions for each octree. Please note that the estimated slope of the dependence of the computation time vs. voxel size for the GPU implementation (Fig. 5) is less than two. The computation time consists of two components. The first component, related to building and maintaining the octree structure of the phantom, is believed to be quadratic function of the inverse voxel size [1]. The second component includes overhead of initializing the OpenCL kernels that has linear or constant complexity as a function of the inverse voxel size. For larger voxel sizes, this linear component becomes dominant, influencing the estimate slope of the regression line.

It is further observed that when the resolution is sufficiently high, the duration increased slightly more than a quadratic as a function of the inverse voxel size. This is caused mainly by the overhead of the data transfers between the host and the devices, which accrue a cost proportional to the cube of the inverse voxel size. For simulations that require resolutions higher than 25 μm, further investigations of performance improvement are needed. Such work should emphasize the reduction of the cost of operations for each sub-volume, such as voxelization and communication between the host and devices. Finally, the frequency of buffer allocation on the devices can be reduced if an accurate maximum buffer size can be estimated in advance for different sets of parameters.

Acknowledgements. This work was supported in part by the US Department of Defense Breast Cancer Research Program (HBCU Partnership Training Award BC083639), and the US National Institutes of Health (grant 1R01CA154444). The content is solely the responsibility of the authors and does not necessarily represent the official views of the funding agency.

References

1. Pokrajac, D.D., Maidment, A.D.A., Bakic, P.R.: Optimized generation of high resolution breast anthropomorphic software phantoms. Medical Physics 39(4), 2290–2302 (2012)
2. Chui, J.H., Pokrajac, D.D., Maidment, A.D.A., Bakic, P.R.: Roadmap for efficient parallelization of breast anatomy simulation. In: Pelc, N.J., Nishikawa, R.M., Whiting, B.R. (eds.) Proc. of SPIE, Medical Imaging 2012: Physics of Medical Imaging, vol. 8313, pp. 83134T-1–83134T-10, SPIE, Bellingham (2012)
3. OpenCL 1.2 Specification, Khronos Group,
   http://www.khronos.org/registry/cl/specs/opencl-1.2.pdf
4. AMD APP SDK v2.6,
   http://developer.amd.com/sdks/AMDAPPSDK/downloads/Pages/default.aspx
5. Harris, M.: Optimizing parallel reduction in CUDA,
   http://developer.download.nvidia.com/compute/cuda/1_1/Website/projects/reduction/doc/reduction.pdf
6. AMD Accelerated Parallel Processing OpenCL Programming Guide (v1.3f),
   http://developer.amd.com/sdks/AMDAPPSDK/assets/AMD_Accelerated_Parallel_Processing_OpenCL_Programming_Guide.pdf

Breast Parenchymal Pattern (BPP) Analysis: Comparison of Digital Mammograms and Breast Tomosynthesis

Jun Wei, Heang-Ping Chan, Yao Lu,
Lubomir Hadjiiski, Chuan Zhou, and Mark A. Helvie

Department of Radiology, University of Michigan,
Ann Arbor, MI, USA 48109
{jvwei,chanhp,yaol,lhadjisk,chuan,mahelvie}@umich.edu

Abstract. We conducted a preliminary study to compare computerized measures of breast parenchymal pattern (BPP) on full field digital mammogram (FFDM) and digital breast tomosynthesis (DBT). A set of 123 subjects who had corresponding clinical FFDM of the same breast was collected from our DBT database. In a retroareolar region on the CC view, texture measures including run-length statistics (RLS), region-size statistics (RSS), and power spectrum were extracted from both modalities. Correlation analysis was performed to evaluate the similarities of the individual BPP measures between FFDM and DBT. It was found that the Pearson's correlation coefficients for the individual BPP measures between the matched pairs of FFDM and DBT ranged from 0.02 to 0.61. Our results indicated that the BPP measures were different between FFDM and DBT in this limited data set.

Keywords: Breast parenchymal pattern, cancer risk, full-field digital mammogram (FFDM), digital breast tomosynthesis (DBT).

1 Introduction

Breast cancer ranks second as a cause of death among women [1]. Currently, women in U.S. have a 12%, or a 1 in 8, lifetime risk of being diagnosed with breast cancer. Dense breast parenchyma is a risk factor for breast cancer [2, 3]. Studies indicated that mammographic density is useful for the prediction of breast cancer risk. Our recent case-control study further showed that computerized mammographic parenchymal pattern (MPP) analysis has the potential to predict breast cancer risk [4].

To date, most of the quantitative methods to evaluate mammographic density are based on digitized screen-film mammograms (SFM). FFDM has become the main modality for breast cancer screening recently. DBT [5] is an emerging breast imaging modality that has the potential to improve the detection and diagnosis of breast cancer. In this study, we compared breast parenchymal pattern (BPP) analysis on the two digital imaging modalities, FFDM and DBT, from the subjects among biopsy population.

A.D.A. Maidment, P.R. Bakic, and S. Gavenonis (Eds.): IWDM 2012, LNCS 7361, pp. 514–520, 2012.
© Springer-Verlag Berlin Heidelberg 2012

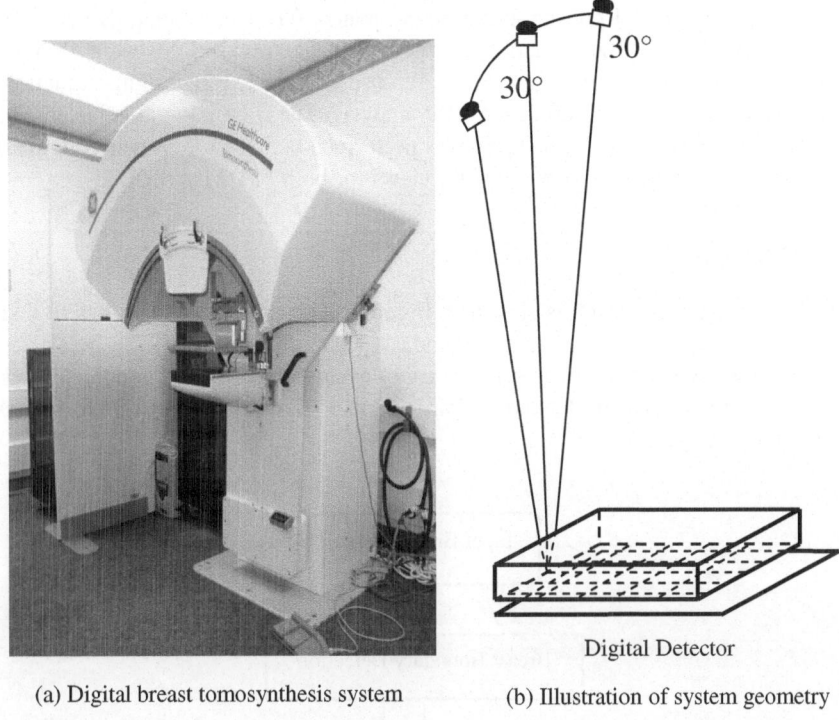

(a) Digital breast tomosynthesis system   (b) Illustration of system geometry

Fig. 1. GE prototype digital breast tomosynthesis system for image acquisition

2   Materials and Methods

2.1   Materials

With IRB approval, we have been collecting DBT from breast imaging patients with written informed consent. Eligible subjects were patients who were recommended for biopsy due to suspicious masses or clustered microcalcifications. For this preliminary study, a total of 123 subjects including 36 with biopsy-confirmed cancer and 87 with benign lesions who had corresponding clinical FFDM of the same breast were collected from our DBT database. The DBTs were acquired with a second generation GE prototype system in the breast imaging research laboratory at the University of Michigan as shown in Figure 1. The DBT system acquired 21 PVs in 3-degree increments over an arc of 60 degrees. The DBT system has a CsI phosphor/a:Si active matrix flat panel digital detector with a pixel size of 100μm x 100μm. We used the simultaneous algebraic reconstruction technique (SART) for DBT reconstruction. BPP was analyzed on the central slice of the reconstructed DBT volume. The clinical FFDMs were collected from patient files retrospectively. The FFDMs were acquired with either GE Senographe 2000D or Essential systems (GE Medical Systems, Milwaukee, Wis). The

516   J. Wei et al.

GE systems have a CsI phosphor/a:Si active matrix flat panel digital detector with a pixel size of 100µm x 100µm and 14 bits per pixel. The raw FFDMs were used in this study, which had an inverted gray scale. We use an inverted logarithmic function [6] to transform the raw data before the BPP analysis. The time interval between FFDM and DBT was 0-28 days. All imaging was performed before biopsy. Our BPP analysis was performed on the craniocaudal (CC) views for both FFDM and DBT.

2.2   Methods

Our BPP analysis approach is shown in Figure 2. For an input FFDM or DBT slice, the first step was to perform breast boundary detection to separate the breast region from the directly exposed area. A previously developed automated boundary tracking technique [7] was used in this study. Parenchymal analysis was then performed only within the breast region.

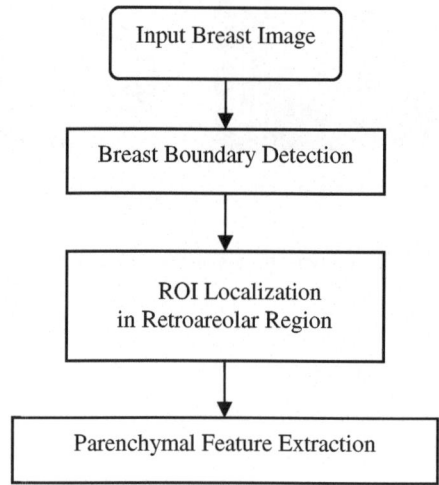

Fig. 2. Block diagram of breast parenchymal pattern analysis

After boundary detection, the image was automatically oriented such that the chest wall would be on the right side of the image in order to simplify the process. The left-most point of the breast boundary was identified as a reference point and the ROI for BPP analysis was centered along a horizontal line from the reference point to the chest wall edge of the image. The ROI was chosen to be a 512 x 512-pixel region in the retroareolar region. If the breast region was too small to accommodate the 512 x 512-pixel ROI, the ROI was reduced to the maximum size that could fit within the breast region. Texture and power spectral analyses were performed within the ROI.

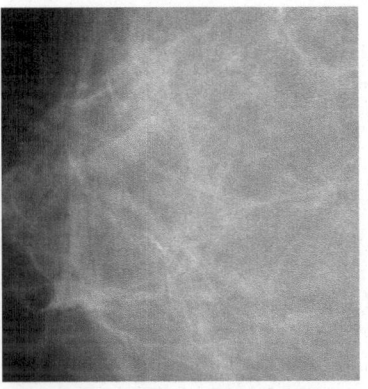 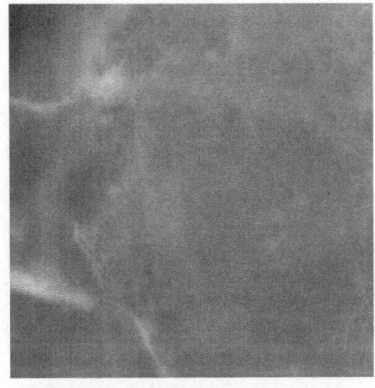

(a) Image examples from a subject with benign finding

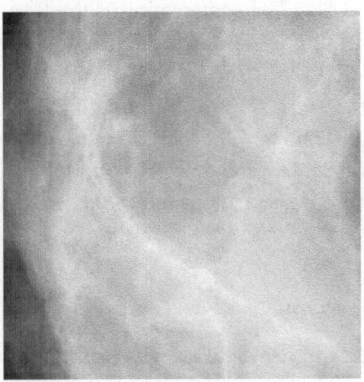 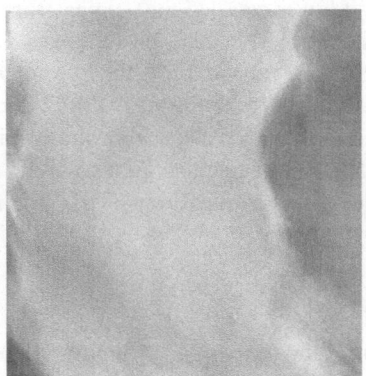

(b) Image examples of a subject with biopsy-proven breast cancer

Fig. 3. Image examples of regions of interest (ROIs) from FFDM (left) and matched DBT (right)

For computerized BPP analysis, two types of texture measures, run-length statistics (RLS) and region-size statistics (RSS), in the spatial domain and power spectral analysis in the frequency domain were extracted to characterize the BPP. The details of texture measures from RLS and RSS for characterizing BPP can be found in our previous study [4]. A total of 20 RLS and 5 RSS features were extracted. For power spectral analysis, we followed the power-law model, $(P(f) = Af^{-\beta})$ of the parenchymal power spectrum as described by Burgess[8]. In short, the 2D power spectral density was first estimated in the frequency domain with discrete Fourier transform in the same ROI as that for texture analysis. The average power spectrum along the radial direction was then calculated from low frequency to the Nyquist frequency. The power-law exponent β was estimated by linear least-squares fit to the average power spectrum in the log-log scale and used as a BPP measure to characterize the complexity of the breast parenchyma.

Correlation analysis was performed to evaluate the similarities of the individual BPP measures between FFDM and DBT. To assess the difference in BPP between subjects with cancer and subjects with benign lesions, the area under the receiver operating characteristic (ROC) curve, A_z, was used to compare the difference in the BPP measures between the two groups.

3   Results

Figure 3 showed examples of ROIs on FFDM and DBT extracted from a subject with breast cancer and a subject with benign lesion. For the entire data set, our analysis found that the Pearson's correlation coefficients for the individual measures between matched pairs of FFDM and DBT ranged from 0.02 to 0.61. The β measure of the power spectrum had the highest correlation while the RLS and RSS texture measures had lower correlation (ranging from 0.02 to 0.31). The scatter plot of the β measures of the power spectra on FFDM and those on DBT is shown in Figure 4. The texture and power spectral measures from DBT had slightly better ability (A_z values of 0.52 - 0.65) than those from FFDM (A_z values of 0.50 - 0.57) in differentiating the BPP of subjects with cancer from those with benign lesions. The best texture measure on FFDM to distinguish the two groups was an RSS feature with A_z value of 0.57 ± 0.03 while the best measure on DBT was an RLS feature with A_z value of 0.65 ± 0.03.

4   Discussion

Our previous study [4] indicated the promise of BPP analysis on mammograms for breast cancer risk prediction. The current study is a preliminary investigation of how BPP measures extracted from DBT may be related to those from mammograms. The initial results demonstrated that the texture and power spectral measures obtained from DBT and FFDM had low correlation, suggesting that the BPP analysis developed for mammograms may not be directly transferrable to DBT. The specific measures and parameters may have to be redesigned based on the characteristics of DBT images. The dependence of the BPP measures and parameters on the various DBT acquisition and reconstruction parameters will also have to be investigated. In addition, although some texture and power spectral measures from DBT appear to show a slightly greater difference between subjects with malignant lesions and subjects with benign lesions than those from FFDM, the differences between the two groups were small. This is probably because subjects with benign lesions may also have an elevated risk of breast cancer, as shown in the Gail risk model. Furthermore, the usefulness of BPP analysis for breast cancer risk prediction will rely on its ability to differentiate subjects who will develop breast cancer from those remaining normal in future years. Such a data set for BPP analysis is not available at present because DBT is a new modality and few prior DBTs a few years before cancer diagnosis exist. Such studies should be conducted to assess the BPP analysis on DBT for breast cancer prediction when a larger set with prior DBT becomes available.

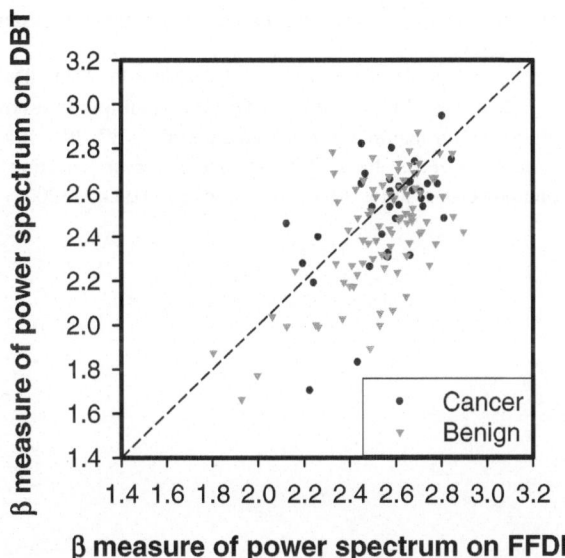

Fig. 4. Scatter plot of the β measures of power spectra from FFDM and DBT of the same breast

Acknowledgements. This work is supported by USPHS grant R01 CA151443. The digital breast tomosynthesis system was developed by the GE Global Research Group, with input and some revisions from the University of Michigan investigators, through the Biomedical Research Partnership (USPHS grant CA91713, PI: Paul Carson, Ph.D.) collaboration. The content of this paper does not necessarily reflect the position of the government and no official endorsement of any equipment and product of any companies mentioned should be inferred.

References

1. American Cancer Society, Cancer Facts & Figures 2010 (2010),
   http://www.cancer.org
2. Kerlikowske, K.: The mammogram that cried wolfe. The New England Journal of Medicine 356, 297–300 (2007)
3. Boyd, N.F., Guo, H., Martin, L.J., Sun, L., Stone, J., Fishell, E., Jong, R.A., Hislop, G., Chiarelli, A., Minkin, S., Yaffe, M.J.: Mammographic density and the risk and detection of breast cancer. New England Journal of Medicine 356, 227–236 (2007)
4. Wei, J., Chan, H.-P., Wu, Y.-T., Zhou, C., Helvie, M.A., Tsodikov, A., Hadjiiski, L.M., Sahiner, B.: A pilot case-control study of the association of computerized mammographic parenchymal pattern (MPP) measure with breast cancer risk. Radiology 260, 42–49 (2011)
5. Niklason, L.T., Christian, B.T., Niklason, L.E., Kopans, D.B., Castleberry, D.E., Opsahl-Ong, B.H., Landberg, C.E., Slanetz, P.J., Giardino, A.A., Moore, R., Albagli, D., DeJule, M.C., Fitzgerald, F.C., Fobare, D.F., Giambattista, B.W., Kwasnick, R.F., Liu, J., Lubowski, S.J., Possin, G.E., Richotte, J.F., Wei, C.Y., Wirth, R.F.: Digital tomosynthesis in breast imaging. Radiology 205, 399–406 (1997)

6. Burgess, A.E.: On the noise variance of a digital mammography system. Medical Physics 31, 1987–1995 (2004)
7. Wu, Y.-T., Zhou, C., Chan, H.-P., Paramagul, C., Hadjiiski, L.M., Daly, C.P., Douglas, J.A., Zhang, Y., Sahiner, B., Shi, J., Wei, J.: Dynamic multiple thresholding breast boundary detection algorithm for mammograms. Medical Physics 37, 391–401 (2010)
8. Burgess, A.E., Jacobson, F.L., Judy, P.F.: Human observer detection experiments with mammograms and power-law noise. Medical Physics 28, 419–437 (2001)

Classification of Microcalcification Clusters Based on Morphological Topology Analysis

Zhili Chen[1,3], Erika R.E. Denton[2], and Reyer Zwiggelaar[1]

[1] Department of Computer Science,
Aberystwyth University, Aberystwyth, SY23 3DB, UK
{zzc09,rrz}@aber.ac.uk
[2] Department of Radiology,
Norfolk and Norwich University Hospital, Norwich, NR4 7UY, UK
erika.denton@nnuh.nhs.uk
[3] Faculty of Information and Control Engineering,
Shenyang Jianzhu University, Shenyang, 110168, China

Abstract. The presence of microcalcification clusters is a primary sign of breast cancer. It is difficult and time consuming for radiologists to diagnose microcalcifications. In this paper, we present a novel method for classification of malignant and benign microcalcification clusters in mammograms. We analyse the connectivity/topology between individual microcalcifications within a cluster using multiscale morphology. A microcalcification graph is constructed to represent the topological structure of clusters. A multiscale topological feature vector is generated by extracting two microcalcification graph properties. The validity of the proposed method is evaluated using a dataset taken from the MIAS database. The performance of including SFS feature selection is investigated. Using a k-nearest neighbour classifier, a classification accuracy of 95% and an area under the ROC curve of 0.93 are achieved. A comparison with existing approaches is presented.

1 Introduction

Breast cancer is currently the most common cancer to affect women worldwide. Mammography is one of the most reliable and effective methods for detecting breast cancer at its early stages [1–10]. The presence of microcalcification clusters is a primary sign of breast cancer, which are small deposits of calcium in breast tissue that appear as small bright spots in mammograms [1, 2, 5, 7]. The radiological definition of microcalcification clusters is that at least three microcalcifications are present within 1 cm^2 region [5, 10]. However, not all microcalcification clusters necessarily indicate the presence of cancer, only certain kinds of microcalcifications are associated with a high probability of malignancy [13]. It is difficult and time consuming for radiologists to distinguish malignant from benign cases, which results in a high rate of unnecessary biopsy examinations [1, 10]. Recently, computer-aided diagnosis (CAD) systems have gained popularity in order to reduce the false positive rate while maintaining sensitivity [1, 8].

A.D.A. Maidment, P.R. Bakic, and S. Gavenonis (Eds.): IWDM 2012, LNCS 7361, pp. 521–528, 2012.

Numerous approaches for the (semi-) automatic analysis of mammographic images have been developed over the last two decades. A variety of features have been used in the literature for the characterisation and classification of microcalcifications, such as shape, morphological, cluster and texture features. Shen et al. [2] developed a set of shape factors to quantitatively measure the roughness of individual microcalcifications. Three shape features including compactness, moments and Fourier descriptors were computed based on the extracted boundaries of regions for microcalcification classification. Ma et al. [5] proposed a novel shape feature on the basis of [2]. A three level wavelet transform was used to analyse the frequency of the normalised distance signature of each closed contour. A novel metric line was defined based on the band pass approximation to quantify the roughness of each microcalcification. Mathematical morphology has also been applied to segment and analyse microcalcifications in the aspect of shape/geometry: Dengler et al. [3] used a morphological filter to reconstruct the original shape of smoothed microcalcifications. Betal et al. [4] used morphological operations to analyse four shape properties of segmented microcalcifications, including infolding, elongation, narrow irregularities and wide irregularities. Chan et al. [6] used morphological features to describe the size, shape, and contrast of individual microcalcifications and their variations within a segmented cluster. Cluster features such as cluster area, number of microcalcifications, average and standard deviation of distances between microcalcifications were used in [4], [7] and [8] to describe the global properties of the whole cluster. Texture features were investigated for malignancy analysis in [7] and [9]. The global texture features were computed based on the spatial grey level dependence (co-occurrence) matrix, and the local texture features were extracted based on the wavelet transform. A comparison of the performance of different types of features for malignant and benign microcalcification classification was presented in [10]. The multiscale representation based on multiwavelet transform was demonstrated to outperform the shape and texture features. In addition, due to the ability of graphs to represent properties and relationships among different parts of an object, graph based techniques have been regarded as a powerful tool for pattern recognition [11]. Moreover, graph based representation has been applied to image classification. In [12], a graph of resulting regions from morphological segmentation was used to represent natural images for classification.

In this paper, we analyse the topology of microcalcification clusters at multiple scales and define a multiscale topological feature vector to discriminate malignant from benign cases. Malignant microcalcifications tend to be small, numerous and densely distributed, while benign microcalcifications are generally larger, smaller in number and more diffusely distributed [13]. The distribution of microcalcifications associated with a malignant process may be different from that associated with a benign process. This forms different topological structure of microcalcification clusters. We investigate the connectivity between individual microcalcifications within a cluster using morphological operations at multiple scales. A graph of microcalcifications connectivity is extracted to represent the topological structure of microcalcifications within the cluster.

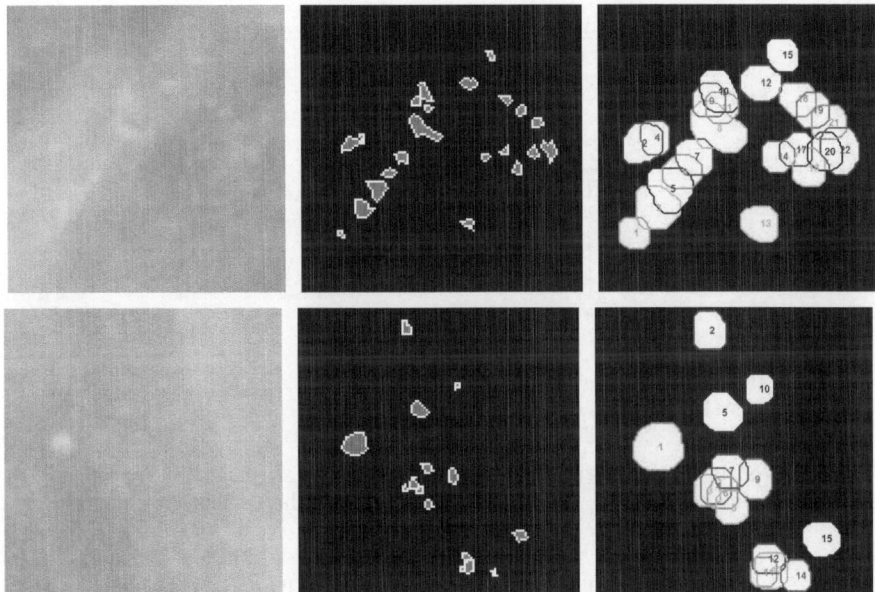

Fig. 1. Example microcalcification clusters: malignant (top row) and benign (bottom row). Left column: mammographic image patches; middle column: manual annotation images; right column: dilated microcalcifications. Note that the microcalcification cluster region is zoomed for better illustration. Microcalcification No. 16 is not displayed in the bottom images as it falls outside the zoomed region.

2   Data and Method

The data used in the experiments are twenty image patches taken from the Mammographic Image Analysis Society (MIAS) database [14], each containing a microcalcification cluster. The size of the image patches is 512×512 pixels, and the spatial resolution is $50 \mu m \times 50 \mu m$ per pixel. This dataset includes biopsy proven nine malignant and eleven benign microcalcification clusters. All the individual microcalcifications have been manually annotated by an expert. The median number of microcalcifications in the clusters is 27. There are a few outliers and 80% of the clusters are within the 6 to 62 range. Example microcalcification clusters and corresponding annotation images are shown in Fig. 1.

2.1   Morphological Operation

Firstly, each individual microcalcification is segmented. For separately located microcalcifications, the boundary pixels are merged with the interior region. For connecting microcalcifications, the boundary pixels between the background and microcalcifications are straightforward merged with the microcalcifications, while the common boundary pixels between two microcalcifications are assigned to either microcalcification. After that, morphological dilation is performed on

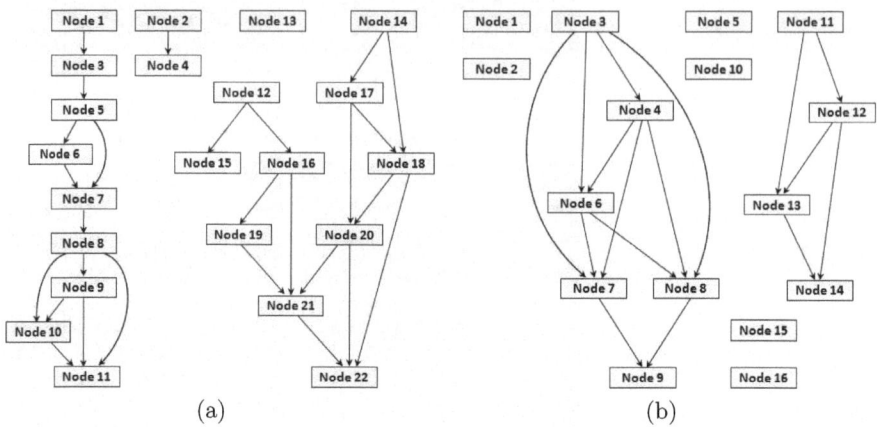

Fig. 2. Microcalcification graphs: (a) malignant ($n_s = 4$, $\delta_s = 1.23$); (b) benign ($n_s = 8$, $\delta_s = 1.00$). The numbering of nodes is consistent with the sequence number in Fig. 1.

each segmented individual microcalcification at multiple scales, using a disk-shaped structuring element with radius equal to the scale. The dilation results of the two example microcalcification clusters are also shown in Fig. 1, where the radius of the structuring element is equal to six pixels. Each individual microcalcification is ordered with a sequence number and the boundaries of dilated microcalcifications are displayed using different colours. It is indicated that the morphological dilation operation adds neighbouring pixels to the boundaries of individual microcalcifications, resulting in a change in the connectivity between individual microcalcifications within clusters.

2.2   Microcalcification Graph

The topology of individual microcalcifications within a cluster can be represented in the form of a microcalcification graph. The microcalcification graph is constructed based on the spatial connectivity relationship between microcalcifications, where each node represents an individual microcalcification, and there is an edge between two nodes if the two corresponding microcalcifications are connected or overlap with each other. Here, we generate a directed graph where the nodes are ordered according to the spatial location of the corresponding microcalcifications in the image patch, and two connected nodes are linked by a directed edge from the smaller to the larger numbered node. The resulting graphs of dilated microcalcifications in Fig. 1 are shown in Fig. 2. The numbering of nodes is consistent with the sequence number in Fig. 1. It is shown that the topological structure of microcalcification clusters is effectively represented by the microcalcification graphs, with useful properties for characterising the distribution of microcalcification clusters. Here, we focus on two properties of the microcalcification graph. The first property is the number of independent connected subgraphs within the graph generated from one microcalcification cluster, which represents the number of independent connected components within the cluster. The second property is the degree of each node defined as the number of edges starting from the node, which describes the connectivity of the corresponding microcalcification with its neighbouring particles.

2.3   Multiscale Topological Feature Vector

We define an upper-triangular adjacency matrix to encode the microcalcification graph, denoted by $A = (a_{ij})$, $a_{ij} \in \{0,1\}$, $i, j = 1, \ldots, m$, where m is the number of nodes within the graph. $a_{ij} = 1$ indicates node i and node j are connected, node i is the *source* node and node j is the *sink* node. A *source* node i is called a *root* node if $\sum_{k=1}^{m} a_{ki} = 0$. A *sink* node j is called a *terminal* node if $\sum_{k=1}^{m} a_{jk} = 0$. A *path* from node i to node j is defined as a sequence of nodes starting from node i and ending with node j. The number of connected subgraphs (denoted by n) is determined by traversing the graph. We traverse the graph starting at each *root* node and explore as far as possible along each *path* until arriving at the *terminal* node. The traversal sequences including common nodes are combined into a single sequence. The number of the final sequences is the number of connected subgraphs. The degree of node i (denoted by $\delta(i)$) is computed by $\delta(i) = \sum_{k=1}^{m} a_{ik}$.

We construct a set of microcalcification graphs $G = (G_0, G_1, \ldots, G_{S-1})$ based on morphologically dilated microcalcifications at multiple scales, which represent the topology of microcalcification clusters at S scales. We analyse the two properties of the resulting microcalcification graphs G using the way described above, which forms two vectors $N = (n_0, n_1, \ldots, n_{S-1})$ and $\Delta = (\delta_1, \delta_2, \ldots, \delta_{S-1})$, where $n_s (s = 0, 1, \ldots, S-1)$ denotes the number of connected subgraphs at scale s, and $\delta_s (s = 0, 1, \ldots, S-1)$ denotes the average node degree at scale s, computed by $\delta_s = \frac{1}{m} \sum_{i=1}^{m} \delta(i)_s$. We normalise N and Δ by n_s/m and $\delta_s / \max \delta(i)_s$, where $\max \delta(i)_s$ is the maximum node degree at scale s. The two normalised vectors are concatenated into a single feature vector. We call such a vector multiscale topological feature vector, representing the multiscale topological characteristics of microcalcification clusters, which can be used for the classification of malignant and benign microcalcification clusters.

3   Experimental Results

To evaluate the potential of the proposed method in discriminating malignant from benign microcalcification clusters, it has been tested using the twenty image patches extracted from the MIAS database [14]. For each cluster, we analysed the morphological topology of microcalcifications at 129 scales ($s = 0, 1, \ldots, 128, S = 129$) by means of computing the number of connected subgraphs n_s and the average node degree δ_s using the corresponding microcalcification graph at scale s. The dimensionality of the multiscale topological feature vectors was 258.

A k-nearest neighbour classifier (kNN) was used for classification. The Euclidean distance was used to measure the similarity between feature vectors.

Table 1. Comparison of our results with those obtained by some related work

Method	Database	# Case	Feature	Classifier	Result
[2]	unknown	18	shape	kNN	$CA = 100\%$
[4]	Liverpool	38	shape/cluster	kNN	$A_z = 0.79\ A_z = 0.84$
[5]	DDSM	183	shape	α_{max}	$A_z = 0.96$
[6]	unknown	145	morphological	LDC	$A_z = 0.79$
[7]	unknown	191	texture & cluster	ANN	$A_z = 0.86$
[8]	MIAS	25	cluster	SVM	$A_z = 0.81$
[9]	unknown	54	texture	ANN	$A_z = 0.88$
[10]	Nijmegen	103	multiwavelet	kNN	$A_z = 0.89$
Our	MIAS	20	multiscale topology	kNN	$CA = 90\%\ A_z = 0.91$
	MIAS	20	SFS selected	kNN	$CA = 95\%\ A_z = 0.93$

Leave-one-out cross validation was used for evaluation. When classifying one cluster, all remaining clusters were used as the training set. Sequential forward selection (SFS) was applied to choose the most discriminating subset of features in the feature space and thus generate a compact multiscale topological representation containing the most meaningful scales. In the feature selection process, SFS was performed based on the training set excluding the testing sample to avoid bias. To quantitatively assess the performance of the multiscale topological features to classify malignant versus benign cases, a ROC curve was constructed and the area under the ROC curve (denoted by A_z) was computed. The ROC curve graphically represents the trade-off between the true positive rate (TPR) against the false positive rate (FPR). Here, TPR is defined as the number of correctly classified malignant cases divided by the total number of malignant cases, and FPR is defined as the number of benign cases incorrectly classified as malignant divided by the total number of benign cases. The construction of the ROC curve is based on a decision criterion which can be regarded as a threshold to decide a testing sample as either positive or negative. We defined a malignancy measure (denoted by M) as the decision criterion based on the kNN classifier. The malignancy measure M of a testing microcalcification cluster was defined to be the number of malignant clusters among its k nearest neighbours, ranging from 0 to k. Thus, a threshold L was set from -1 to k, and the testing cluster was classified as malignant if M was larger than L. When $L = -1$, all the microcalcification clusters were classified as malignant with TPR and FPR equal to 1. At the other extreme, when $L = k$, all the microcalcification clusters were classified as benign with TPR and FPR equal to 0. The remaining TPR and FPR were obtained by varying L from 0 to $k-1$. This produced $k+2$ points of TPR and FPR. Finally, A_z was computed using the trapezoidal rule.

We tested a range of k values in the kNN classifier. Using the unreduced dimensionality of the feature space, the best overall classification accuracy (CA) was 90% obtained with $k = 3$ where 9 of the 11 benign cases were classified correctly without misclassifying any malignant cases, and the largest A_z value was 0.91 obtained when $k = 5$. Using the reduced feature space, the best overall CA was increased to 95% for $k = 3$, while the largest A_z value was increased to 0.93

for $k = 5$. We compared our proposed method with some related publications. Table 1 shows a summary of the comparison. Note that the various approaches use different images taken from different databases, and therefore it is a qualitative comparison. In [2], the 100% CA was obtained by classifying 143 individual calcifications from 18 biopsy proven cases (and a leave-one-calcification-out approach was used), which is different from the goal of our classification of microcalcification clusters. In [5], the classification of microcalcification clusters was based on the maximum feature value obtained by a selected microcalcification rather than the whole cluster (and some manual aspects were involved in the extraction process). It is shown that our classification results are comparable to or better than the various approaches in Table 1.

4   Discussion and Conclusions

To our knowledge, this work is a first attempt to analyse microcalcifications in terms of the connectivity and topology for discriminating malignant from benign clusters. Unlike most features in previous publications extracted at a single scale, a representation covering the multiscale characteristics was developed in this paper. The obtained results demonstrate the extracted features based on the morphological topology are useful for the classification of microcalcification clusters. When analysing the topology of microcalcification clusters, we focused on two microcalcification graph properties, the number of connected subgraphs and the degree of nodes. A range of other properties can be investigated to generate a more sophisticated representation. Other features such as shape and texture of individual microcalcifications and the whole cluster can be incorporated to build a complete microcalcification analysis framework. Weighted graphs may be applied to involve the spatial distance between two microcalcifications. The definition of a similarity measure between graphs can be investigated in order to realise classification using the graph based representation directly without generating feature vectors. On the other hand, alternative approaches to feature selection (e.g. genetic algorithm) will be investigated to select the best subset of features. Moreover, other classifiers (e.g. decision tree, artificial neural network, and support vector machine) will also be investigated.

One limitation of this method is that it cannot provide a reliable classification for the case where the cluster is structureless or few microcalcifications are segmented within the cluster. An extreme is that if only a single microcalcification is detected from the cluster by the CAD detection method, it will fail to discriminate malignant from benign based on the topology and tend to classify this kind of cases as benign. The evaluation of the method is currently based on manually segmented microcalcifications from twenty cases. A further extension of the current work will be straightforward using CAD detection results instead of using manual segmentation results. In addition, further evaluation using a large dataset taken from the DDSM database and a dataset of full-field digital mammograms to confirm the validity of the method is in progress.

In summary, we have presented a novel method for classifying malignant and benign microcalcification clusters in mammograms. The topological structure of microcalcification clusters was analysed using the multiscale morphology. Using manual annotations of microcalcifications, good classification results have been achieved, which indicates the potential of the proposed method for the analysis and classification of mammographic microcalcification clusters.

References

1. Cheng, H.D., Cai, X., Chen, X., Hu, L., Lou, X.: Computer-Aided Detection and Classification of Microcalcifications in Mammograms: A Survey. Pattern Recognition 36(12), 2967–2991 (2003)
2. Shen, L., Rangayyan, R.M., Desautels, J.E.L.: Application of Shape Analysis to Mammographic Calcifications. IEEE Transactions on Medical Imaging 13(2), 263–274 (1994)
3. Dengler, J., Behrens, S., Desaga, J.F.: Segmentation of Microcalcifications in Mammograms. IEEE Transactions on Medical Imaging 12(4), 634–642 (1993)
4. Betal, D., Roberts, N., Whitehouse, G.H.: Segmentation and Numerical Analysis of Microcalcifications on Mammograms Using Mathematical Morphology. British Journal of Radiology 70(837), 903–917 (1997)
5. Ma, Y., Tay, P.C., Adams, R.D., Zhang, J.Z.: A Novel Shape Feature to Classify Microcalcifications. In: IEEE 17th International Conference on Image Processing, pp. 2265–2268 (2010)
6. Chan, H.P., Sahiner, B., Lam, K.L., Petrick, N., Helvie, M.A., Goodsitt, M.M., Adler, D.D.: Computerized Analysis of Mammographic Microcalcifications in Morphological and Texture Feature Spaces. Medical Physics 25(10), 2007–2019 (1998)
7. Dhawan, A.P., Chitre, Y., Kaiser-Bonasso, C.: Analysis of Mammographic Microcalcifications Using Gray-level Image Structure Features. IEEE Transactions on Medical Imaging 15(3), 246–259 (1996)
8. Papadopoulos, A., Fotiadis, D.I., Likas, A.: Characterization of Clustered Microcalcifications in Digitized Mammograms Using Neural Networks and Support Vector Machines. Artificial Intelligence in Medicine 34(2), 141–150 (2005)
9. Chan, H.P., Sahiner, B., Petrick, N., Helvie, M.A., Lam, K.L., Adler, D.D., Goodsitt, M.M.: Computerized Classification of Malignant and Benign Microcalcifications on Mammograms: Texture Analysis Using an Artificial Neural Network. Physics in Medicine and Biology 42, 549–567 (1997)
10. Soltanian-Zadeh, H., Rafiee-Rad, F., Pourabdollah-Nejad, D.S.: Comparison of Multiwavelet, Wavelet, Haralick, and Shape Features for Microcalcification Classification in Mammograms. Pattern Recognition 37(10), 1973–1986 (2004)
11. Conte, D., Foggia, P., Sansone, C., Vento, M.: Thirty Years of Graph Matching in Pattern Recognition. International Journal of Pattern Recognition and Artificial Intelligence 18(3), 265–298 (2004)
12. Harchaoui, Z., Bach, F.: Image Classification with Segmentation Graph Kernels. In: IEEE Conference on Computer Vision and Pattern Recognition, pp. 1–8 (2007)
13. Sickles, E.A.: Breast Calcifications: Mammographic Evaluation. Radiology 160(2), 289–293 (1986)
14. Suckling, J., Parker, J., Dance, D.R., Astley, S., Hutt, I., Boggis, C., Ricketts, I., Stamatakis, E., Cerneaz, N., Kok, S.L., Taylor, P., Betal, D., Savage, J.: The Mammographic Image Analysis Society Digital Mammogram Database. In: Excerpta Medica. International Congress Series, vol. 1069, pp. 375–378 (1994)

Spectral Volumetric Glandularity Assessment

André Gooßen[1], Harald S. Heese[1],
Klaus Erhard[1], and Björn Norell[2]

[1] Philips Research, Röntgenstr. 24-26, 22335 Hamburg, Germany
[2] Philips Healthcare – Women's Healthcare,
Smidesvägen 5, 17141 Solna, Sweden
{andre.goossen,harald.heese,klaus.erhard,bjorn.norell}@philips.com

Abstract. Breast density is associated with an increased risk of developing breast cancer, and several methods have been proposed recently for the fully-automatic assessment of volumetric breast density. However, conventional algorithms require an accurate estimation of the breast shape and thickness for the separation into adipose and glandular tissue within the breast. Here, a spectral extension of a recently developed automatic volumetric breast density algorithm is investigated. The proposed approach measures the adipose and glandular tissue content without any additional breast thickness model. The feasibility of the spectral glandularity assessment is illustrated with measurements from an energy-resolving photon-counting mammography system using reference materials including the BR3D phantom.

Keywords: volumetric breast density, breast cancer risk assessment, mammography, spectral imaging, material decomposition.

1 Introduction

Breast density is associated with an increased risk of developing breast cancer [21,16,3]. Recently, regulation authorities have acted by requiring the enlisting of breast density in the mammographic report with a recommendation for subsequent ultra-sound or MRI examinations for women with dense breasts [20].

However, in current clinical practice, breast density is evaluated as mammographic percent density on basis of a 2D mammogram with high inter-reader variability [5,6]. Therefore, various methods for automatically estimating breast density as *mammographic percent density* and *volumetric breast density* have been proposed.

Two-dimensional methods [15,7,14] mimic the behaviour of mammographic readers and compute the fraction of the projected glandular tissue on the projected breast area from the mammogram, whereas volumetric methods [10,19] estimate the absolute volume of glandular tissue inside the breast using a physical model of the mammographic image formation process.

Accurate estimation of both mammographic percent density and volumetric breast density on full-field digital mammography devices requires a thorough

A.D.A. Maidment, P.R. Bakic, and S. Gavenonis (Eds.): IWDM 2012, LNCS 7361, pp. 529–536, 2012.

calibration of the detector as well as a good model of the breast shape being compressed between support and compression plate. An error in the estimation of the compression height will result in an equal relative error in the estimation of the linear attenuation coefficient within the breast, but in a two to three times higher error in the estimate of the glandular fraction [1].

This effect becomes even stronger in the peripheral regions of the breast, where the breast height is not equal to the compression thickness, i.e. the distance between the support and the compression plate. In these peripheral regions, a breast shape model has to be used to estimate the local breast height, and any error in this estimate will additionally effect the accuracy of the glandular fraction computation. Furthermore, the compression plate itself can be tiltable and bend significantly along the breast contact area [13], which requires additional correction steps [18].

To overcome these problems of breast thickness estimation, additional information has to be acquired along with the mammogram. One possible solution is to acquire a second mammogram at a different X-ray energy at the cost of increasing the mean glandular dose level. Another option is to perform the energy-separation in a photon-counting detector after the X-ray beam has traversed the breast. In this case, a single exposure with the same mean glandular dose as a conventional mammogram suffices.

In the following, a feasibility study of spectral glandularity assessment on a Philips MicroDose prototype system using a photon-counting silicon strip detector with two energy bins [12] is presented. Compared to previous work on spectral breast density assessment [8,17], the new approach does not require a dual-energy exposure. Moreover, the geometry of the MicroDose mammography device yields virtually scatter-free X-ray images [2] and thus enables a direct material separation without additional scatter correction steps.

While the conventional approach uses one measurement and an estimation of the compression thickness to compute a 2D or 3D breast density value, the spectral method acquires two measurements from which both a thickness and a glandularity map can be computed. Hence, with spectral mammography the breast thickness is measured and does not need to be estimated.

2   Methods and Materials

The suggested approach for spectral volumetric breast density assessment has been developed using pre-processed data ($0.05 \times 0.05\,\mathrm{mm}^2$ resolution), from a prototype Philips MicroDose spectral X-ray mammography systems (Philips Healthcare, Solna, Sweden) as input data.

For the spectral separation of adipose and glandular tissue, the mammography device has been calibrated using adipose and glandular equivalent material (CIRS, Norfolk, VA), see Fig. 1a. To demonstrate the feasibility of the spectral

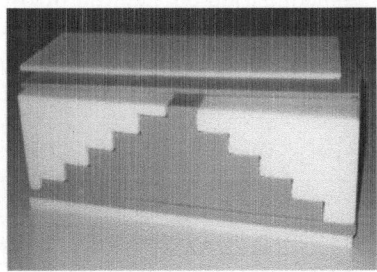
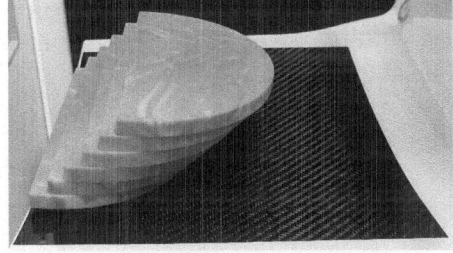

(a) calibration phantom   (b) BR3D phantom

Fig. 1. Adipose and glandular equivalent material. (a) A calibration phantom consisting of adipose and glandular tissue equivalent material, assembled in a step wedge. With a constant height, the phantom contains steps with 0, 10, ..., 100 % of either tissue type. (b) Stack of misaligned CIRS Model 020 BR3D Mammography Phantom (BR3D phantom) as used for the evaluation of the spectral tissue separation.

material separation, both the glandularity and the thickness of a mis-aligned stack of a BR3D phantom (CIRS, Norfolk, VA – cf. Fig. 1b) have been measured and evaluated.

2.1 Spectral Material Decomposition

The expected counts of the photon-counting silicon strip detector of the Micro-Dose system are modelled as

$$S_i = N_0 \int_0^\infty \phi(E) \cdot e^{-(\mu_{\mathrm{gland}}(E) \cdot h_{\mathrm{gland}} + \mu_{\mathrm{adp}}(E) \cdot h_{\mathrm{adp}})} \Gamma_i(E) \eta_i \, dE \,, \quad i = 1, 2 \,, \quad (1)$$

where N_0 is the incident number of photons, $\phi(E)$ is the normalized incident energy spectrum, $\mu_{\mathrm{adp}}(E)$ and $\mu_{\mathrm{gland}}(E)$ are the linear attenuation coefficients of adipose and glandular tissue, respectively. Furthermore, $\Gamma_i(E)$ denotes the bin sensitivity function for the two energy bins $i = 1, 2$, which measure the signal of the low and high energy photons, respectively, and η_i denotes the quantum efficiency for the two energy bins.

For the material separation of adipose and glandular tissue, the forward model (1) of the system, can be used to generate lookup tables directly mapping high and low energy photon counts to breast thickness and breast glandularity. Such an approach was employed to measure breast density and glandularity variations in breast tissue using the forward model (1) for the MicroDose mammography system [11].

Instead of modelling the detector response, we decided to use a calibration based approach similar to [9]. However, an additional scatter correction step could be omitted due to the virtually scatter-free acquisition on the MicroDose system. In contrast to the iterative approach presented in [9], the material decomposition could be performed directly in one step using the nonlinear eight-term rational functions

$$h_{\text{adp}}\left(L_1, L_2\right) = \frac{\alpha_0 + \alpha_1 L_1 + \alpha_2 L_2 + \alpha_3 L_1^2 + \alpha_4 L_1 L_2 + \alpha_5 L_2^2}{1 + \beta_1 L_1 + \beta_2 L_2}, \qquad (2)$$

$$h_{\text{gland}}\left(L_1, L_2\right) = \frac{\gamma_0 + \gamma_1 L_1 + \gamma_2 L_2 + \gamma_3 L_1^2 + \gamma_4 L_1 L_2 + \gamma_5 L_2^2}{1 + \delta_1 L_1 + \delta_2 L_2}, \qquad (3)$$

where L_1 and L_2 denote the line-integral value of the low and high energy signal, i.e. $L_i = -\ln\left(S_i/S_i^{\text{air}}\right)$, for $i = 1, 2$, with the low and high energy signal S_i^{air} of the spectrum without any object. The eight-term rational forms (2) and (3) of the conic surface equation are known to provide a fast and accurate material decomposition [4]. The coefficients α_p, γ_q, $p, q = 0, \ldots, 5$ and β_r, δ_s, $r, s = 1, 2$ have been determined from calibration measurements with the adipose and glandular equivalent phantoms as depicted in Fig. 1a and explained in the following.

2.2   Spectral Calibration

A spectral mammogram consisting of a low-energy and a high-energy image, can be separated into its adipose and glandular contributions by evaluation of (2) and (3), once the calibration coefficients $\alpha_p, \beta_r, \gamma_q, \delta_s$ have been identified. To this end, a collection of calibration phantoms has been used to measure the log-signal in the low and high energy bin for various tissue compositions and phantom heights.

The tissue compositions have been realized using adipose and glandular equivalent materials that constitute complementary step phantoms. Each single phantom comprises 11 cuboid volumes of glandularity $0\%, 10\%, \ldots, 100\%$ and have been manufactured for the heights $\hat{h} = 2\,\text{cm}$ and $\hat{h} = 4\,\text{cm}$ in the configuration depicted in Fig. 1a as well as with interchanged adipose and glandular compartments.

Additional adipose and glandular equivalent material slabs are used for sampling the intermediate heights $\hat{h} = 3\,\text{cm}$ and $\hat{h} = 5\,\text{cm}$ in the original and the complementary phantom configuration. The maximum height in this measurement was $\hat{h} = 6\,\text{cm}$ with the two calibration phantoms on top of each other. Therefore, 55 non-redundant data samples were available. Together with the corresponding samples from the complementary phantoms, this results in a total of $N = 110$ calibration points that could be used for the calibration procedure at one specific X-ray spectrum, given by the tube settings.

With the known material heights $\hat{h}_{\text{adp}}^{(j)}$ and $\hat{h}_{\text{gland}}^{(j)}$ of the adipose and glandular calibration phantoms and the corresponding measured line integral values $L_1^{(j)}$

and $L_2^{(j)}$ in the low and high energy bin for the calibration points $j = 1, \ldots, N$, we derive the non-linear least-squares minimization problems

$$\underset{\alpha_p, \beta_r}{\operatorname{argmin}} \sum_{j=1}^{N} \left(\hat{h}_{\mathrm{adp}}^{(j)} - h_{\mathrm{adp}} \left(L_1^{(j)}, L_2^{(j)} \right) \right)^2 , \qquad (4)$$

$$\underset{\gamma_q, \delta_s}{\operatorname{argmin}} \sum_{j=1}^{N} \left(\hat{h}_{\mathrm{gland}}^{(j)} - h_{\mathrm{gland}} \left(L_1^{(j)}, L_2^{(j)} \right) \right)^2 . \qquad (5)$$

Finally, the calibration coefficients α_p, γ_q, $p, q = 0, \ldots, 5$ and β_r, δ_s, $r, s = 1, 2$ are computed solving (4) and (5) using the Levenberg-Marquardt algorithm.

Since it is possible to perform acquisitions with different X-ray spectra, a separate set of calibration coefficients is stored for each X-ray spectrum, i.e. tube voltages $U \in \{26 \, \mathrm{kV}, 29 \, \mathrm{kV}, 32 \, \mathrm{kV}, 35 \, \mathrm{kV}, 38 \, \mathrm{kV}\}$ for the examined system.

The quality of the presented approach has been evaluated in two complementing experiments. In a first experiment, the slabs of the BR3D phantom, each consisting a mixture of adipose and glandular tissue with a height of 10 mm, are arranged as depicted in Fig. 1b, such that they form a step wedge. Computing the calibration coefficients via (4) and (5), and evaluating the material separation (2) and (3), we derive a height map $h(x, y) = h_{\mathrm{adp}}(x, y) + h_{\mathrm{gland}}(x, y)$ of 0.5 mm resolution that we compare to the true heights $\hat{h} = 10, \ldots, 60 \, \mathrm{mm}$ of the different combinations of slabs.

In a second experiment we demonstrate the feasibility of accurate tissue decomposition using additional layers of adipose and glandular tissue on top of four slabs of the BR3D phantom. We compute $h_{\mathrm{adp}}(x, y)$ and $h_{\mathrm{gland}}(x, y)$ as well as the total height $h(x, y) = h_{\mathrm{adp}}(x, y) + h_{\mathrm{gland}}(x, y)$. From the heights of the two components we derive the total volume of glandular tissue and compute the glandularity

$$g(x, y) = \frac{h_{\mathrm{gland}}(x, y)}{h_{\mathrm{adp}}(x, y) + h_{\mathrm{gland}}(x, y)} . \qquad (6)$$

3   Results

Comparing true heights $\hat{h} = 10, \ldots, 60 \, \mathrm{mm}$ of the BR3D step wedge to the measured heights we achieve absolute errors between 0.2 mm and 0.6 mm corresponding to relative errors of 0.4 % to 3.0 %. The standard deviation σ from the measured height increases with the total height as a result of the increasing quantum noise.

The measurements show excellent correlation with the true heights with small standard deviations and non-overlapping extremal values. Experiments with different configurations in terms of tissue heights and X-ray spectra indicate a strong robustness of the height measurement. Refer to Fig. 2 for two examples and a quantitative analysis of the height map for a setting with six shifted BR3D slabs.

Figure 3 depicts an example decomposition as part of the second experiment. It is evident, that all additional stripes add a constant height offset to the total

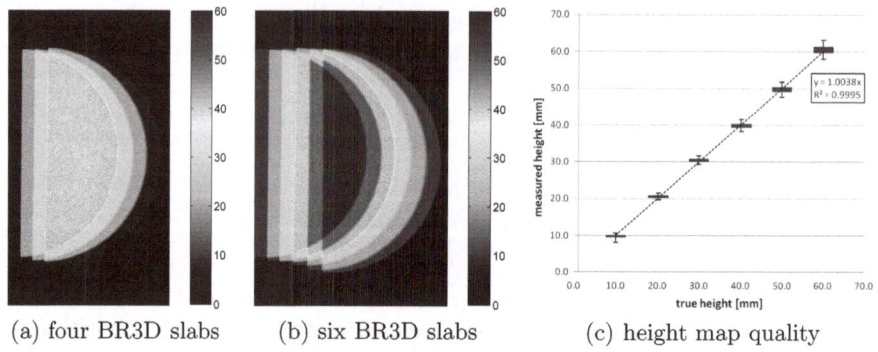

(a) four BR3D slabs   (b) six BR3D slabs   (c) height map quality

Fig. 2. Total tissue height reconstruction using spectral imaging for (a) four slabs of the BR3D phantom, i.e. $\hat{h} = 10, \ldots, 40\,\text{mm}$, $U = 32\,\text{kV}$, (b) six slabs of the BR3D phantom, i.e. $\hat{h} = 10, \ldots, 60\,\text{mm}$ total height, $U = 35\,\text{kV}$, and (c) box-whisker plot depicting the accuracy of the height map with 0.5 mm resolution, boxes correspond to $\pm 1\sigma$, whiskers denote the minimum and maximum values, the correlation of measured heights h with true heights $\hat{h}$ is $r = 0.9997$

height map, whereas they separate well in the adipose and glandular tissue height maps, even on top of the highly textured BR3D phantom slabs. The measured heights of the stripes are $h_{\text{adp}} = 9.5\,\text{mm}$ and $h_{\text{gland}} = 9.6\,\text{mm}$ compared to $\hat{h}_{\text{adp}} = 9.8\,\text{mm}$ and $\hat{h}_{\text{gland}} = 9.9\,\text{mm}$ determined via mechanical measurement. The total volume of the phantom arrangement for this example is $V = 755\,\text{cm}^3$ with volume of glandular tissue is $V_{\text{gland}} = 438\,\text{cm}^3$ corresponding to a mean glandularity $\bar{g} = 58\,\%$.

4   Discussion

The assessment of conventional volumetric breast density aims at *estimating* two physical quantities at the same time and therefore requires at least two independent measurements for its physical quantification. So far, a priori information is incorporated in conventional volumetric breast density estimation algorithms to overcome this problem at the cost of a decreased accuracy, particularly in the peripheral regions of the breast and when using flexible compression plates. The presented work demonstrates the feasibility of accurately *measuring* the volume of glandular tissue using two independent measurements by exploiting the spectral information of an energy-discriminating detector unit. Using the virtually scatter-free Philips MicroDose prototype device enabled a straightforward material decomposition without the need for a second pass scatter correction step.

The presented examples illustrate the benefit of spectral glandularity assessment that simultaneously measures the height and the composition of the phantom without any a priori knowledge. An accurate measurement of mis-aligned slabs of the BR3D phantom could be achieved in both height and tissue composition, which would otherwise not be possible with conventional methods.

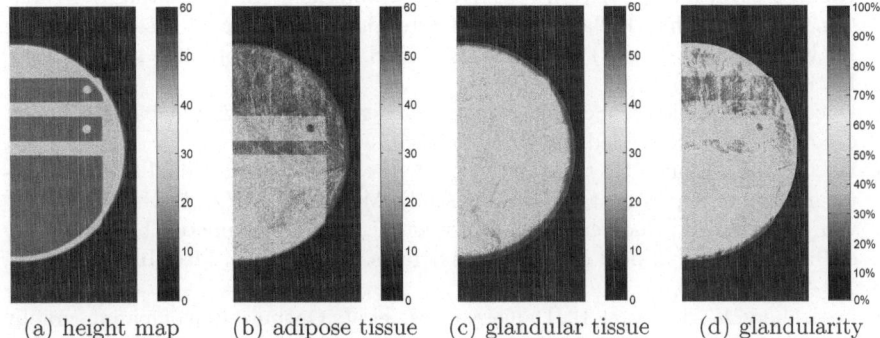

(a) height map   (b) adipose tissue   (c) glandular tissue   (d) glandularity

Fig. 3. Decomposition of a phantom scan consisting of four BR3D slabs and additional pieces of $\hat{h}_{adp} = 10\,\text{mm}$ pure adipose and $\hat{h}_{gland} = 10\,\text{mm}$ pure glandular tissue, respectively. (a) Total tissue height $h(x,y)$, (b) adipose tissue height $h_{adp}(x,y)$, (c) glandular tissue height $h_{gland}(x,y)$, and (d) resulting glandularity $g(x,y)$

In clinical practice, the accuracy of conventional volumetric breast density assessment depends on the precision of the system model or system calibration as well as on the quality of the underlying breast shape or height model. The spectral approach reduces these dependences to only one system calibration and will be used in our future work for a clinical comparison study of conventional breast density and spectral glandularity.

Acknowledgement. We would like to thank Hanns-Ingo Maack of Philips Healthcare, Hamburg, Germany and Mats Lundqvist of Philips Healthcare, Solna, Sweden for performing the image acquisition of the calibration and evaluation phantoms.

References

1. Alonzo-Proulx, O., Tyson, A.H., Mawdsley, G.E., Yaffe, M.J.: Effect of Tissue Thickness Variation in Volumetric Breast Density Estimation. In: Krupinski, E.A. (ed.) IWDM 2008. LNCS, vol. 5116, pp. 659–666. Springer, Heidelberg (2008)
2. Åslund, M., Cederström, B., Lundqvist, M., Danielsson, M.: Scatter rejection in multislit digital mammography. Med. Phys. 33, 933–940 (2006)
3. Boyd, N.F., Martin, L.J., Rommens, J.M., et al.: Mammographic density: a heritable risk factor for breast cancer. Methods Mol. Biol. 472, 343–360 (2009)
4. Cardinal, H.N., Fenster, A.: An accurate method for direct dual-energy calibration and decomposition. Med. Phys. 17(3), 327–341 (1990)
5. Ciatto, S., Houssami, N., Apruzzese, A., et al.: Categorizing breast mammographic density: intra- and interobserver reproducibility of BI-RADS density categories. Breast 14(4), 269–275 (2005)
6. Ciatto, S., Houssami, N., Apruzzese, A., et al.: Reader variability in reporting breast imaging according to BI-RADS assessment categories (the Florence experience). Breast 15(1), 44–51 (2006)

7. Diffey, J., Hufton, A., Astley, S., Mercer, C., Maxwell, A.: Estimating Individual Cancer Risks in the UK National Breast Screening Programme: A Feasibility Study. In: Krupinski, E.A. (ed.) IWDM 2008. LNCS, vol. 5116, pp. 469–476. Springer, Heidelberg (2008)

8. Ducote, J.L., Molloi, S.: Scatter correction in digital mammography based on image deconvolution. Phys. Med. Biol. 55(5), 1295–1309 (2010)

9. Ducote, J.L., Molloi, S.: Quantification of breast density with dual energy mammography: an experimental feasibility study. Med. Phys. 37(2), 793–801 (2010)

10. van Engeland, S., Snoeren, P.R., Huisman, H., et al.: Volumetric breast density estimation from full-field digital mammograms. IEEE Trans. Med. Imaging 25(3), 273–282 (2006)

11. Fredenberg, E., Svensson, B., Danielsson, M., et al.: Optimization of mammography with respect to anatomical noise. In: Proc of SPIE, Physics of Medical Imaging, vol. 7961, pp. 796112–11 (2011)

12. Fredenberg, E., Lundqvist, M., Cederström, B., et al.: Energy resolution of a photon-counting silicon strip detector. Nucl. Instrum. Meth. A 613(1), 156–162 (2010)

13. Hauge, I.H.R., Hogg, P., Szczepura, K., et al.: The readout thickness versus the measured thickness for a range of screen film mammography and full-field digital mammography units. Med. Phys. 39(1), 263–271 (2012)

14. Heese, H., Erhard, K., Gooßen, A.: Fully-automatic breast density assessment from full field digital mammograms. In: Proc. Workshop on Breast Image Analysis, pp. 113–120 (2011)

15. Kallenberg, M.G.J., Lokate, M., van Gils, C.H., Karssemeijer, N.: Automatic breast density segmentation: an integration of different approaches. Phys. Med. Biol. 56(9), 2715–2729 (2011)

16. Saftlas, A.F., Hoover, R.N., Brinton, L.A., et al.: Mammographic densities and risk of breast cancer. Cancer 67(11), 2833–2838 (1991)

17. Shepherd, J.A., Kerlikowske, K.M., Smith-Bindman, R., et al.: Measurement of breast density with dual X-ray absorptiometry: feasibility. Radiology 223(2), 554–557 (2002)

18. Snoeren, P.R., Karssemeijer, N.: Thickness correction of mammographic images by means of a global parameter model of the compressed breast. IEEE Trans. Med. Imaging 23(7), 799–806 (2004)

19. Tromans, C., Brady, M.: An Alternative Approach to Measuring Volumetric Mammographic Breast Density. In: Astley, S.M., Brady, M., Rose, C., Zwiggelaar, R. (eds.) IWDM 2006. LNCS, vol. 4046, pp. 26–33. Springer, Heidelberg (2006)

20. U.S. Connecticut Senate (ed.): Bill No. 458. Public Act No. 09-41 (2009)

21. Wolfe, J.N.: Breast patterns as an index of risk for developing breast cancer. AJR Am. J. Roentgenol. 126(6), 1130–1137 (1976)

Power-Law, Beta, and (Slight) Chaos in Automated Mammography Breast Structure Characterization

Joep J.M. Kierkels[1,3,*], Wouter J.H. Veldkamp[2,3],
Ramona W. Bouwman[3], and Ruben E. van Engen[3]

[1] TweeSteden Hospital, Medical Physics Department, Tilburg, The Netherlands
[2] Leiden University Medical Centre, Radiology Department, Leiden, The Netherlands
[3] LRCB, National Expert & Training Center, Nijmegen, The Netherlands
{j.kierkels,w.veldkamp,r.bouwman,r.vanengen}@lrcb.nl

Abstract. "Power-law" characterization of breast tissues can be achieved in different ways, as can be found in literature. The outcomes of all such characterizations appear to be in line with early observations stating that the power-law exponent β has a value between two and four for mammography images. Ambiguous aspects of power-law characterization and their implementation are addressed in this paper, including data representation, filtering, frequency range and ROI size. It is shown how different implementations have an effect on computed β values, using three different datasets (mammography images, chest x-ray images, and non-medical images). It is found that differences in computed β value within the mammography image dataset can be even larger than the differences between the mammography image dataset, chest x-ray images, and the non-medical images. A clear description of the used methodology is therefore essential for the interpretation and relevance of any power-law characterization.

Keywords: Mammography, Image Processing, Power Spectrum.

1 Background

In recent years, a growing number of papers is referring to "power-law" characterization as a means to classify breast structure and as a means to quantifying the detectability of lesions and calcifications in breasts. The key-point of the power-law characterization is that a 1D power spectrum (1DPS) of an image is of a form similar to

$$P(f) = \frac{c}{f^\beta} \, ,$$ (1)

in which f represents spatial frequency (lp/mm), C is an (arbitrary) constant, P is the power spectrum and β is a factor that determines the slope of the resulting graph. By calculating the optimal fit between the derived 1DPS and equation (1) parameters β and C can be determined.

Initially, Burgess [1] used the power-law characterization to understand statistical properties of breast structure and their effects on lesion detectability. To achieve this, β estimation was performed on digitized films that were mathematically adjusted in

A.D.A. Maidment, P.R. Bakic, and S. Gavenonis (Eds.): IWDM 2012, LNCS 7361, pp. 537–544, 2012.

order to reflect true breast attenuation properties. Furthermore only a specific region-of-interest (ROI) in the image was used to construct the 1DPS and it was stated that the power-law characterization should be limited to a small range of frequencies due to quantum noise and due to the desired frequency resolution. If power-law characterization was performed in this way, breast structure could be characterized by a β in the range of two to four, average three. Following this publication, many researchers have used power-law characterization to classify breast structure. Other papers have also used this characterization for breast-tomosynthesis images and/or breast-CT images (e.g., [2]). However, not all papers rigorously stick to the restrictions mentioned in [1]. Nevertheless, the outcomes always appear to be in line with early observations stating that β is between two and four for mammograms.

Literature results are based on different sets of data, obtained using different equipment and different methodological approaches. Assuming that β is a characteristic of breast-structure (and hence does not depend on equipment type) it remains unclear how the exact methodology of computing β appears to have little or no effect on the final result.

In this paper, relevant issues concerning these restrictions on power-law characterization of breast images are addressed. It will be shown that different implementations have been chosen and how all these implementations in literature lead to very similar values of β.

2   Method

The following subsections will cover aspects of power-law characterization that should (more or less chronologically) be considered when computing β. The sequence of   aspects to be covered is illustrated in Figure 1.

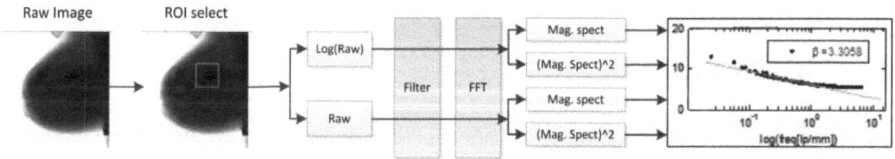

Fig. 1. Illustration of β-computation, showing computational sequence with some variants

2.1   Image Selection

Because power-law characterization requires digital image analysis, the image should be in a digital format. This can e.g. be achieved by directly using full-field digital mammography (FFDM) images or by using digitized films. One should be aware of what the pixels in the image actually reflect, which is certainly not as trivial as it appears. Pixel values can be proportional to exposure at the detector-level for image A, proportional to breast-attenuation properties for image B, or related to some film-characteristics for Image C. In [1] it was argued that proportionality to breast-attenuation properties should be favoured, since this is the physical property of interest. This would imply that anyone using images with different pixel representations should either convert their images through some mathematical procedure (e.g. log(..)) or be well aware (and state explicitly) their pixel representation. In this context it is also important to consider image post-processing. FFDM images are typically available as "for processing" and "for presentation". The first one represents the un-edited image whereas the second is the result of some image-enhancement software that typically makes the image suitable for viewing by a radiologist. Using the same argument of proportionality to breast-attenuation it would appear most appropriate to use the "for processing" images, although a recent study claims adequate results on "for presentation" images [3]. There are to our knowledge no pros and cons for using either Medio Lateral Oblique (MLO)   or Cranio Caudal (CC) views.

2.2   ROI Selection

Power-law analysis is never performed on the image as a whole but always on one or more ROIs in the image. In literature, square shaped ROIs are most common but some use a rectangular shape. A square shape is mathematically straightforward to process and hence often used. ROI size varies greatly in literature. Restrictions on size are given by the requirement that the ROI should have statistical uniform properties (not too large), and the requirement of a certain resolution in the frequency domain (not too small). ROIs of either 128*128 pixels or 256*256 pixels are often used. In [1] a ROI of at least 1024*1024 was used. The location of an ROI in the image can be chosen freely to zoom in on a certain aspect of the image. If the goal is to characterize the breast as a whole, it is common to use multiple ROIs (which may or may not overlap), covering the whole breast area and use the statistics of all ROIs to characterize the whole breast-area. In some papers special care is given to characterize only breast area that is compressed to equal thickness and to exclude muscle tissue from further analysis.

2.3   Filtering

Before computing the Fourier transform of an image it is common to perform filtering in order to avoid spectral leakage due to discontinuities at the edges of the image. For this purpose 2D-Hamming and 2D-Hanning filters are used in literature. Although most appear to use the Hanning filter (which fully eliminates discontinuities), there are to our knowledge no strong arguments against the Hamming filter.

2.4   2D-Power Spectrum

Commonly, a 2D implementation of the fast Fourier transform (hence the ROI size 2^N) is used to compute the 2D-power spectrum (2DPS) of the filtered ROI. The result of this Fourier operation is a complex matrix, from which a magnitude plot, a phase plot or a power plot (spectrum) may be constructed. The power spectrum is the square of the magnitude plot.

2.5   1D-Power Spectrum

In order to arrive at a more intuitive representation of the Power spectrum, the 2DPS is commonly converted to a 1DPS. Under the assumption that any orientations of breast structures in the ROI are random, most power-law related studies use "radial averaging" to perform this conversion. For each index in the 2DPS, the radial frequency is determined based on the root of the sum of squared 2DPS frequencies. This results in the 1DPS, in which power is plotted against frequency.

It should be noted that breast structures are not entirely randomly oriented, e.g. ducts run towards the nipple. Currently such orientations are mostly ignored in power-law characterization. This appears a valid initial approach, with possible future improvements.

2.6   Power-Law Fit

The key-point of the power-law characterization is the fit between the 1DPS and equation (1). To allow for an easy computation of this fit, log(power) is displayed against log(frequency), the result of which should resemble a line as

$$\log(P(f)) = \log\left(\frac{C}{f^{\beta}}\right) = \log(C) - \log(f^{\beta}) = \log(C) - \beta * \log(f). \quad (2)$$

The slope of this equation equals $-\beta$ and can be determined by fitting the 1DPS curve to this equation, this is usually performed in a least-squares approach. The range of frequencies over which the fit is computed varies greatly in literature. Some include all available frequencies (as determined by the ROI size) whereas others use a limited range, e.g. 0.15-0.7 lp/mm. The motivation behind limiting the frequency range lies in the fact that power at very high frequencies is dominated by quantum noise and hence does not reflect breast structures, whereas power at very low frequencies is difficult to assess because of the limited information available in the 2DPS on these frequencies.

3   Data Analysis

Three different sorts of data analysis have been performed to illustrate the versatility of data that can be used for computing β. Firstly, a literature review is conducted in which 15 papers have been analyzed and they are characterized by the way in which β is computed. Secondly, β computations are performed following different definitions in the process of determining β. For this purpose, a dataset was used containing 80 mammograms (20 women, bilateral, MLO and CC views). All imaging was performed using an IMS Giotto direct mammography system with a 0.085 mm/pixel size. For this system, pixel value in the raw image is proportional to exposure at the detector. Thirdly, in order to compare mammographic β computations to other classes of images, β is computed for 16 ROIs taken from a chest x-ray image (being other medical images, previously used and described in [4]) and for a set of 10 cartoon images (being unrelated non-medical images, obtained using a Google image search, converted to grayscale 256*256 images and assuming system-resolution equal to the mammography images). Our mammography-related computations were performed using raw digital images, using 256*256 ROIs covering the whole breast with an overlap of 128 pixels. ROIs outside the breast area and close to the contour of the breast were automatically excluded from further analysis. Bilateral breast images were included as well as both CC and MLO views. Figure 2 shows an example of how one image is divided into multiple ROIs.

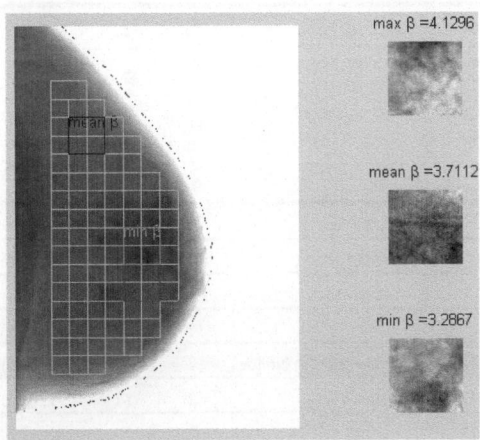

Fig. 2. Illustration of β computations for one mammogram divided into many ROIs with each their own β. Three ROIs (max, mean, min β) are zoomed in on (purely for illustration).

A Hanning filter was applied prior to computing the Fourier transform. The 2DPS was radially averaged and β was determined over a frequency range from 0.15 lp/mm to X lp/mm. X was determined for each ROI separately based on the best linear fit (R^2) to the 1DPS. This approach to determining the upper-frequency of the β range was also used in [2], but was not originally implemented in [1]. Typical examples of the ROIs that are used are shown in Table 1.

Table 1. Illustration of typical ROIs taken from the datasets of images

	Mammography	Chest X	Cartoon
Nr. images	20*2*2	16	10
Example			

The effect of applying a log-transform to the data as well as the use of either the power or the magnitude of the Fourier transformed image will be examined. Results will be shown for both options.

4   Results

The results of our literature review are shown in Table 2.

Table 2. Different approaches to computing β as found in literature[1]

Author (Year)		Analog/digital	Raw/Processed	Modality	Log(image)/No log	Power/Magnitude	Window	Beta(std)	Freq.band (lp/mm)	ROI size (pixels)
Bliznakova (2010)	[5]	A	?	Mammo	?	?	Hann	2.96 (0.009)	0.156-5	256*256
	[5]	A	P[2]	Mammo	?	?	Hann	2.78 (0.07)	0.156-5	400*400
Burgess (1999)	[1]	A	R	Mammo	Log	P	Hann	2 - 4	0.1-1	>1024
Burgess (2007)	[6]	?	?	?	Log	?	?	?	?	?
Chen (2011)	[2]	D	?	Mammo	No log	?	Hamm	3.06 (0.25)	F1-F2[3]	?
	[2]	D	?	Mam-Tom	?	?	?	2.91 (0.35)	F1-F2	?
	[2]	D	?	CT	?	?	?	1.8 (0.23)	F1-F2	?
Engstrom (2009)	[7]	D	R	Mam-Tom	No log	P	Hann	3.06 (0.21) 2.87 (0.24)	0.15-0.7	128*128
	[7]	A	?	Mammo	?	?	?	2.74 (0.19)	0.15-1	?
Fredenberg (2011)	[8]	D	R	Mammo	No Log	P	Hann	2.7(0.06)	0.1-	256*256
Gang (2010)	[9]	D	?	Phantom	No Log	P	Hann	2.0-4.0	0.063-0.31	50*50
Heine (2002)	[10]	D	?	Mammo	Log	?	Hann	2β= 2.8-3	All	69*96 (mm)
Lau (2011)	[11]	D	R+P	Mam-Tom	[Burgess]	[Burgess]	Hann	2.4-3.2	[Engstrom]	128*128/ 256*256/ 320*320
Li (2008)	[12]	A	?	Mammo	No Log	P	Hann	HR 2.92(0.28) LR 2.47(0.2)	All	256*256
Metheany (2008)	[13]	D	?	CT	No Log	P	Hann	2	0.07-0.5	128*128
	[13]	A	?	Mammo	?	?	Hann	3.01 (0.32)	?	256*256
Reiser (2006)	[14]	A	R	Mammo	Log	?	?	2.6-3.0	?	256*256
Reiser (2010)	[15]	D	(3D)	Mam-Tom	No Log	P	Hann	3.1 (model)	?	?
Reiser (2011)	[16]	D	?	?	No Log	P	?	?	?	?
Zheng (1996)	[17]	A	?	Mammo	?	?	?	1.8-2.0	1.0-4.0	128*128

[1] Only methodological issues included. Equipment specs. (manufacturer) should not affect β computation (unless used for image post-processing).
[2] Processed using General Electric post-processing software.
[3] Upper and lower frequency determined based on optimal fit (R^2).

Results on β computations are shown in Table 3.

Table 3. β computations for mammography images, chest x ray images and cartoon images computed using four different approaches

		Mammo		Chest X		Cartoon	
		β	Std(β)	β	Std(β)	β	Std(β)
Log	Power	3.80	0.13	4.75	1.27	2.76	0.30
Log	Magnitude	1.90	0.07	2.37	0.64	1.38	0.15
No log	Power	3.14	0.18	3.25	0.53	2.67	0.17
No log	Magnitude	1.57	0.09	1.62	0.26	1.33	0.09

5   Discussion

For four different methodologies, β was computed. It was shown that the methodologies using log-transformed data result in a significantly higher β compared to methodologies using untransformed data. The two methodologies using the power of the Fourier spectrum result in a β in the range of {2-5}. Results for six out of twelve computations could be described as being between two and four (as often stated in literature for expected β values). Results for the mammography log transformed power data and the mammography untransformed power data differ by as much as ~17%.

To illustrate the importance of this: the difference in computed β values between untransformed mammography images and log-transformed cartoon images is only ~12% and the difference in computed β values between untransformed mammography images and untransformed chest x-ray images is only ~4%. This implies that inter-study comparisons of β values require a thorough description of the used methodology. If such a description is lacking, results are no more similar than a comparison to unrelated images.

Using magnitude instead of power halves the computed β. Because $\log(x^2) = 2*\log(x)$ this result was to be expected. This factor 2 difference can however not be seen in the results from literature. Results showing a β below 2 are not reported. It should be mentioned here that most papers state the use of the 'power spectrum' and hence implicitly indicate the use of power instead of magnitude without directly stating the quadratic term. It often remains unclear as to whether the quadratic term is introduced prior to radial averaging or following radial averaging.

The high β value for chest X ray images can be explained by the fact that many of the 16 ROIs were positioned over lung-structures (as in Table 1). In such structures there are few small structures and hence there are less high frequency components in the power spectrum, resulting in a steep descending curve and hence a high β. The chest X ray ROIs which were not placed over the lungs, had a lower β, which resulted in a large standard deviation overall.

It is the authors opinion that adequate β computation on mammographic images should be based on images reflecting breast-attenuation properties (which may or may not involve applying the log-transform), using either a 2D-Hanning or 2D-Hamming filter, computing the power spectrum followed by (radial) averaging to obtain a 1D power spectrum and using a frequency range roughly from 0.15 – 0.8 lp/mm. The upper frequency limit could also be iteratively determined by fitting equation 2 to the obtained data (R^2) for multiple upper frequency limits and selecting the best fit. Such an approach appears methodologically correct and leads to reproducible results.

References

1. Burgess, A.E.: Mammographic structure: data preparation and spatial statistics analysis. In: Proceedings of SPIE, vol. 3661, pp. 642–653 (1999)
2. Chen, L., Boone, J.M., Nosratieh, A., Abbey, C.K.: NPS comparison of anatomical noise characteristics in mammography, tomosynthesis, and breast CT images using power law metrics. Physics 7961, 79610F–79610F-4 (2011)
3. Li, D., Gavenonis, S., Conant, E., Kontos, D.: Comparison of breast percent density estimation from raw versus processed digital mammograms. Imaging 7963, 79631X–79631X-6 (2011)
4. Kroft, L., Veldkamp, W., Mertens, B.: Detection of Simulated Nodules on Clinical Radiographs: Dose Reduction at Digital Posteroanterior Chest Radiography. Radiology 241 (2006)
5. Bliznakova, K., Suryanarayanan, S., Karellas, A., Pallikarakis, N.: Evaluation of an improved algorithm for producing realistic 3D breast software phantoms: Application for mammography. Medical Physics 37, 5604 (2010)
6. Burgess, A.E., Judy, P.F.: Signal detection in power-law noise: effect of spectrum exponents. Journal of the Optical Society of America A 24, 52–60 (2007)
7. Engstrom, E., Reiser, I., Nishikawa, R.: Comparison of power spectra for tomosynthesis projections and reconstructed images. Medical Physics 36, 1753 (2009)
8. Fredenberg, E., Svensson, B., Danielsson, M., Lazzari, B., Cederstr, B., Ab, M.: Optimization of mammography with respect to anatomical noise. In: SPIE, pp. 1–11 (2011)
9. Gang, G.J., Lee, J.: Anatomical background and generalized detectability in tomosynthesis and cone-beam CT. Medical Physics 37, 1948–1965 (2010)
10. Heine, J.J., Velthuizen, R.P.: Spectral analysis of full field digital mammography data. Medical Physics 29, 647 (2002)
11. Lau, B.A., Reiser, I., Nishikawa, R.M.: Issues in characterizing anatomic structure in digital breast tomosynthesis. Physics 7961, 796113–796113-8 (2011)
12. Li, H., Giger, M.L., Olopade, O.I., Chinander, M.R.: Power spectral analysis of mammographic parenchymal patterns for breast cancer risk assessment. Journal of Digital Imaging: The Official Journal of the Society for Computer Applications in Radiology 21, 145–152 (2008)
13. Metheany, K.G., Abbey, C.K., Packard, N., Boone, J.M.: Characterizing anatomical variability in breast CT images. Medical Physics 35, 4685 (2008)
14. Reiser, I., Nishikawa, R.M.: Identification of simulated microcalcifications in white noise and mammographic backgrounds. Medical Physics 33, 2905 (2006)
15. Reiser, I., Nishikawa, R.M.: Task-based assessment of breast tomosynthesis: Effect of acquisition parameters and quantum noise. Medical Physics 37, 1591 (2010)
16. Reiser, I., Lee, S., Nishikawa, R.M.: On the orientation of mammographic structure. Medical Physics 38, 5303 (2011)
17. Zheng, B., Chang, Y.H., Gur, D.: Adaptive computer-aided diagnosis scheme of digitized mammograms. Academic Radiology 3, 806–814 (1996)

Breast Density Measurement in Full-Field Digital Mammography: System Calibration and Stability

Charlotte Kerrison[1], Oliver Putt[1], Jamie C. Sergeant[2], Tina Dunn[3], Jennifer Diffey[4], Susan M. Astley[2], and Alan Hufton[2]

[1] School of Physics and Astronomy, The University of Manchester,
Oxford Road, Manchester, M13 9PL, UK
charlotte.kerrison@student.manchester.ac.uk,
oliver.putt@gmail.com
[2] School of Cancer and Enabling Sciences, The University of Manchester,
Oxford Road, Manchester M13 9PT, UK
{jamie.sergeant,sue.astley}@manchester.ac.uk,
alan.hufton@btinternet.com
[3] The Nightingale Centre and Genesis Breast Cancer Prevention Centre, University Hospital of
South Manchester NHS Foundation Trust, Southmoor Road,
Wythenshawe, Manchester M23 9LT, UK
tina.dunn@uhsm.nhs.uk
[4] Department of Medical Physics, Westmead Hospital,
P.O. Box 533, Wentworthville, NSW 2145, Australia
jennifer.diffey@swahs.health.nsw.gov.au

Abstract. Breast density calibrations and stability measurements were undertaken on digital mammography systems to investigate whether a single calibration could be used for extended periods. The results indicated that the calibration did not change over time and was the same for two units investigated. The daily mean pixel value per mAs (MPV/mAs) for five systems was recorded over 22 months and showed varying periods of stability up to more than a year. However, step changes in MPV/mAs were noted and resulted from, for example, detector re-calibration or replacement. During stable periods the MPV/mAs for the static units varied mostly by <±5%, excluding outliers. This corresponds to <±2mm error on dense tissue thickness. The stability was worse for the mobile units. These results indicate that it should be possible to use a single calibration over extended periods of time, provided allowance is made for changes in stability exceeding 5%.

Keywords: Breast density, digital mammography, calibration, stability.

1 Introduction

Breast density is a well-established risk factor and modifiable marker for breast cancer [1]. Consequently, in recent years considerable effort has been made to introduce objective and quantitative ways of measuring breast density. In particular, methods have been developed for determining the volume of dense (glandular) tissue in the

A.D.A. Maidment, P.R. Bakic, and S. Gavenonis (Eds.): IWDM 2012, LNCS 7361, pp. 545–552, 2012.

breast, originally for screen-film mammography and now for full-field digital mammography (FFDM). The different methods fall broadly into two categories: those based primarily on an imaging physics approach [2-4], and 'calibration' methods in which the detector signal is calibrated in terms of dense tissue thickness above each pixel, using suitable tissue equivalent materials [5-10].

Our calibration method for measuring volumetric breast density (VBD) in screen-film mammography involved imaging a step-wedge alongside the breast in every mammogram [5-6]. While this had the advantage of taking into account variations in film processing and drifts in x-ray tube potential (kV) or product of tube current and exposure time (mAs), the use of a step-wedge was cumbersome and it would be more convenient to avoid such a procedure. With the advent of FFDM and the need to modify our method, the intention was to try and eliminate the need for the step-wedge.

The aim of this investigation was therefore to determine whether an initial calibration of an FFDM system (in this study the GE Senographe Essential) can be used during routine mammography for extended periods without the need to re-calibrate. Three calibrations were performed on two systems between 2009 and 2012 to see whether the calibration data sets differed in either absolute or relative terms. In addition, the daily mean pixel value per mAs (MPV/mAs), measured as part of routine quality control (QC) procedures, was examined for five FFDM systems over a period of 22 months to quantify the performance stability of each system.

Similar work to that reported here has been published for the earlier GE Senographe 2000D system [10-12].   Although a direct comparison is difficult due to differences in the presentation of results, the conclusions appear to be broadly similar.

2   Methods

2.1   Calibration

All calibration and stability measurements were undertaken on equipment used in the Greater Manchester Breast Screening Programme, part of the UK National Health Service Breast Screening Programme (NHSBSP). Calibrations were carried out on two GE Senographe Essential FFDM systems used mainly for symptomatic and assessment work at the Nightingale Centre and Genesis Prevention Centre. The first unit, denoted by Room 1, was calibrated in January 2012 and again in March 2012, while the second unit, Room 3, had previously been calibrated in January 2009. It was originally intended to also calibrate Room 3 in January 2012 but this proved impossible due to a detector failure.

The procedure followed was similar to that used previously [5], except that the step-wedge was omitted and MPV was recorded instead of digitised film density. In summary, semi-circular phantoms composed of adipose and glandular tissue equivalent materials were used to simulate a range of breast compositions and thicknesses. Epoxy-resin based tissue substitutes AP6 and WT1 were used to simulate adipose and glandular tissue respectively [13]. The total breast phantom thicknesses (T) ranged from 20-70mm, with compositions of 0-100% glandular tissue. Each composition and thickness combination was then imaged under the same manual exposure factors: kV, mAs and target/filter combination, as used by Kaufhold et al [10]. MPV/mAs for each image was obtained over a 200x200 pixel region-of-interest (ROI) near the centre of the image of the phantom, similar to that used in the QC measurements. The first two calibrations used only glandular tissue proportions of 0, 50 and 100% for 11 combinations of kV/target/filter [10]. The third calibration was made in March 2012 as a repeat of that performed in January 2012. However, the main purpose of this calibration was to generate a comprehensive calibration dataset of all possible breast compositions, given the available phantom thicknesses (i.e. 5mm steps of glandular tissue), as opposed to the limited values of 0, 50 and 100% used in the earlier calibrations. Time constraints prevented measurements being made at more than one combination of kV, target and filter. For this calibration 29kV and a target/filter of Rh/Rh was used. This target/filter is by far the most commonly selected automatically by the GE equipment at the Nightingale Centre for clinical mammograms across all breast thicknesses and compositions, while 29kV is typical for an average breast.

From these data, calibration curves were constructed relating the glandular tissue thickness (t_g) to measured MPV/mAs and total breast thickness, for each combination of kV and target/filter.

2.2   Performance Stability

Stability measurements were undertaken on five GE Senographe Essential FFDM systems. Three of these were static units used for symptomatic and assessment work and included the two units on which calibrations were performed. The remaining two units were mounted on mobile breast cancer screening vans. The system stability was investigated through analysis of daily quality control (QC) measurements, performed according to manufacturer's requirements and national QC protocols [14]. The QC test utilised for this work was the 'SNR daily system check', designed to detect changes in the performance of the x-ray set or image receptor. The test involves imaging a 40mm thick Perspex block using exposure factors for the kV, mAs and target/filter given by the clinically used automatic setting. The MPV and standard deviation are calculated from the raw QC image by means of a 200x200 pixel ROI drawn on the midline, 6cm from the edge of the image furthest from the gantry. For QC purposes a tolerance level of ±10% of the baseline value for mAs and MPV is used, so no remedial action would be taken unless these limits were exceeded.

The daily MPV/mAs values over a period of 22 months, beginning 1 January 2010, were analysed to determine if the system performance was stable over long periods, and to identify any daily deviations from the mean value. The system service reports, completed by the manufacturer's engineer and stored at the Nightingale Centre, were scrutinised to identify possible causes for deviations from, or changes to, the mean MPV/mAs. Such events might have included system re-calibrations, software upgrades, routine service visits or replacement of faulty parts.

Following analysis of the data, an attempt was made to locate the original images from PACS for any outliers, defined as individual MPV/mAs values more than 1.5 times the inter-quartile range outside the upper or lower quartiles. This was not always possible, as raw images are not required to be kept on the system, but those that could be retrieved had their MPV/mAs recalculated from the raw image data to investigate possible causes.

3   Results

3.1   Calibration

Figure 1 shows an example set of calibration data for Room 1, obtained in March 2012 for 29kV, rhodium target and rhodium filter (29kV, Rh/Rh). The measured data points are well described by a log function of the form:

$$t_g = a*\ln(MPV/mAs) + b \tag{1}$$

where t_g is the thickness of glandular tissue (mm) and the fitted parameters a and b are functions of T, kV and target/filter. Equation (1) gives values of t_g to within 1mm of the known phantom thicknesses. The values for the fitted parameters are given in Table 1, along with those for the earlier calibrations.

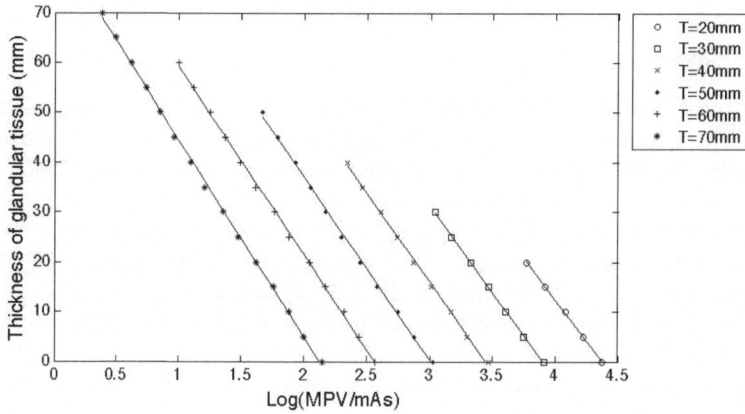

Fig. 1. Calibration data for 29kV, Rh/Rh and total phantom thicknesses (T) from 20-70mm, obtained in March 2012 for Room 1

Table 1. Comparison of fitted parameters for 29kV, Rh/Rh for the three sets of calibration data. Also shown is the MPV/mAs for the T = 40mm, t_g = 40mm exposure

T (mm)	Jan 2009 (Room 3)		Jan 2012 (Room 1)		Mar 2012 (Room 1)	
	a	b	a	b	a	b
20	-32.81	142.7	-32.93	144.4	-32.66	143.1
30	-34.42	133.3	-34.40	134.7	-34.68	135.2
40	-35.34	120.8	-35.51	122.9	-35.79	123.3
50	-36.75	108.9	-36.74	110.8	-36.84	110.7
60	-38.42	96.52	-38.28	98.39	-37.88	97.24
70			-39.61	84.49	-39.45	83.92
MPV/mAs	9.99		10.47		10.41	

There is very little difference between the three calibration sets. On average the gradients of the fits agree to within 1%, with the maximum difference being 1.4%, while the intercepts differ by <2%.

In order to investigate whether one of these calibrations could be used to calculate t_g on the two other dates, an adjustment has to be made to allow for any differences in performance, as indicated by the differences in MPV/mAs obtained under standardised conditions (see last row in Table 1). Denoting these MPV/mAs by S_1, S_2 and S_3 for Jan 2009, Jan 2012 and March 2012, the MPV/mAs values used in Jan 2009 and Jan 2012 were multiplied by S_3/S_1 and S_3/S_2 to calculate the MPV/mAs values that would have been obtained had the measurements been undertaken in March 2012. The two sets of adjusted MPV/mAs were then inserted into equation (1) and t_g calculated. It was found that the March 2012 calibration predicted t_g to within 1mm of the known values on the other dates.

Figure 1 can also give an indication of the errors incurred if the system stability changes. Differentiating equation (1) gives:

$$\delta t_g = a * \delta(MPV/mAs)/(MPV/mAs) \tag{2}$$

Thus, for example, a 5% change in MPV/mAs would give an error of 1.5-2mm for the glandular tissue thickness. This would seem to be a reasonable target to aim for as it is approximately the same, or better than, the magnitude of the error incurred by uncertainties in the measurement of total breast thickness [7,10].

3.2   Stability

The performance stability of each mammography unit is shown in figure 2. A number of outliers are evident, but those exceeding an MPV/mAs of 30 have been omitted from the plots for clarity. The numbers of such cases involved were one for Room 1, one for Room 2, none for Room 3, eight for Van 1 and none for Van 2. Some outliers were resolved by reference to those original raw images still available, and were found to be due to errors in data input. The reasons for the remaining outliers and the generally worse stability for the mobile units need further investigation to identify the causes and whether they represent genuine variations in performance. It may be noted that temperature, rate of temperature change and humidity can affect detector performance, although we are not aware of any publications in the literature quantifying these effects.

For the static units, the mean MPV/mAs was remarkably stable over long periods, whereas the variations were much greater for the mobile units. Discontinuities were evident where there were systematic changes in MPV/mAs. Apart from three occasions where the cause was unknown, these were traced to the installation of a new detector (Room 1, day 472), bucky changes and/or detector re-calibrations (Room 1, day 277; Room 2, day 260; Van 1, day 224), routine service (Room 1, day 83) or raising input voltage (Van 1, day 553).

Table 2 summarizes the mean MPV/mAs during each stable period and the number of days where the MPV/mAs exceeded ± 5% and ± 10% from the mean. These figures are relevant in view of the effects such changes have on the glandular tissue thickness errors (see section 3.1).

For the most part, the daily MPV/mAs does not vary from the mean by more than ± 5%, but there are significant exceptions to this, notably for the mobile vans. Further work is needed to investigate these outliers.

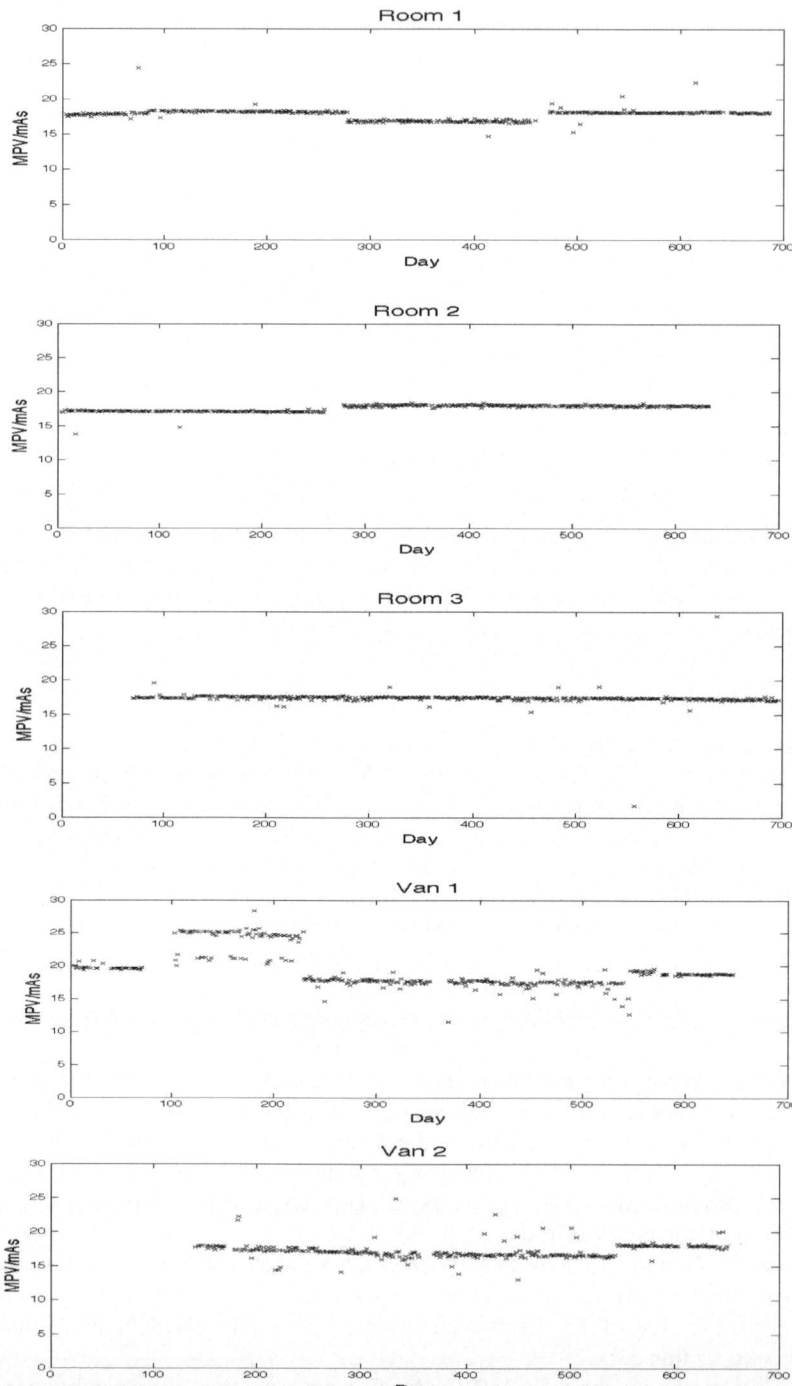

Fig. 2. Daily MPV/mAs values for the five mammography units investigated

Table 2. Summary of stability data for each unit

	Day range	No. days with data	Mean MPV/mAs	No. days MPV/mAs outside ±5% of mean	No. days MPV/mAs outside ±10% of mean
Room 1	4-83	56	17.91	1	1
	84-277	132	18.19	1	0
	278-472	124	16.83	1	1
	473-686	144	18.14	5	3
Room 2	4-260	178	17.15	3	3
	279-631	244	18.00	0	0
Room 3	70-697	427	17.39	11	5
Van 1	4-71	38	19.65	2	0
	103-224	84	23.99	36	20
	225-553	207	17.56	27	14
	554-569	11	19.12	0	0
	578-645	44	18.76	0	0
Van 2	141-543	260	17.01	29	19
	546-649	69	18.01	3	3

4   Conclusions

Breast density calibrations performed on two GE Senographe Essential FFDM systems indicate that the relative calibration does not change with time or with equipment, although similar measurements performed on more systems would be desirable to confirm this. A simple correction derived from daily QC measurements of MPV/mAs can take into account changes in equipment performance and allow a single absolute calibration to be applied. Excluding uncertainties in total breast thickness, this allows the thickness of glandular tissue above each pixel in a mammogram to be determined to within 1mm.

An analysis of QC records showed that there were long periods where the MPV/mAs did not vary by more than ± 5% from the mean, implying a glandular tissue thickness error of up to ± 2mm. Nevertheless, there were a significant number of deviations much greater than this, especially for systems installed on mobile vans. In addition, step changes in mean MPV/mAs were observed, corresponding to the installation of new components or other actions by the service engineer. Such step changes could relatively easily be taken into account. However, further work is needed to resolve the large apparent variations in MPV/mAs that occurred on 118 out of 2018 days.

References

1. Boyd, N.F., Martin, L.J., Yaffe, M.J., Minkin, S.: Mammographic density and breast cancer risk: current understanding and future prospects. Breast Cancer Research 13 (223) (2011)

2. Hartman, K., Highnam, R., Warren, R., Jackson, V.: Volumetric Assessment of Breast Tissue Composition from FFDM Images. In: Krupinski, E.A. (ed.) IWDM 2008. LNCS, vol. 5116, pp. 33–39. Springer, Heidelberg (2008)
3. Highnam, R., Brady, S.M., Yaffe, M.J., Karssemeijer, N., Harvey, J.: Robust Breast Composition Measurement - Volpara™. In: Martí, J., Oliver, A., Freixenet, J., Martí, R. (eds.) IWDM 2010. LNCS, vol. 6136, pp. 342–349. Springer, Heidelberg (2010)
4. Highnam, R.P., Pan, X., Warren, R., Jeffreys, M., Davey Smith, G., Brady, M.: Breast composition measurements using retrospective SMF. Phys. Med. Biol. 51, 2695–2713 (2006)
5. Hufton, A., Astley, S., Marchant, T., Patel, H.: A method for the quantification of dense breast tissue from digitised mammograms. In: Proceedings of the 7th IWDM (2004)
6. Diffey, J., Hufton, A., Astley, S.: A New Step-Wedge for the Volumetric Measurement of Mammographic Density. In: Astley, S.M., Brady, M., Rose, C., Zwiggelaar, R. (eds.) IWDM 2006. LNCS, vol. 4046, pp. 1–9. Springer, Heidelberg (2006)
7. Yaffe, M.J., Boone, J.M., Packard, N., Alonzo-Proulx, O., Huang, S.-Y., Peressotti, C.L., Al-Mayah, A., Brock, K.: The myth of the 50-50 breast. Med. Phys. 36(12), 5437–5443 (2009)
8. Pawluczyk, O., Augustine, B.J., Yaffe, M.J., Rico, D., Yang, J., Mawdsley, G.E.: A volumetric method for estimation of breast density in digitised screen-film mammograms. Med. Phys. 30(3), 352–364 (2003)
9. Malkov, S., Wang, J., Kerlikowske, K., Cummings, S.R., Shepherd, J.A.: Single x-ray absorptiometry method for the quantitative mammographic measure of fibroglandular tissue volume. Med. Phys. 36(12), 5525–5536 (2009)
10. Kaufhold, J., Thomas, J.A., Eberhard, J.W., Galbo, C.E., Gonzalez Trotter, D.E.: A calibration approach to glandular tissue composition estimation in digital mammography. Med. Phys. 29(8), 1867–1880 (2002)
11. Heine, J.J., Cao, K., Beam, C.: Cumulative sum quality control for calibrated breast density measurements. Med. Phys. 36(12), 5380–5390 (2009)
12. Heine, J.J., Thomas, J.A.: Effective x-ray attenuation coefficient measurements from two full field digital mammography systems for data calibration applications. BioMedical Engineering OnLine 7(13) (2008)
13. International Commission on Radiation and Units. Tissue substitutes in radiation dosimetry and measurement. ICRU Report 44 (1989)
14. NHSBSP Equipment Report 0702 Version 1. Routine Quality Control Tests for Full Field Digital Mammography Systems. NHS Cancer Screening Programmes (2007)

A Method for Lesion Visibility Prediction in Mammograms by Local Analysis of Spectral Anatomical Noise

Stephanie Simbt[1], Hanns-Ingo Maack[1], and Harald S. Heese[2]

[1] Philips Medical Systems DMC GmbH, Röntgenstr. 24, 22335 Hamburg, Germany
{hanns-ingo.maack,harald.heese}@philips.com
[2] Philips Research, Röntgenstr. 24-26, 22335 Hamburg, Germany

Abstract. Detection of mass lesions in mammograms via visual readings is a challenging task, and the radiographic density of the breast tissue or its strong anatomical structure may render lesions completely invisible. In order to assess visibility of lesions of a certain size in a given mammogram, we propose a measure for prediction of lesion visibility that complements established approaches for breast density assessment by taking also local structure into account. This measure is based on the analysis of spectral anatomical noise in terms of local standard deviation values for several frequency bands of the mammogram. The resulting values are used to generate two dimensional visibility maps for different lesion sizes. Phantoms of structured tissue equivalent materials were imaged using a full-field digital mammography (FFDM) system, and spherical lesions of different sizes were artificially added to the images. In an observer study with ten observers visibility thresholds were determined from a total of 290 simulated lesions. The resulting nonlinear threshold curve was verified in a second observer study, where 66 lesions were artificially added in clinical mammograms of varying breast density according to BI-RADS classification. A prediction accuracy of 92% was obtained, suffering mostly from different image characteristics in the breast tissue regions near the skinline or the pectoral muscle.

Keywords: Lesion visibility, tissue structure, digital mammography, anatomical noise, nodule.

1 Introduction

Image-based indicators for breast cancer risk increasingly gain importance in mammography [7,13,15]. These indicators cover both statistical (or lifetime) risk [13], and oversight risk (or mammographic sensitivity) [1] as two major attention points in assessing breast cancer risk. Although these effects are not independent [1], they characterize different aspects of breast cancer risk.

Today, mammographic breast density assessment is an accepted measure for assessing breast cancer risk [11] without addressing these two risk factors distinctively, fostering the impression that radiographic density is the dominant factor

A.D.A. Maidment, P.R. Bakic, and S. Gavenonis (Eds.): IWDM 2012, LNCS 7361, pp. 553–560, 2012.

for reduced sensitivity. Nevertheless, a mass lesion may not only be obscured by the global level of density of the breast, but also by the inherent anatomical structure or pattern of the breast tissue. In consequence, low contrast lesions may not be visible inside strongly structured breast tissue of rather low radiographic density. At the same time, it may well be that a lesion is clearly visible inside a region of dense but homogenous tissue.

In both situations, approaches that estimate oversight risk solely from radiographic density will be misleading. On the one hand, oversight risk for small regions of strongly structured tissue is underestimated, while, on the other hand, oversight risk is overestimated for large regions of dense, but homogeneous tissue.

The concept of *anatomical noise* has also been extensively studied in the academic literature for at least a decade [2,3,5,6,10,12]. Nevertheless, localized information about *anatomical noise* has not yet been employed in the context of breast cancer risk assessment.

Hence, we propose a local measure of mass lesion visibility in order to adequately capture the oversight risk arising from the inherent tissue structure. The approach uses simple thresholding techniques on localized parameter maps in the space domain that are equivalent to concentric regions in frequency domain, which are usually employed in the analysis of anatomical noise. Thresholds for visibility of mass lesions were empirically derived in a first observer study using phantom images, and validated in a second observer study using clinical image data.

2   Methods and Materials

The proposed approach has been developed using image data from a Philips MammoDiagnost DR 2.0 X-ray FFDM system (Philips Medical Systems DMC GmbH, Hamburg, Germany), presented as dose-proportional signal intensity with a resolution of $0.085 \times 0.085\,\mathrm{mm}^2$ and a matrix size of 2084×2800 pixels.

According to [6], the characteristics of breast tissue structure can be described by *anatomical noise* σ^2 using an approximated power-law function

$$\sigma^2 = \mathrm{NPS}(f) = \alpha f^{-\beta} + A, \tag{1}$$

where f is the radial frequency, α and β are constants, and A is a residual term describing high frequency system noise. The lower frequency anatomical noise, which is described by α and β can be determined in the Fourier domain by calculating the squared modulus on concentric rings (cp. [2,3,10,12]). Equivalently, a spectral decomposition of the mammogramm can be obtained using a bank of bandpass filters. Consequently, α and β can be approximated by employing variance or standard deviation as measure on the each bandpass image [2], thus approximating the squared modulus in the Fourier domain.

The flow of the presented approach is depicted in Figure 1 for an exemplary case. Each of its steps will be described in more detail in the following.

To measure the local strength of structure of the breast tissue, we at first decompose the mammogram into several frequency bands analogous to [14], by

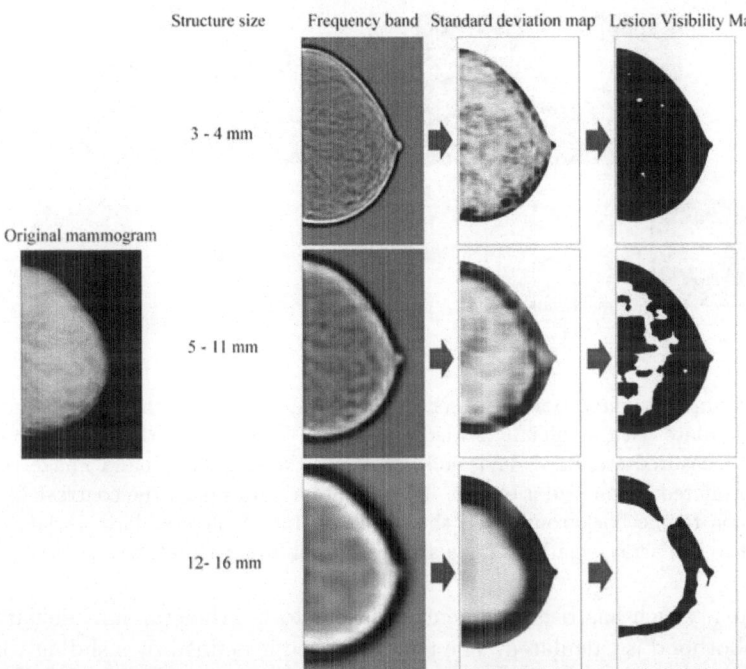

Structure size   Frequency band   Standard deviation map   Lesion Visibility Map

3 - 4 mm

Original mammogram

5 - 11 mm

12- 16 mm

Fig. 1. Exemplary depiction of algorithm flow for creation of lesion visibility maps. Original X-ray image (far left) is decomposed in several frequency band images (third column) relating to different structure sizes (second column). Local *structuredness* is measured by calculating local standard deviation (fourth column) on each of the frequency band images. Binary lesion visibility maps (right column) for each structure size are finally generated from the standard deviation maps by appropriate thresholding.

using a Laplacian image pyramid (Figure 1, third column). At first, the original image I is convolved with a small box kernel of 3×3 pixels. By subtracting the result I'_0 from the original image a high-frequency image I_{-1} is generated. This image is disregarded for the remaining analysis as it is assumed that this image is dominated by high frequency system noise A as described in (1). Now, band pass images I_k, $k \geq 0$ of decreasing spatial frequencies are generated iteratively by the following process. In order to generate the next pyramid level image I'_{k+1}, the current image I'_k is convolved with a smoothing filter kernel and subsequently subsampled in each direction by a factor of 2. The band pass image I_k is obtained by upsampling I'_{k+1} and subtracting it from I'_k. Usually, this process is stopped after eight frequency band images have been obtained. In each frequency band image I_k, only structural information of a certain size range (e.g. 0.25 mm, 0.5 mm, 1 mm, 2 mm, 4 mm, 8 mm, 16 mm and 32 mm median structure size) relating to the frequency band are retained.

For each of the frequency band images $I_3, \ldots, I_7$, that carry information equivalent to the sizes of anatomical soft tissue structures $(2, \ldots, 32\,\text{mm})$, the standard deviation is measured locally in a second step. For each pixel inside the

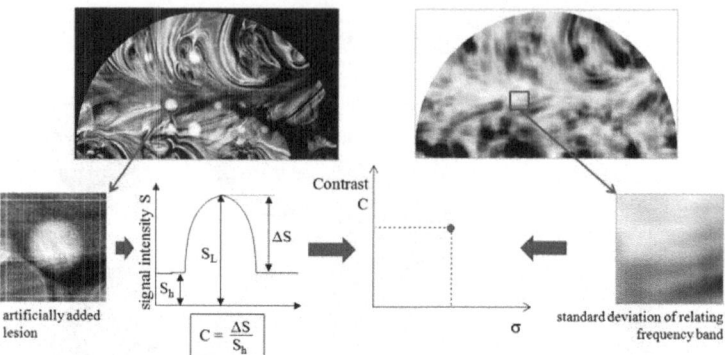

Fig. 2. Data point generation for observer study evaluation. On the top left, an X-ray of a BR3D plate with artificially added lesions can be seen. On the top right, a map of locally measured standard deviation values for the frequency band image relating to the considered lesion size is shown. To generate a data point, the contrast C of the added lesion to the background and the median value of the standard deviation map restricted to the array position of the artificial lesion are calculated.

breast area, which has been segmented similar to [9], the standard deviation of its neighborhood is calculated. The neighborhood is defined by a sliding window of 5×5 pixels, which corresponds to a neighbourhood that scales with structure size of the current frequency band, e.g. $2\,\text{mm} \times 2\,\text{mm}$ for structure sizes with a diameter of $2\,\text{mm}$. In that way, a two dimensional standard deviation map for each frequency band image is produced (see Figure 1, fourth column). These maps can already be interpreted as a continuous measure corresponding to the likelihood that a lesion of size corresponding to the frequency band is obscured by the surrounding tissue structure.

In order to increase the usability of this measure, thresholds are applied to each standard deviation map, dividing the parameter space into three categories (*surely visible, visibility uncertain, surely obscured*). The thresholds were modeled as nonlinear threshold curves of a form similar to (1) with respect to lesion size, and calibrated in an observer study with 10 observers (2 image processing specialists, 3 application specialists for mammography, 3 software tester for mammography systems, 1 clinical scientist, 1 student). The setup of the threshold estimation process is summarized in Figure 2.

In this study, X-ray images of randomly structured plates of tissue equivalent material (BR3D phantom, CIRS Inc.) representing an equal mixture of fatty and glandular tissue were imaged using an FFDM system, and differently sized spherical lesions (diameter ranging from 1 mm to 20 mm) with attenuation coefficients of muscle tissue were simulated into the structured regions (see Figure 2, top left image, for an exemplay arrangement). The observers had to decide whether or not they can detect a lesion in an array of possible lesion positions. In total, 413 array positions had to be evaluated containing a total of 290 simulated lesions. For each array position containing a simulated lesion, the following data was recorded: Firstly, the local contrast C of the simulated lesion to the structured background as described by

$$C = \frac{S_L - S_H}{S_H}, \tag{2}$$

where S_L, S_H are the average signal intensities of the lesion and the surrounding background. And secondly, the median of the local standard deviation (corresponding to simulated lesion size) of the structured background at the array location of the lesion (see Figure 2, top right image).

A threshold curve was computed in the form of

$$\sigma_{threshold} = [a \cdot l(h) \cdot C]^{\frac{1}{b}} \tag{3}$$

by correlating these parameters to the observer results, while considering the increasing contrast loss l with increasing compression height h. In this way, a lesion lying inside of a region with a standard deviation above the given threshold is categorized as *surely obscured*.

In Figure 1, far right column, exemplary lesion visibility maps are shown for three different structure sizes, where regions of the standard deviation maps with parameter values above the threshold curve, i.e. where lesions are *surely obscured*, are marked black and regions, where lesions may be visible, are indicated in white. With a second threshold curve, all lesions that were *surely visible* can be predicted in an additional visibility map.

3   Results

To characterize the image data of the observer study, results were analyzed using kappa statistics between the visibility decisions of each single observer and the visibility decision of the majority, revealing an agreement ranging between 0.59 and 0.88 (average: 0.78) with actual agreements ranging between 0.79 and 0.94 (average: 0.89) and per chance agreement between 0.49 and 0.53. See Table 1 for details.

Table 1. Reader agreement from observer study for threshold estimation. Numbers of lesions classified as visible or non-visible for each individual reader are given in top rows, kappa score against majority vote is given in bottom row.

Reader	R1	R2	R3	R4	R5	R6	R7	R8	R9	R10	maj
visible	194	130	160	201	179	216	166	171	116	184	178
non-visible	219	283	253	212	234	197	247	242	297	229	235
kappa vs majority	0.84	0.71	0.87	0.84	0.82	0.59	0.88	0.81	0.68	0.73	n/a

Corresponding threshold curves are shown in Figure 3 in a plot of local standard deviation versus contrast with logarithmic scaling of both axes. Each simulated lesion is marked by a square colored according to the size of the lesion.

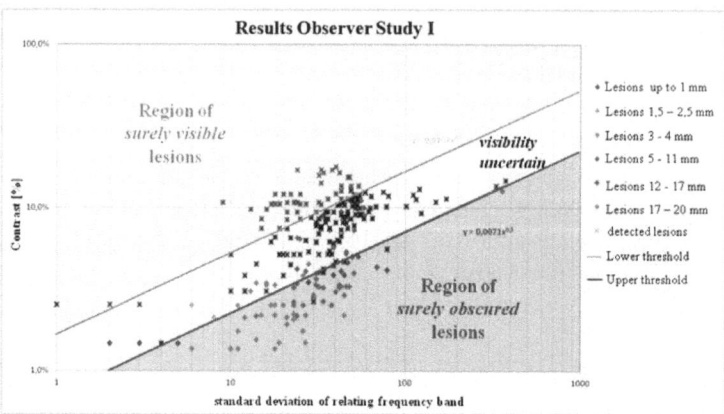

Fig. 3. Estimation of threshold curves for visibility prediction of lesions. Data points marked with a black cross are detected by the majority of observers. Data point colors indicate corresponding structure sizes. Two curves can be estimated for dividing data points in three categories: *surely visible, visibility uncertain* and *surely obscured*.

If the lesion is detected by the majority of observers, the square is overlaid by a black cross. The estimated threshold curve dividing *surely obscured* lesions from all others is given as red line, the curve dividing *surely visible* lesions from all others is given as a green line, with the corresponding regions being colored respectively.

To verify these lesion visibility threshold curves, a second observer study with clinical mammograms and simulated spherical lesions of different size was carried out. The same 10 observers were asked to detect 66 differently sized lesions from 2 to 17 mm in 16 different mammograms of different breast density categories according to the BI-RADS standard [4] (ACR class I-IV). In the first study, lesions bigger than 17 mm were always detected and therefore not considered in this second study. The mammograms were using the vendor's standard postprocessing to ensure a setup that is comparable to the clinical workflow.

The observers had to specify, if and in which quadrant of a quadratic area a lesion was located. Reader agreement characteristics were again calculated using kappa statistics (see Table 2) with respect to the majority voting, revealing similar performance of the readers.

The prediction with the aid of the threshold curves was *surely visible* for 12 lesions and *surely obscured* for 13 lesions. All *surely visible* lesions were correctly detected by at least 5 observers and only 2 of 13 *surely obscured* lesions were detected by more than 4 observers. A prediction accuracy of 92% for lesion visibility was computed for this study. For lesions of category *visibility uncertain*, a detection probability can be given by appropriately transforming the continuous measure derived from the local standard deviation between the two threshold curves. Between this probability and the percentage of observers who correctly detected a lesion, a correlation of 0.67 for all lesions was computed.

Table 2. Reader agreement from observer study for threshold validation. Numbers of lesions classified as visible or non-visible for each individual reader are given in top rows, kappa score against majority vote is given in bottom row.

Reader	R1	R2	R3	R4	R5	R6	R7	R8	R9	R10	maj
visible	22	31	27	34	37	24	45	26	30	32	29
non-visible	44	35	39	32	29	42	21	40	36	34	37
kappa vs majority	0.71	0.82	0.94	0.79	0.64	0.85	0.54	0.91	0.79	0.73	n/a

4   Discussion

The results of the second observer study show that it is possible to predict the visibility of soft tissue lesions through spectral standard deviation maps and to determine clinically meaningful threshold curves. The applicability of the developed method is verified by the high prediction accuracy obtained in the second observer study.

It has to be noted that the proposed method provides information from a single image that is multi-dimensional in terms of the frequency spectrum, which needs careful interpretation. For example, some aspects of the results displayed in Figure 1 may seem implausible on first glance as they indicate that a lesion of approx. 4 mm will be *obscured* almost in the entire breast, while a lesion of approx. 8 mm will be *visible* almost everywhere. But if we add a hazelnut and a pea in bag of coffee beans and produce an X-ray image of the bag, we expect to detect the hazelnut much more easily than the pea, as the structural pattern of the former is distinct from structural pattern of the coffee beans, whereas the structural pattern of the latter is rather indistinct from the coffee beans.

In both studies, we observed that big lesions lying in the region of the breast boundary or in the vicinity of the pectoral muscle led to false predictions. This is attributed to the strong gradient in low frequency bands which is present in both of these regions. By omitting lesions in breast boundary regions (only one in the second observer study) the prediction accuracy increases to 95.8%. Hence, future work will address to incorporate inclusion of segmentation methods for the pectoral muscle as well as modeling approaches for the breast boundary regions (as presented in e.g. [8,9]) to further improve the robustness of the developed method in the entire breast region.

Moreover, the clinical use case of the method needs to be investigated further. Although the proposed measure is invariant with respect dose as it depends on contrast rather than signal strength (see eq. (2)), contrast may be influenced to some extent by the choice of tube voltage. This may allow to use the proposed method as an additional feature for the optimization of individualized image acquisition parameter settings. At the same time, visual comparisons to existing breast density assessment solutions [8] show that the information derived from the proposed method contains additional or even complementary aspects.

Hence, larger observer studies with more images and experienced observers are needed to investigate and demonstrate usability and benefit of the approach for automated image acquisition parameter optimization and as an adjunct to mammographic breast density assessment in daily clinical routine.

References

1. Berg, W.A., Gutierrez, L., NessAiver, M.S., et al.: Diagnostic accuracy of mammography, clinical examination, US, and MR imaging in preoperative assessment of breast cancer. Radiology 233(3), 830–849 (2004)
2. Burgess, A.E.: Mammographic structure: data preparation and spatial statistics analysis. In: Hanson, K.M. (ed.) Proc. SPIE, Medical Imaging 1999, vol. 3661, pp. 642–653 (1999)
3. Burgess, A.E., Jacobson, F.L., Judy, P.F.: Human observer detection experiments with mammograms and power-law noise. Med. Phys. 28(4), 419–437 (2001)
4. D'Orsi, C.J., Bassett, L.W., Berg, W.A., et al.: BI-RADS: Mammography. In: D'Orsi, C.J., Mendelson, E.B., Ikeda, D.M., et al. (eds.) Breast Imaging Reporting and Data System: ACR BI-RADS - Breast Imaging Atlas, 4th edn. American College of Radiology, Reston (2003)
5. Engstrom, E., Reiser, I., Nishikawa, R.: Comparison of power spectra for tomosynthesis projections and reconstructed images. Med. Phys. 36(5), 1753–1758 (2009)
6. Fredenberg, E., Svensson, B., Danielsson, M., et al.: Optimization of mammography with respect to anatomical noise. In: Pelc, N.J., Samei, E., Nishikawa, R.M. (eds.) Proc. SPIE, Medical Imaging 2011, vol. 7961, p. 796112 (2011)
7. Gram, I., Bremnes, Y., Ursin, G., et al.: Percentage density, Wolfe's and Tabar's mammographic patterns: agreement and association with risk factors for breast cancer. Breast Cancer Res. 7(5), R854–R861 (2005)
8. Heese, H., Erhard, K., Goossen, A.: Fully-automatic breast density assessment from full field digital mammograms. In: Tanner, C., et al. (eds.) Proc. BIA 2011, pp. 113–120. Dept. of Computer Science (DIKU), University of Copenhagen (2011)
9. Heese, H.S., Erhard, K., Goossen, A., et al.: Robust estimation of mammographic breast density: a patient-based approach. In: Haynor, D.R., Ourselin, S. (eds.) Proc. SPIE, Medical Imaging 2012, vol. 8314, p. 83140T (2012)
10. Heine, J.J., Velthuizen, R.P.: Spectral analysis of full field digital mammography data. Med. Phys. 29(5), 647–661 (2002)
11. Houssami, N., Kerlikowske, K.: The impact of breast density on breast cancer risk and breast screening. Curr. Breast Cancer Rep. (in print, 2012)
12. Li, H., Giger, M.L., Olopade, O.I., et al.: Power spectral analysis of mammographic parenchymal patterns for breast cancer risk assessment. J. Digit. Imaging 21(2), 145–152 (2008)
13. McCormack, V.A., dos Santos Silva, I.: Breast density and parenchymal patterns as markers of breast cancer risk: A meta-analysis. Cancer Epidem. Biomar. 15(6), 1159–1169 (2006)
14. Stahl, M., Aach, T., Dippel, S.: Digital radiography enhancement by nonlinear multiscale processing. Med. Phys. 27(1), 56–65 (2000)
15. Wolfe, J.N.: Breast patterns as an index of risk for developing breast cancer. Am. J. Roentgenol. 126(6), 1130–1137 (1976)

Adapting Breast Density Classification from Digitized to Full-Field Digital Mammograms

Meritxell Tortajada[1], Arnau Oliver[1], Robert Martí[1], Mariona Vilagran[2], Sergi Ganau[2], Lidia Tortajada[2], Melcior Sentís[2], and Jordi Freixenet[1]

[1] Computer Vision and Robotics,
University of Girona, Girona, Spain
txell@eia.udg.edu
[2] Department of Breast and Gynecological Radiology,
UDIAT-Diagnostic Center, Parc Taulí Corporation, Sabadell, Spain

Abstract. Mammographic density is strongly associated with breast cancer, being considered one of the most important risk indicators for the development of this type of disease. Likewise, the sensitivity of automatic breast lesion detection systems is significantly dependent on breast tissue characteristics. Therefore, the measurement of density is definitely useful for detecting breast cancer. The aim of this work is to adapt our previously developed automatic breast tissue density classification methodology for digitized mammograms to full-field digital mammograms (FFDM), as well as to evaluate the possible improvements and the classification results. After breast area extraction and peripheral enhancement, the method segments the breast area into fatty and dense tissue, then morphological and texture features from each class are extracted and finally FFDM are classified according to a standard qualitative criteria. Results show a strong correlation ($\kappa = 0.88$) between automatic and expert assessments and a better classification correction percentage (CCP = 92%) compared to our earlier work.

Keywords: Breast density classification, full-field digital mammography, feature extraction and selection, peripheral enhancement.

1 Introduction

Mammographic density represents the amount of radiodense tissue within the breast and it is one of the strongest risk factors for breast cancer. Most of the studies about the relationship between breast density and breast cancer report that women with high dense breast have greater risk of breast cancer than those with low dense breast [2]. Besides risk of developing breast cancer, density is also related to the difficulty of detecting breast cancer [13]. The latest studies show that even though breast density does not affect the sensitivity of microcalcification detection Computer Aided Detection (CAD) systems, it significantly affects mass detection, so the sensitivity of CAD systems for mass detection decreases

A.D.A. Maidment, P.R. Bakic, and S. Gavenonis (Eds.): IWDM 2012, LNCS 7361, pp. 561–568, 2012.

in dense mammograms [15]. Therefore, breast density assessment is regarded as an important tool to help radiologists and CAD systems to detect breast cancer.

Mammographic density can be measured both quantitatively and qualitatively. Quantitative studies use the estimation of the percentage of breast density (dense area divided by total area), the absolute dense area or the breast density volume [8]. Whereas for qualitative assessment, the Wolfe categories, the Tabár grade or the Breast Imaging Reporting and Data System (BIRADS) score [12] can be used. However, BIRADS classification is becoming a standard on the evaluation of mammographic density where four patterns are used: (I) the breast is almost entirely fat ($< 25\%$ glandular), (II) there are scattered fibroglandular densities ($25 - 50\%$ glandular), (III) the breast tissue is heterogeneously dense ($51 - 75\%$ glandular) and (IV) the breast tissue is extremely dense ($> 75\%$ glandular).

We have previously presented a breast tissue density classification methodology for digitized mammograms [14]. The main purposes of this work are to extend our method for digitized mammograms to FFDM, to assess the benefits of the updates, and finally to classify digital mammograms according to the BIRADS score.

2   Original Methodology

The classification method is based on our previously developed algorithm for breast tissue density classification [14]. The original method consisted in: (1) preprocessing, (2) segmentation in fatty and dense tissue, (3) feature extraction from both classes, and (4) classification according to BIRADS categories.

(1) **Preprocessing:** During the preprocessing step, the breast skin-line and the pectoral muscle are detected using the approach of Kwok et al. [11]. Mammograms are divided in breast area, background and pectoral muscle, and only the breast area is kept.
(2) **Segmentation:** Gray-level information in combination with the fuzzy C-means (FCM) clustering approach is used to group the pixels of the breast area into fatty and dense tissue classes.
(3) **Feature extraction:** Once the breast area is divided into two classes, a set of morphological and texture features for fatty and dense tissue are extracted. As morphological features, the relative area and the first four moments of the histogram are calculated and as texture features, the ones derived from co-occurrence matrices.
(4) **Classification:** BIRADS classification of mammograms is performed using three classifiers: K-Nearest Neighbor (KNN), the C4.5 decision tree and a Bayesian classifier based on the combination of KNN and C4.5.

3   Updated Methodology

Although the general idea of the methodology is preserved, some changes have been done to adapt the method to FFDM. The main differences are: (1) a peripheral enhancement is applied during the preprocessing stage and (2) additional feature selection techniques and classifiers are tested during the classification stage.

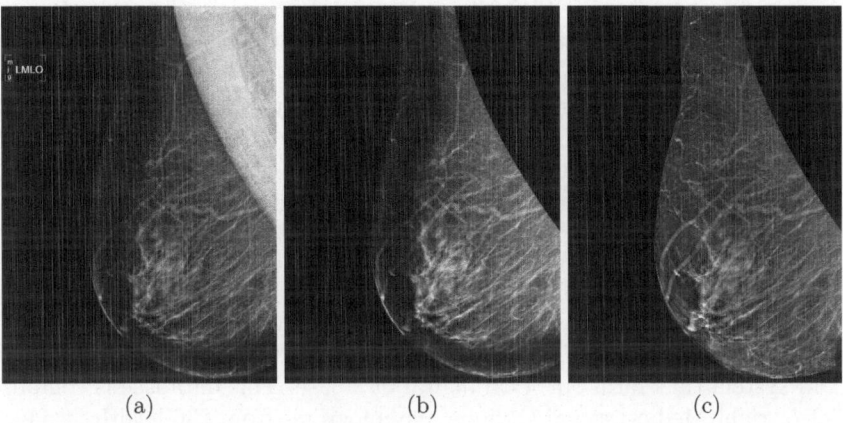

(a)   (b)   (c)

Fig. 1. Example of the preprocessing process: (a) original image, (b) breast area segmentation and (c) peripheral enhancement

3.1 Peripheral Enhancement

The first results of the FCM segmentation were not accurate enough due to the presence of an overexposed area in the majority of mammograms (see Fig. 1(a)-(b) and Fig. 2(a)). This is a known issue that happens during mammographic acquisition because of breast thickness changes. During mammographic acquisitions, breast is compressed with a tilting compression paddle, so the breast thickness can be non uniform, being lower in the periphery and overexposing this area. We decided to compensate the thickness variations in the periphery of the breast by a peripheral enhancement method that is similar to the work of Karssemeijer et al. [10] but using a multiplicative model. After extracting the breast boundary and the pectoral muscle, the overexposed area is determined by Otsu's thresholding and a correction factor is applied over each pixel of the detected region. To calculate the correction factor, firstly a distance map is generated using the distance from each point (x) in a mammogram (M) to the breast skin line. From the furthest peripheral pixel to the closest, each pixel value $M(x)$ at distance i is divided by the mean value of its neighborhood at distance i $(N_i(x))$ and multiplied by the mean value of its neighborhood at distance $i+1$ $(N_{i+1}(x))$, where $N_i(x) = \{t \in M \ at \ distance \ i : distance(t,x) \leq k\}$, being k an experimentally set parameter (100 for our case). An example of the overall process can be seen in Fig.1.

3.2 Feature Selection and Classification

Due to the large number of features, a feature-selection step is included selecting the most effective subset of features. Various feature selection techniques are evaluated (using WEKA [18] data mining software) such as Principal Component Analysis [9], Gain Ratio attribute evaluation [17] or Support Vector Machine (SVM) [6]. The classification of mammograms according to BIRADS categories is also performed with WEKA. We used more recent classifiers like Random Forest [3] or SVM [4] and some combinations of classifiers as AdaBoost [5] or a binary tree of SVM. The binary tree consists in firstly, classification of digital mammograms in low or high breast density category and then low dense cases are classified in BIRADS I or II and independently, high dense cases in BIRADS III or IV. The reason was to convert our multiclass classification problem into multiple binary classification problems as SVM is originally a binary classifier [1].

4   Results

The method was applied to the whole set of 236 FFDM acquired with a Selenia FFDM system that form our local digital database. This database is composed of left or right Medio-Lateral Oblique mammograms from 236 healthy women.

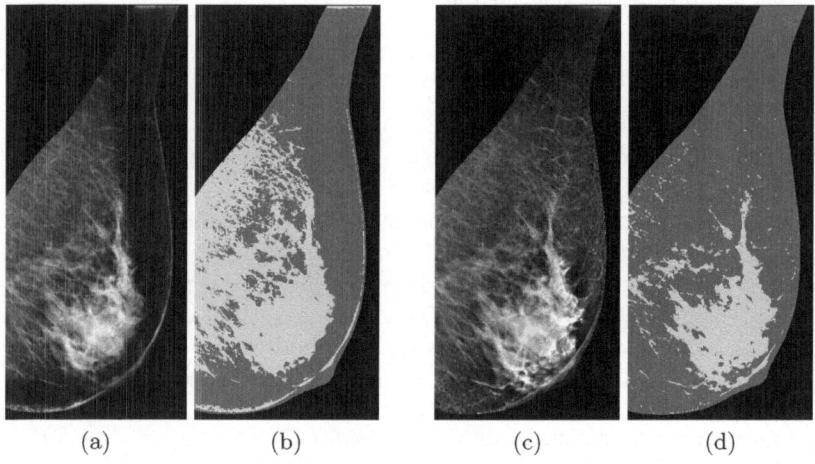

(a)   (b)   (c)   (d)

Fig. 2. Example of the segmentation process: (a) original breast area, (b) FCM without previous peripheral enhancement, (c) breast area after peripheral enhancement and (c) FCM with previous peripheral enhancement.

4.1   Preprocessing and Segmentation

To determine not only the quality of the preprocessed images but also the segmentation results, visual assessment was performed by one observer with more than 10 years of experience in mammographic images. To evaluate the enhancement process, the observer labeled the images as correctly enhanced or not and a total of 83% of the images were considered to be improved with the peripheral enhancement. An example of the enhancement results can be seen in Fig. 1(c). To assess the segmentation improvements, the observer evaluated the differences in the segmentation results when images were enhanced or not. Around 92% of the segmentations obtained after image enhancement were considered similar or better than the ones obtained before enhancement. Specifically, the 45% were regarded as strictly better, therefore results show that there is a clear improvement in the segmentation results when images are previously peripheral enhanced (see Fig. 2).

4.2   Classification

Experts Classification. Four expert mammographic readers classified all the images using BIRADS (current readers are different from the ones that participated in the study [14]). The ground truth was determined by majority vote. In case of tie, the median value was considered as the consensus opinion (like in [14]).

Table 1(A)-(D) shows the confusion matrices for the classification of FFDM for the four readers and the consensus opinion in year 2011. Like in our previous work [14], the results show an evident interobserver variability, illustrating the difficulty of the breast tissue density classification task. In low dense breasts categories {BIRADS I & II}, expert B tends to classify in BIRADS I (17 mammograms were classified as BIRADS I being BIRADS II) whereas experts C and D tend to classify in BIRADS II (31 and 34 mammograms respectively were classified as BIRADS II being BIRADS I). Note also that expert B repeats this underestimation assignment when classifying in BIRADS II (8 mammograms were classified as BIRADS II being BIRADS III) and expert C repeats the overestimation appointment when classifying in BIRADS III (11 mammograms were classified as BIRADS III being BIRADS II). In high dense categories {BIRADS III & IV}, expert D differs from the rest considering a few BIRADS III mammograms (18/46) and a lot of BIRADS IV (27 mammograms were classified as BIRADS IV being BIRADS III). When considering the individual BIRADS classes, the correct classification percentage (CCP) values for expert A are really high (99%, 98%, 85%, 100%, respectively). The results of the other experts are less homogeneous and lower, except for expert C in BIRADS III with CCP = 91%. Using the Cohen's kappa coefficient (κ) values, the agreement of expert A with the consensus opinion belongs to the *almost perfect* category ($\kappa = 0.94$) whereas the agreement of experts B, C and D with the consensus opinion belong to the *substantial* category ($\kappa = 0.78, 0.70, 0.61$ respectively).

Furthermore, a few years ago, one of the experts classified the same database according to BIRADS. Table 1(D)-(E) shows the confusion matrices for the classification of FFDM for one reader and the consensus opinion, in two different periods of time. Results reveal intraobserver variability in BIRADS II and III classification. In the past the reader classified 88 mammograms as BIRADS II whereas now the number increases to 120. On the other hand, 52 mammograms were considered BIRADS III opposite to the current 20. Examining each class, there are no significant variations in CCP values for BIRADS I (before: 58%, after: 60%), BIRADS III (before: 37%, after: 39%), and BIRADS IV (before: 94%, after: 100%), opposite to the CCP values for BIRADS II (before: 59%, after:97%).

Table 1. (A)-(D) Confusion matrices for four expert radiologists and their consensus opinion and (E) confusion matrix for one expert radiologist and the consensus opinion in 2005.

		Expert A (Year 2011) $\kappa = 0.94$ $CCP = 96\%$				Expert B (Year 2011) $\kappa = 0.78$ $CCP = 86\%$				Expert C (Year 2011) $\kappa = 0.70$ $CCP = 79\%$				Expert D (Year 2011) $\kappa = 0.61$ $CCP = 73\%$				Expert D (Year 2005) $\kappa = 0.41$ $CCP = 57\%$			
		I	II	III	IV	I	II	III	IV	I	II	III	IV	I	II	III	IV	I	II	III	IV
Consensus	I	84	1	0	0	85	0	0	0	54	31	0	0	51	34	0	0	49	36	0	0
	II	1	86	1	0	17	67	4	0	0	77	11	0	0	85	2	1	0	52	35	1
	III	0	0	39	7	0	8	36	2	0	2	42	2	0	1	18	27	0	0	17	29
	IV	0	0	0	17	0	0	4	13	0	0	3	14	0	0	0	17	1	0	0	16

        (A)   (B)   (C)   (D)   (E)

Automatic Classification. To evaluate our algorithm, we used a leave-one-out methodology, i.e., each digital mammogram is analyzed by a classifier trained using the mammograms of all other women in the database. Table 2(C) shows the best confusion matrix after analyzing different feature selection and classification methods. Specifically the confusion matrix is obtained using SVM feature selection followed by binary tree of SVM classification and this combination achieved a κ of 0.88 and a CCP of 92% (216/236). These values are higher than the values of experts B, C and D although they are lower than the ones of the expert A. When considering each BIRADS classes, the CCP for BIRADS I is 93% (79/85), for BIRADS II is 89% (78/88), for BIRADS III is 93% (43/46) and for BIRADS IV is 94% (16/17). Note that BIRADS III reaches the highest CCP value in comparison with the ones reached by the experts (A: 85%, B: 78%, C: 91%, D: 39%).

Table 2. Confusion matrices for MIAS, DDSM and digital databases classification and their respectively consensus opinion: (A) Bayesian combination of KNN and C4.5 classifiers in MIAS, (B) Bayesian combination of KNN and C4.5 classifiers in DDSM and (C) SVM Selection (SVS) + Binary Tree of SVM classification (BTSVC) in digital database.

		Bayesian MIAS $\kappa = 0.81$ $CCP = 86\%$				Bayesian DDSM $\kappa = 0.67$ $CCP = 77\%$				SVS + BTSVC $\kappa = 0.88$ $CCP = 92\%$			
		I	II	III	IV	I	II	III	IV	I	II	III	IV
Consensus	I	79	1	3	4	58	25	23	0	79	6	0	0
	II	3	86	6	8	15	295	26	0	5	78	5	0
	III	0	2	85	8	12	46	196	1	0	2	43	1
	IV	0	6	4	27	5	18	18	93	0	0	1	16

        (A)   (B)   (C)

Table 2(A)-(B) also shows the best confusion matrices of our work in [14]. In this case the used classifier was a Bayesian combination of KNN and C4.5 classifiers and the classification method was tested using two public databases: the Mammographic Image Analysis (MIAS) database [16] and the Digital Database for Screening Mammography (DDSM) [7] which were obtained from scanned or digitized film images. Although a direct comparison with our previous results is difficult because the datasets used are different, in principle, the confusion matrix of the digital database (Table 2(C)) seems to be better than the others because there are less non-zeros off-diagonal elements. When comparing κ and CCP values in digital and digitized databases ($\kappa = 0.81$, CCP $= 86\%$ (277/322) for MIAS and $\kappa = 0.67$, CCP $= 77\%$ (642/831) for DDSM), they are slightly better in the digital case. Examining the individual BIRADS classes, the CCP for MIAS data set were 91%, 84%, 89% and 73% (respectively) and for DDSM were 55%, 88%, 77% and 69% (respectively). All these values are also somewhat better in the digital case (93%, 89%, 93% and 94%), although the highest difference is in BIRADS IV. Using the two-class classification (low vs high density), the CCP for low case is 97% for digital, 89% for MIAS and 89% for DDSM, whereas for high case is 97% for digital, 94% for MIAS and 79% for DDSM, so in both cases, the percentage is higher for digital database. These results make explicit the improvement reached with the updated method.

5   Conclusions

We have provided a breast density classification method that can be applied to both digitized and digital mammograms. For our digital database we obtained a κ of 0.88 and a CCP of 92% that represents a better agreement in 3 out of 4 radiologists. Results are also better than our previous work using MIAS and DDSM, which indicates that the included changes improve the overall method. In the future, we plan to work in two directions: (1) although the segmentation results are qualitatively better when including peripheral enhancement, other segmentation algorithms will be investigated; and (2) regions of interest will be described using other texture features.

Acknowledgment. M. Tortajada holds a UdG grant BRGR10-04. This work was partially supported by the Spanish Science and Innovation grant TIN2011-23704.

References

1. Allwein, E.L., Schapire, R.E., Singer, Y.: Reducing multiclass to binary: A unifying approach for margin classifiers. J. Mach. Learn. Res. 1, 113–141 (2000)
2. Boyd, N.F., Lockwood, G.A., Byng, J.W., Tritchler, D.L., Yaffe, M.J.: Mammographic densities and breast cancer risk. Cancer Epidem. Biomarkers Prev. 7(12), 1133–1144 (1998)
3. Breiman, L.: Random forests. Mach. Learn. 45(1), 5–32 (2001)

4. Cortes, C., Vapnik, V.: Support-vector networks. Mach. Learn. 20(3), 273–297 (1995)
5. Freund, Y., Schapire, R.E.: Experiments with a new boosting algorithm. In: Int. Conf. Mach. Learn. / Conf. Uncert. Art. Intell. / Conf. Learn. Theory, pp. 148–156 (1996)
6. Guyon, I., Weston, J., Barnhill, S., Vapnik, V.: Gene selection for cancer classification using support vector machines. Mach. Learn. 46, 389–422 (2002)
7. Heath, M., Bowyer, K., Kopans, D., Moore, R., Kegelmeyer, P.J.: The Digital Database for Screening Mammography. In: Int. Work. Dig. Mammography, pp. 212–218 (2000)
8. Highnam, R., Brady, S.M., Yaffe, M.J., Karssemeijer, N., Harvey, J.: Robust Breast Composition Measurement - Volpara^{TM}. In: Martí, J., Oliver, A., Freixenet, J., Martí, R. (eds.) IWDM 2010. LNCS, vol. 6136, pp. 342–349. Springer, Heidelberg (2010)
9. Jolliffe, I.T.: Principal Component Analysis, 2nd edn. Springer (2002)
10. Karssemeijer, N., te Brake, G.M.: Combining single view features and asymmetry for detection of mass lesions. In: Int. Work. Dig. Mammography, pp. 95–102 (1998)
11. Kwok, S.M., Chandrasekhar, R., Attikiouzel, Y., Rickard, M.T.: Automatic pectoral muscle segmentation on mediolateral oblique view mammograms. IEEE Trans. Med. Imag. 23(9), 1129–1140 (2004)
12. American College of Radiology. Illustrated Breast Imaging Reporting and Data System BIRADS, 3rd edn. American College of Radiology (1998)
13. Oliver, A., Freixenet, J., Martí, J., Pérez, E., Pont, J., Denton, E.R.E., Zwiggelaar, R.: A review of automatic mass detection and segmentation in mammographic images. Med. Image Anal. 14(2), 87–110 (2010)
14. Oliver, A., Freixenet, J., Martí, R., Pont, J., Pérez, E., Denton, E.R.E., Zwiggelaar, R.: A novel breast tissue density classification methodology. IEEE Trans. Inform. Technol. Biomed. 12(1), 55–65 (2008)
15. Romero, C., Varela, C., Cuena, R., Almenar, A., Pinto, J.M., Botella, M.: Impact of mammographic breast density on computer-assisted detection (CAD) in a breast imaging department. Radiología 53(5), 456–461 (2011)
16. Suckling, J., Parker, J., Dance, D.R., Astley, S.M., Hutt, I., Boggis, C.R.M., Ricketts, I., Stamatakis, E., Cerneaz, N., Kok, S.L., Taylor, P., Betal, D., Savage, J.: The Mammographic Image Analysis Society digital mammogram database. In: Int. Work. Dig. Mammography, pp. 211–221 (1994)
17. Witten, I.H., Frank, E.: Data Mining Pactical Machine Learning Tools and Technique, 3rd edn. Morgan Kaufmann (2005)
18. Witten, I.H., Frank, E., Hall, M.A.: Data Mining: Practical machine learning tools and techniques, 3rd edn. Morgan Kaufmann (2011)

Improvements and Performance of Diagnostic Compositional Imaging Using a Novel Dual-Energy X-ray Technique

Fred Duewer[1], Chris I. Flowers[1], Karla Kerlikowske[2], Serghei Malkov[1],
Bonnie N. Joe[1], and John A. Shepherd[1]

[1] University of California, San Francisco: Department of Radiology
[2] University of California, San Francisco: Department of Medicine and Epidemiology
Frederick.duewer@ucsf.edu

Abstract. Determine whether or not improvements to the calibration procedure for a novel dual-energy x-ray mammography technique improve the uniformity, accuracy, and/or reproducibility of the measured breast composition. The long-term goal of this project is to develop a technique that will improve the specificity of mammography diagnosis. Energy dependent corrections for light-field, dark-field, and Heel effect were made for each measurement. A total of 20 women who were scheduled for additional imaging prior to biopsy underwent an additional dual-energy/low dose full-field digital mammography scan as part of a pilot study investigating the use of breast composition measures in mammography. The estimated water/lipid/protein content of suspicious lesions were measured. The modified x-ray calibration procedure resulted in over a 3-fold improvement in the uniformity of a flat-field calibration phantom with known breast density. Some preliminary results from women are available and show that different types of breast lesions have different compositions.

Keywords: mammography, dual-energy x-ray imaging, breast cancer.

1 Introduction

Since 2002, cancer has been the leading cause of death in US adults under 85 years old, and breast cancer is the most prevalent cancer among women accounting for 31% of all cancers (1). In 2005 alone, there were an estimated 200,000+ new breast cancer cases diagnosed in the US and 41,000 deaths from breast cancer second only to lung cancer. X-ray mammography is currently the primary diagnostic tool for early breast cancer detection. However, one third of all women who are screened with mammography have abnormal results even though no breast cancer is present increasing the cost of mammographic screening by 33% (2). Thus, there is an urgent need for techniques to decrease false positive results while maintaining high sensitivity. Newer methods being evaluated to improve mammographic sensitivity and specificity include the use of intravenous (IV) contrast such as iodine dual-energy methods to

A.D.A. Maidment, P.R. Bakic, and S. Gavenonis (Eds.): IWDM 2012, LNCS 7361, pp. 569–574, 2012.

increase the contrast of breast lesions (3). But IV contrast procedures have limited applicability because of potentially severe side effects associated with iodine-based contrast agents (4) and because they increase the cost of mammography and would require the presence of a radiologist at the time of imaging. In addition, IV contrast may potentially turn well women off screening if they are averse to injections.

We have developed a dual-energy x-ray mammography technique that allows the estimation of the lipid, water, and protein content of the breast. The technique is based on the measurement of the low-energy x-ray attenuation (standard screening mammography image), the high-energy x-ray attenuation (high-energy x-ray mammography image in combination with three millimeter aluminum filter), and the breast thickness using a geometric phantom (Figure 1) and software code used to model the breast edges. Given these three independent measurements, and the assumption that the density of water, lipid, and protein remain constant in the breast, the water, lipid, and protein content of the breast may be estimated independently.

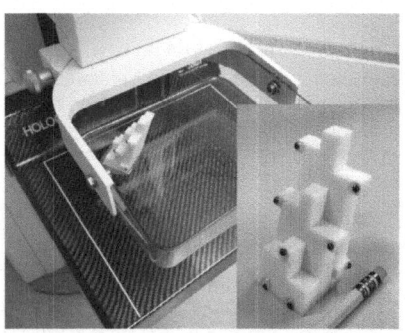

Fig. 1. Image of geometric used for breast thickness estimation

While theoretically straightforward, developing a method enabling accurate estimation of the water, lipid, and protein content has been challenging because of both temporal and spatial variations in the performance of the mammography system. The largest source of error that we have observed is spatial dependence of the detector illumination owing to spatial and temporal variation of the system properties. To remove spatial dependence in detector illumination, we have developed a multistep calibration procedure that removes spatial variations in both illumination and x-ray spectrum. That work is described in this manuscript.

2   Methods

A 3-compartment compositional model was defined for the breast using specific compositional definitions. First, the mass of the breast was defined to be exclusively composed of protein, lipid, and water with all other residual components (soft-tissue mineral, glycogen, etc.) representing less than 1% of breast mass (5). For each compartment, well-described stoichiometries that others have found to be representative of human compositional compartments (6) were used: water without salinity (H_2O), standard protein, $C_{100}H_{159}N_{26}O_{32}S_{0.7}$ (7,8), human fatty acid, $C_{51}H_{98}O_6$, and soft tissue mineral as calcium hydroxyapatite ($[Ca_3(PO_4)_2]_3Ca(OH)_2$). Phantom materials were chosen that mimicked the X-ray attenuation properties in the mammographic range (10-50 keV) of the above molecules using standard techniques and tables. We found that solid water (CIRS, Inc, Norfolk, VA), machinable wax for lipid (McMaster Carr, Inc, Elmhurst, IL), and Delrin plastic as protein (McMaster Carr) were good approximations for X-ray imaging. Following previous work, (9) the three mass components were solved assuming the following three measures were known: tissue thickness, and two X-ray attenuations at a low and high-energy. For example, the low-energy attenuation equation is written as:

$$A_{LE} = \ln\left(\frac{I}{I_0}\right)_{LE} = \ln\left(\int_{E_{1,LE}}^{E_{2,LE}} I_0^{'}(E)\exp\left(-\mu_w(E)t_w - \mu_p(E)t_p - \mu_f(E)t_f\right)dE \right) \tag{1}$$

A similar equation can be derived for the high-energy attenuation, AHE. Lastly, the sum of the three compositional thicknesses, T, equals the total thickness of tissue projected into a pixel. T is found using the SXA phantom method as described in (10,11). Prior work demonstrated the ability to separately estimate the water, lipid, and protein content of breast tissue. (11)

2.1   Imaging Procedure

The low-energy x-ray attenuation was obtained from a standard screening mammogram. The high-energy x-ray attenuation was obtained from a high-energy mammogram taken immediately after the standard screening mammogram without releasing the patient's breast from the compression paddle. The x-ray acceleration voltage for the mammogram was 39 kVp and the exposure was 40 µAs. A 3 mm thick aluminum filter was added to filter out low-energy x-ray from the high-energy mammogram. The high-energy mammogram increased the dose by roughly 10% compared to a standard mammogram. All images were taken on a Hologic Selenia digital mammography unit.

2.2   Analysis Procedure

The pioneering work described in Laidevant et al estimated low-energy and high-energy x-ray attenuation using spatially constant detector offsets and light-field corrections. Unfortunately, spatial variations in detector offset, x-ray illumination over the detector, and x-ray spectrum resulted in significant non-uniformity (>10%) across the field of view for estimates of water, lipid, and protein content of a plastic calibration phantom. This nonuniformity is problematic for estimation of lesion composition because the typical lesion comprises less than 20% of breast thickness and lesion protein content is expected to comprise less than 10% of that lesion thickness.

We developed a calibration procedure to remove this nonuniformity. Quantitative estimates of low-energy and high-energy x-ray attenuation were obtained in the following fashion. First, local variations in the detector offset were measured. The detector offset with no x-ray exposure across the entire CCD was measured three times and the average exposure value for each pixel was selected. This detector offset image was subtracted from detector results. Second, local variations in the average x-ray intensity, detector sensitivity, and x-ray incidence angle were measured using a uniform four centimeter thick phantom chosen to have 50% breast density (CIRS) at the voltages chosen for the low-energy and high-energy mammograms. For each measured image, the total image attenuation relative to the four centimeter thick phantom was estimated by taking the ratio of the measured image to the appropriate light field image. Finally, spatial variations owing to changes in the x-ray incident angle in the x-ray spectrum were compensated by measurement of the incremental attenuation from a uniform one centimeter thick phantom applied to the four centimeter phantom. The measured incremental attenuation was normalized to the estimated attenuation in a two centimeter strip adjacent to the breast edge. The measured normalized incremental attenuation was smoothed using a five pixel Gaussian filter and applied to the measured relative attenuation from each patient image.

2.3   Patient Population

Twenty women scheduled for repeat imaging with suspicious mammography findings were recruited and imaged with 3-component breast imaging before their biopsies. Four had no mammographically identifiable findings and were excluded. In addition, two women did not generate usable data owing to irretrievable protocol failures. Of the 14 remaining women, 18 lesions were identified by a trained radiologist. Of those findings, three CC (cranio-caudal) and one MLO (mediolateral-oblique) view were excluded either because of poor compositional results owing to proximity to the breast edge or because of superposition of the chest wall. Of those four lesions, only one was not available in the other view direction and was excluded. The results for CC and MLO views were averaged for those lesions for which both views were available. Seventeen lesions had usable findings. There were 4 benign breast tissue findings (BBT), 7 fibroadenomas (FA), 2 ductal carcinoma-in-situ (DCIS), and 4 intraducal carcinoma (IDC). This study was conducted with approval from the Institutional Review Board at the University of California, San Francisco. All women received both CC and MLO views of the affected breast or breasts. All received a biopsy of the suspicious area and breast biopsies were clinically reviewed by our Pathology Department. Inclusion Criteria: Only women receiving a breast biopsy were included in the study. Exclusion Criteria: Women with prior biopsy of the affected breast or history of breast cancer were excluded from the study. In addition, findings that were on the breast edge were excluded from the analysis because the thickness model used for the analysis was not sufficiently accurate at the breast edge. Finally, images with no mammographically identifiable region of interest that could be delineated by the

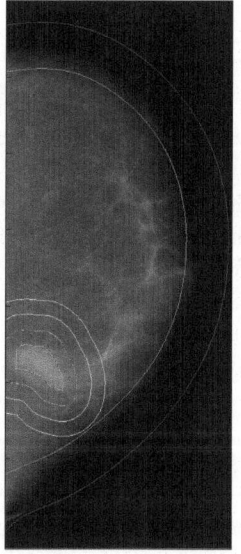

Fig. 2. Delineated regions for patient with invasive ductal cancer. The innermost region indicates the cancer and the region surrounding the region immediately surrounding the cancer indicates the chosen background region.

radiologist were excluded from the analysis. All lesions were delineated by an experienced MQSA certified radiologist. Lesion composition was estimated as the difference between the median value inside the delineated lesion and the median value in the region 2.5 to 5 millimeters distant from the edge of the delineated lesion.

Table 1. Average lesion compositions (5th - 95th %centiles shown in brackets). Negative values indicate the compartment is below the surrounding tissue averages.

Finding (n)	Water(cm)	Protein (cm)	Lipid (cm)
Invasive cancer(n=4)	0.19	0.21	-0.46
	(-0.17-0.62)	(-0.03-0.77)	(-0.88—0.15)
Ductal carcinoma in situ (n=2)	0.31	0.038	-0.34
	(0.095-0.52)	(0.00-0.075)	(-0.53—0.16)
FA (n=7)	0.83	0.096	-1.03
	(0.11-1.80)	(-0.13-0.47)	(-1.88—0.097)
BBT (n=4)	0.19	0.22	-0.46
	(-0.17-0.62)	(-0.027-0.77)	(-0.88--0.16)

3   Results

Breast thickness uniformity was determined using a four centimeter plastic calibration phantom of known composition. Images were taken using the standard three-component image protocol described above and analyzed using both the prior image protocol and the newly implemented protocol. The spatial uniformity was measured corner to corner.

$$Uniformity = \frac{T_{max} - T_{min}}{T_{max} + T_{min}} * 100 \qquad (2)$$

where T_{max} is the highest measured compositional thickness and T_{min} is the lowest measured compositional thickness on a line drawn corner to corner in the image. The spatial uniformity of the water, lipid, and protein measurement improved from >10% to <3% for a uniform plastic calibration phantom designed to mimic breast tissue.

We categorized findings as either benign (fibroadenoma, benign breast tissue) or malignant (invasive cancer, DCIS) findings and then constructed a logistic model. To reduce sample-size dependent bias and eliminate complete separation problems, we used Firth's method to reduce likelihood bias.(12) We found that the Beta coefficient (the regression coefficient and intercepts) for lesion water content was close to statistically significant even at this small sample size (P=0.064).

4   Discussion

Improvements to the breast thickness model and to the x-ray calibration procedure resulted in significant improvement to both the accuracy of the thickness measure and the spatial uniformity of the compositional estimate. We are encouraged by the low P-value with this limited sample size and expect that further data acquisition will better characterize the biological variance in different lesion types and improve the predictive models. In addition, larger sample number will allow the incorporation of lesion characteristics that are typically indicative of malignancy, such as calcifications.

Potential advantages associated with improved visualization of the protein compartment include fewer missed cancers, clearer visualization of subtle structures used to differentiate benign and malignant lesions (e.g. spiculations) and thus reductions in false positive findings and screening cost. The image acquisition, analysis, and reconstruction techniques used in FFDCM could be integrated into existing FFDM units following inexpensive modifications. With the infrastructure necessary for the implementation of FFDM largely in place, the application of compositional imaging to clinical studies would be swift.

References

1. Jemal, A., Siegel, R., Ward, E., Murray, T., Xu, J., Smigal, C., Thun, M.J.: Cancer statistics. CA Cancer J. Clin. 56(2), 106–130 (2006)
2. Elmore, J.G., Barton, M.B., Moceri, V.M., Polk, S., Arena, P.J., Fletcher, S.W.: Ten-year risk of false positive screening mammograms and clinical breast examinations. N. Engl. J. Med. 338(16), 1089–1096 (1998)
3. Dromain, C., Balleyguier, C., Adler, G., Garbay, J.R., Delaloge, S.: Contrast-enhanced digital mammography. Eur. J. Radiol. 69(1), 34–42 (2009)
4. Mishkin, M.M.: Contrast media safety: what do we know and how do we know it? Am. J. Cardiol. 66(14), 34F–36F (1990)
5. Allison, D.B., Zannolli, R., Faith, M.S., Heo, M., Pietrobelli, A., VanItallie, T.B., Pi-Sunyer, F.X., Heymsfield, S.B.: Weight loss increases and fat loss decreases all-cause mortality rate: results from two independent cohort studies. Int. J. Obes. Relat. Metab. Disord. 23(6), 603–611 (1999)
6. Wang, Z.M., Heshka, S., Pierson Jr., R.N., Heymsfield, S.B.: Systematic organization of body-composition methodology: an overview with emphasis on component-based methods. Am. J. Clin. Nutr. 61(3), 457–465 (1995)
7. Heymsfield, S.B., Waki, M., Kehayias, J., Lichtman, S., Dilmanian, F.A., Kamen, Y., Wang, J., Pierson, R.N.: Chemical and Elemental Analysis of Humans Invivo Using Improved Body-Composition Models. American Journal of Physiology 261(2), E190–E198 (1991)
8. Yang, J., Rico, D., Augustine, B., Mawdsley, G., Yaffe, M.: An optical method for measuring compressed breast thickness. In: 6th Int. Workshop on Digital Mammography, pp. 569–573 (2002)
9. Michael, G.J., Henderson, C.J.: Monte Carlo modelling of an extended DXA technique. Phys. Med. Biol. 43(9), 2583–2596 (1998)
10. Shepherd, J.A., Herve, L., Landau, J., Fan, B., Kerlikowske, K., Cummings, S.R.: Clinical comparison of a novel breast DXA technique to mammographic density. Med. Phys. 33(5), 1490–1498 (2006)
11. Laidevant, A., Malkov, S., Au, A., Shepherd, J.A.: Dual-Energy X-Ray Absorptiometry Method Using a Full Field Digital Mammography System. In: Krupinski, E.A. (ed.) IWDM 2008. LNCS, vol. 5116, pp. 108–115. Springer, Heidelberg (2008)
12. Heinze, G., Schemper, M.: A solution to the problem of separation in logistic regression. Stat. Med. 21(16), 2409–2419 (2002)

Monte Carlo Simulation of a-Se X-ray Detectors for Breast Imaging: Effect of Nearest-Neighbor Recombination Algorithm on Swank Noise

Yuan Fang[1,2,*], Diksha Sharma[1], Andreu Badal[1],
Karim S. Karim[2], and Aldo Badano[1]

[1] Division of Imaging and Applied Mathematics,
Office of Science and Engineering Laboratories,
Center for Devices and Radiological Health, U.S. Food and Drug Administration
10903 New Hampshire Avenue, Silver Spring, MD 20993-0002
[2] Department of Electrical and Computer Engineering, University of Waterloo,
Waterloo, ON, N2L3G1
yuan.fang@fda.hhs.gov

Abstract. We study the effect on Swank noise of different recombination algorithms for secondary carriers implemented in ARTEMIS, a detailed Monte Carlo transport that simulates the three-dimensional spatial and temporal transport of electron-hole pairs in semiconductor x-ray detectors. Two modeling approaches for recombination are compared including a first-hit (FH) algorithm that recombines the first pair from the list of candidate carriers, and a more realistic nearest-neighbor algorithm (NN). We report simulated pulse-height spectra (PHS) in a Se detector for two clinical mammography spectra, and use the entire PHS distribution to calculate Swank noise. We found that the FH and NN recombination results in terms of pulse-height spectra and Swank noise agree within the mammography energy range. The NN algorithm increased the simulation time by 30% compared to FH at 4 V/μm applied bias and 10% at 30 V/μm.

Keywords: Recombination, Swank, ARTEMIS, Monte Carlo simulation, amorphous Selenium.

1 Introduction

X-ray medical imaging has grown to become one of the most widely used techniques for medical diagnosis. Digital x-ray detectors have demonstrated performance superior to traditional film-based detectors, and amorphous selenium (a-Se) direct digital x-ray detectors have shown great promise in improving performance and lowering costs. Digital imagers using stabilized a-Se as the photoconductive material can be used for a wide range of applications[1], including digitial mammgraphy[2,3].

---

* Corresponding author.

A.D.A. Maidment, P.R. Bakic, and S. Gavenonis (Eds.): IWDM 2012, LNCS 7361, pp. 575–582, 2012.

In direct digital x-ray detectors, the incident x-ray photons lead to creation of high energy electrons and large numbers of electron-hole pairs. This high concentration of oppositely charged carriers leads to recombination of many electron-hole pairs, and significantly degrades the detector performance. It has been shown that this recombination process occurs in the nanometer scale, where drift and diffusion of electron-hole pairs plays a significant role[4]. Essentially, electron-hole pairs recombine due to the Coulomb attraction of oppositely charged carriers. Practically, a high applied electric field has been used to separate the electron-hole pairs to improve detector performance. However the high electric field causes higher leakage and break down of the photoconductor. We study the effect of different recombination algorithms on Swank noise taking into account detailed Monte Carlo (MC) transport of electron-hole pairs.

2   Method

2.1   Swank Noise

The Swank factor[5], also known as the information factor is a critical performance parameter of x-ray imaging detectors[6]. Swank noise represent the statistical variation in the detected signal per primary quantum, defined as:

$$I = \frac{M_1^2}{M_0 M_2} \ . \tag{1}$$

These statistical fluctuations can be due to random events such as Compton scattering, K-fluorescence, photoelectric and Compton electron range, and transport of electron-hole pairs, where M_n is the n_{th} moment of the electron-hole pair PHS distribution:

$$M_n = \sum_m p(m) m^n \ , \tag{2}$$

and the fluctuations in m (number of detected electron-hole pairs) are given by the probability distribution, $p(m)$. In semiconductor x-ray detectors, the Swank factor, I, is a statistical factor that arises from the fluctuations in the number of electron-hole pairs detected per absorbed x-ray. Alternatively, the definitions of the mean (μ) and standard deviation (σ) of the distribution can be used to estimate I,

$$\mu = \frac{M_1}{M_0}, \sigma^2 = \frac{M_2}{M_0} - \left(\frac{M_1}{M_0}\right)^2, I = \frac{\mu^2}{\mu^2 + \sigma^2} \ . \tag{3}$$

2.2   Monte Carlo Simulations

This work utilizes a custom Monte Carlo transport code, ARTEMIS (pArticle transport, Recombination, and Trapping in sEMiconductor Imaging Simulations) specifically developed for detailed simulation of electron-hole-pair transport in direct x-ray detectors[4]. The simulation of the signal formation process in ARTEMIS is based on PENELOPE[7] for the simulation of photon and secondary-electron transport coupled with a novel transport code for the spatiotemporal simulation of electron-hole pair transport. We modeled an a-Se detector with a thickness of 150 μm with a pencil beam source.

We consider two recombination algorithms, first-hit (FH) and nearest-neighbor (NN), in the simulation model. In an array of electron-hole pairs, the FH algorithm recombines the first candidate that are within the recombition radius where the Coulomb attraction between the electron and hole are considered too strong for escape. For one carrier at a time, the NN algorithm calculate the distance between electrons and holes and recombines the pair that has the smallest distance apart. The NN algorithm provides a more accurate physical model recombining the electron and hole that is the closest to each other but requires longer simulation time. The two recombination algorithms considered in this study are described in detail in previous work[8]. The probability of recombination for electron-hole pairs, recombination fraction (f_R), is calculated as the ratio between the number of recombined and generated electron-hole pairs.

2.3   Signal Formation Process

X rays can interact with the atoms of the semiconductor material through various mechanisms. In the energy range of medical imaging applications, an incident photon can interact through the following main mechanisms: Rayleigh scattering, Compton scattering, and photoelectric absorption. The interaction cross-sections are a function of the energy and the material, and for a-Se, photoelectric absorption is the dominant photon interaction mechanism in the diagnostic energy range. In the case of photoelectric absorption, a secondary electron is created with most of the energy of the initial x ray and therefore capable of producing many electron-hole pairs. This high-energy secondary electron gradually loses energy through inelastic scattering as it travels through the detector material, and the energy lost, E_d, is deposited in the semiconductor material.

The energy deposited, E_d, in the semiconductor can lead to either phonon emission or ionization. The number of electron-hole pairs created, N_{EHP}, is modeled using a Poisson random variable utilizing a semi-empirical formula developed by Que and Rowlands[9], for the ionization energy, W_0. When an electron-hole pair is created, it has been postulated[10] that the electron and the hole lose their initial kinetic energy in a thermalization process, after which they are separated by a finite distance r_0. We defined the concept of a burst as the cloud (spatiotemporal distribution) of electrons and holes generated after a local deposition of energy given an assumed thermalization distance r_0[8]. In this work, the shape of the burst is modeled as a spherical shell.

2.4   Clinical Spectra

We used two known mammography beam qualities generated with methods described by Boone *et al.*[11] Both beam qualities are taken from the table of radiation qualities in IEC document 62220-1-2 (2007). The spectra chosen include tungsten and molybdenum anodes and a tube voltage of 28 kVp shown in Fig. 1. The molybdenum spectrum (RQA-M 2) includes a molybdenum filter of 32 μm and an additional 2 mm aluminum filter and the tungsten spectrum includes an aluminum filter of 2.5 mm.

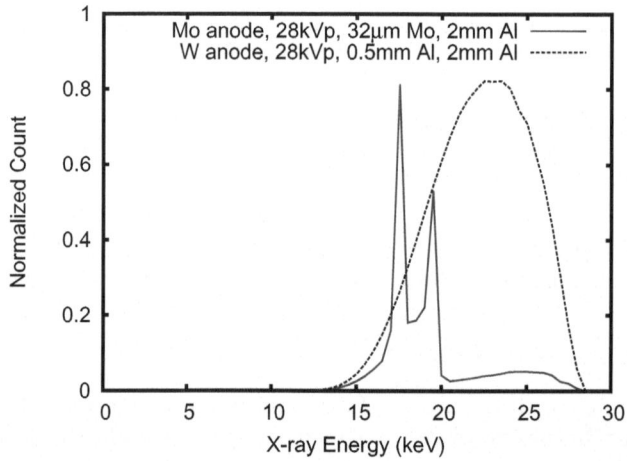

Fig. 1. Mammography beam qualities used in the Swank factor simulations

3   Results and Discussions

The simulated PHS for both radiation qualities are shown in the following figures. The x axis is in number of electron-hole pairs detected per incident x ray. For molybdenum, Fig. 2 shows the PHS for transport at 4 V/μm applied electric field with the FH and NN models, and Fig. 3 shows the PHS for transport at 30 V/μm. The Swank factor calculated from the PHS, and the recombination fraction are listed in Table 1. Comparing the two applied bias conditions, the number of detected electron-hole pairs signficantly increased from the 4 to 30 V/μm case, while maintaining the general shape of the PHS. The simulation results are comparable for the FH and NN recombination algorithms, with an increase in the simulation time from approximately 10 to 30 percent.

For tungsten, Fig. 4 shows the PHS for transport at 4 V/μm applied electric field with the FH and NN models, and Fig. 5 shows the PHS for transport at 30 V/μm. The tungsten PHS have higher Swank factor because the molybdenum input spectrum have two characteristic peaks at 17.5 and 19.5 keV, much closer to the K-edge of a-Se at 12.6 keV causing degradations in the Swank factor, while the tungsten spectrum is centered around 23.5 keV, farther from the a-Se K-edge.

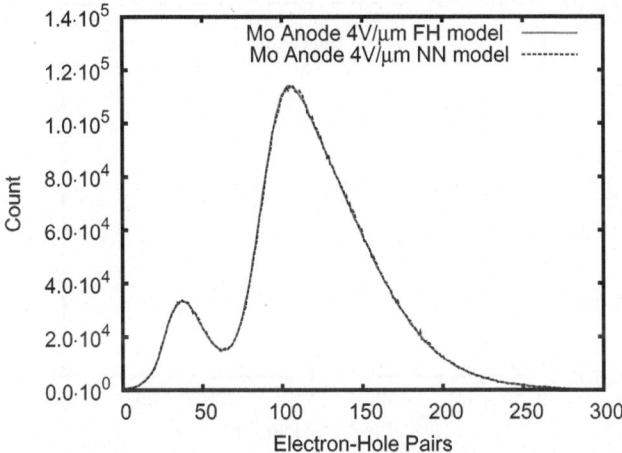

Fig. 2. Simulated PHS with molybdenum mammography spectrum as a function of electron-hole pair transport for 4 V/μm applied electric field using FH and NN recombination algorithms

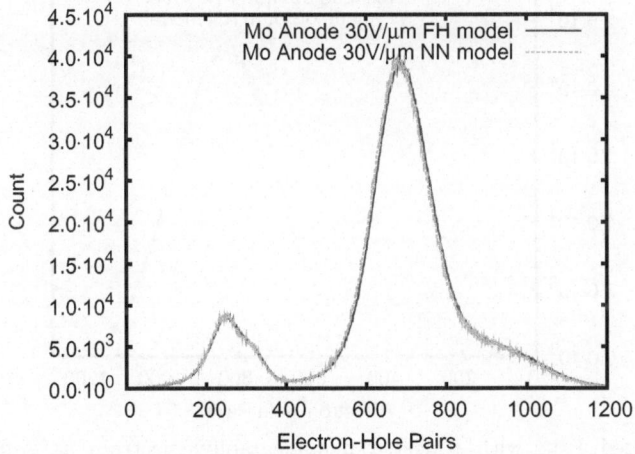

Fig. 3. Simulated PHS with molybdenum mammography spectrum as a function of electron-hole pair transport for 30 V/μm applied electric field using FH and NN recombination algorithms

Table 1 lists the Swank factors and recombination fractions with the two recombination algorithms for the molybdenum and tungsten spectra. The total simulation time is reported for ten million incident x-ray photons. Both the Swank noise and recombination results agree well between the FH and NN algorithm, while the simulation time increases for lower applied bias because electron-hole pairs take more time to separate and therefore, recombination is more likely to occur.

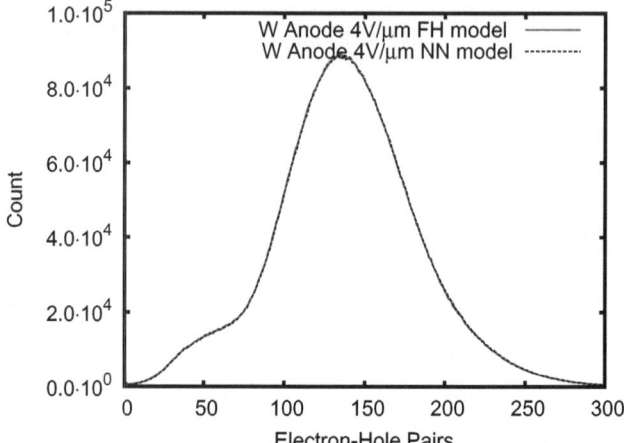

Fig. 4. Simulated PHS with tungsten mammography spectrum as a function of electron-hole pair transport for 4 V/μm applied electric field using FH and NN recombination algorithms

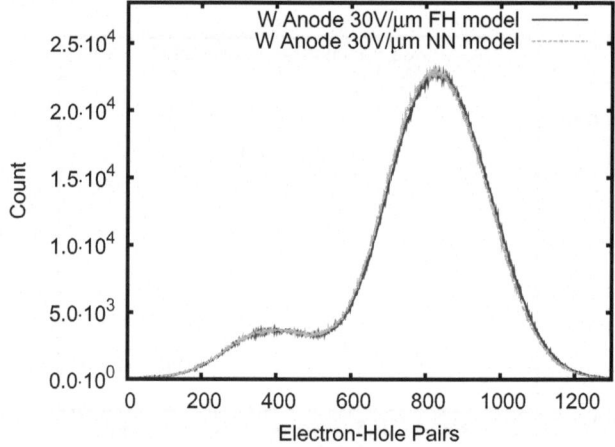

Fig. 5. Simulated PHS with tungsten mammography spectrum as a function of electron-hole pair transport for 30 V/μm applied electric field using FH and NN recombination algorithms

A detailed MC code taking into account spatial and temporal transport of electron-hole pairs is used to study the effect of different recombination algorithms on Swank noise for a-Se x-ray detectors. The results show that the incident photon energy and the bias voltage affect the magnitude of Swank noise and that results for FH and NN recombination algorithms agree reasonably well in their prediction of PHS, Swank noise and recombination fraction.

Table 1. Simulated Swank factor and recombination fraction for Mo/Mo (RQA-M 2) and W/Al standard radiation qualities with varying transport conditions

Radiation Quality		$4V/\mu m$		$30V/\mu m$	
(IEC 61267)		FH	NN	FH	NN
Mo/Mo (RQA-M 2)	$I(E)$	0.878	0.878	0.922	0.922
	f_R	96.5%	96.5%	80.0%	80.1%
	Time (s)	1.18×10^7	1.51×10^7	7.75×10^6	8.66×10^6
W/Al	$I(E)$	0.903	0.904	0.937	0.937
	f_R	96.5%	96.4%	79.6%	80.1%
	Time (s)	1.38×10^7	1.80×10^7	9.29×10^6	1.03×10^7

4   Conclusion and Future Work

The effect on Swank noise from different carrier recombination algorithms is studied by implementing a more realistic NN algorithm in ARTEMIS and comparing the results to those obtained with the faster FH algorithm. PHS results for a-Se detector show that Swank noise and recombination fraction computed with the two algorithms are consistent within the clinical mammography energy range with an approximate 10% to 30% increase in simulation time for the cases of 4 and 30 $V/\mu m$ applied electric field.

The distribution of electron-hole pairs and their spatial proximity upon creation can affect the recombination fraction. Different burst models can be explored to examine its effect on the recombination models. For this work, a constant carrier mobility is used for both holes and electrons. The effect of different carrier mobilities and detector thicknesses on the recombination models can be explored in the future. We are also currently working on validation of the simulation results with pulse-height spectroscopy experimental measurements.

Acknowledgments. The authors would like to thank Dr. Robert J. Jennings for the computer software used for generation of standard beam qualities. Y.F. acknowledges funding by an appointment to the Research Participation Program at the Center for Device and Radiological Health administered by the Oak Ridge Institute for Science and Education through an interagency agreement between the U.S. Department of Energy and U.S. Food and Drug Administration. This work was also financially supported in part by the Natural Sciences and Engineering Research Council of Canada (NSERC).

References

1. Rowlands, J.A., Yorkston, J.: Chapter 4: Flat panel detectors for digital radiography. Handbook of Medical Imaging, vol. 1. SPIE Press, Washington (2000)
2. Irisawa, K., Yamane, K., Imai, S., Ogawa, M., Shouji, T., Agano, T., Hosoi, Y., Hayakawa, T.: Direct-conversion 50 μm pixel-pitch detector for digitial mammography using amorphous selenium as a photoconductive switching layer for signal charge readout. In: Proc. SPIE, vol. 7258, p. 725811 (2009)

3. Zentai, G., Partain, L., Richmond, M., Ogusu, K., Yamada, S.: 50 μm pixel size a-Se mammography imager with high DQE and increased temperature resistance. In: Prof. SPIE., vol. 7622, p. 762215 (2010)
4. Fang, Y., Badal, A., Allec, N., Karim, K.S., Badano, A.: Spatiotemporal Monte Carlo transport methods in x-ray semiconductor detectors: Application to pulse-height spectroscopy in a-Se. Med. Phys. 39, 308–320 (2012)
5. Swank, R.K.: Absorption and noise in x-ray phosphors. J. App. Phys. 44, 4199–4203 (1973)
6. Ginzburg, A., Dick, C.: Image Information transfer properties of x-ray intensifying screens in the energy range from 17 to 320 keV. Med. Phys. 20, 1013–1021 (1993)
7. Salvat, F., Fernandez-Varea, J.M., Sempau, J.: PENELOPE 2006: A code system for Monte Carlo Simulation of Electron and Photon Transport. Issy-les-Moulineaux. France: OECD/NEA Data Bank (2006)
8. Sharma, D., Fang, Y., Zafar, F., Karim, K.S., Badano, A.: Recombination models for spatio-temporal Monte Carlo transport of interacting carriers in semiconductors. App. Phys. Let. 98, 242111 (2011)
9. Que, W., Rowlands, J.A.: X-ray photongeneration in amorphous selenium: Geminate versus columnar recombination. Phys. Rev. B 51, 10500–10507 (1995)
10. Knight, J., Davis, E.: Photogeneration of charge carrier in amorphous selenium. J. Phys. Chem. Solids 35, 543–554 (1975)
11. Boone, J.M., Fewell, T.R., Jennings, R.J.: Molybdenum, rhodium, and tungsten anode spectral models using interpolating polynomials with application to mammography. Med. Phys. 24, 1863–1874 (1997)

Initial Result of a Prospective Study: Comparison between a Low Dose 3D Stereo Mammography and FFDM

Andreas Lohre[1], Dirk Stoesser[1], Akira Hasegawa[2], and Cord Neitzke[1]

[1] Gemeinschaftspraxis für Radiologie, Dinslaken, Germany
uhu_5@live.de, d.stoesser@radiologieduisburg.de,
cord.neitzke@arcor.de
[2] Fujifilm Medical Systems, USA, San Jose, CA, USA
ahasegawa@fujifilm.com

Abstract. This report describes the initial result of a prospective clinical trial to compare 3D stereoscopic mammography (3DSDM) and standard full-field digital mammography (FFDM) for detection of biopsy proven cancers in a diagnostic population. In 3DSDM exam, an additional low-dose image is taken from 4 degree right after taking standard FFDM images in left/right CC and MLO. A total of 2,016 patients underwent 3DSDM exams since February, 2011 through March, 2012, which were read by different radiologists independently. Compared to FFDM, 3DSDM significantly reduced false positive detection by 29.4% ($p=0.007$). Cancer detection was slightly improved by 3D 4% although there was no statistical significance ($p=0.317$).

Keywords: 3D mammography, stereoscopic, prospective study.

1 Introduction

Over the last decade, there has been a progressive shift in breast imaging. Two-dimensional full-field digital mammography (FFDM) took over film-screen mammography (FSM) in this digital era. Superior performance as indicated by the ACRIN DMIST results [1], image acquisition workflow, improved technologist productivity, reading features, sharing, storage and retrieval were the main factors for technology adoption. However, like FSM, diagnostic outcomes were limited by overlapping tissues, especially in dense breasts, due to the two-dimensional nature of the projection images.

3D stereo digital mammography (3DSDM) is expected to help radiologists overcome this limitation, leading to potential reduction of false readings and thereby further improving diagnoses of breast cancer. Getty, et al. conducted a large prospective study [2] and reported that 3DSDM could provide higher sensitivity and specificity compared to FFDM and that 3DSDM reading time could be shorter than FFDM. However, Getty, et al. used double dose for 3DSDM acquisition compared to FFDM and it was not clear if some improvements came from 3D effect or dose increase.

A.D.A. Maidment, P.R. Bakic, and S. Gavenonis (Eds.): IWDM 2012, LNCS 7361, pp. 583–588, 2012.
© Springer-Verlag Berlin Heidelberg 2012

The purpose of this study is to prospectively identify a potential clinical benefit of a low-dose 3DSDM compared to FFDM as an initial result of an ongoing prospective study.

2   Methods and Materials

Patients had undergone 3DSDM exams since February 3, 2011. All patients had some kind of clinical reasons such as pain or suspect palpation and all exams were for diagnostic purposes. There was no screening examination.

The FFDM system with a 3DSDM option used in this study (Amulet, FUJIFILM Corporation) has received MDD and CE marking in European market. All examinations were performed under informed consent by participants.

In 3DSDM exam, an additional low-dose image is taken from 4 degree immediately after taking 0 degree images in left/right CC and MLO which are standard FFDM exams (Figure 1). A standard mammography image (0 degree image) and its corresponding 4 degree images are treated as a stereo-pair in the 3DSDM. The acquired stereo-pair images are sent to a 3D mammography workstation with a stereo 3D monitor (RadiForce GS521-ST, EIZO Nanao Corporation). The stereo 3D monitor consists of two 5 mega pixel grayscale monitors for mammography with a half mirror as shown in Figure 2.

Without any reconstruction processes, one of the paired images is displayed on one of the 5 mega pixel grayscale monitors and the other image is on the other monitor. The light coming from the top monitor reflected on the half mirror and the light from the bottom monitor comes through the half mirror. The polarization of the light coming through the half mirror rotates 90 degree. By wearing a pair of polarized glasses, viewer's visual system fuses the stereo-paired images into a single instant, in-depth, 3D image of a breast.

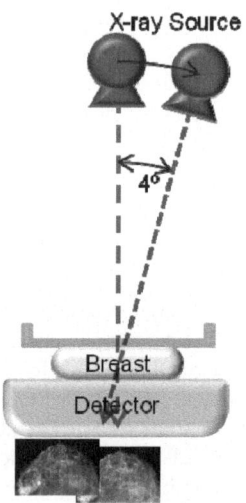

Fig. 1. Stereosopic image acquisition. Additional 4 degree image is taken after a standard mammography image is taken.

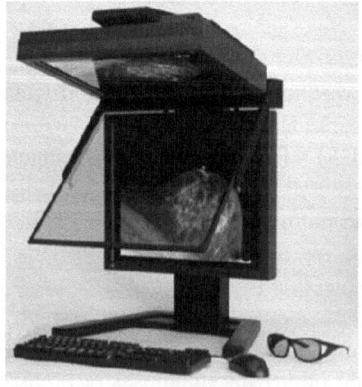

Fig. 2. 3D display consisting of 5 mega pixel grayscale monitors with a half mirror

The spatial resolution of both 0 and 4 degree images acquired for this study is 50μm/pixel. The target/filter combination used is W/Rh. The average glandular dose used for this study is 1.04 mGy for 0 degree images and 0.35 mGy for 4 degree as shown in Figure 3. These AGD was measured with a 45 mm (50/50) PMMA phantom.

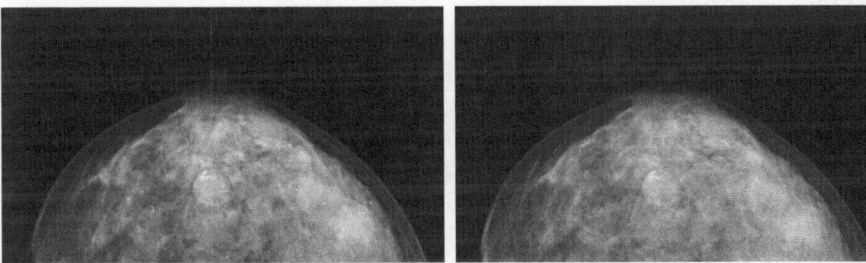

Fig. 3. Sample stereopair mammograms; (a) 0 degree image for left eye, which is the same as FFDM and (b) 4 degree image for right eye

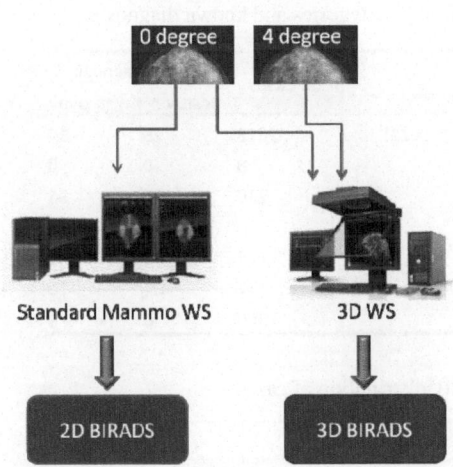

Fig. 4. Reading workflow. Zero degree images were sent to a standard mammography WS and both 0 and 4 degree images to 3D WS.

As shown in Figure 4, each day one radiologist read only 0 degree images as FFDM on 2D workstation with two 5 mega pixel grayscale monitors. He reads FFDM with prior films/digital images if available. In a ddition, he access patients for palpation if necessary. Then, he comes up with BI-RADS categories. In the same day, another independently read stereo-pair images (0 and 4 degree images) of the same cases on a 3D workstation with prior films or prior digital images if available. So far, roughly 80% priors are accessible by films and only remaining 20% are in digital images. Findings from palpation exams done by FFDM readers are shared with 3DSDM readers by writing if available. Then, 3DSDM reader comes up with his own BI-RADS categories.

The 3D workstation has a function to display 2D mammograms on the 3D monitor and can switch between 2D and 3D display modes. But, the 2D display mode is not used in reading 3DSDM in this study to compare purely FFDM and 3DSDM.

Four experienced radiologists with experience ranging from 15 to 25 years of reading mammograms participate to the study. To minimize inter-reader variability, these four radiologists take turns at FFDM and 3DSDM reading. A reader never reads both FFDM and 3DSDM of the same cases.

All of BI-RADS categories 4 and 5 in at least one of FFDM and 3DSDM reading and some of BI-RADS category 3 patients were recommended biopsy. Based on the recommendation, patients are referred to other hospitals/clinics to get biopsy. Biopsy results are collected as many as possible by following up these hospitals/clinics or patients. Based on biopsy results, BI-RADS categories between FFDM and 3DSDM reading were compared in terms of sensitivity and specificity.

Bennett's χ^2 test [4] was employed to compare sensitivity and specificity between 2D FFDM and 3DSDM.

3   Results

From February 3, 2011 through March 30, 2011, a total of 2,016 patients underwent 3DSDM exams. Patients' age ranging was from 19 to 89 years old. Out of these 2,018 cases, 8 cases were excluded mainly because of motion artifacts during 3DSDM acquisitions and 2,010 cases were used for the analysis.

BI-RADS categories of FFDM and 3DSDM and the number of cases in each category are shown in Table 1. Of the 2,010 cases, 210 cases were rated BI-RADS category 3, 4 or 5 by at least one of FFDM and 3DSDM, and 1,800 cases BI-RADS category 1 or 2 by both FFDM and 3DSDM.

Table 1. The number of cases in BI-RADS categories and known diagnosis

BI-RADS Categories	Total Cases	Known Diagnosis	
		positive	negative
A total number of cases (Feb. 3, 2011 - Nov. 17, 2011)	2018	25	34
Excluded Cases	8	0	0
BIRADS 3, 4 or 5 (by FFDM or 3DSDM)	210	25	31
BIRADS 3, 4 or 5 only by FFDM	74	0	11
BIRADS 3, 4 or 5 only by 3DSDM	19	1	1
BIRADS 3, 4 or 5 both by FFDM and 3DSDM	117	24	19
BIRADS 1 or 2 (by FFDM and 3DSDM)	1800	0	3

Table 2. Breast density distribution of cases

ACR BI-RADS classification for breast density	Total
A total number of cases (Feb. 3, 2011 – Mar 30, 2012)	2018
Excluded Cases	8
Type 1	235
Type 2	961
Type 3	753
Type 4	52
Not Recorded	9

By March 30, 2012, fifty nine histology results were collected. As shown in Table 1, out of these 59 cases, 25 cancer and 34 cancer-free cases were identified. Out of 25 cancer cases, one was categorized as BI-RADS category 4 only by 3DSDM but BI-RADS category 2 by FFDM although all other 24 cancer cases were detected by both. On the other hand, 11 out of 34 cancer-free cases were classified as BI-RADS category 2 by 3DSDM whereas they were classified as BI-RADS category 3 or 4 only by FFDM. Of the remaining 23 cancer-free cases, one case was categorized as BI-RADS 4 only by 3DSDM and BIRADS 2 by FFDM. Of the remaining 22 cancer-free cases, 19 cases were detected as false positives by both FFDM and 3DSDM and the remaining 3 cases were classified to BI-RADS category 1 or 2 by both FFDM and 3DSDM.

Distribution of the ACR BI-RADS classification for breast density was shown in Table 2. The breast density types were made by FFDM only.

By taking only cases with known diagnosis including cancer and cancer-free cases, sensitivity and specificity of FFDM and 3DSDM were calculated and are shown in Table 3. As shown in this table, sensitivity was 100% for 3DSDM and 96% for FFDM. Obviously there is no difference in sensitivity between FFDM and 3DSDM. On the other hand, specificity was 41.2% for 3DSDM and 11.8% for FFDM.

Table 3. FP, TN, TP, FN, sensitivity and specificity of 3DSDM and FFDM on cases with known results

Results on cancer-free cases

	FP	TN
3DSDM	20	14
FFDM	30	4

Results on biopsy proven cancer cases

	TP	FN
3DSDM	25	0
FFDM	24	1

Sensitivity and specificity

	Sensitivity	Specificity
3DSDM	100%	41.2%
FFDM	96%	11.8%

The null hypothesis of equal specificities was tested by using Bennett's χ^2 test and it turned out p-value = 0.007. By this result, it is able to say that there is a statistically significant difference between specificities between 3DSDM and FFDM. The null hypothesis of equal sensitivities was tested, too. It turned out p-value=0.317 and there is no statistical difference in sensitivities.

4   Discussions

We analyzed BI-RADS category distribution of FFDM and 3DSDM to find out whether or not there are different reading trends between two. Both distributions are shown in Figure 5. As shown in this figure, the number of BI-RADS category 3 by 3DSDM is about half of FFDM. This result may indicate that 3DSDM may help to reduce the BI-RADS category 3 compared to the FFDM.

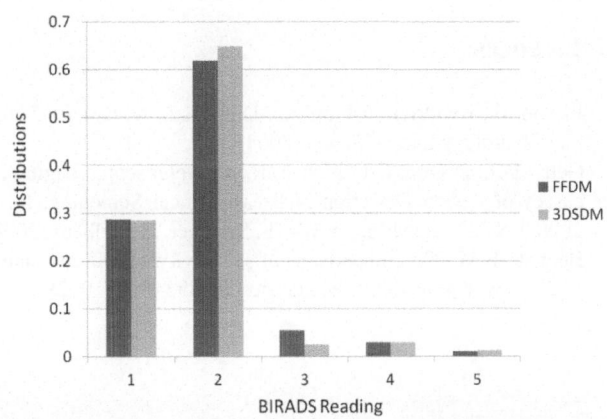

Fig. 5. BI-RADS category distribution of FFDM and 3DSDM. The number of BI-RADS 3 by 3DSDM is about half compared to FFDM.

FFDM findings in cases with different BI-RADS in FFDM and 3DSDM were also analyzed. There were a total of 12 negative those cases. Out of 12 cases, 11 were turned out to FP by FFDM and TN by 3DSDM and their breakdowns are as follows; 6 masses, 2 calcs, 1 mass+calc and 1 unknown. The remaining one case, which was a FP by 3DSDM and a TN by FFDM, was a calcification case. Although there are too few cases, 3DSDM might help readers to categorize masses.

Only mammography exams are performed in this hospital and all patients who need additional exams are referred to other breast clinics, breast centers, or hospitals. Mostly these patients go to special breast centers for biopsy. They bring their mammograms on a CD and take them to referred breast centers. Normally, additional ultrasound would be done in breast centers, especially if a suspect mass or architecture distortion were found by FFDM/3DSDM. The correlation between FFDM/3DSDM and US are normally done at the breast centers. If there is clear correlation, the biopsy normally is done assisted by ultrasound control, otherwise a stereotactic biopsy. In case of microcalcification, normally a vacuum biopsy is used assisted by mammography. The concordance/discordance of biopsy results are normally discussed in tumor-conferences at the breast centers.

According to Table 1, biopsies were performed to some of cases with BI-RADS 3, 2 and 1. These could be caused by some of the following reasons; (a) a clinical hint, e. g. some palpable mass, (b) outside made ultrasound by the assigning doctor (outside our clinic) or a breast center with a suspect result or (c) the explicit wish of some patients for the biopsy, because they were fearful and didn´t want to wait for a control mammography.

There is a special guideline, called S3 guidance, in Germany for negative biopsy cases. These patients have to go through 6 month follow-up.

Although diagnostic population has been used in this study, this initial result indicates that a low dose 3DSDM may have great potential in a substantial reduction of the recall rate.

References

1. Pisano, E., Hendrick, R.E., et al.: Diagnostic Accuracy of Digital verses Film Mammography. Radiology 246, 376–383 (2008)
2. Getty, D.J., D'Orsi, C.J., Pickett, R.M.: Stereoscopic Digital Mammography: Improved Accuracy of Lesion Detection in Breast Cancer Screening. In: Krupinski, E.A. (ed.) IWDM 2008. LNCS, vol. 5116, pp. 74–79. Springer, Heidelberg (2008)
3. Bennett, B.M.: On comparisons of sensitivity, specificity, and predictive Value of a number of diagnostic procedures. Biometrics 28, 793–800 (1972)

Volumetric and Area-Based Measures of Mammographic Density in Women with and without Cancer

Leila Nutine[1], Jamie C. Sergeant[2], Julie Morris[3], Paula Stavrinos[4], D. Gareth Evans[4], Tony Howell[4], Caroline Boggis[4], Mary Wilson[4], Nicky Barr[4], and Susan M. Astley[2]

[1] Manchester Medical School, University of Manchester, Oxford Road,
Manchester, M13 9PT, UK
[2] School of Cancer and Enabling Sciences, University of Manchester,
Oxford Road, Manchester M13 9PT, UK
[3] Department of Medical Statistics, University Hospital of South Manchester,
Manchester M23 9LT, UK
[4] Nightingale Centre and Genesis Prevention Centre,
University Hospital of South Manchester, Manchester M23 9LT, UK
sue.astley@manchester.ac.uk

Abstract. We compare mammographic density in 44 women with screen-detected breast cancer and a control group of 923 women with normal screening mammograms. Multiple regression was used to compare the effects of case-control status on breast density of the contra-lateral breast. Two breast density measures were investigated: the average visual assessment, recorded on a visual analogue scale (VAS), for the two views and two independent readers; and volumetric percentage density measured by Quantra[TM]. We adjusted for confounding factors of BMI, HRT use, age and menopausal status. Initially there was no significant difference in mean percentage density between cases and controls using either measure of density: VAS (cases 27.5%, controls 26.9%) and Quantra[TM] (cases 17.2%, controls 18.2%). However, when confounding factors were controlled for, case-control status had a statistically significant effect on breast density as measured by Quantra[TM] (adjusted means: cases 19.2%, controls 14.8%; $p = 0.002$) but not by VAS.

Keywords: Breast density, breast cancer, Visual Analogue Scale, volumetric, mammography, Quantra.

1   Introduction

Mammographic breast density, measured as the proportion of the breast area occupied by dense fibro-glandular tissue, has a well-established link with the risk of developing breast cancer [1]. Much of the previous research in this area has used either visual estimation of density [2] or semi-automated assessment [3]. With the advent of full-field digital mammography (FFDM), fully automated methods of quantifying density have become available, and with them, an interest in establishing the relationship of such measures with risk. These methods compute breast density in a volumetric way, and in addition to a relative measure of percentage density, they can also output the

A.D.A. Maidment, P.R. Bakic, and S. Gavenonis (Eds.): IWDM 2012, LNCS 7361, pp. 589–595, 2012.
© Springer-Verlag Berlin Heidelberg 2012

breast volume and the volume of glandular tissue within the breast. Since they are fully automatic they are suitable for mass screening.

This work forms part of a larger trial, PROCAS (Predicting Risk Of Cancer At Screening) aiming to identify women attending routine breast screening who are at higher than average risk of developing breast cancer, so they can be offered risk-reducing interventions including lifestyle advice [4-5]. Those with dense breasts may also benefit from alternative forms of screening such as Digital Breast Tomosynthesis or Magnetic Resonance Imaging. Women recruited to the PROCAS trial have provided risk information via a questionnaire at the time of screening, and the density of their digital screening mammograms was both subjectively assessed using a visual analogue scale (VAS) and computed by Hologic's Quantra™ software. This paper describes the first reported case-control study in the screening age group that uses both VAS and Quantra™, and allows adjustment for confounding factors.

2   Methods

2.1   Selection of Cases and Controls

The PROCAS study invites the participation of all women in the Greater Manchester Breast Screening Programme, part of the UK nationwide National Health Service Breast Screening Programme (NHSBSP). Consenting women undergo routine mammography either on a mobile unit or at a static site. Data from the first 109 consenting women with screen-detected cancer were obtained; of the mammograms, 64 were images obtained on a GE Senographe Essential FFDM system that were amenable to processing with Hologic's Quantra™ software. The remainder were analogue mammograms, images obtained on a Fischer Senoscan FFDM system to which Quantra™ could not be applied, or images for which raw digital data were not available. Out of the 64 cases for which volumetric measures of density were available, 13 had not been visually assessed as part of the PROCAS study and were excluded. A further seven cases were excluded because of missing questionnaire data relating to confounding factors. Of 1207 women with normal screening mammograms, 110 were excluded due to lack of Quantra™ or VAS data and 174 were excluded due to incomplete questionnaire data. This resulted in a set of 44 cases (screen-detected cancers) and 923 controls (women with normal screening mammograms). All the cancers were uni-lateral.

2.2   Assessment of Mammographic Density

A visual assessment of breast density was made by two independent expert mammographic film readers as part of the PROCAS study. Readers were drawn from a pool of 7 Consultant Radiologists, 2 Advanced Practitioner Radiographers and 2 Breast Physicians. All are readers within the NHSBSP and interpret an annual volume of between 5000 and 10000 mammograms. Experience in reading mammograms ranged from <1 year to 22 years, and in assessing density experience ranged from <1 year to 8 years. Reader performance on synthetic images with known density has previously been characterized [6] and observations of differences in reader performance described [7]. Pairing of readers in PROCAS is done on a pragmatic basis.

Each reader marked a 10cm visual analogue scale for each of the four radiographic projections obtained during screening. The scales were scanned and automatically converted to percentages according to the positions of the marks. An average percentage density per breast was obtained for each woman from the two readers' assessments of the two views.

One of the aims of the PROCAS study is to establish the relationship of volumetric density measures with risk of developing breast cancer. Full validation has not yet been achieved because of the relatively recent introduction of FFDM and the need to acquire suitable longitudinal data for analysis, but validation data are encouraging [8]. In this study we use Quantra^{TM} (Version 1.3; Hologic Inc.); although this software was developed for use on Hologic FFDM data, it is also commercially available for other FFDM systems including the GE Senographe Essential.

For each woman, the density of only one breast was used. In the cancer group, density values were obtained for the contra-lateral breast. In the control group, left or right breast values were selected randomly subject to the constraint that the proportion should be similar to that in the cancer group. Body Mass Index (BMI) was calculated from self-reported weight and height, and age at the time of screening was determined to the nearest day.

2.3   Analysis

Independent samples t-tests were conducted to compare the percentage breast density, by VAS and Quantra^{TM}, of the contralateral breasts of cases and controls. A standard multiple regression model was used to assess the effect of case-control status on percentage density as measured by VAS and Quantra^{TM} once age, menopausal status, current HRT use and BMI were controlled for.

3   Results

The characteristics of the women in the case and control groups are illustrated in Table 1. These data were taken from, or computed from, the self-reported information in the completed questionnaires.

Table 1. Characteristics of the case and control populations

	Cases n=44	Controls n=923
	Mean (SD)	Mean (SD)
Age	63.1(5.7)	59.6 (7.0)
BMI	27.6 (4.5)	27.2 (5.4)
Postmenopausal (%)	86.4	70.7
HRT ever used (%)	40.9	33.4
Years of HRT use	7.0 (5.8) n=18	6.8 (6.1) n=309
Still on HRT(%)	6.8	7.9

Table 2. Summary of density of case and control populations

	Cases n=44		Controls n=923	
	Mean	(SD)	Mean	(SD)
Quantra average density (L+R) %	16.8(7.2)		17.2(6.7)	
Quantra glandular volume R	101.1(46.7)		102.4(65.1)	
Quantra glandular volume L	98.2(57.3)		100.5(56.0)	
VAS average density (L+R) %	28.7(17.9)		27.0(17.1)	
Contralateral breast VAS % dens.	26.9(19.0)		27.5(19.1)	
Contralateral breast Quantra % dens.	18.2(7.2)		17.2(6.9)	

The mean percentage density of the contralateral breast, as measured by VAS, was 27.5% for controls and 26.9% for cases, but the standard deviations were very large (see Table 2). Conversely, breast density as measured by Quantra^{TM} was 18.2% for the contralateral breasts of cases and 17.2% for controls. The density values are summarised in Table 2.

There was no significant difference in the percentage density of the contralateral breasts of cases and controls, with density measured by VAS ($p > 0.05$) and by Quantra^{TM} ($p > 0.05$). In the regression model for percentage density as measured by Quantra^{TM}, the variable that made the biggest contribution was BMI ($p < 0.001$). In addition, case-control status ($p = 0.002$), menopausal status ($p = 0.032$) and current use of HRT ($p = 0.036$) were all found to have a statistically significant effect on density. Age made no statistically significant contribution towards the variation in breast density. The model explained 19.2% of the variation in breast density. Standardized coefficients from the model are presented in Table 3.   Once adjusted for the

Table 3. The multiple regression modèl coefficients illustrating the strength of the contribution towards the outcome of the dependent variable (Beta) and the statistical significance of the contribution (Sig.) to the dependent variable which is contralateral breast density % as measured by Quantra^{TM}

	Dependent Variable: Contralateral breast density % Quantra	
	Standardized Coefficients	
	Beta	Sig.
Cases vs. controls	0.148	0.002
Age	0.045	0.411
Menopausal status	0.117	0.032
BMI	-0.376	0.000
Currently on HRT	0.109	0.036

confounding variables in the regression model, the mean percentage densities by Quantra^{TM} for cases (19.2%) and controls (14.8%) were significantly different ($p = 0.002$). In the regression model for percentage density as measured by VAS, case-control status was found not to be a significant predictor of density ($p = 0.160$).

4   Discussion

Visual analogue scales provide an accessible, quantitative method of recording subjective area-based density assessments. A relationship between VAS density and risk of developing cancer was demonstrated in a study in which readers assigned densities to film-screen mammograms that were followed up for six years [9]. In that study, the association matched that of the best computer-assisted method. There is, however, no such evidence for a similar visual assessment of full-field digital mammograms, and in our research we have found that visual assessments recorded using visual analogue scales depend on reader, on modality (digital vs. film-screen) and to a lesser extent on FFDM manufacturer. The results obtained in this study show no significant difference between the VAS density of the contralateral breast of women with cancer and of controls; this is unsurprising given the relatively small number of cancer cases available and subjective nature of assessment. Furthermore, this study differs from that conducted by Duffy et al. in that we are only able to examine images from one screening round, rather than measuring density in prior mammograms.

In this work, all the women were imaged on similar FFDM systems. Visual assessments were made by readers from a pool of experienced density assessors, and it is likely that inter-observer variability may have contributed to the lack of significance of the visually assessed results [7], [10]. With large cohorts it is not feasible to have the same assessors for every case; we adopted a pragmatic design with a view to correcting assessments post-hoc based on an ongoing analysis of individual reader performance. Where visual assessment is used clinically such analysis is crucial; it is interesting to note that in many of the key research papers in which mammograms have been assessed subjectively a very small number of highly experienced assessors were used [11], [12].

Fully automated volumetric breast density measures offer a number of benefits over visual assessment: there is no disruption to normal screening workflow; values obtained are repeatable; differences in imaging parameters are accounted for; and absolute (rather than relative) density measures are possible, eliminating inaccuracies due to temporary weight gain [13].

Our results using Quantra^{TM} are promising, yielding a statistically significant relationship with case-control status, with the contra-lateral breasts of cases having a higher density than those of controls. Our results became significant only when BMI, HRT use, menopausal status and age were accounted for. This is of clinical significance because in many screening programmes not all of these data are routinely collected. It would be interesting to explore the possibility of using breast volume (as output by automated volumetric methods such as Quantra^{TM}) as a surrogate for weight as there is doubt over the reliability of self-reported weight [14], and such an approach would provide a snapshot at the time of imaging and risk assessment. In order to properly assess the validity of this, an objective measure of weight would be necessary. This is, however, difficult within the context of routine screening on mobile units where space and privacy are limited. It is of concern that reliability of self-reported weight and height is reduced in overweight women, since this group comprises a significant part of the screening population.

In this study it was not practical to exactly match the case and control groups with respect to all prognostic factors, however the small disparities between the case and control groups (mainly for age and menopausal status) were adequately adjusted for in the statistical analysis ensuring that these differences could not have confounded the breast density comparisons. Future research will focus on assessing the utility of volumetric measures for risk prediction as longitudinal data become available.

Acknowledgements. We acknowledge the support of the National Insitute for Health Research (NIHR) and the Genesis Breast Cancer Prevention Appeal for their funding of the PROCAS trial. We would like to thank the study radiologists and advanced practitioner radiographers for VAS reading. We would also like to thank the many radiographers involved in the Greater Manchester Breast Screening Programme, the study staff for recruitment and data collection, and Hologic Inc. for providing the Quantra™ software. This paper presents independent research commissioned by the National Institute for Health Research (NIHR) under its Programme Grant (Reference Number RP-PG-0707-10031). The views expressed are those of the author(s) and not necessarily those of the NHS, the NIHR or the Department of Health.

References

1. McCormack, V.A., dos Santos Silva, I.: Breast density and parenchymal patterns as markers of breast cancer risk: a meta-analysis. Cancer Epidemiol. Biomarkers Prev. 15, 1159–1169 (2006)
2. Wolfe, J.N.: Breast patterns as an index of risk for developing breast cancer. Am. J. Roentgenol. 126, 1130–1139 (1976)
3. Byng, J.W., Boyd, N.F., Fishell, E., Jong, R.A., Yaffe, M.J.: The quantitative analysis of mammographic densities. Phys. Med. Biol. 39, 1629–1638 (1994)
4. Evans, D.G., Warwick, J., Astley, S.M., et al.: Assessing individual breast cancer risk within the UK National Health Service Breast Screening Programme: a new paradigm for cancer prevention. Cancer Prevention Research (forthcoming)
5. Howell, A., Astley, S., Warwick, J., et al.: Prevention of breast cancer in the context of a national breast screening programme. Journal of Internal Medicine 271, 321–330 (2012)
6. Makaronidis, J., Berks, M., Sergeant, J., et al.: Assessment of breast density: reader performance using synthetic mammographic images. In: Medical Imaging 2011: Image Perception, Observer Performance and Technology Assessment. SPIE, vol. 7966, p. 796603 (2011)
7. Sergeant, J.C., Warwick, J., Gareth Evans, D., Howell, A., Berks, M., Stavrinos, P., Sahin, S., Wilson, M., Hufton, A., Buchan, I., Astley, S.M.: Volumetric and Area-Based Breast Density Measurement in the Predicting Risk Of Cancer At Screening (PROCAS) Study. In: Maidment, A.D.A., Bakic, P.R., Gavenonis, S. (eds.) IWDM 2012. LNCS, vol. 7361, pp. 228–235. Springer, Heidelberg (2012)

8. Hartman, K., Highnam, R., Warren, R., Jackson, V.: Volumetric Assessment of Breast Tissue Composition from FFDM Images. In: Krupinski, E.A. (ed.) IWDM 2008. LNCS, vol. 5116, pp. 33–39. Springer, Heidelberg (2008)

9. Duffy, S.W., Nagtegaal, I.D., Astley, S.M., et al.: Visually Assessed Breast Density: the need for two views. Breast Cancer Research 10, R64 (2008)

10. Astley, S., Swayamprakasam, C., Berks, M., Sergeant, J., Morris, J., Wilson, M., Barr, N., Boggis, C.: Assessment of change in breast density: reader performance using synthetic mammographic images. In: Proc. SPIE (forthcoming)

11. Cuzick, J., Warwick, J., Pinney, E., Duffy, S.W., Cawthorn, S., Howell, A., Forbes, J.F., Warren, R.: Tamoxifen-induced reduction in mammographic density and breast cancer risk reduction: a nested case-control study. J. Natl. Cancer Inst. 103, 744–752 (2011)

12. Mitchell, G., Antoniou, A.C., Warren, R., et al.: Mammographic density and breast cancer risk in BRCA1 and BRCA2 mutation carriers. Cancer Research 66(3), 1866–1872 (2006)

13. Patel, H.G., Astley, S.M., Hufton, A.P., Harvie, M., Hagan, K., Marchant, T.E., Hillier, V., Howell, A., Warren, R., Boggis, C.R.M.: Automated Breast Tissue Measurement of Women at Increased Risk of Breast Cancer. In: Astley, S.M., Brady, M., Rose, C., Zwiggelaar, R. (eds.) IWDM 2006. LNCS, vol. 4046, pp. 131–136. Springer, Heidelberg (2006)

14. Rowland, M.L.: Self-reported weight and height. American Journal of Clinical Nutrition 52, 1125–1133

Mammographic Parenchymal Texture Analysis for Estrogen-Receptor Subtype Specific Breast Cancer Risk Estimation

Gopal Karemore[1,2], Brad M. Keller[1], Huen Oh[1], Julia Tchou[1], Mads Nielsen[2], Emily F. Conant[1], and Despina Kontos[1]

[1] University of Pennsylvania, PA 19104, USA
Gopal.Karemore@uphs.upenn.edu
[2] University of Copenhagen, Copenhagen 2100, Denmark
karemore@diku.dk

Abstract. We investigate the potential of mammographic parenchymal texture as a surrogate marker of the risk to develop Estrogen Receptor (ER) sub-type specific breast cancer. A case-control study was performed, including 118 cancer cases stratified by ER receptor status and 354 age-matched controls. Digital mammographic (DM) images were retrospectively collected and analyzed under HIPAA and IRB approval. The performance of the texture features was compared to that of the standard mammographic density measures. We observed that breast percent density PD% and parenchymal texture features can both distinguish between cancer cases and controls (A_z >0.70). However, for ER subtype-specific classification, PD% alone does not provide sufficient classification ($A_z = 0.60$), while texture features have significant classification performance ($A_z = 0.70$). Combining breast density with texture features achieves the best performance ($A_z = 0.71$). These findings suggest that mammographic texture analysis may have value for sub-type specific breast cancer risk assessment.

Keywords: Breast cancer, sub-type specific risk, mammogram parenchymal texture.

1 Introduction

Growing evidence suggests etiologic and risk profile differences between women who tend to develop estrogen receptor ER+ and ER- breast cancer. Higher risk of ER+ breast cancer appears to be associated with increased endogenous overall exposure to estrogen and cycling reproductive hormones [1]. Biomarkers of such hormonal exposure could be used during screening procedures to identify women at high risk of ER+ breast cancer, implementing targeted chemoprevention strategies [2]. Increased breast density has been shown to strongly associate with the risk of breast cancer, however, data with respect to subtype-specific risk (e.g., ER+ vs ER-) are still inconclusive [3,4]. Growing evidence in literature shows a potential causal association between risk and mammographic texture

A.D.A. Maidment, P.R. Bakic, and S. Gavenonis (Eds.): IWDM 2012, LNCS 7361, pp. 596–603, 2012.

[5,6]. Mammographic parenchymal patterns are also shown to reflect the change of their structure in response to hormonal exposure [3,7]. Here we investigate the potential role of mammographic texture analysis for ER sub-type specific breast cancer risk assessment.

2 Materials

Digital mammographic (DM) images were retrospectively collected and analyzed under HIPAA and IRB approval. Cases included the contralateral (i.e., unaffected) images of women diagnosed with unilateral breast cancer ($n = 118$), stratified by ER-positive ($n = 88$) and ER-negative ($n = 30$) receptor status after pathology confirmation. Controls included DM images randomly selected from our screening program during the same time period at 3:1 ratio to cases ($n = 354$) and side and age-matched based on 5-yr intervals. Images were aquired using GE Senographe 2000D and DS machines with a pixel depth of 12 bit and 10 pixel/mm resolutions. Post-processed $Premium View^{TM}$ images (GE Healthcare) with MLO views were analyzed. All images were normalized prior to sub-sequent analysis with Z-score normalization.

3 Methods

3.1 Texture Feature Extraction

For each mammogram, three broad categories of texture features are extracted namely Gaussian derivatives (n-jet), coherence properties of structure tensor and structure enhancing diffusion tensor, representing the orientation and heterogeneity of the parenchymal tissue within breast [8,9].

Gaussian Derivatives. Physiological evidence suggests that the visual receptive fields in the primate eye are shaped like the sum of a Gaussian function and its Laplacian generating Gaussian derivative-like fields [10]. Based on these fields, it can be expected to provide an assessment similar to the human visual system in image processing algorithms. For every pixel in the mammogram, Gaussian derivative features are extracted at four different Gaussian scales, namely 2, 4, 8, and 16 mm considering the typical resolution of mammogram (i.e. 10 pixel/mm). In addition, 10 different combinations of partial derivatives of the image intensities with respect to x-y coordinates at particular scale σ are extracted. This contributes to a total of 40 jet features per pixel for four different scales in each mammogram.

Structure Tensor and Structure Enhancing Diffusion. Structure tensor is a second-moment matrix, derived from the gradient of a function. It summarizes the predominant directions of the gradient in a specified neighborhood of a point, and the degree to which those directions are coherent [11]. Features based on structure tensors are invariant to affine intensity transformations and rotationally invariant. In addition, point-wise robustness is provided through convolution with Gaussian kernel of scales σ. Computation of structure tensor S for a mammogram image $I_{(x,y)}$ is shown in Equation 1

$$S_\sigma(I_{(x,y)}) = G_\sigma * \begin{bmatrix} \frac{\partial I^2}{\partial x^2} & \frac{\partial^2 I}{\partial x \partial y} \\ \frac{\partial^2 I}{\partial x \partial y} & \frac{\partial I^2}{\partial y^2} \end{bmatrix} \tag{1}$$

Structure Enhancing Diffusion acts as a denoising model that suppresses the noise as well as preserves the flow-like structure, which has special interest in mammography, since mammographic parenchymal pattern has flow-like, thin, linear structures within breast vasculature representing significant textural information [12]. It adapts its Eigenvalues to enhance the structure, hence the Eigenvalues are related to the anisotropy of the image represented by two conductivity terms β_1 and β_2 in the direction of gradient and isophote at a given scale respectively. Detailed information can be found in [11,13]. Structure enhancing diffusion tensor D is defined in the following Equation 2 as

$$D_\sigma(I_{(x,y)}) = G_\sigma * \frac{1}{\sqrt{l_2 - norm(I_x^\sigma, I_y^\sigma)}} \begin{bmatrix} \beta_1 \frac{\partial I^2}{\partial x^2} + \beta_2 \frac{\partial I^2}{\partial y^2} & (\beta_2 - \beta_1)\frac{\partial I}{\partial x}\frac{\partial I}{\partial y} \\ (\beta_2 - \beta_1)\frac{\partial I}{\partial x}\frac{\partial I}{\partial y} & \beta_1 \frac{\partial I^2}{\partial y^2} + \beta_2 \frac{\partial I^2}{\partial x^2} \end{bmatrix} \tag{2}$$

where $\beta_2 = e^{-\frac{\frac{\partial I^2}{\partial x^2} + \frac{\partial I^2}{\partial y^2}}{\eta^2}}$, $\beta_1 = \frac{1}{5} * \beta_2$, and G_σ denotes the Gaussian with standard deviation σ (aperture size over which the orientation information is averaged).

Both S and D can be decomposed by Eigen analysis. Eigensystem of these 2D tensors carries orientation information of the image that allows us to separate the image into constant areas, corners and straight edges according to number of non-zero Eigenvalues. The parameter to measure the spread of the Eigenvalues is the coherence C. For every sampled pixel, coherence features C based on Eigenvalues of structure tensor matrix S at four different scales σ of 2, 4, 8, and 16 mm are computed as shown in Equation 3

$$C_\sigma = (\frac{\lambda_1 - \lambda_2}{\lambda_1 + \lambda_2 + \eta})^2 \tag{3}$$

Where, λ_1 and λ_2 are eigen values of the tensor at specific scale σ and $\lambda_1 > \lambda_2$. η is a small positive number to avoid numerical stability problems in a the planner region of an image where $\lambda_1 \approx \lambda_2 \approx 0$.

In this way, the extracted texture features includes 48 features in total for each pixel location from three aforementioned feature categories, contributing 40 features for Gaussian derivative, and 4 coherence features each from structure tensor and structure enhancing diffusion as shown in Figure 1. In addition to these 48 features a position feature of each pixels from the centroid of the breast is added.

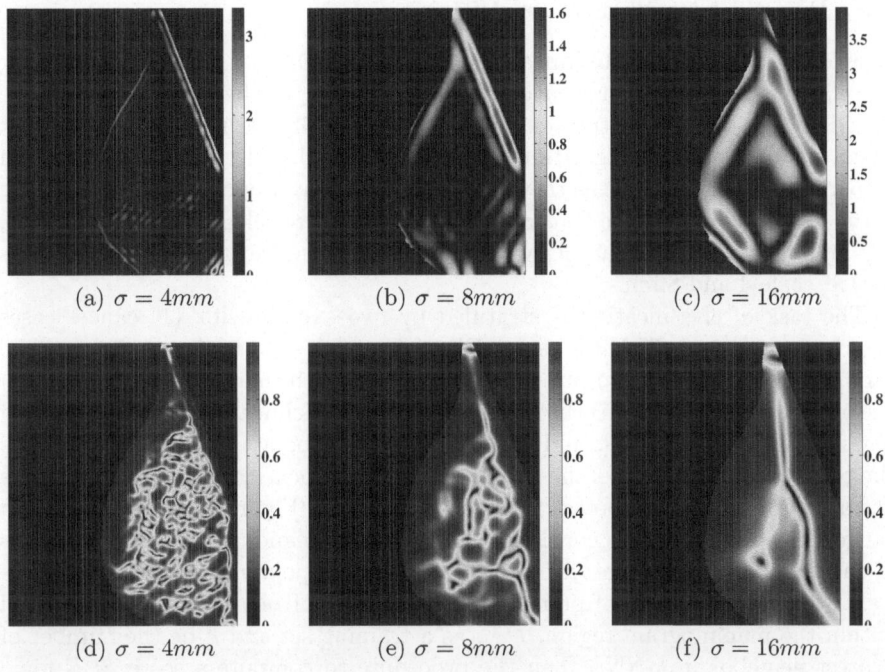

Fig. 1. (a-c) Representative 3-jet features at three different scales, (d-f) Examples of Coherence feature map of structure tensor at three different scales

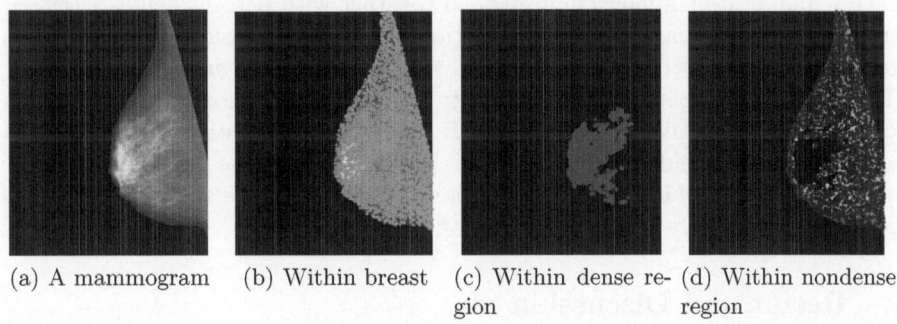

Fig. 2. Illustration of the feature sampling process (e.g., pixel locations) within various region of mammogram, considered for texture analysis, representing the total breast area, and specifically the dense and the fatty (e.g., non-dense) tissue regions

Breast percent density PD% of a mammogram is computed by a multi-class fuzzy c-means (FCM) algorithm based on an optimal number of clusters derived by the tissue properties of the specific mammogram as described in Keller et al. [14].

3.2 Feature Classification and Scoring

A pixel based approximate k-nearest neighbor (k-NN) classifier [15] is used for the classification of texture features. Dimensionality of the feature space is reduced to a maximum feature of 6 from the initial 48 features by using a rank based feature selection algorithm [16] followd by 10 fold cross validation with recognition rate quantified as the area under the receiver operating characteristic curve (AUC). The texture features selected by feature selection mostly include, 2nd and 3rd order Gaussian derivatives and coherence features of structure tensors at scale 4 and 8mm.

The task of classification is stratified by two experiments: (1) cancer cases versus controls and (2) ER+ versus ER- cancer cases. In both experiments, we sample pixel locations from three different regions of the mammogram namely, (i) the entire breast region, (ii) the dense breast region delineated by the automated segmentation method [14], and (iii) the non-dense breast region, calculated as the total breast area minus the dense region. Pixel locations selected for feature extraction from various breast regions are shown in Figure 2. We investigate a range for the set of points consisting 500, 1000, 2000 and 3000 number of pixels in each region. We average the score from all set of points as explained below.

Let AP be the array of point set with number of pixel location considered within the mammogram region, D_{TR} as a training set and k be the number of nearest neighbor in k-NN , then the procedure to compute a score SCR for a mammogram is explained in Algorithm 1.

Initial analysis was done within each region of the breast separately (namely, entire breast, dense region, non-dense region, and PD%). Scores obtained from each region of a mammogram are added together with percent dentsity (PD%) to make a multivariate model and a series of logistic regression analysis is done to identify variable that were associated with the class label in each experiment. To measure the sensitivity and specificity of each region, the c-statistics i.e. area under receiver operator characteristic (ROC) curve for logistic regression model was calculated. Standard error of AUC is computed using the methods of Hanley and McNeil [18], which guide in determining the size of the sample required to provide a sufficiently reliable estimate of this area.

4 Result and Discussion

Figure 3 shows the performance of the texture measures extracted from the various regions of the mammogram for the task of both (1) cancer vs controls and (2) ER subtype specific classification. Breast (PD%) and parenchymal texture features can both distinguish between cancer cases and controls (A_z >0.70, see Figure 3(a)). These results supports previous research findings by Kerlikowske et al. [19] where women with high mammographic density are reported to have increased risk of both ER-positive and ER-negative breast cancers $A_z =$ 0.70. However, for ER subtype-specific discrimination (see Figure 3(b)), PD% alone does not provide sufficient information ($A_z = 0.61$), while texture features

Algorithm 1. Mammogram scoring procedure

Input: $AP = \{500, 1000, 2000, 3000\}$, Training set D_{TR}, $k = 100$, $SCR = 0$

Output: The summary of mammogram score.

  for $ps = 1$ to size of AP **do**
    for $n = 1$ to size of ps **do**
      Extract fourty eight texture features and one position feature of nth pixel within specified region of a given mammogram.
      Do Rank based feature selection on D_{TR}.
      Compute the class label probability of nth pixel using k-NN with k number of nearest neighbour.
      Store the class label probability in array SC
    end for
    $SCR_{ps} = \overline{SC}$
  end for
  $SCR = \overline{SCR_{ps}}$

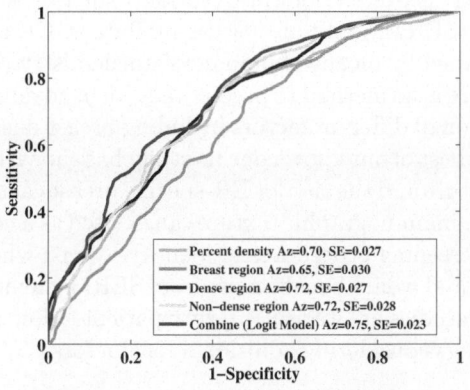

(a) Cancer vs Control classification

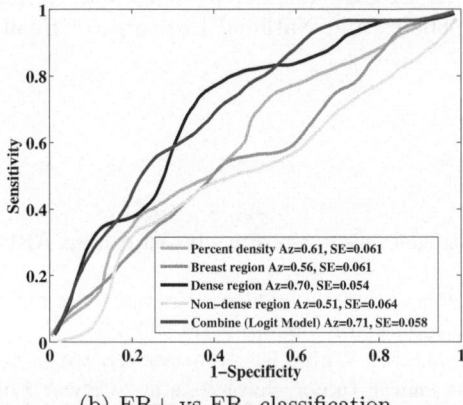

(b) ER+ vs ER- classification

Fig. 3. Area under Receiver Operative Characteristic Curve (A_z) and standard error (SE) required to compute statistical significance by DeLong test[17] for various experiments

independently discriminate with significant classification accuracy ($A_z = 0.70$). Combining breast PD% with texture features achieves the best performance ($A_z = 0.71$). In addition, we observe that the discrimination between ER subtypes becomes better while considering the dense region only than the non-dense region (see Figure 3). Further investigation is underway to help better understand the link between percent density, mammographic parenchymal texture features and ER specific subtype risk.

5   Conclusion

Our study suggests that mammographic texture potentially has value for ER specific breast cancer risk assessment. To the best of our knowledge our study is the first to explore the potential of mammographic parenchymal texture analysis for ER subtype-specific breast cancer risk assessment. This could have significant impact in personalized risk-reduction interventions, such as selective estrogen receptor modulators (SERMs) and aromatase inhibitors. Currently, evaluation of ER-status is performed by means of immunohistochemistry (IHC) at the time of diagnosis, while there is no method to predict the risk in advance [20]. Studies have shown the association of different factors including breast density with ER status [21]. To date, to the best of our knowledge no study has shown the association with mammographic texture and the risk for ER-specific breast cacncer. If our hypothesis proves to be true, mammographic texture can be used as a non-invasive imaging biomarker during screening procedures to identify women who are at high risk of ER+ breast cancer and would benefit most from SERM chemoprevention. Larger prospective clinical studies are warranted, with patient follow-up, to prospectively validate these findings considering additional risk factors.

Acknowledgement. This work was supported in part by American Cancer Society Grant RSGHP-CPHPS-119586, United States Department of Defense Concept Award BC086591, and National Institutes of Health PROSPR Grant 1U54CA163313-01.

References

1. Shelley Hwang, E., Chew, T., Shiboski, S., Farren, G., Benz, C.C., Wrensch, M.: Risk factors for estrogen receptor-positive breast cancer. ARCH SURG 140, 58–62 (2005)
2. Savage, L.: Researchers wonder why high-risk women are not taking chemoprevention drugs. J. Natl. Cancer Inst. 99, 913–914 (2007)
3. Aiello, E.J., Buist, D.S.M., White, E.: Association between mammographic breast density and breast cancer tumor characteristics. Cancer Epidemiol. Biomarkers Prev. 14, 662–668 (2005)
4. Boyd, N.F., Melnichouk, O., Martin, L.J., Hislop, G., Chiarelli, A.M., Yaffe, M.J., Minkin, S.: Mammographic density, response to hormones, and breast cancer risk. J. Clin. Oncol. 29, 2985–2992 (2011)

5. Heine, J.J., Malhotra, P.: Mammographic tissue, breast cancer risk, serial image analysis and digital mammography. part 1 tissue and related risk factors. Academic Radiology 9(3), 115–122 (2002)
6. Li, H., Giger, M.L., Olopade, O.I., Margolis, A., Lan, L., Chinander, M.R.: Computerized texture analysis of mammographic parenchymal patterns of digitized mammograms. Acad. Radiol. 12(7), 863–873 (2005)
7. Yerushalmi, R., Woods, R., Kennecke, H., Speers, C., Knowling, M., Gelmon, K.: Patterns of relapse in breast cancer: changes over time. Breast Cancer Res. Treat 120, 753–759 (2010)
8. Nielsen, M., Karemore, G., Loog, M., Raundahl, J., Karssemeijer, N., Otten, J.D., Karsdal, M.A., Vachon, C.M., Christiansen, C.: A novel and automatic mammographic texture resemblance marker is an independent risk factor for breast cancer. Cancer Epidemiol. 35, 381–387 (2011)
9. Karemore, G., Brandt, S., Sporring, J., Nielsen, M.: Anisotropic diffusion tensor applied to temporal mammograms: an application to breast cancer risk assessment. In: Conf. Proc. IEEE Eng. Med. Biol. Soc. (2010)
10. Young, R.A.: The gaussian derivative model for spatial vision: I. retinal mechanisms. Spat. Vis. 2(4), 273–293 (1987)
11. Weickert, J.: Coherence-enhancing diffusion filtering. Int. J. Comput. Vision 31, 111–127 (1999)
12. Karahaliou, A., Skiadopoulos, S., Boniatis, I., Sakellaropoulos, P., Likaki, E., Panayiotakis, G., Costaridou, L.: Texture analysis of tissue surrounding microcalcifications on mammograms for breast cancer diagnosis. Br. J. Radiol. (2007)
13. van den Boomgaard, R.: Algorithms for non-linear diffusion. Technical report, Intelligent Sensory Information Systems, University of Amsterdam, Kruislaan 403, 1098 SJ Amsterdam,The Netherlands
14. Keller, B., Nathan, D., Wang, Y., Zheng, Y., Gee, J., Conant, E., Kontos, D.: Adaptive multi-cluster fuzzy c-means segmentation of breast parenchymal tissue in digital mammography. Med. Image Comput. Comput. Assist. Interv. 14(3), 562–569 (2011)
15. Arya, S., Mount, D.M., Netanyahu, N.S., Silverman, R., Wu, A.Y.: An optimal algorithm for approximate nearest neighbor searching fixed dimensions. J. ACM 45, 891–923 (1998)
16. Geng, X., Liu, T.-Y., Qin, T., Li, H.: Feature Selection for Ranking, vol. (49), pp. 407–414. ACM Press (2007)
17. DeLong, E.R., DeLong, D.M., Clarke-Pearson, D.L.: Comparing the areas under two or more correlated receiver operating characteristic curves: a nonparametric approach. Biometrics 44(3), 837–845 (1988)
18. Hanley, J.A., McNeil, B.J.: The meaning and use of the area under a receiver operating characteristic (roc) curve. Radiology 143, 29–36 (1982)
19. Ziv, E., Tice, J., Smith-Bindman, R., Shepherd, J., Cummings, S., Kerlikowske, K.: Mammographic density and estrogen receptor status of breast cancer. Cancer Epidemiology Biomarkers Prevention 13(12), 2090–2095 (2004)
20. Kostopoulos, S., Cavouras, D., Daskalakis, A., Kalatzis, I., Bougioukos, P., Kagadis, G.C., Ravazoula, P., Nikiforidis, G.: Assessing Estrogen Receptors' Status by Texture Analysis of Breast Tissue Specimens and Pattern Recognition Methods. In: Kropatsch, W.G., Kampel, M., Hanbury, A. (eds.) CAIP 2007. LNCS, vol. 4673, pp. 221–228. Springer, Heidelberg (2007)
21. Hines, L.M., Risendal, B., Slattery, M.L.: Differences in estrogen receptor subtype according to family history of breast cancer among hispanic, but not non-hispanic white women. Cancer Epidemiol. Biomarkers Prev. 17, 2700–2706 (2008)

A Phantom Study for Assessing the Effect of Different Digital Detectors on Mammographic Texture Features

Yan Wang, Brad M. Keller, Yuanjie Zheng, Raymond J. Acciavatti,
James C. Gee, Andrew D.A. Maidment, and Despina Kontos

Department of Radiology, University of Pennsylvania, Philadelphia, PA USA
wangyan1@sas.upenn.edu

Abstract. Digital mammography (DM) is commonly used as the breast imaging screening modality. For research based on DM datasets with various sources of x-ray detectors, it is important to evaluate if different detectors could introduce inherent differences in the images analyzed. To determine the extent of such effects, we performed a study to compare the effects of two DM detectors, the GE 2000D and DS, on texture analysis using a validated breast texture phantom (Yaffe et. al, University of Toronto). DM images are acquired in Cranio-Caudal (CC) view, and texture features are generated for both raw and post-processed DM images. Image intensity profiles and texture features are compared between the two detector systems. Our results suggest that there are inherent differences in the images. For raw and processed images, the image intensity cumulative distribution function (CDF) curves reveal that there is a scaling and shifting factor respectively between the two detectors. Image normalization with z-score can reduce detector differences for grey-level intensity and the histogram-based texture features. The differences between co-occurrence and run-length texture features persist after intensity normalization, suggesting that simple z-scoring cannot alleviate all the detector effects, potentially also due to differences in the spatial distribution of the intensity values between the two detectors.

Keywords: Digital mammography, detectors, breast phantom, texture analysis.

1 Introduction

Breast cancer is considered a major health problem in western countries, as it comprises 10.4% of the cancer incidence among women, making it the second most common type of cancer. Early screening and proper treatment after diagnosis for individual women are both important aspects of current breast cancer research, and digital mammography (DM) is the main screening tool for cancer detection [1].

The Gail Model [2] has been shown be able to estimate breast cancer at the population level, however with limited capacity at the individual level. There's intensive research for individual breast cancer risk estimation, and mammographic density, estimated as the percent of dense tissue area within the breast, has been shown to be the strongest risk factor for breast cancer after age [3, 4]. Studies [5-8] also support a relationship between mammographic texture and breast cancer risk, as mammographic texture features may be able to quantify the local distribution of the

A.D.A. Maidment, P.R. Bakic, and S. Gavenonis (Eds.): IWDM 2012, LNCS 7361, pp. 604–610, 2012.

parenchymal pattern, potentially providing complementary information for breast cancer risk estimation.

In the process of developing proper imaging biomarkers for risk estimation, it is commonly the case that studies use DM images acquired with different imaging systems and different x-ray detectors. It may be important and necessary to treat the detector source as an additional parameter in the analysis, as different detectors may possibly introduce inherent differences in the DM images [9]. To determine the effects of x-ray detectors in mammographic texture analysis, we designed a physical breast phantom study. The image intensity and extracted texture features [10-12] from the breast phantom are compared between two x-ray detectors for both raw and the vendor post-processed (a.k.a., processed) images. The rationale is that since images are generated from the same phantom, quantitative imaging features should be consistent between the images (e.g., affected only minimally by noise). Instead of limiting to a square of region of interest (ROI) behind the nipple as has been done in prior work [6, 8], the textures of the whole breast region are used for the analysis. The results of this comparison study could guide the proper choice of more robust texture features that are less sensitive to detector differences. Our study can be potentially helpful for any studies utilizing texture analysis in digital mammography, including breast cancer risk assessment, breast tissue classification and computed aided lesion detection, as a method for assessing potential detector differences.

2   Methods

The Gammex 169 "Rachel" breast phantom was used in our experiments (Yaffe. et al, University of Toronto) [13]. Image acquisition was performed on GE Healthcare 2000D and DS FFDM system at 0.1mm/pixel resolution, 14 bit gray-levels. On each machine, the clinically optimized phototimed setting of (kVp, mAs) was chosen, which was 29 kVp, 71 mAs for the 2000D; and 29 kVp, 90 mAs for the DS system. The image acquisition process was repeated 5 times for both machines. The average of the 5 images was used to reduce the effects of noise in the imaging process.

In the original phantom image, the outer bounding case appeared in the image (Figure. 1). Therefore, as an additional preprocessing step, in order to avoid the operational artifacts (e.g. the phantom may not be centered perfectly on the two detectors and the outer case artifacts), we cropped a region of interest (ROI) corresponding to the breast area, as shown in the middle of Figure 1, and used a synchronic threshold scheme to generate the breast masks for the two detectors. Based on the assumption that the breast area in the image is the same using the two detectors, we optimize the thresholds of post-processed image intensity by solving the optimization problem:

$$\arg\min_{(t_1,t_2)} |BA(2000D, t_1) - BA(DS, t_2)| \tag{1}$$

here breast area is denoted as BA, t_1, t_2 as the intensity threshold for the post-processed images from the two detectors. $BA(\text{detector}, t) =$ the cardinal of the set $\{p|$ the pixel p is in the ROI and the post-processed image intensity at $p >= t\}$.

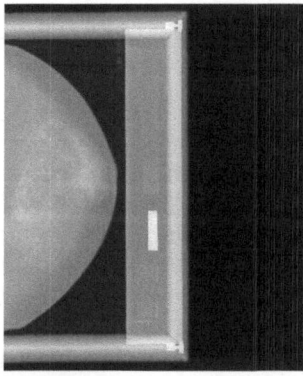 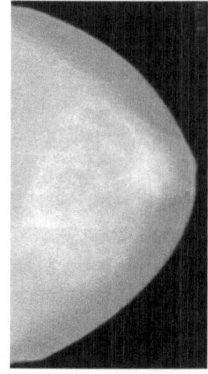 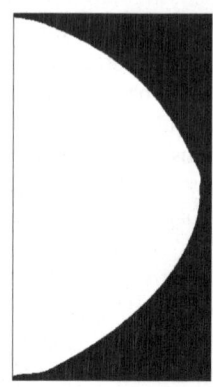

Fig. 1. Processed DM image acquired on the 2000D system; Left: original phantom image, Middle: manually cropped ROI, Right: the final breast region mask

Multiple texture features are extracted using an automated breast image analysis software pipeline [14], including 1) grey-level histogram features, 2) co-occurrence texture features, and 3) run-length features. These features have been shown in previous studies to have value in breast cancer risk estimation [5-7]. The texture images are generated by calculating texture features within a series of adjacent square regions covering the original breast region, with the side length of the square equals to 16 pixels. A total of 26 texture features were computed. A summary of these texture features is shown in Table 1.

Table 1. Texture descriptors included in parenchymal texture analysis

Grey-Level Histogram	5th /5thmean/95th/95thmean/ max/mean/min/sum entropy/kurtosis/sigma/skewness
Co-occurrence	cluster shade/ inverse difference moment correlation/energy/entropy/inertia Haralick correlation
Run-Length	grey level nonuniformity/ run length nonuniformity high grey level run emphasis/ long run emphasis low grey level run emphasis/short run emphasis run percentage

Our comparison study is based on comparing the image intensity and texture feature profiles of both the raw and processed DM phantom images, where the cumulative distribution function (CDF) curves of each image feature are computed and compared between the two x-ray detectors. All features in Table 1 are generated for both original images and the z-scored images, and the effects of z-scoring on detector differences are also evaluated. The Kolmogorov-Smirnov distance, which defined as the maximum of the absolute vertical difference between two CDF curves [15, 16], is used as the distance between two CDF curves in the result.

3   Results

The size of the ROI is 1842×775 pixels for the images of both detectors, with optimized threshold of $(t_1^*, t_2^*) = (1068, 456)$, with $BA(2000D, t_1^*) = 939916$ (pixels), and BA(DS, t_2^*)=940598 (pixels). The |breast area difference|/$BA(2000D, t_1^*) = 0.07\%$.

On the 2000D system, for raw and processed images, the standard deviation of the 5 times of phototimed imaging in terms of the maximum/minimum/standard deviation of the image intensity is 2.25/7.29/0.52 and 9.4/4.2/0.0821 respectively. On the DS system, the corresponding values are 24.4/5.39/1.1 and 5.1/4.3/0.12. In the following analysis, the average of the 5 phototimed images was used for each detector to reduce the effects of noise in the imaging process. The cumulative distribution function (CDF) of the image intensity within the breast region is shown for the two detectors (Fig. 2).

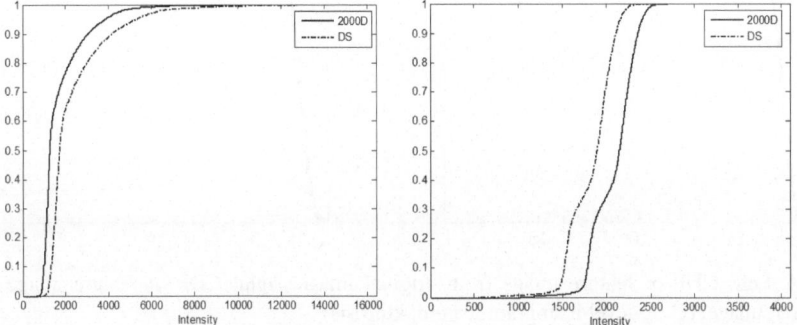

Fig. 2. The image intensity CDF of the original image. Left: raw, right: processed images.

The CDF comparison in the raw/processed images indicates that the intensity differences between the images from two detectors may be affected by a scaling/shifting factor respectively. After z-scoring the image intensity within the breast area, the differences in the CDF of the image intensity are alleviated, as shown in Figure 3. The distance between CDF curves of the two detectors are reduced from 0.4730/0.4731 to 0.0249/0.0263 for raw/processed images respectively.

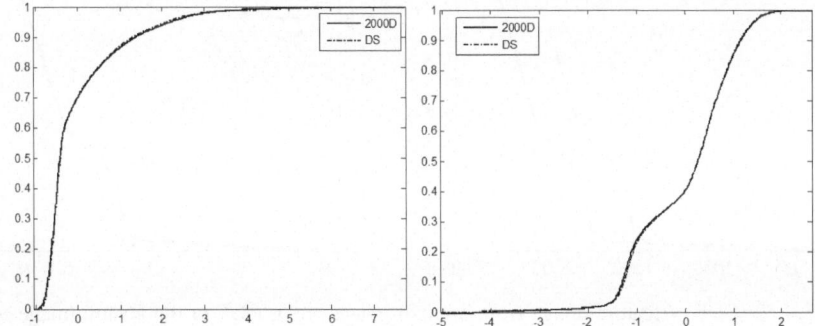

Fig. 3. The image intensity CDF of z-scored image. Left: raw, Right: processed image.

Comparisons are also done for all the texture features listed in Table 1. Our results indicate that texture features can be broadly categorized into three groups, according to how they are affected by the detector differences and z-scoring. Certain features are not affected by detectors, others are affected but compensated by z-score, and some are affected regardless.

Specifically, the first group of features that is minimally affected by detectors includes the grey-level histogram features (e.g., entropy, kurtosis, sigma, skewness). The CDF curves of the texture feature kurtosis is shown as an example in Figure 4, for which the distance between the CDF curves is 0.0839/0.0732 for the original raw and processed images, after z-scoring, the distance remains the same 0.0839/0.0732.

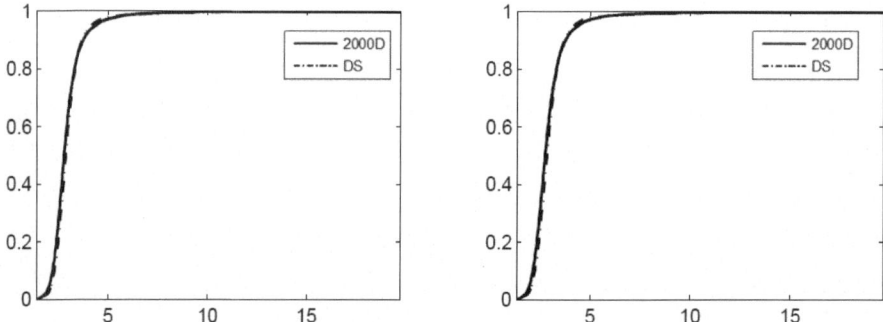

Fig. 4. Left: CDF of feature image from original image, right: CDF of feature image from z-scored image. (Grey-level histogram feature: kurtosis)

The second group of features is affected by detectors, but the differences in the CDF can be alleviated by z-scoring the original image. This includes the remaining grey-level histogram features and the cluster shade co-occurrence feature. As an example in Figure 5, for the grey-level histogram feature mean, the distance between the CDF curves of the two detectors is 0.4732/0.4728 for raw and processed images, after z-scoring, the distance is decreased to 0.0255/0.0328.

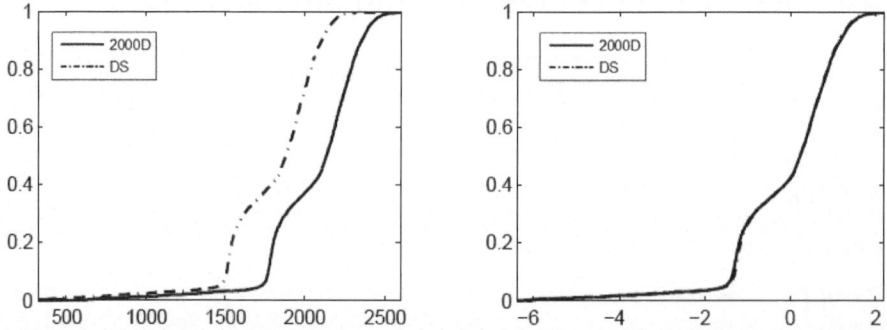

Fig. 5. Left: CDF of feature image from original image, right: CDF of the feature image from z-scored image. (Grey-level histogram feature: mean)

The third group of features is affected by detectors; however simple z-scoring cannot reduce the observed differences. This group mainly includes the co-occurrence texture features (except cluster shade) and run-length features. As an example in Figure 6, for the co-occurrence feature inverse difference moment, the distance between the CDF curves between two detectors is 0.2331/0.2301 for raw and processed images, however after z-scoring, the distance is increased to 0.3229/0.4145.

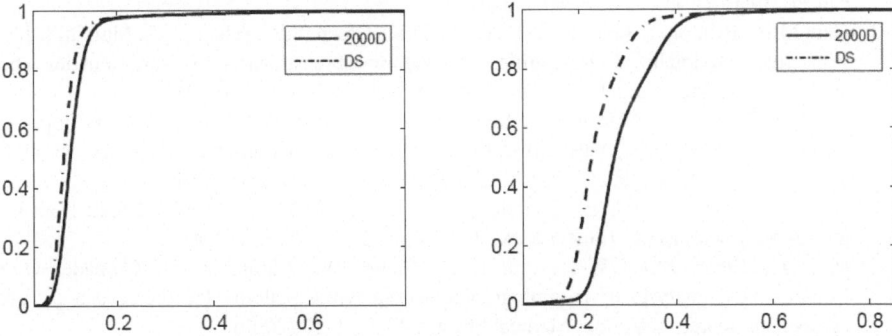

Fig. 6. Left: CDF of feature image from original image, right: CDF of feature image from z-scored image (Co-occurrence texture feature: inverse difference moment)

4   Discussion and Conclusion

In this study, we compared the image intensity and texture profiles of two GE DM x-ray detectors using a physical breast phantom. The rationale is that since images are generated from the same phantom, the resulting image features should remain very similar (e.g., effected only minimally by noise). Our results show that the CDF curves for processed and raw image intensity values between two detectors reveal a shifting and scaling pattern respectively. Comparing the different texture features suggests that the texture features can be broadly categorized into three groups. In summary, after z-scoring the image intensity of the original phantom images, the differences in the intensity values and the grey-level histogram features are alleviated, however the differences in texture features may depend not only on absolute gray-level intensity values in the image, but also on the spatial distribution of the image intensity values, such as most of the co-occurrence and run-length texture features differences between the two detectors, which are not reduced by simple intensity normalization z-scoring.

The CDF curve information studied in this study is used as the first step comparison study on how different x-ray detectors may affect the image intensity and texture. Further work is underway to fully-investigate such differences, and to develop a comprehensive feature standardization scheme that can be potentially used to reduce effects introduced by the imaging system on the subsequent image analysis process.

Acknowledgement. This work was supported in part by American Cancer Society Grant RSGHP-CPHPS-119586, United States Department of Defense Concept Award BC086591, and National Institutes of Health PROSPR Grant 1U54CA163313-01.

References

1. Smith, K.L., Isaacs, C.: Management of women at increased risk for hereditary breast cancer. Breast Disease 27, 51–67 (2006)
2. Gail, M.H., Brinton, L.A., Byar, D.P., Corle, D.K., Green, S.B., Schairer, C., Mulvihill, J.J.: Projecting individualized probabilities of developing breast cancer for white females who are being examined annually. J. Natl. Cancer 81(24), 1879–1886 (1989)
3. Boyd, N.F., Guo, H., Martin, L.J., Sun, L., Stone, J., Fishell, E., Jong, R.A., Hislop, G., Chiarelli, A., Minkin, S., Yaffe, M.J.: Mammographic density and the risk and detection of breast cancer. New England Journal of Medicine 356(3), 227–236 (2007)
4. Harvey, J.A., Bovbjerg, V.E.: Quantitative Assessment of Mammographic Breast Density: Relationship with Breast Cancer Risk. Radiology 230(1), 29–41 (2004)
5. Huo, Z., Giger, M.L., Wolverton, D.E., Zhong, W., Cumming, S., Olopade, O.I.: Computerized analysis of mammographic parenchymal patterns for breast cancer risk assessment: feature selection. Medical Physics 27(1), 4–12 (2000)
6. Li, H., Giger, M.L., Olopade, O.I., Margolis, A., Lan, L., Chinander, M.R.: Computerized Texture Analysis of Mammographic Parenchymal Patterns of Digitized Mammograms. Academic Radiology 12(7), 863–873 (2005)
7. Manduca, A., Carston, M.J., Heine, J.J., Scott, C.G., Pankratz, V.S., Brandt, K.R., et al.: Texture Features from Mammographic Images and Risk of Breast Cancer. Cancer Epidemiol. Biomarkers Prev. 18(3), 837–845 (2009)
8. Kontos, D., Bakic, P.R., Carton, A.K., Troxel, A.B., Conant, E.F., Maidment, A.D.A.: Parenchymal texture analysis in digital breast tomosynthesis for breast cancer risk estimation: A preliminary study. Academic Radiology 16(3), 283–298 (2009)
9. Williams, M.B., Yaffe, M.J., Maidment, A.D., Martin, M.C., Seibert, J.A., Pisano, E.D.: Image quality in digital mammography: image acquisition. Journal of the American College of Radiology 3(8), 589–608 (2006)
10. Haralick, R.M., Shanmugam, K., Dinstein, I.: Textural features for image classification. IEEE Transactions on Systems, Man and Cybernetics 3, 610–621 (1973)
11. Galloway, M.D.: Texture classification using gray level run length. Computer Graphics and Image Processing 4, 172–179 (1975)
12. Amadasum, M., King, R.: Textural features corresponding to textural properties. IEEE Transactions on Systems Man and Cybernetics 19, 1264–1274 (1989)
13. Caldwell, C.B., Yaffe, M.J.: Development of an anthropomorphic breast phantom. Medical Physics 17(2), 273–280 (1990)
14. Zheng, Y., Keller, B., Wang, Y., Tustison, N., Song, G., Bakic, P.R., Maidment, A.D., Conant, E.F., Gee, J.C., Kontos, D.: A Fully-Automated Software Pipeline for Parenchymal Pattern Analysis in Digital Breast Images: Toward the Translation of Imaging Biomarkers in Routine Breast Cancer Risk Assessment. In: Quantitative Imaging Reading Room, the 97th Scientific Assembly and Annual Meeting of the Radiological Society of North America (RSNA) 2011, Chicago, IL (software exhibit) (2011)
15. Smirnov, N.V.: Tables for estimating the goodness of fit of empirical distributions. Annals. of Mathematical Statistics 19, 279–281 (1948)
16. Rachev, S.T.: Probability Metrics and Stability of Stochastic Models. JohnWiley & Sons (1991)

Reduction of Patient Dose in Digital Mammography: Simulation of Low-Dose Image from a Routine Dose

Yuki Saito[1], Aya Kawai[2], Naotoshi Fujita[3], Maki Yamada[1], and Yoshie Kodera[1]

[1] Department of Radiological Sciences,
Nagoya University Graduate School of Medicine, Nagoya, Japan
saitoh.yuuki@e.mbox.nagoya-u.ac.jp
[2] Department of Radiological Technology, Toyota Regional Medical Center, Toyota, Japan
[3] Department of Radiological Technology, Nagoya University Hospital, Nagoya, Japan

Abstract. Several low-dose images are necessary to obtain an image that can be used for diagnosis. However, it is clinically undesirable to expose a patient to multiple exposures in order to obtain an optimal image. The purpose of this study was to simulate a low-dose image from the image generated by a routine dose. Images of acrylic steps were obtained using multiple doses in digital mammography with computed radiography to generate additional noise. This noise was added to take into account the resolution of the X-ray detector using the some filters. The image simulated using the filter based on the WS was similar to an actual low-dose image. The image simulated using the presampled MTF filter was less similar to an actual low-dose image. By using the proposed method, we were able to obtain a simulated low-dose image from an image generated by a routine dose.

Keywords: simulation, computed radiography, dose reduction.

1 Introduction

To reduce patients' exposure to radiation during digital mammography, it is preferable to acquire images using a minimum dose. Recently, owing to the developments of X-ray detectors, the exposure dose required for acquiring a digital image has been re-examined. It is necessary to assess several low-dose images in order to establish a diagnosis. However, it is clinically undesirable to expose a patient to several exposure conditions for determining an optimal image. Even if the technique involves the use of a phantom, considerable time is required for obtaining several images. Therefore, it is necessary to generate a low-dose image through simulation. The purpose of this study is to simulate a low-dose image from the image generated using a routine dose. The noise in an image varies because the detected photons pass through materials consisting of different substances and having varying thicknesses. Hence, it is necessary to add a different noise to each pixel value in the image. In previous studies, the noise was not changed for pixel by pixel [1] or the resolution of the X-ray detector on noise differed from actual measurement [2]. The aim of this study is the addition of a different noise for each pixel by considering the resolution of the X-ray detector.

A.D.A. Maidment, P.R. Bakic, and S. Gavenonis (Eds.): IWDM 2012, LNCS 7361, pp. 611–618, 2012.

2   Methods and Materials

2.1   Simulation Process

Fig. 1 shows a flow-chart of the simulation process. The noise image that accounts for the pixel value of the low-dose image is generated from the relationship between the pixel value and the standard deviation (SD), which serves as the noise index. The noise is calculated for each pixel value, based on the variation in detected photons of a routine-dose image. The noise is blurred by the resolution of the X-ray detector in a spatial frequency domain. The blurred noise image is added to the routine-dose image to generate the simulation image.

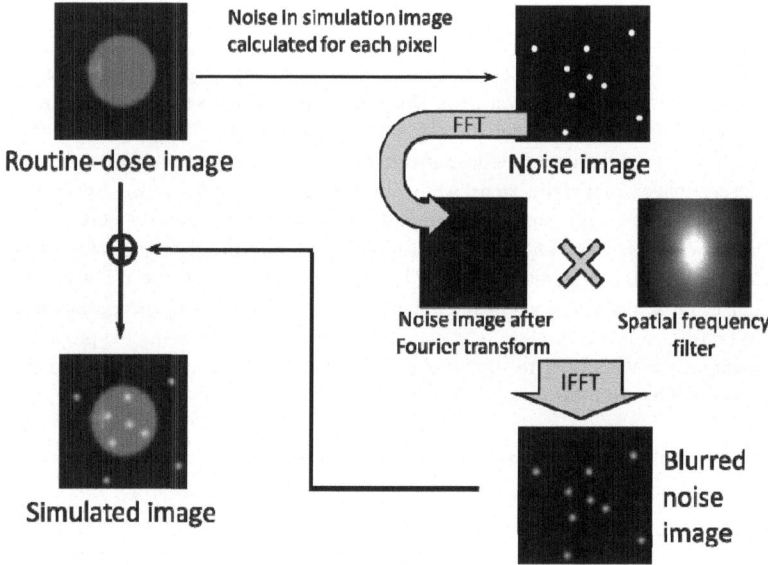

Fig. 1. Flow-chart of the simulation process

2.2   Materials

The digital mammography system was used in this study. The CR reader used was a REGIUS V stage, Model 190. The CR plate used was CP1M200. These were manufactured by Konica Minolta MG.

2.3   Generation of Additional Noise

Images of the acrylic steps were obtained to examine the relationship between the pixel value and the noise. The experimental setup is shown in Fig. 2.

It included 10 acrylic steps spaced at 1 mm intervals and four acrylic plates spaced at 1 cm intervals. By employing both acrylic steps and acrylic plates, images with up

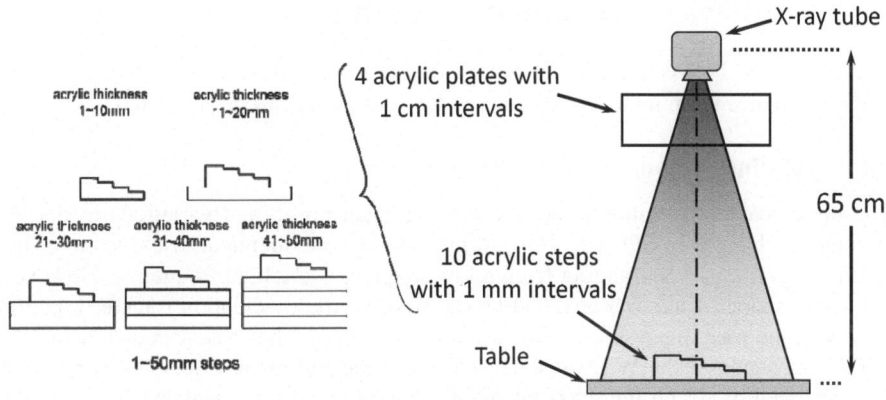

Fig. 2. Experimental setup

to 50 acrylic steps placed at 1mm intervals were obtained. Ten different exposure doses were established through digital mammography with computed radiography. Next, the images were generated under 500 different exposure conditions. We measured the pixel value under each exposure condition and calculated the SD as the noise index. Under all exposure conditions, the tube voltage was 28 kV and the target/filter was Mo/Mo.

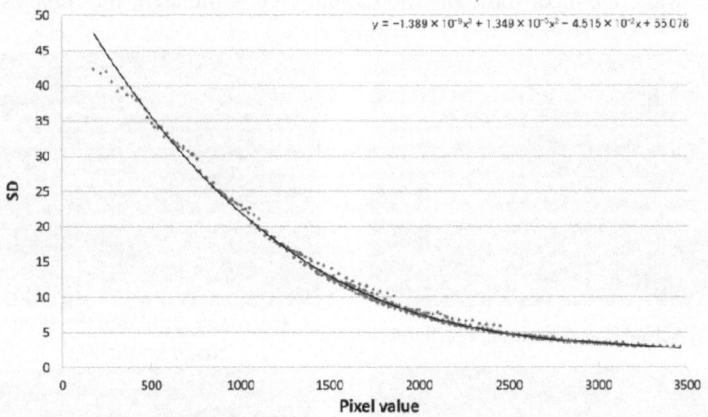

Fig. 3. Relationship between SD and pixel value

Next, we determined relationship between the pixel value and the SD of the acrylic steps. This relationship is shown in Fig. 3 the horizontal axis represents the pixel value and the vertical axis represents the SD. It can be seen from the figure that the SD decreases as the pixel value increases. In other words, the noise in an image decreases as the exposure dose increases. The SD of a routine-dose image is $\sigma_{routine}$, whereas that of the low-dose image is σ_{low}. Moreover, the additional noise SD σ_x can be described by equation (1).

$$\sigma^2_{low} = \sigma^2_{routine} + \sigma^2_x \tag{1}$$

The difference between the pixel values of the routine-dose and low-dose images freely fluctuates with the mAs value of the low-dose image to be simulated.

2.4   Take into Account Detector Resolution

The noise made was approximated to the Gaussian noise, and variations in dosage resulted in changes in SD. The simulation noise became identical to the value of the Wiener spectrum (WS) ranging from a low frequency to a high frequency. However, the actual shape of the WS changed on the basis of the modulation transfer function (MTF) of the imaging system. Thus, a spatial frequency filter was designed using the MTF. The shape of the WS was corrected using the following filters. The first filter was designed based on the presampled MTF, the second was designed based on the digital MTF containing aliasing, and the third was designed based on the measured value of the WS.

3   Result

3.1   Comparison of Phantom Images

The 50 mAs image was used as the routine-dose image, and the low-dose image of 2.5 mAs was obtained through simulation. We simulated the images using a

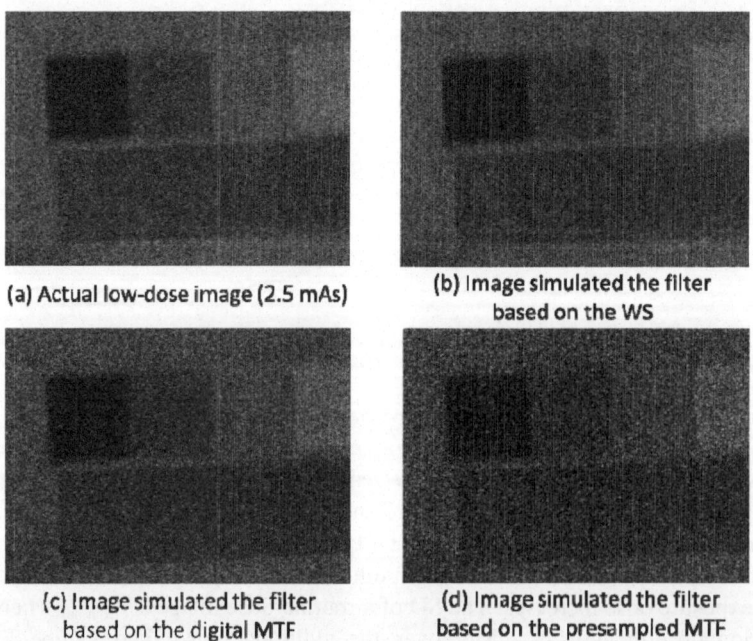

(a) Actual low-dose image (2.5 mAs)

(b) Image simulated the filter based on the WS

(c) Image simulated the filter based on the digital MTF

(d) Image simulated the filter based on the presampled MTF

Fig. 4. Phantom images

tissue-equivalent mammography phantom of CIRS Model 011A. Figure 4 (a) shows the images actual low-dose image of 2.5 mAs, Fig. 4 (b) the image simulated using the filter based on the WS, Fig. 4 (c) the image simulated using the filter based on the digital MTF, and Fig. 4 (d) the image simulated using the filter based on the presampled MTF. The image simulated using the filter based on the WS is similar to the actual low-dose image. The noise suitable for the generation of the low-dose image could be easily transferred to the routine-dose image.

3.2   Comparison of Wiener spectra for various filters

The WS of the simulations and the actual low-dose are shown Fig. 5. The WS of the image simulated using the presampled MTF filter is very different from the WS of the actual low-dose image. Next, we consider the image simulated using the digital MTF filter. In this case, the shape of the WS was closer to an actual low-dose image compared to the image simulated using the presampled MTF filter. Finally, the WS of the image simulated using the filter based on the WS is found to similar to the WS of an actual low-dose image.

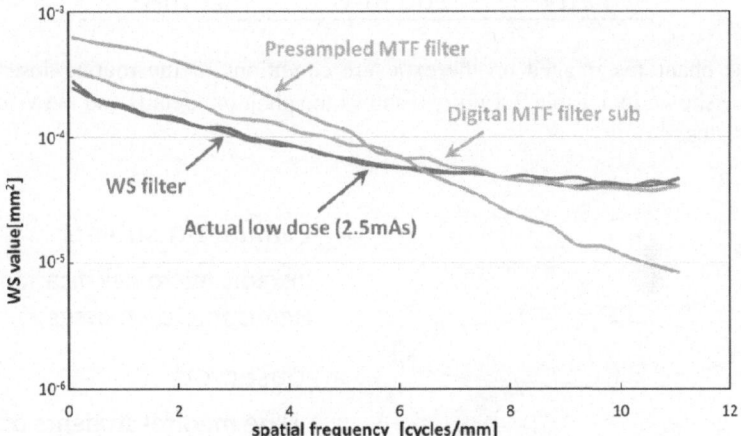

Fig. 5. Wiener spectra of simulations and actual low-dose image (sub scan direction)

3.3   Comparison between Visual Evaluations

We generated the images simulated using the mammography research set Model 012A of CIRS. This research set includes tissue equivalent phantoms that are 4, 5 and 6 cm thick. The glandular contents of the phantoms are 50%, 30%, and 20%, respectively, and these phantoms are referred to a Dense, Normal, and Fatty. The phantoms contain embedded micro-calcifications and hemispherical masses. For the evaluation, we referred to the method used by the Central Committee on Quality Control of Mammographic Screening in Japan [3]. A valuation basis is shown in Table 1.

Table 1. Valuation basis of mammography phantom

subject	valuation	score
Micro-calcification	6-4 observable	1
	2-3 observable	0.5
	only one observable, no observation	0
Hemispherical masses	observable as a circle	1
	poorly defined edge, but observable	0.5
	no observation	0

Table 2. Exposure conditions

phantom	routine-dose	low-dose
Dense	50 mAs	10 mAs
Normal	80 mAs	25 mAs
Fatty	100 mAs	32 mAs

These phantoms imaged on the exposure conditions of the routine-dose and the low-dose shown in a Table 2. Figure 6 shows the phantom details and the visual evaluation status.

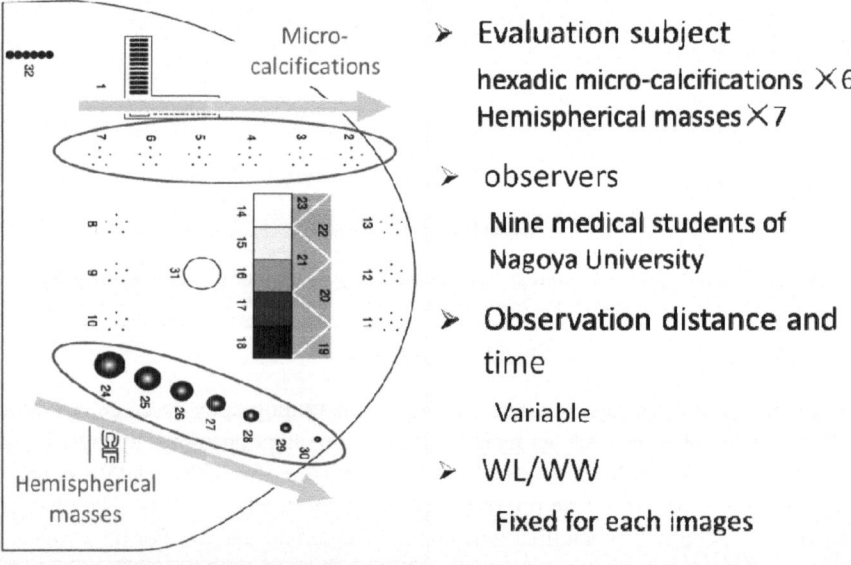

Micro-calcifications

Hemispherical masses

➤ **Evaluation subject**
hexadic micro-calcifications ×6
Hemispherical masses ×7

➤ observers
Nine medical students of Nagoya University

➤ **Observation distance and time**
Variable

➤ WL/WW
Fixed for each images

Fig. 6. Mammography phantom of CIRS and visual evaluation status

The actual low-dose image and the simulation image were displayed at random. The score in each object was summed for each observer and the difference in the average is compared between actual image and simulation image. Statistical significance test used Wilcoxon signed-rank test. The result of the test is shown in Figs. 7 and 8.

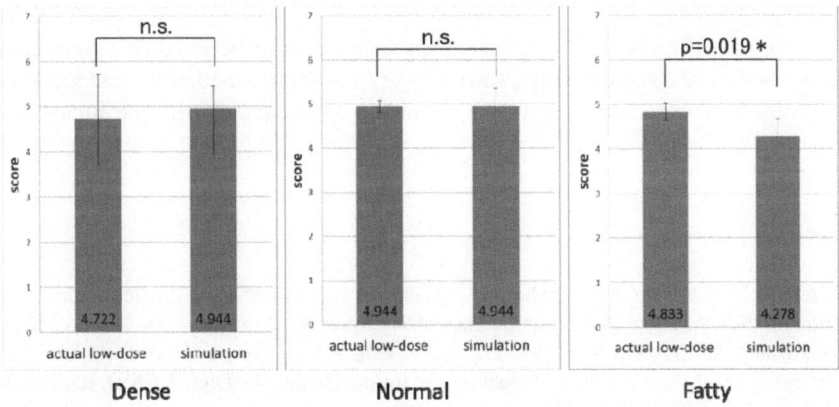

Fig. 7. Micro-calcification score

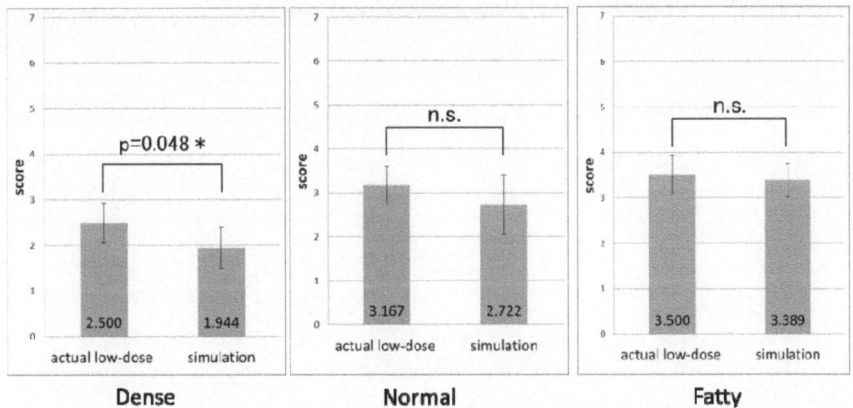

Fig. 8. Hemispherical masses score

In part of micro-calcification and hemispherical masses were significant difference at 5%, and others were no significant difference at 1%.

4   Discussion

The image simulated using the presampled MTF filter is less similar to the actual low-dose image. Since the MTF value is high, the CR plate used in this case was developed for mammography and influences the aliasing in the image. Therefore, the image simulated using the digital MTF filter is close to an actual low-dose image. In addition, when using the digital MTF filter, it is necessary to divide noise into components. This is because certain noise is influenced by the resolution of the X-ray detector (e.g., quantum noise) while certain other noise is not (e.g., structure noise). In addition, the dominant noise component depends on the amount of photons absorbed by the X-ray detector. We believe that the simulation becomes even more precise when the additional noise is also divided into noise component. We consider that the reason for the difference in the vision evaluation is change between observers and the setting interval of a score is large. I would like to examine whether dose reduction can henceforth be focused on as a viable technique as compared with the image in the auto mode.

References

1. Båth, M., Håkansson, M., Tingberg, A., Månsson, L.G.: Method of simulating dose reduction for digital radiographic systems. Radiation Protection Dosimetry 114, 253–259 (2005)
2. Veldkamp, W.J.H., Kroft, L.J.M., Pieter, J., Delft, A.V., Geleijns, J.: A Technique for Simulating the Effect of Dose Reduction on Image Quality in Digital Chest Radiography. Journal of Digital Imaging 22(2), 114–125 (2009)
3. The Central Committee on Quality Control of Mammographic Screening in Japan, Digital mammography quality control manual (2009)

Comparison of Hologic's Quantra Volumetric Assessment to MRI Breast Density

Jeff Wang, Ania Aziz, David Newitt, Bonnie N. Joe,
Nola Hylton, and John A. Shepherd

Department of Radiology and Biomedical Imaging, University of California, San Francisco
jeff.wang2@.ucsf.edu

Abstract. Interest in measuring breast tissue density due to its association with breast cancer risk grows, though the majority of studies use qualitative density measures manually reported by radiologists, which are time-consuming and costly. The purpose of this study was to compare the accuracy of Hologic's FDA-approved, commercially available automatic quantitative Quantra technique to a semi-automatic quantitative MRI-based Fuzzy C-Means technique in a screening population.

MRI and mammographic images were retrospectively analyzed from 123 women who had both types of exams within four years, a BIRADs diagnosis outcome of 1 or 2, and no history of breast cancer or surgery. Both techniques produced three measures: total breast volume, fibroglandular tissue volume, and percent fibroglandular tissue, which were compared.

Correlations between the three measures produced by the two techniques were mixed, with total volume having the highest correlation ($R2=0.8909$), percent fibroglandular density having moderate correlation ($R2=0.5015$), and fibroglandular tissue volume having the lowest correlation ($R2=0.3853$). Quantra results for percent fibroglandular density were significantly compressed in comparison with that of MRI, by about two-fold.

Keywords: Volumetric breast density, MRI segmentation, Fuzzy C-Means, Hologic Quantra.

1   Introduction

There is growing interest in measuring breast tissue density due to its association with breast cancer risk. The majority of studies up until now link breast density to breast cancer risk using qualitative mammographic density measures manually reported by radiologists, which are time-consuming and costly to obtain. The purpose of this study is to compare the accuracy of Hologic's automatic quantitative Quantra technique (Hologic, Inc., Bedford, MA) to a semi-automatic quantitative MRI-based Fuzzy C-Means technique in a screening population.

2   Background

The measure of dense breast tissue volume from mammograms has been shown to be a strong risk factor for breast cancer [1]. Tissue volume, however, is most accurately

A.D.A. Maidment, P.R. Bakic, and S. Gavenonis (Eds.): IWDM 2012, LNCS 7361, pp. 619–626, 2012.

described by three-dimensional imaging techniques such as MRI or CT. Techniques reconstructing the breast in three-dimensions from two-dimensional mammograms have been developed in recent years as mammography is foreseen to remain the most prevalent screening modality and digital systems are much more conducive to a method that is both automated and quantitative.

3   Methods

Our study design was a retrospective analysis to compare breast density measured from MRI exams to that from digital mammograms on a screening population of women. The methods used to assess volumetric breast density are a fuzzy clustering segmentation method on the MRI images [2] and the Quantra method on Full-Field Digital Mammography (FFDM) images [3].

3.1   Subjects

For a woman to have been included in our study, she must have had a set of screening digital mammograms and a screening MRI exam acquired within 4 years of each other (majority being within 2 years, visits alternating between mammography and MRI from being at high-risk), a completed breast health questionnaire, no previous history of breast cancer or breast surgery, and a BI-RADS diagnostic outcome of either 1 or 2. 123 women seen at the University of California, San Francisco (UCSF) Medical Center's Breast Health Clinic between April 2007 and November 2010 met these criteria.

3.2   MRI Imaging and Breast Density Analysis

MRI imaging was performed on either a 1.5 or 3 Tesla GE scanner (General Electric Medical Systems, Milwaukee, WI) using a bilateral phased array breast coil (Medical Devices, Madison, WI) in a prone position. T1-weighted precontrast images of the left laterality were analyzed using a quantitative Fuzzy C-Means (FCM) technique previously described by Klifa et al [2]. Briefly, a region of interest corresponding to the breast volume was identified per slice on T1 fat-saturated images using a semi-automated method. Segmentation at first is adjusted manually, then for subsequent slices, voxels are automatically segmented into one of six clusters depending on intensity. Voxels of higher intensity corresponded to fibroglandular tissue and those of lower intensity corresponded to fat. Percent dense volume was calculated as the ratio of fibroglandular tissue volume to total breast volume.

3.3   Mammographic Imaging and Density Analysis

All mammograms were acquired on one of six Hologic Selenia FFDM systems at UCSF. These systems use a molybdenum anode x-ray tube and have a pixel spatial resolution of 70 μm x 70 μm. The raw (unprocessed) format images of the left

Cranial-Caudal (CC) view were archived and processed through Hologic's Quantra algorithm. Quantra is an FDA-approved, commercially-available, and fully-automated software for quantifying volumetric breast density estimation previously described by Harman et al [3]. The method estimates the thickness of fibroglandular breast tissue associated with each pixel in the image and aggregates these values to compute the total breast volume. The fibroglandular tissue volume is found by referencing each pixel's attenuation to the attenuation of pixels that are labeled exclusively as fat. The estimated fibroglandular tissue volume is then divided by the total breast volume to calculate the volumetric percentage of fibroglandular tissue in the breast.

3.4   Statistics

Basic statistics were performed on results from the two methods. As the distributions were not observed to be normal, sign tests were used to determine difference between medians of Quantra and MRI. Linear regression was performed between Quantra results and those of MRI. Pearson's correlation coefficients were calculated from these relationships. Regression equation parameters were calculated and tested for significance with t-tests. A similar analysis carried out in 2010 by Kontos comparing low and high Quantra values with MRI density in 32 women was also studied here with this dataset [4].

4   Results

Basic statistics seen in table 1 reveal no significant differences between the medians of three measures produced by Quantra and MRI. The range of Quantra's percent fibroglandular volume is significantly compressed in comparison to MRI's, however, by about two-fold. A boxplot of the two method's percent fibroglandular volume distributions can be seen in figure 1 which diagrams this difference and both methods being skewed toward higher densities.

Table 1. Basic statistics of three measures from two techniques. Medians and interquartile ranges shown instead of means and standard deviations as distributions are not normal.

	MRI			FFDM Quantra		
	Median (Quartile range)	Min	Max	Median (Quartile range)	Min	Max
Left Breast Volume (ml)	480.0 (400.1)	49.9	1828.4	465.0 (352.0)	51.0	1870.0
Left Breast Dense Volume (ml)	111.8 (107.5)	14.3	338.1	101.0 (96.0)	9.0	425.0
Left Breast Percent Density (%)	24.0 (33.0)	2.0	85.0	21.0 (15.0)	9.0	49.0

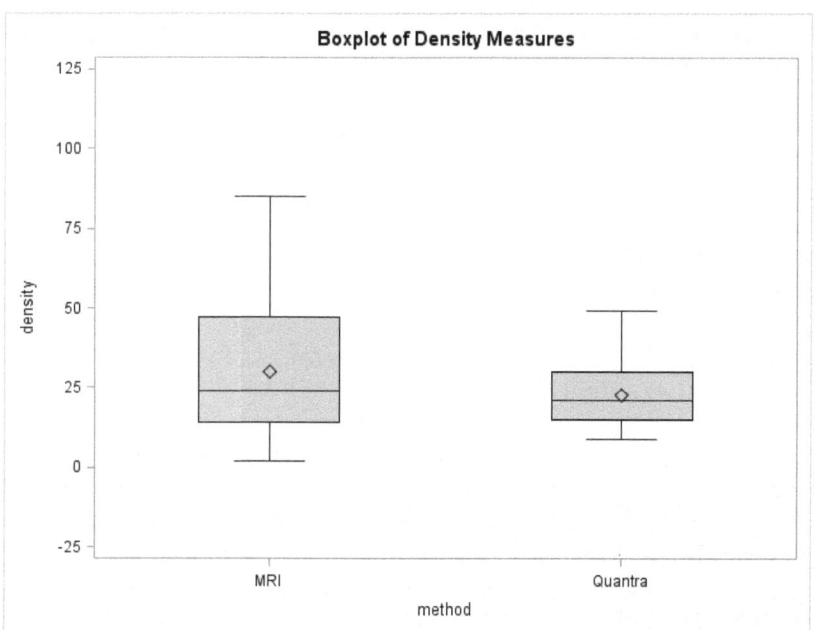

Fig. 1. Box of two techniques' percent fibroglandular density distributions, both showing skewness toward higher densities

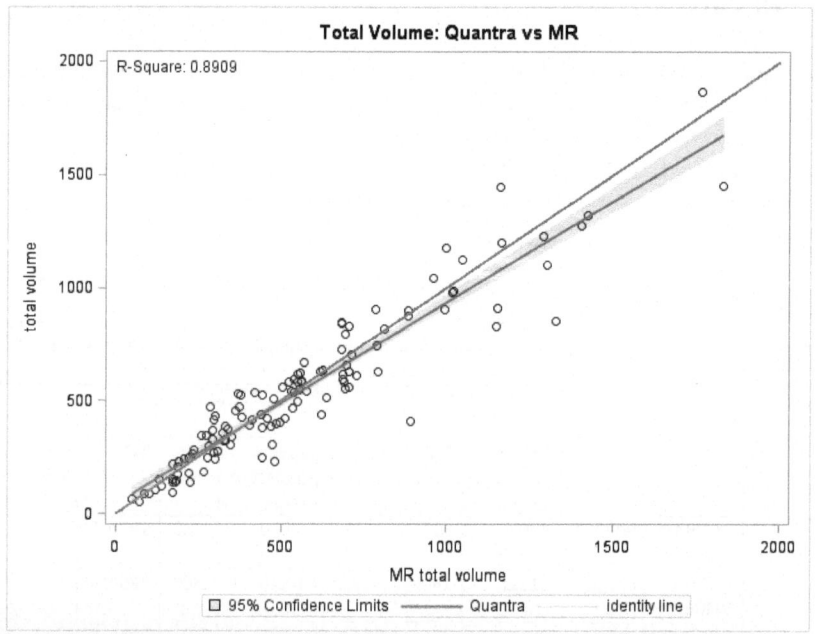

Fig. 2. Linear regression of total volume measure between Quantra and MRI

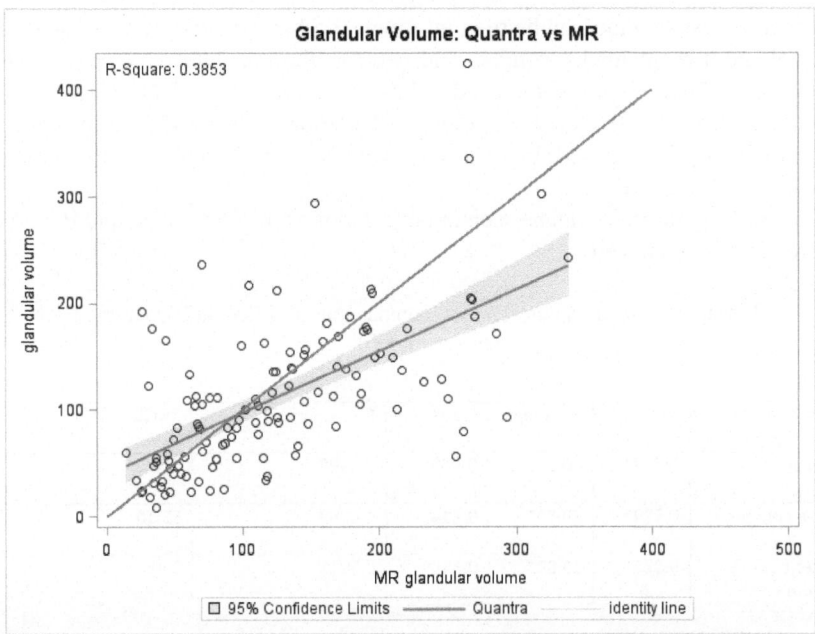

Fig. 3. Linear regression of fibroglandular volume measure between Quantra and MRI

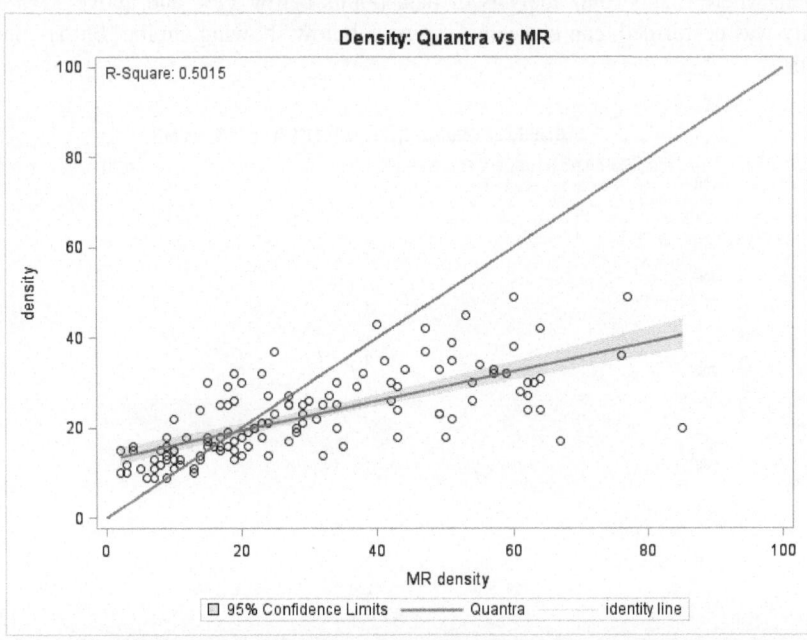

Fig. 4. Linear regression of percent fibroglandular volume measure between Quantra and MRI

Linear regression plots can be seen in figures 2-5 below. Pearson's coefficients for total volume, fibroglandular volume, and percent fibroglandular volume are 0.9439, 0.6207, and 0.7082 respectively. Total volume measures were highly correlated with each other ($R2=0.8909$). Glandular volume calculations between the two methods had low correlation ($R2=0.3853$). Percent fibroglandular density values were moderately correlated ($R2=0.5015$).

Regression parameters can be seen in table 2 along with R-Squared and Root Mean Squared Errors calculated.

Table 2. Linear regression parameters in comparison of MRI and Quantra. From t-test: *Significantly different than 1, P-value < 0.0001. ** Significantly different than 0, P-value<0.0001.

MR = Quantra × Slope + Intercept	Slope	Intercept	Slope (int=0)	R^2	RMSE
Total volume	0.897*	40.2**	0.949	0.8909	110.55
Dense volume	0.579*	39.7**	0.814	0.3853	55.10
Percent dense volume	0.326*	13.0**	0.628	0.5015	6.48

A reproduction of Kontos' 2010 comparison of Quantra and MRI density in 32 women, where a subgroup analysis of data points below 11% and above 11% MRI density was performed, can be seen in figure 5 below showing similar, but attenuated results.

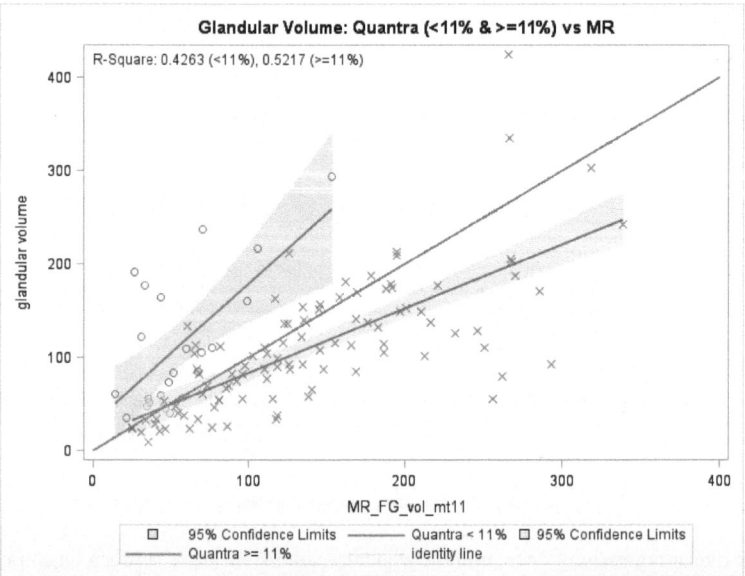

Fig. 5. Linear regression fits for the Quantra and MRI measures of fibroglandular tissue volume for women with ≥ 11% and < 11% MRI density

5   Discussion

Correlations between Quantra and MRI measures were mixed. The total volume measure had the highest correlation out of the three between the methods, with Quantra and MRI being highly correlated. This ability to abstract volume from a two-dimensional image is highly encouraging that the mammographic approach of volumetric breast density is possible. The differences seen are likely to be largely a product of different amounts of the breast tissue being imaged by the two modalities. MRI delineation of breast tissue up to the pectoral muscle may extend well beyond what is captured within CC views in mammography. Also, Quantra's reconstruction of total volume from two-dimensional images will inevitably have some noise given the modeling necessary to accomplish this.

Fibroglandular volume saw the lowest correlation out of the three measures, showing the two methods having a low correlation. Quantra and MRI fibroglandular tissue density are moderately correlated, with persistently lower density values seen with Quantra, whose range is significantly compressed. The fundamental difference in the approach between the two techniques is apparent here. Quantra's dependence on a particular image's pixel distribution for calculation of percent density can be seen in figure 4, where data points associated with higher MRI density compare to Quantra values that span nearly its entire range. The fat references selected by Quantra from images of predominantly fibroglandular tissue appear to produce more noise in the percent fibroglandular density results, and even more so fibroglandular volume results.

Regression equation slope parameters were all significantly different than one, and intercepts significantly different than zero. Quantra appears able to find dense tissue in breasts that appear completely fatty to a segmentation technique like the Fuzzy C-Means technique. Perhaps skin is being misinterpreted as dense tissue with the former. Root Mean Squared Errors are of similar magnitudes for total volume and dense volume, though Quantra measures were, in general, half the magnitude of MRI measures.

Subgroup analysis to mimic that of Kontos produced similar, but attenuated results. It is not clear whether 11% MRI fibroglandular density should be the threshold for this set of data. It would be worthwhile to pursue such subgroup analysis further, however, as clinical significance will be dependent upon being able to better separate those that are at higher risk of cancer due to having denser breasts.

6   Conclusion

Agreement between the measures produced by the two techniques was mixed. The two techniques agree well in the measure of total breast volume, which is encouraging for the pursuit of a quantitative mammographic measure of volumetric breast density. The measures of fibroglandular tissue volume and density produced by the two techniques studied here have agreements to lesser degrees, likely as a result of Quantra's method in selection of fat references.

References

1. Shepherd, J.A., Kerlikowske, K., Ma, L., Duewer, F., Fan, B., Wang, J., Malkov, S., Vittinghoff, E., Cumming, S.: Volume of Mammographic Density and Risk of Breast Cancer. Cancer Epidemiol. Biomarkers Prev. 20, 1473–1482 (2011)
2. Klifa, C., Carballido-Gamio, J., Wilmes, L., Laprie, A., Lobo, C., DeMicco, E., Watkins, M., Shepherd, J., Gibbs, J., Hylton, N.: Quantification of Breast Tissue from MR data using Fuzzy Clustering. In: Proc. of 26th Annual International Conference of IEEE: Engineering in Medicine and Biology Society 2004, San Francisco, CA, vol. 1, pp. 1667–1670 (2004)
3. Hartman, K., Highnam, R., Warren, R., Jackson, V.: Volumetric Assessment of Breast Tissue Composition from FFDM Images. In: Krupinski, E.A. (ed.) IWDM 2008. LNCS, vol. 5116, pp. 33–39. Springer, Heidelberg (2008)
4. Kontos, D., Xing, Y., Bakic, P.R., Conant, E.F., Maidment, A.D.A.: A comparative study of volumetric breast density estimation in digital mammography and magnetic resonance imaging: Results from a high-risk population. In: Karssemeijer, N., Summers, R. (eds.) Proc. of SPIE, Medical Imaging 2010: Computer-Aided Diagnosis, San Diego, CA, vol. 7624, p. 762409 (2010)

2D/3D Registration for Localization of Mammographically Depicted Lesions in Breast MRI

Torsten Hopp and Nicole V. Ruiter

Karlsruhe Institute of Technology, Germany
torsten.hopp@kit.edu

Abstract. X-ray mammography (XRM) and Magnetic Resonance Imaging (MRI) are likely to provide complementary diagnostic information for early breast cancer detection. However, topographic correlation of both modalities is challenging due to different dimensionality of images, patient positioning and compression state of the breast. In this paper we present an automated registration method, which allows prediction of the position of a lesion in the contrary modality. It is based on a FEM simulation mimicking the mammographic compression and is carried out using a patient-specific biomechanical model. An intensity-based optimization of the registration parameters is proposed to incorporate with the clinical variability of datasets. After registration, the position of a point of interest can be estimated within the three-dimensional MRI volume based on two mammograms acquired from different projection angles. The method was evaluated with 47 datasets from clinical routine. The mean registration error for localizing a lesion in the 3D MRI volume was 14.3 mm. The automatic registration method enables localization of e.g. microcalcifications which are only visible in XRM, within the corresponding MRI volume. It is therefore likely to assist radiologists in multimodal diagnosis.

Keywords: 2D/3D Registration, Magnetic Resonance Imaging, X-ray Mammography, Multimodal Diagnosis, Lesion Localization.

1 Introduction

It is widely known that breast cancer is the most common cancer among women in Europe and North America [1,2]. Currently, the established screening method to detect breast cancer is X-ray mammography (XRM). Yet, it frequently provides poor contrast for tumors located within glandular tissue [3]. Additionally, Magnetic Resonance Imaging (MRI) can be used for diagnosis. It offers a high contrast of soft tissue and high diagnostic accuracy [4].

Due to their different physical basis, XRM and MRI are likely to provide complementary diagnostic information and hence are often read in combination for definite diagnosis. However, topographic correlation of both modalities is challenging and requires a high level of training due to different dimensionality of images, patient positioning and compression states of the breast.

A.D.A. Maidment, P.R. Bakic, and S. Gavenonis (Eds.): IWDM 2012, LNCS 7361, pp. 627–634, 2012.

Image registration may help reduce the complexity of multimodal diagnosis by providing a mapping between both modalities. In previous work we presented a method which is capable to predict the position of a lesion in the contrary modality (e.g. [5,6]). It is based on biomechanical simulation of the mammographic compression to register XRM images with MRI volumes [7]. For example, contrast-enhancing regions depicted by MRI can be located within the mammogram [6]. In this work we extended the method to map lesions vice versa: e.g. microcalcifications, which are only visible in XRM, can be located within the MRI volume. In contrast to approaches in literature (e.g. [8,9,10,11,12]), our registration method is fully automated and was evaluated with a significantly larger number of datasets (47) which represent the variability of clinical routine images.

2   Methods

The general idea of our registration method is mimicking the compression which is applied to the breast during XRM by a Finite Element Simulation. The underlying patient specific biomechanical Finite Element Method (FEM) model is built on the basis of the pre-processed (i.e. segmented and cropped) MRI volume. Material parameter from literature as well as metadata and geometric information from the mammogram is used to parameterize the deformation process. Afterwards the FEM simulation is carried out, resulting in a compressed configuration of the MRI volume. The deformed MRI volume is comparable to the compressed configuration of the breast imaged during XRM. Hence by projecting the deformed MRI volume along the mammographic projection axis, an artificial mammogram can be created. The position of a lesion which is visible in the MRI volume can directly be transferred to the mammogram and the corresponding region in the mammogram can be retrieved (Fig. 1).

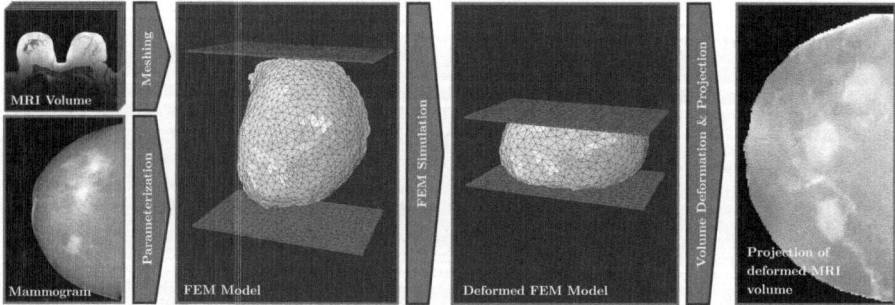

Fig. 1. Simplified illustration of the registration process

2.1   Preprocessing

Images of both modalities have to be preprocessed. They are rotated to fit the internally used coordinate system and the XRM is downsampled to match the resolution of the MRI. An interpolation between slices is applied to the MRI volume in order to obtain isotropic voxels. Images are segmented automatically into background and object using a toolbox of thresholding, morphological operations, active contours, de-islanding and three-dimensional smoothing methods. In the same fashion, fatty and glandular tissue are segmented in the MRI volume in order to model the characteristics of these predominant structures individually. In an automatic global alignment, the amount of breast tissue imaged in XRM and the MRI volume is matched by estimating the breast volumes based on the segmented images.

2.2   Registration

To simulate the compression, which is applied to the breast during XRM, a biomechanical model is generated. FEM is used for numerical solution of the deformation process. To describe the geometry of the biomechanical model, the segmented volume image is passed to a meshing algorithm [13] resulting in a mesh with approximately 25,000 tetrahedral elements. Nodes at the back of the model are held in position to model the fixation of the breast at the chest wall.

The physical behavior of the model is described by the material model and the boundary conditions of the compression simulation. The stress-strain relationship of the breast tissue is approximated by a Neo-Hookean model using material parameters of Wellman [14]. The stiffness parameters for fatty respectively glandular tissue are assigned to each Finite Element based on the MRI volume segmentation by a majority decision. Isotropic behavior of the material is assumed.

The mammographic compression is mimicked by a two-step approach. Both steps are computed using the commercial FEM package Abaqus [15]. In the first step, compression plates are added to the simulation, which are moved closer until the individual compression thickness is achieved. The thickness of the breast during mammography is readout from the mammogram's metadata. The contact between compression plate and breast surface is assumed to undergo only small frictions and therefore modeled in Abaqus by a small-sliding interface.

Due to uncertainties and simplifications in the biomechanical model, the circumferences of the deformed volume image and the XRM usually do not overlay completely after the first simulation step. Therefore, in the second step, a three-dimensional target model of the deformed configuration of the breast during XRM is estimated on basis of the mammogram. This model is compared to the deformed volume image derived from the first simulation step. Displacement vectors between surface nodes of the FEM mesh and the target model are defined by a nearest neighbor measure and used to describe the boundary conditions for the second simulation step. It results in a configuration of the MRI volume which shows congruently overlaying circumferences with the mammogram. All

FEM simulations are solved using non linear solvers for large deformations [16]. A detailed description of the registration algorithm can be found in [6].

Variability in patient positioning and mammographic projection angle might cause less accurate results than proposed by the original method [7]. We approximate this misregistration by iteratively rotating the MRI volume around the anterior/posterior axis. For each rotation step, the registration process is carried out. The optimal rotation angle is estimated by an intensity-based optimization. An X-ray mimicking projection of the deformed MRI volume after the second simulation step and the corresponding mammogram are compared using a image similarity metric S. The registration R using rotation angle α delivering the best value S_{max} is used as final result:

$$S_{max} = \max(S(R(\alpha))) \tag{1}$$

2.3 Localization of a Lesion in the MRI Volume

Based on two mammograms acquired from different projection angles, the position of a point of interest can be estimated within the three-dimensional MRI volume (Fig. 2). To retrieve the 3D position, the center point of the mammogram lesion is mapped to the third dimension, i.e. a straight line perpendicular to the mammogram plane is mapped into the deformed MRI volume. The deformation field calculated by the described registration method is inverted ("decompression"), converting the line into a curve within the undeformed MRI volume. Ideally, curves from two different mammographic projection angles intersect in a point, which is defined as the estimated 3D center of the lesion. In case of non-intersecting curves, the two points on both lines with the smallest Euclidean distance, i.e. the smallest distance between the curves, is calculated. The center position of these points is is then used as the estimated 3D center of the lesion.

3 Results

The method was evaluated by 47 datasets from clinical routine, acquired at University Hospital of Jena, Germany. Each dataset consists of a MRI volume and the corresponding mammograms of the patient from cranio-caudal and medio-lateral oblique projection angle. MRI volumes were acquired on 1.5 T scanners (Siemens Magnetom Symphony, Sonata and Avanto). The measurement parameters followed the internal guidelines (T1-weighted spoiled gradient echo scans, matrix size $= 384 \times 384$ pixel, slices $= 33$ - 44 depending on scanner, in-plane resolution $= 0.9 \times 0.9$ mm, slice thickness $= 3$-4 mm). XRM images were acquired digitally with a resolution of 0.094×0.094 mm.

Datasets included in this study had to depict clearly at least one lesion in the MRI volume and both mammograms for evaluation of the registration accuracy. Center points of theses lesions were identified by two experienced radiologists in consensus.

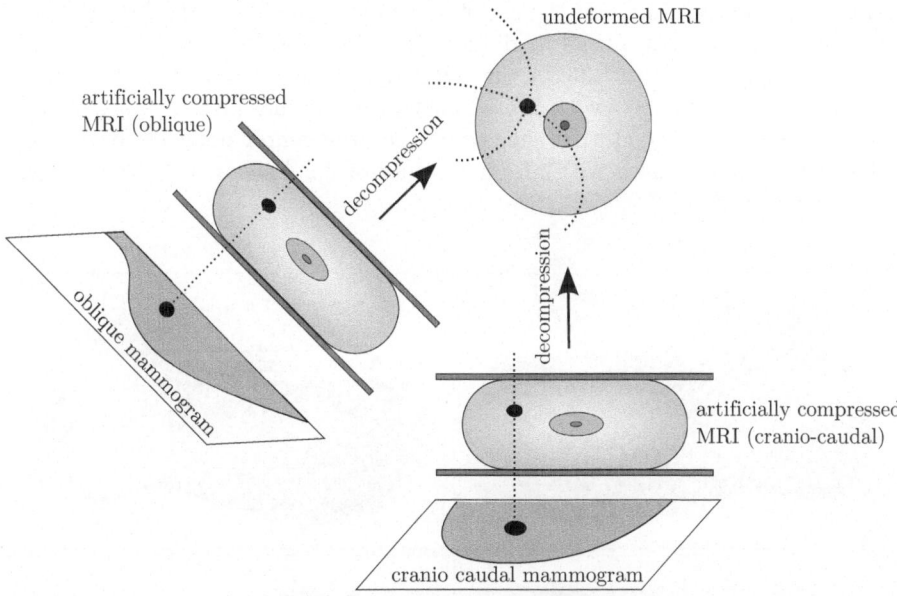

Fig. 2. Estimation of a lesion position in the three-dimensional MRI volume based on two mammograms from cranio-caudal respectively oblique projection angle

The registration was carried out for cranio-caudal and medio-lateral oblique mammograms using the intensity-based optimization approach. MRI volumes were rotated around the anterior/posterior axis in a range of $-20°$ to $+20°$ from the mammographic projection angle recorded by the XRM device in order to account for rotation of images against each other. Maximization of Normalized Mutual Information was used as optimization criterion. Afterwards the lesion localization within the MRI volume was carried out according to the described method.

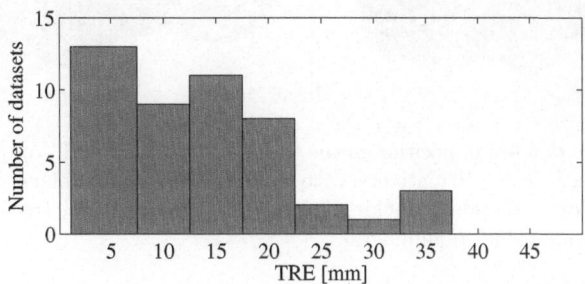

Fig. 3. Histogram of the target registration error (TRE)

The target registration error (TRE) of the lesion localization within the MRI was calculated by the three-dimensional Euclidean distance between the estimated lesion position and the annotated lesion position in the MRI volume. The mean displacement for all 47 datasets was 14.3 mm (median: 13.4 mm, SD: 8.8 mm). For 17 datasets (36 %) the TRE was below 10 mm, for 26 datasets (55 %) the TRE was below 15 mm. A histogram of the TRE is illustrated in Figure 3. The transversal MRI slice containing the center point of the marked lesion could be estimated with an uncertainty of ±2.4 slices. Resulting images are shown in Fig. 4.

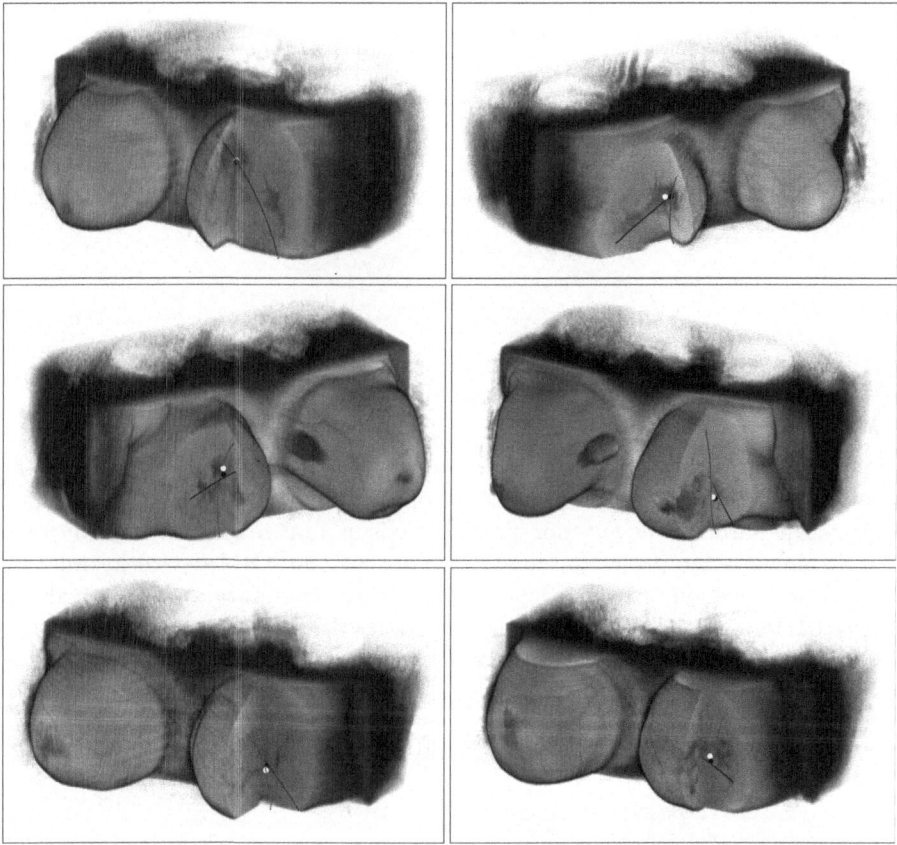

Fig. 4. Estimation of a lesion position in the three-dimensional MRI. Volume rendering of the MRI dataset from six patients with estimated position (black dot), marked position (white dot) and point tracking curve from cranio-caudal (red) respectively medio-lateral oblique (blue) mammogram.

4   Conclusion

In this work we presented a novel automated approach to localize lesions depicted in XRM images within a three-dimensional MRI volume. Even though the method is completely automated, the mean registration accuracy evaluated by 47 datasets from clinical routine was in a clinically valuable range below 15 mm. Reducing uncertainties in marking the same center of the lesion in both modalities correctly may increase registration accuracy further. With the mean registration accuracy presented, we believe that the method is likely to benefit multimodal diagnosis. The registration accuracy is currently limited by the pre-deformations of the datasets, which are likely to occur by patient-specific positioning on the MRI breast coils and the XRM compression plates. Improving the algorithm to deal with the pre-deformations is subject to our current research, e.g. extending the parameter search space of the intensity-based optimization might reduce the TRE.

The presented method enables localizing small-scale structures like microcalcifications which are only visible in XRM within the corresponding MRI volume. It is therefore likely to assist radiologists in combined reading. The estimated position may give hints where to have a closer look in the MRI, even in cases with a suboptimal registration accuracy. Furthermore the method allows for evaluating upcoming MRI protocols, which e.g. focus on the imaging of calcifications [17]. Due to the automation of the software, no manual steps have to be carried out by radiologists. Because of the use of standard devices and standard imaging parameters, no additional non-routine-imaging has to be carried out.

References

1. Fischer, T., Bick, U., Thomas, A.: Mammographie-Screening in Deutschland. Visions Journal 15, 62–67 (2007)
2. American Cancer Society: Breast Cancer Facts and Figures 2011- 2012. American Cancer Society, Inc., Atlanta (2011)
3. Pisano, E.D., et al.: Diagnostic Accuracy of Digital Versus Film Mammography: Exploratory Analysis of Selected Population Subgroups in DMIST1. Radiology 246(2), 376–383 (2008)
4. DeMartini, W., Lehman, C.: A Review of Current Evidence-Based Clinical Applications for Breast Magnetic Resonance Imaging. Topics in Magnetic Resonance Imaging 19(3), 143–150 (2008)
5. Hopp, T., et al.: Configurable Framework for Automatic Multimodal 2D/3D Registration of Volume Datasets with X-Ray Mammograms. In: Proceedings Workshop on Breast Image Analysis in conjunction with MICCAI 2011, pp. 145–152 (2011)
6. Hopp, T., et al.: 2D/3D image fusion of X-ray mammograms with breast MRI: visualizing dynamic contrast enhancement in mammograms. International Journal of Computer Assisted Radiology and Surgery (2011) (in press)
7. Ruiter, N.V., et al.: Model-Based Registration of X-ray Mammograms and MR Images of the Female Breast. IEEE Transactions on Nuclear Science 53(1), 204–211 (2006)
8. Rajagopal, V., et al.: Mapping Microcalcifications Between 2D Mammograms and 3D MRI Using a Biomechanical Model of the Breast Computational Biomechanics for Medicine, pp. 17–28. Springer, New York (2010)
9. Lee, A.W.C., et al.: Breast X-ray and MR Image Fusion Using Finite Element Modeling. In: Proceedings Workshop on Breast Image Analysis in conjunction with MICCAI 2011, pp. 129–136 (2011)

10. Reynolds, H.M., et al.: Mapping Breast Cancer Between Clinical X-Ray and MR Images. In: Computational Biomechanics for Medicine, pp. 81–90. Springer, New York (2011)
11. Mertzanidou, T., Hipwell, J.H., Cardoso, M.J., Tanner, C., Ourselin, S., Hawkes, D.J.: X-ray Mammography – MRI Registration Using a Volume-Preserving Affine Transformation and an EM-MRF for Breast Tissue Classification. In: Martí, J., Oliver, A., Freixenet, J., Martí, R. (eds.) IWDM 2010. LNCS, vol. 6136, pp. 23–30. Springer, Heidelberg (2010)
12. Mertzanidou, T., et al.: MRI to X-ray Mammography Registration Using an Ellipsoidal Breast Model and Biomechanically Simulated Compressions. In: Proceedings Workshop on Breast Image Analysis in conjunction with MICCAI 2011, pp. 161–168 (2011)
13. Fang, Q., Boas, D.: Tetrahedral Mesh Generation from Volumetric Binary and Grayscale Images. In: Proceedings IEEE International Symposium on Biomedical Imaging, pp. 1142–1145 (2009)
14. Wellman, P.S., et al.: Breast Tissue Stiffness in Compression is Correlated to Histological Diagnosis. Technical Report, Harvard BioRobotics Laboratory (1999)
15. Dassault Systèmes: Abaqus 6.11 Online Documentation (2011)
16. Dassault Systèmes: Abaqus Theory Manual v 6.9 (2009)
17. Fatemi-Ardekani, A., et al.: Identification of Breast Calcification using Magnetic Resonance Imaging. Medical Physics 36(12), 5429–5436 (2009)

Application of a Protocol for Constancy Control of Digital Breast Tomosynthesis Systems: Results and Experiences

Kristin Pedersen[1], Robin L. Hammond[2], and Bjørn H. Østerås[3,4]

[1] Norwegian Radiation Protection Authority, P.O. Box 55, NO-1332 Østerås, Norway
[2] Department of Radiology, Oslo University Hospital, Oslo, Norway
[3] The Intervention Centre, Oslo University Hospital, Oslo, Norway
[4] Faculty Division of Clinical Medicine, University of Oslo, Oslo, Norway
kristin.pedersen@nrpa.no

Abstract. A simple protocol for routine technical quality control of digital breast tomosynthesis (DBT) systems of the type Hologic Selenia Dimensions was developed from a national protocol for FFDM systems and the manufacturer's QC manual. The protocol was implemented in conjunction with a clinical DBT study. Analyzing test results collected over a 13 month period we found a 100 % pass rate for the majority of tests. Some deviations were seen in dose level (mAs), Signal-to-Noise Ratio and for the review monitors. Based on our results and experiences a revised test regimen is suggested.

Keywords: Mammography, tomosynthesis, quality control, constancy control.

1   Introduction

In mammography it is paramount to obtain images with sufficient image quality at acceptable dose levels. Quality control (QC) of the imaging equipment is among the tools to achieve this. In established mammography environments, such controls are usually divided between annual and semi-annual controls by physicists, and more frequent tests performed by technologists, sometimes referred to as constancy tests.

Standard projection (conventional) mammography is considered the method of choice for breast cancer screening. With this technique, the three-dimensional breast is projected into a two-dimensional image plane, and overlaying tissue may obscure actual lesions. This can make the images difficult to interpret, and lead to cancers being missed.

Recently, digital breast tomosynthesis (DBT) has been introduced as a breast imaging alternative with a potential to reduce the problem with overlaying tissue. In DBT, multiple images of millimeter thickness are reconstructed from x-ray exposures made with the x-ray tube at a limited range of angles.

The actual performance of DBT in a clinical environment can only be assessed through clinical trials. When a trial of DBT was planned in our breast screening program, a protocol for technical quality control was also developed. The purpose of this

A.D.A. Maidment, P.R. Bakic, and S. Gavenonis (Eds.): IWDM 2012, LNCS 7361, pp. 635–641, 2012.
© Springer-Verlag Berlin Heidelberg 2012

636   K. Pedersen, R.L. Hammond, and B.H. Østerås

paper is to report results and experiences from the constancy control program performed by the technologists, and to suggest revisions to the protocol, if indicated.

2   Method

The mammography x-ray units used in our study were two systems of the type Hologic Selenia Dimensions (Hologic, Inc., Bedford, MA, USA). The units allow both 2D (full field digital mammography – FFDM) and 3D (DBT) imaging. Softcopy reading of mammograms was done using three dedicated workstations in separate rooms. The protocol developed for constancy tests included elements from the protocol used in our national screening program for conventional FFDM units [1] and procedures suggested in the manufacturer's QC manual for this particular system. A summary of the tests performed is given in Table 1, followed by a brief description of each test.

Table 1. Summary of test items in the constancy control protocol. The following abbreviations are used: SP: Standard national protocol for FFDM systems. HP: Hologic protocol for Selenia Dimensions. Q: quantitative test assessment. S/V: subjective/visual test assessment.

Procedure	Source	Frequency	Evaluation
Daily Control of AEC	SP	Daily	Q
Ambient Light (reading room, mammography lab)	SP	Daily	S/V
Monitors	SP	Daily	S/V
Detector Flat-Field Calibration (Gain Calibration)	HP	Weekly	Q
Artifact Evaluation	HP	Weekly	S/V
Phantom Image Quality Evaluation	HP	Weekly	S/V
Signal-To-Noise/Contrast-To-Noise Measurements	HP	Weekly	Q
Detector Uniformity	SP	Weekly	Q
Diagnostic Review Workstation Quality Control	HP, SP	Weekly	S/V
Compression Thickness Indicator	HP	Biweekly	Q
Unit Assembly Evaluation	SP	Quarterly	V
Reject Analysis	HP	Quarterly	S/V/Q
Geometry Calibration	HP	Semi-annually	Q

- Daily Control of AEC: 45 mm PMMA imaged with "clinical" settings. mAs recorded, mean pixel value and standard deviation determined for ROI with standard size and position, SNR calculated. mAs and SNR required to be within +/- 10 % of reference value.
- Ambient Light: Desired conditions in reading rooms described in checklist.
- Monitors: Quick visual assessment of the AAPM TG18 QC image, focus on obvious defects like flicker, large distortions or dead pixels.

- Artifact Evaluation: Images of 40 mm PMMA phantom evaluated visually for the presence of i.e. bad pixels or sharp lines of demarcation. 2D: Images with Rh and Ag filter. 3D: Al filter used, projection images evaluated.
- Phantom Image Quality Evaluation: The ACR Mammographic Accreditation Phantom imaged in "combo" mode (a combined mode where a 3D acquisition is directly followed by 2D acquisition without changing the compression or positioning between acquisitions) with system settings. Images scored according to the 1999 ACR Mammography Quality Control Manual.
- Signal-To-Noise/Contrast-To-Noise measurements: SNR and CNR values computed manually or automatically (our study) by the system on the image of the ACR phantom with a small acrylic disk. Recommended performance criteria given in the QC manual.
- Detector Uniformity: Mean pixel values from ROIs placed in the center and corners of the image from the daily AEC test registered. The ROI with the largest pixel value deviation compared to the central ROI is determined and the percentage deviation calculated. The largest deviation not to exceed 10 %.
- Diagnostic Review Workstation Quality Control: The AAPM TG18-QC test image loaded onto the viewing monitors from the PACS and evaluated according to a checklist derived from the AAPM TG18 report [2]. In addition, results from tests run by the application MediCal QAWeb Agent, installed on the review stations, confirmed to be OK or repeated if not OK..
- Compression thickness indicator: The ACR phantom compressed to approximately 133 dN using the 7.5 cm spot contact compression paddle. Measured thickness should be within +/- 5 mm from the actual thickness.
- Unit assembly evaluation: Performed according to checklist.
- Reject Analysis.

In addition, "Detector Flat-Field Calibration" and "Geometry Calibration", two procedures described in the vendor's QC manual, were routinely performed. Simple spreadsheets for recordkeeping, calculation of certain parameters, and graphic rendering of results were developed in MS Excel.

3   Results

Test data for a total of 13 months from November 2010 through December 2011 are included in our analyses. During this period up to 50 patients were imaged per system per day. A majority of these examinations were in so called "combo" mode, i.e. both 2D and 3D mammography in the same compression. Results from the analyses of tests performed on the x-ray systems and review monitors are summarized in Table 2 and Table 3 respectively. We do not report any results from the reject analysis, as collection of data for this procedure did not start until towards the end of the data collection period specified above. No data was collected for the protocol item Ambient Light.

In the daily AEC test, mAs (equivalent to dose level) and signal-to-noise ratio (SNR) are tracked over time. For one of the x-ray systems, intentional interventions by the manufacturer, like adjustment of dose level, software upgrades, and tube re-placement, occasionally gave a shift in mAs level. These shifts are clearly visible on plots of mAs versus time. Other than this, mAs failed to fall within the designated limits a total of ten times for the two systems combined. For SNR the total number of failed tests was four.

Table 2. Summary of results of tests on the x-ray units. In Daily Control of AEC, two parameters (mAs and SNR) are tracked. *Number of failed tests for this procedure is given as failed mAs tests/failed SNR tests.

Procedure	Frequency	Number of tests performed	Number of failed tests
Daily Control of AEC	Daily	466	10/4*
Detector Flat-Field Calibration (Gain Calibration)	Weekly	97	0
Artifact Evaluation	Weekly	93	0
Phantom Image Quality Evaluation	Weekly	93	0
Signal-To-Noise/Contrast-To-Noise Measurements	Weekly	89	0
Detector Uniformity	Weekly	93	0
Compression Thickness Indicator	Biweekly	53	0
Unit Assembly Evaluation	Quarterly	10	1
Geometry Calibration	Semi-annually	6	0

Table 3. Summary of results of tests of the review station monitors

Procedure	Frequency	Number of tests performed	Number of failed tests	Percentage of failed tests
Monitors	Daily	110	10	9.1%
Diagnostic Review Workstation Quality Control (Standard protocol)	Weekly	74	0	0%
Diagnostic Review Workstation Quality Control (Hologic protocol)	Weekly	71	3	4.2%

4   Discussion

Among the test procedures performed on the x-ray systems, failed test results were only recorded for two: The Daily Control of AEC, and the Unit Assembly Evaluation. The one deviating test result recorded for the latter was due to the buttons on the gantry not working properly. One failed test result for the Daily Control of AEC pro-cedure was due to a genuine problem which prompted a service intervention. The remaining failed test instances seem to be caused by random variation.

The AEC test procedure highlighted shifts in dose level (mAs level) following in-terventions by the manufacturer. As these interventions were not always announced, the test procedure contributed to alerting the technologists to when such deliberate changes in dose (mAs) level were made. In addition to providing daily information on dose level and SNR, the daily procedure revealed a problem with the compression assembly. It also showed artifacts caused by a filter at an earlier stage than would have been the case if only relying on the weekly or bi-weekly Artifact and Compression Thickness Indicator tests. Summing up, we found the daily test of the AEC to be valuable, quick and easy to perform. Further, it yielded daily information about features covered in the two above mentioned, less frequently performed, test procedures.

The majority of the failed monitor tests (Table 3) were attributable to improper lighting conditions. On closer inspection, the deviating results were seen to occur in two separate clusters, indicating that this was a systematic rather than random problem.

The implementation of a constancy control regimen requires time and effort on part of the technologists. It should therefore only include procedures that are considered necessary and useful. The nearly perfect pass rates for the tests performed on the x-ray systems raises the question of whether the systems simply performed without fault with regard to the features tested, or if the test procedures were not sensitive enough to detect potential system problems. When considering answer to these questions one should keep in mind that constancy tests are designed to monitor the stability of the system performance. Our data indicates that these were indeed two x-ray systems that performed stably with regard to technical parameters including dose level and detector output. Close inspection of our data, and recommendations published by others, lead us to believe that some test procedures can be omitted or replaced, and test frequencies changed.

Artifacts and problems with the compression assembly were occasionally picked up by the daily test. This could indicate that a more frequent evaluation of artifacts and the compression assembly is warranted. We suggest to include evaluation of artifacts as part of the daily test, and only performing the specific procedures for Artifact Evaluation, and Compression Thickness Indicator as diagnostic tools if the daily artifact evaluation indicates a problem might exist.

For digital mammography, Yaffe et al. [3] recommend that routine use of the ACR accreditation phantom should be replaced by more discriminative tests, including signal-difference-to-noise ratio (SDNR), which is equivalent to contrast-to-noise ratio (CNR). In our study we did not record any failed test instances for the Phantom Image Quality Evaluation test. This supports the conclusion of Yaffe et al. We therefore suggest that this test is omitted.

A weekly evaluation of CNR was included in our test regimen. The test results were very stable throughout the study period, thus a reduced test frequency could be considered. We suggest that the CNR assessment be made monthly, and after changes to hardware or software. Based on our results it also seems sufficient to make monthly assessments of detector uniformity. Feedback from the technologists leads us to suggest that the quarterly Unit Assembly Evaluation be replaced by continuous registration, reporting, follow-up and repair of findings for a specifically defined selection of relevant system features.

Daily test procedures were proposed both for the x-ray systems and monitors. Tables 2 and 3 show that the number of daily monitor tests performed is less than 50 % of the number of daily tests on the x-ray systems. This could be a reflection of the fact that while the technologists were responsible for performing the tests, reading rooms and monitors are mainly used by the radiologists. It could therefore be better if the radiologists assumed responsibility for making sure the criteria in the daily assessment of ambient light and monitor quality are met. We do not propose changing the frequency of the daily Monitors test. However, we think the low failure rate found for the weekly monitor tests could warrant a reduced test frequency for these. Table 4 show suggested test items and frequencies for a revised protocol for constancy tests.

Table 4. Suggested test items and frequencies. Q: quantitative test assessment. S/V: subjective/visual test assessment.

Procedure	Frequency	Evaluation
Daily AEC, Artifact and Compression Assembly Evaluation	Daily	Q
Ambient Light (reading room, mammography lab)	Daily	S/V
Monitors	Daily	S/V
Detector Flat-Field Calibration (Gain Calibration)	Weekly	Q
Artifact Evaluation	If indicated by results of daily evaluation	S/V
Signal-To-Noise/Contrast-To-Noise Measurements	Monthly; after changes in hard- or software	Q
Detector Uniformity	Monthly	Q
Diagnostic Review Workstation Quality Control	Monthly	S/V
Compression Thickness Indicator	If indicated by results of daily evaluation	Q
Unit Assembly Evaluation	Revised: Continuous registration	V
Reject Analysis	Not evaluated in study	S/V/Q
Geometry Calibration	Semi-annually	Q

Our study included data from one system model only. This model is designed for both 2D and 3D mammography. Some tests in the protocol included 3D specific elements: Artifact Evaluation (for which images with the filter only used in 3D are among those evaluated), Phantom Image Quality Evaluation, and Geometry Calibration. In the suggested revision of the test protocol, the evaluation of ACR phantom images is omitted. Based on the arguments presented above, we believe the exclusion of this particular test item is warranted for all 2D and 3D full field digital mammography (FFDM) systems. With regard to routine tests for the 3D element of mammography systems, our advice is to consult the quality control manual developed by the manufacturer for the system in question. Because systems differ in design, specifically tailored test procedures might be called for.

The remaining test items are not particular to 3D systems. Experience with other 2D system models indicates that this selection of tests and limiting values can be suitable for any FFDM system. For tests that are not performed daily, it might be advisable to investigate what the optimal test frequency is for a particular system before settling on a final protocol.

References

1. Pedersen, K., Landmark, I.D.: Trial of a proposed protocol for constancy control of digital mammography systems. Medical Physics 36(12), 5537–5546 (2009)
2. Samei, E., et al.: American Association of Physicists in Medicine (AAPM), Assessment of display performance for medical imaging systems, Task Group 18, Madison, WI (April 2005)
3. Yaffe, M.J., et al.: Quality control for digital mammography: Part II recommendations from the ACRIN DMIST trial. Medical Physics 33(3), 737–752 (2006)

Design and Evaluation of a Phantom with Structured Background for Digital Mammography and Breast Tomosynthesis

Lesley Cockmartin[1,*], Nicholas Marshall[1,2], and Hilde Bosmans[1,2]

[1] Catholic University Leuven, Belgium
[2] University Hospital Gasthuisberg, Department of Radiology, Leuven, Belgium
{lesley.cockmartin,nicholas.marshall,hilde.bosmans}@uzleuven.be

Abstract. The presence of anatomical structure in 2D mammograms and digital breast tomosynthesis (DBT) images impacts cancer detection. Previous work has shown that the low frequency range of the power spectrum (PS) of breast structure in mammograms can be characterized by a power law with exponent (β). This work reports our experience with the development of a self-similar phantom that produces a structured background in both 2D mammography and breast tomosynthesis. Theory predicts that this phantom produces a PS with power law exponent related to its fractal dimension. Results of a phantom with acrylic spheres in air and in water respectively, evaluated on a Siemens mammographic system with tomosynthesis option, show power law exponents of 2.90 and 3.18 for 2D, 2.91 and 2.45 for DBT projections and, 2.06 and 1.66 for DBT reconstructions. These values were within the range of the exponents measured in patient data.

Keywords: 2D digital mammography, digital breast tomosynthesis, phantom, anatomical breast structure, power spectrum analysis.

1 Background

Two-dimensional (2D) digital mammography is the standard imaging modality for breast cancer screening and diagnostics. A major drawback of this technique is the projection of three-dimensional (3D) overlying tissues, a factor which 3D techniques such as digital breast tomosynthesis (DBT) attempt to overcome. In order to justify the application of this technique, performance testing of the system including an investigation of the removal or the reduction of overlying tissue is required. In contrast with 2D mammography, where image quality is expressed in terms of contrast thresholds at specific diameters, the quality of DBT is determined by the visualization of details in the focal plane and its efficiency of suppressing the overlying tissue. The presence of a structured background surrounding the details is therefore crucial for performance test methods. Burgess *et al* investigated breast structure in radiographic images via power spectrum (PS) measurements and found that structure was characterized by a power law of the form κ/f^{β}, where f is the radial spatial frequency and β

A.D.A. Maidment, P.R. Bakic, and S. Gavenonis (Eds.): IWDM 2012, LNCS 7361, pp. 642–649, 2012.

the power law exponent [1]. A number of researchers have used the power law model to generate images with textured backgrounds [2-4].

The hypothesis for the present study was that a test object producing a similar PS to patient cases has potential for the development of a performance testing phantom. We therefore present results of PS analyses of images acquired with a physical phantom that was developed using the work of Gang *et al.* These authors have shown that the distribution of spherical self-similar objects, a special class of which are fractals, obeys a power law in frequency space and the power law exponent β is related to the fractal dimension [4]. The phantom data from 2D mammography, DBT projections and reconstructed images were compared against patient data.

2   Methods and Materials

2.1   Design of a Phantom with Structural Background

Gang showed that equal volumes of differently sized spheres provide a fractal dimension of 3 as well as a power law exponent β equal to 3 [4] and hence we created a phantom consisting of equal volumes of acrylic spheres of six different diameters (15.88, 12.70, 9.52, 6.35, 3.18 and 1.58 mm) (United States Plastic Corp, Ohio, USA). The spheres were placed within an acrylic semi-circular container of thickness 58 mm and diameter 200 mm, resembling a compressed breast. As an alternative to spheres placed in air, the space between the spheres was also filled with water, a material with X-ray properties closer to breast tissue. However, air bubbles were visible at the upper side of the phantom because of the practical difficulties in completely filling the phantom with water (Figure 1). Measurements were performed under automatic exposure control (AEC) control on a digital mammographic system with tomosynthesis option - the Siemens Inspiration Tomosynthesis unit. The system utilizes a version of the filtered back projection (FBP) reconstruction algorithm to generate the DBT volume [5].

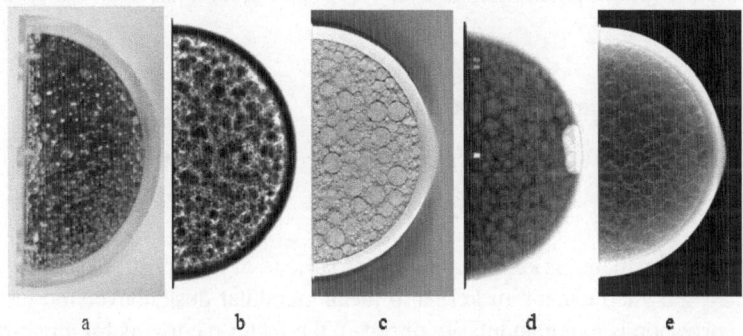

a   b   c   d   e

Fig. 1. Images of the sphere-phantom filled with (b,c) air and (d,e) water. (a) photograph, (b,d) raw 2D mammograms and (c,e) DBT reconstructed planes, imaged on a Siemens Inspiration TOMO mammographic system.

2.2   Patient Dataset

The patient dataset consisted of 50 lesion-free patient cases with 80 mammograms and DBT image series in cranio-caudal (CC) and/or medio-lateral oblique (MLO) view. Breast thickness varied between 28 and 86 mm and all density classes were represented. Given that our hospital only performs DBT for further investigation of BIRADS 3, 4 or 5 cases, requiring a diagnostic workup for an asymmetry or a suspected lesion, the majority of the lesion-free breasts contained dense fibroglandular structures.

2.3   Measurement of Power Spectral Density

Power spectra were measured in 2D, DBT projections and DBT reconstruction images of the sphere-phantom and patients. The PS was calculated at a fixed, approximately central position (x-y) within the breast for all projection images and reconstructed planes. Square regions adapted to the size of the breast were extracted from the centre of the breast and records of size 128 x 128 pixels were taken from this region, overlapping by 64 pixels in both x and y directions. Records were input to a standard 2D PS calculation with a Hann window applied to each record. The final PS was the radial average of the ensemble, including the $0°$ and $90°$ spatial frequency axes. Normalization of the projection image PS was effected by dividing the ensemble by the square of the signal mean from the linearized image *i.e.* by (air kerma)^2. This form of normalization for x-ray signal was not applied to the PS calculated from the reconstructed planes as the pixel value (PV) in reconstructed planes is independent of dose used for the acquisition. Additionally radial averaged PS were compared with PS calculated in both horizontal and vertical direction in the reconstructed planes since radial non-isotropy was noted in the majority of the reconstructed breast images. Different spatial frequency ranges have been proposed for the curve fit from which β is determined [1, 6-7]; a typical range of 0.2 to 0.7 mm^{-1} was used for both the patient images and the sphere-phantom in this study. A least squares method was used for the curve fit.

2.4   Mean Glandular Dose Calculation

Mean glandular dose (MGD) was calculated using Dance's method [8]:

$$MGD = Kgcs$$

where K is the incident air kerma at the upper surface of the breast, measured without backscatter, g is the incident air kerma to mean glandular dose conversion factor (the g-factor corresponds to a glandularity of 50%), the factor c corrects for any difference in breast composition from 50% glandularity and the factor s corrects for the x-ray spectrum used.

3   Results and Discussion

3.1   Reproducibility of Power Law Exponents in Sphere-Phantom

Short and long term reproducibility of the power law exponents of the 'sphere-phantom with air' background was tested by scanning the phantom multiple times on different days while shaking the phantom between each image acquisition. Shaking was done to ensure that the smallest spheres did not remain on the bottom of the phantom, limiting the self-similarity and introducing bias to the PS calculations. As the spheres were free to move inside the phantom, the background changed slightly but remained unchanged in terms of ensemble statistics. Short term reproducibility of power law exponents was assessed with the coefficient of variation (COV); mean COVs were 6%, 5% and 9% for 2D, DBT projections and reconstructed images respectively. Long term variations were slightly higher, with a COV from 4% to 13%.

3.2   Measurement of Power Law Characteristics in Phantom and Patient Images

In order to validate the structure in the sphere-phantom for mammographic purposes, we compared its PS results and power law exponents with those from patient breast images. The frequency region of the PS, expected to follow a power law characteristic, is delimited by the largest and smallest diameters of the spheres in the phantom [4]. These frequencies cover almost the complete range that was used for the fitting, namely from 0.06 to 0.63 mm^{-1}. In figure 2a, log(PS) plots of patient data (grey curves) are shown, together with the curve of an acquisition of the 'sphere-phantom with air' (black curve, squares), the 'sphere-phantom with water' (black curve, dots) and a homogeneous PMMA phantom of 4 cm thickness (black curve, triangles) for 2D mammography images. Additionally, figure 2b illustrates the log(PS) of the DBT central projection images. The patient and sphere-phantom PS curves are reasonably parallel, suggesting some agreement in texture in the images, however the noise magnitude is higher in the phantom with spheres in air. This can be due to the higher attenuation differences between acrylic spheres and air and therefore higher contrast in the images, increasing the noise magnitude. Another reason for the difference in noise magnitude is the lower AEC controlled dose for the 'spheres in air phantom' when compared to the 'spheres in water phantom'. As a reference, the figure also includes the analysis performed on homogenous PMMA. The flat region of the PS curve of the PMMA phantom extends down to approximately 0.5 mm^{-1}, probably due to absence of structure in the PMMA test object. Figure 2c shows the un-normalized PS curves of the central reconstructed planes of patients, the sphere-phantoms and PMMA. The difference in noise magnitude between that for the sphere-phantom with air and those of the patients is reduced when compared to the projection images and this may be due to a global reduction in image contrast by the reconstruction algorithm. The PS curve for PMMA increases as a function of spatial frequency (until ~2mm^{-1}). This is more obvious with this radially averaged PS than in a 0° or 90° power spectrum (results not shown) since this increase of power is only seen in tube-travel direction; greater non-isotropy will be seen in images of homogeneous objects as this object-type clearly shows the influence of the various filters used in the reconstruction

[9]. The texture is mainly characterized by the power law exponent; exponents are tabulated in table 1, where power law exponents for 2D and DBT patient and phantom images can be compared.

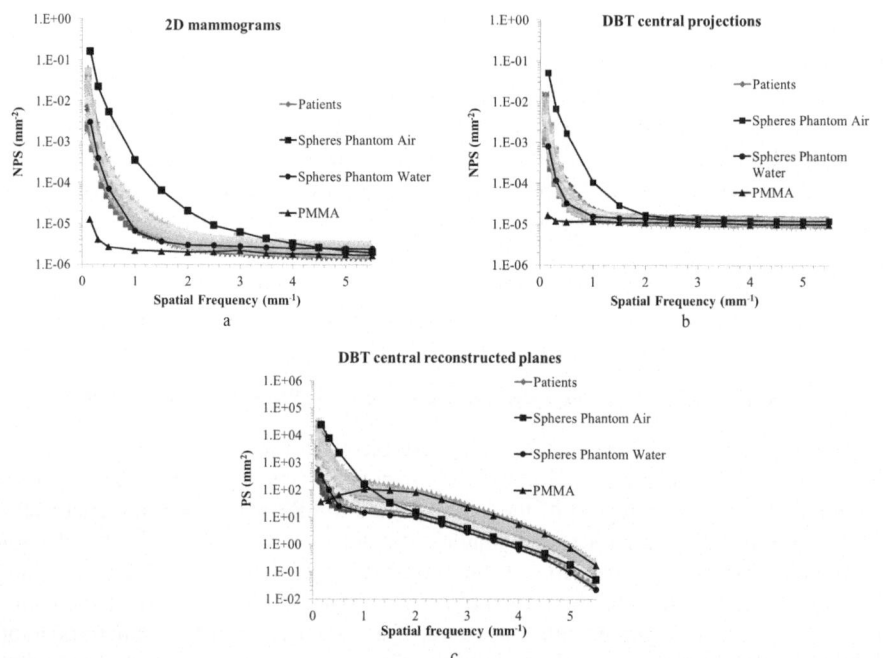

Fig. 2. Power spectrum curves for (a) 2D projection mammography, (b) DBT central projection images and (c) DBT central reconstructed planes. Data are shown for patients (grey curves), sphere-phantom with air (black curve, squares), sphere-phantom with water (black curve, dots) and homogeneous PMMA (black curve, triangles).

Table 1. Power law exponents of 2D and DBT images of patients and sphere-phantoms

	2D			DBT projection			DBT reconstruction		
	Patients	Spheres in air	Spheres in water	Patients	Spheres in air	Spheres in water	Patients	Spheres in air	Spheres in water
min	2.63	2.61	2.93	2.09	2.71	2.22	1.11	1.06	1.49
max	3.94	3.34	3.48	3.45	3.26	2.72	3.23	2.55	1.76
mean	3.37	2.90	3.18	2.92	2.91	2.45	2.41	2.06	1.66
stdev	0.29	0.22	0.18	0.34	0.17	0.23	0.41	0.29	0.09

3.3   Radial (an)isotropy in Power Spectrum Analysis

Potential radial (an)isotropy in the low frequency range of the PS of structured backgrounds was further investigated. Since horizontal (chest wall-nipple direction) and vertical (tube-travel direction) PS are different for reconstructed planes, the radial average for each plane is not a correct or complete representation of the PS. This anisotropy is a characteristic of volumes reconstructed using (cone-beam like) FBP methods [10]; this effect is seen strongly in images of homogeneous PMMA. Figure 3 shows the difference between horizontal (full lines) and vertical (dashed lines) PS for a reconstructed plane of the sphere-phantoms and for a patient image. For very low frequencies, the PS curves are fairly isotropic, possibly indicating that anatomical structure fills this small frequency region. The influence of reconstruction filters is illustrated in figure 4. The strongly curved shape of the PS is due to the reconstruction filters (*e.g.* related to interpolation sinc functions used in FBP) and the peak in the lower frequencies indicates anatomical structure. As with the projection data, the PS of the central reconstructed plane of the sphere-phantom with water (Figure 4c) is more similar to the PS of the patient image compared to the phantom with air. Finally, the anisotropy of the PS results in different power law exponents in horizontal and vertical directions. These exponents also differ from the exponents of the radial averaged PS. Power law exponents of radial, horizontal and vertical PS of the central reconstructed planes were calculated for a subset of ten patients and compared to the exponents of the sphere-phantom (Table 2). These exponents are different from each other and the meaning of this difference in quantifying the texture in reconstructed planes of breast tomosynthesis images is not yet fully understood [11].

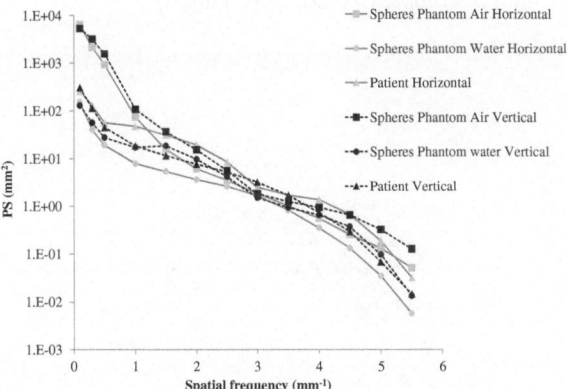

Fig. 3. Horizontal (full lines) and vertical (dashed lines) power spectra of the central reconstructed planes of a sphere-phantom acquisition with air and with water compared with a patient image

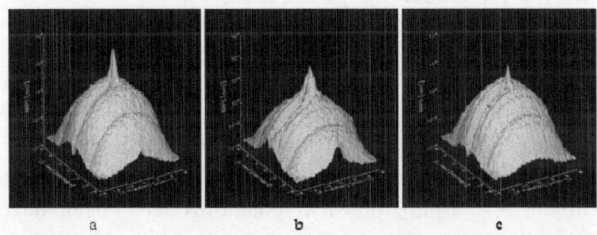

Fig. 4. PS of the central reconstructed plane of (a) a patient, (b) sphere-phantom with air and (c) sphere-phantom with water

Table 2. Power law exponents of radial averaged PS and, horizontal and vertical PS separately for a subset of ten patients compared to the phantom with spheres in air and in water

	Radial	Horizontal	Vertical
Patients	2.41	1.68	1.35
Spheres in air	1.88	2.12	1.75
Spheres in water	1.92	1.45	1.17

3.4   Phantom and Patient Dosimetry

Testing of clinical performance of 2D digital mammography and DBT systems includes the investigation of the mean glandular dose (MGD). In order to produce a clinically relevant test object, the dose of the phantom should be similar to patient doses. Phantom doses with air were 1.1 mGy and 1.7 mGy for 2D and DBT respectively and, 1.9 mGy and 3.1 mGy for the phantom filled with water. The results of the sphere-phantom with air are in good agreement with patient doses of our dataset (average: 1.0 mGy and 1.6 mGy) for a breast equivalent thickness of 75 mm, assuming that the sphere-phantom and PMMA thickness of 60mm can be treated the same and are equivalent to 75mm of compressed breast (Figure 5).

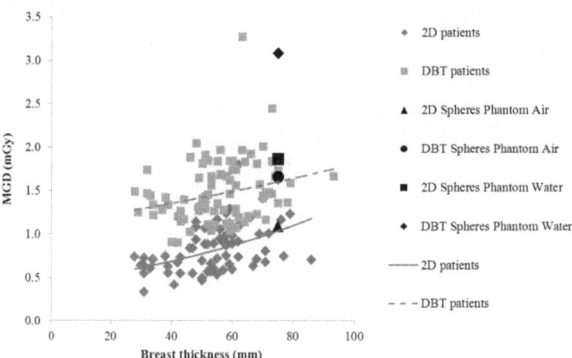

Fig. 5. Mean glandular doses (MGD) of sphere-phantom filled with air exposures are in good agreement with 2D and DBT patient doses of the dataset. Doses of the phantom filled with water are significantly higher compared to patient doses.

4   Conclusion

Development of three-dimensional techniques in breast imaging have increased the need for a more clinically relevant phantom with structures that simulate breast anatomy in three dimensions. Many physical phantoms have been developed for 2D mammography, usually embedding details in a homogeneous background or possibly with a thin layer of two-dimensional structure projected on top of the details. Computerized Imaging Reference Systems (CIRS), Incorporated (Virginia, USA), have produced a phantom with lesions that vary in size embedded within a breast tissue equivalent, complex, heterogeneous background, showing a swirl pattern. Recently, Park *et al* have developed a physical phantom with spheres of different sizes and densities for simulating tissue compositions and textures similar to those of the breast for testing performance [12]. However, evidencing clinical relevance of these backgrounds is more difficult. The proposed phantom in this paper does not aim for an exact simulation of anatomical breast structures. However, the relative position of the PS curves of the sphere-phantom with air and with water to the patient curves, expressed also by overlapping confidence intervals of the power law exponents, suggests the viability of the sphere-phantom as a 3D heterogeneous background: the self-similar spheres background mimics the texture and the statistical properties of the power spectrum of patient breast images in low frequencies. As the phantom allows the insertion of target details simulating microcalcifications, fibrils or masses, it is a potential candidate for close-to-clinically relevant detection tasks for 2D and (pseudo) 3D breast imaging.

References

1. Burgess, A.E., Jacobson, F.L., Judy, P.F.: Human observer detection experiments with mammograms and power-law noise. Med. Phys. 28, 419–436 (2001)
2. Grosjean, B., Muller, S.: Impact of Textured Background on Scoring of Simulated CDMAM Phantom. In: Astley, S.M., Brady, M., Rose, C., Zwiggelaar, R. (eds.) IWDM 2006. LNCS, vol. 4046, pp. 460–467. Springer, Heidelberg (2006)
3. Bliznakova, K., Bliznakov, Z., Bravou, V., Kolitsi, Z., Pallikarakis, N.: A three-dimensional breast software phantom for mammography simulation. Phys. Med. Biol. 48, 369–3719 (2003)
4. Gang, G.J., Tward, D.J., Siewerdsen, J.H.: Anatomical background and generalized detectability in tomosynthesis and cone-beam CT. Med. Phys. 37, 1948–1965 (2010)
5. Mertelmeier, T., Orman, J., Haerer, W., Dudam, M.K.: Optimizing filtered backprojection reconstruction for a breast tomosynthesis prototype device. In: Proceedings of SPIE (2006)
6. Engstrom, E., Reiser, I., Nishikawa, R.: Comparison of power spectra for tomosynthesis projections and reconstructed images. Med. Phys. 36, 1753–1758 (2009)
7. Metheany, K.G., Abbey, C.K., Packard, N., Boone, J.M.: Characterizing anatomical variability in breast CT images. Med. Phys. 35, 4685–4694 (2008)
8. Dance, D.R., Skinner, C.L., Young, K.C., Beckett, J.R., Kotre, C.J.: Additional factors for the estimation of mean glandular breast dose using the UK mammography dosimetry protocol. Phys. Med. Biol. 45, 3225–3240 (2000)
9. Zhao, B., Zhao, W.: Three-dimensional linear system analysis for breast tomosynthesis. Med. Phys. 35, 5219–5232 (2008)
10. Siewerdsen, J.H., Cunningham, I.A., Jaffray, D.A.: A framework for noise-power spectrum analysis of multidimensional images. Med. Phys. 29, 2655–2671 (2002)
11. Reiser, I., Lee, S., Nishikawa, R.M.: On the orientation of mammographic structure. Med. Phys. 38, 5303–5306 (2011)
12. Park, S., Jennings, R., Liu, H., Badano, A., Myers, K.: A statistical, task-based evaluation method for three-dimensional x-ray breast imaging systems using variable-background phantoms. Med. Phys. 37, 6253–6270 (2010)

An Experimental Comparison of Continuous Motion and Step-and-Shoot Modes in Digital Breast Tomosynthesis

Rui Peng, Rongping Zeng, Eugene O'Bryan, Cecilia Marini Bettolo,
Berkman Sahiner, Kyle J. Myers, and Robert J. Jennings[*]

Division of Imaging and Applied Mathematics, OSEL, CDRH,
U.S. Food and Drug Administration, 10903 New Hampshire Avenue,
Silver Spring, MD, USA
RobertJ.Jennings@fda.hhs.gov

Abstract. There are two basic tomosynthesis data acquisition modes: step-and-shoot. Most experimental research on tomosynthesis has been done using commercial breast tomosynthesis systems, which can operate in only a single mode, either step-and-shoot or continuous motion. Thus the only studies that have been done to compare these two imaging modes for otherwise identical systems have been simulation studies. In this paper we describe a versatile, bench-top 3D breast imaging system that can acquire tomosynthesis data using either mode. Preliminary experimental studies of in-plane blur and artifact propagation using different acquisition protocols are discussed. Our initial results indicate that, noticeable difference was observed in system MTF from projection views between step-and-shoot mode and continuous motion mode while there was little difference in other measures from reconstruction slices. This system provides great flexibility for studying breast imaging and image quality under different acquisition protocols.

Keywords: breast tomosynthesis, step-and-shoot, continuous motion, angular sampling protocol.

1 Introduction

For the past few decades, 2D mammography has been the accepted imaging modality for breast cancer screening. However, due to the nature of 2D projection imaging, mammography has limitations in both sensitivity and specificity that are thought to be caused at least in part by the effects of superimposed normal breast structures.[1] Volumetric techniques such as tomosynthesis, because they reduce or remove the superimposition of tissue structures, may improve the ability to distinguish malignant

---

[*] Corresponding author.

A.D.A. Maidment, P.R. Bakic, and S. Gavenonis (Eds.): IWDM 2012, LNCS 7361, pp. 650–657, 2012.
© Springer-Verlag Berlin Heidelberg 2012

lesions from normal structures. They may also improve the specificity of cancer diagnosis by revealing features that distinguish malignant from benign lesions.

Currently there are two available acquisition modes for x-ray tube motion during tomosynthesis data acquisition: step-and-shoot and continuous motion. While much research effort has been directed to acquisition mode, geometry optimization, detector performance and reconstruction algorithms, [1-5] most studies have been based on commercial breast tomosynthesis systems, which, to the authors' knowledge, use either step-and-shoot or continuous motion, but not both. Researchers have studied the differences between the two modes, but due to the lack of an experimental imaging system capable of acquiring data in both modes, these studies have been limited to simulation investigations.[6]

Previously, we reported on the development of a flexible 3D breast imaging system using step-and-shoot mode, and included some sample images.[7] This paper describes the current status of this system, which can now perform tomosynthesis acquisition in both step-and-shoot and continuous motion modes. With this system we have conducted a preliminary experimental comparison of in-plane blur and the propagation of reconstruction artifacts generated by signals in the focal plane to off-focus planes, for both acquisition modes.

2   Materials and Methods

The system consists of three major components: x-ray source, motion control system, and image acquisition system. The x-ray source has a changeable configuration of high voltage generator and x-ray tube. In our breast tomosynthesis studies, a Varian RAD71SP mammography tube (Varian, Inc., Palo Alto, CA) with tungsten target, Be window, and both 0.1 mm and 0.3 mm focal spots is used in combination with a Sedcal SHF-1030-M mammographic x-ray generator (Sedecal USA, Inc., Buffalo Grove, IL). The system can also operate with a general-purpose radiographic generator and x-ray tube capable of producing x-ray spectra suitable for breast CT.

The motion control system provides the geometry and acquisition mode versatility. It comprises three rotary stages (axes 5, 6 and 7 in Figure 1) and four linear stages (axes 1, 2, 3 and 4 in Figure 1), all driven by stepper motors and controlled by a "6k Compumotor" motion controller (Parker Hannifin Corp., Rohnert Park, CA).

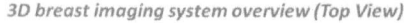

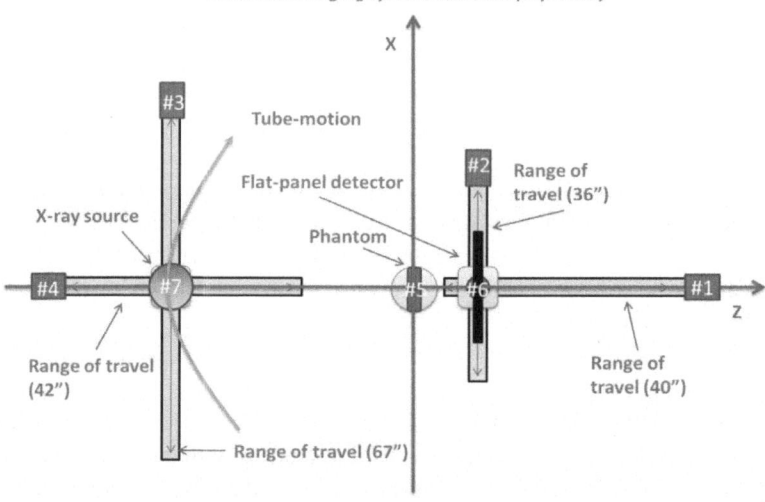

Fig. 1. Schematic diagram of the 3D breast imaging system. The in-plane direction normal to the direction of motion is perpendicular to the plane of the diagram.

The image acquisition system is a flat-panel x-ray detector (Pixium 4343RF, Thales USA, Inc., Arlington, VA). The detector has a 2880×2881 pixel array with 148 μm pixels. The hardware components have been integrated with custom control circuitry and a LabVIEW software user interface. The software also handles automatic image transfer and storage in the control workstation (Dell Precision T3400 running Microsoft Windows Vista OS).

To investigate the impact on image quality of the tube motion, pre-sampled MTFs were calculated for both acquisition modes from images of a 0.001 inch silver edge placed about 50mm away from the detector. Images were acquired at 28kV with 1 mm Al added filtration. The exposure time was 400 ms, the tube current was 25 mA, and the 0.1 mm focal spot was used. The tangential velocity of the focal spot was 10 mm/sec in continuous motion mode. Images were acquired at the 0 degree position with the pivot 70 mm from the detector and radius of the tube arc 605 mm.

In order to compare in-plane object blur and artifact propagation into different reconstruction planes for the two tomosynthesis acquisition modes, a customized phantom with uniform background was used. The phantom consists of the wax insert from an ACR phantom, sandwiched between layers of epoxy-based material simulating 50% glandular and 50% adipose breast-tissue (CIRS, Norfolk, VA). The thickness of the phantom was 42.94 mm with the wax insert located approximately 15.65 mm from the front surface (facing the x-ray source) and 19.93 mm from the back surface (facing detector). The back surface of the phantom was 15 mm away from the detector.

In order to minimize the effects of quantum noise, a relatively high x-ray exposure level was used to image the phantom. The x-ray projection acquisition parameters were 28 kVp, 1 mm Al added filtration, 400 ms exposure time and 125 mA tube current. The 0.3 mm focal spot was used. The tangential speed for x-ray tube motion was 10 mm/s in the continuous motion acquisition mode. This combination of tube velocity and exposure time produces a focal spot displacement of 4 mm during each projection image exposure.

Using the flexibility of the system, we varied geometric parameters to explore their impacts on image quality. As a preliminary study, the distance from pivot (center of the tube's circular trajectory) to detector surface was varied from 0 to 70 mm. All other geometric parameters were kept constant, for both step-and-shoot mode and continuous motion modes. The detector to object center distance (DOD) was 36.5 mm. The distance between x-ray source and pivot was 675 mm. Three sets of 11 projection views were acquired with 15°, 30° and 60° angle spans for each acquisition mode. The projection data sets were reconstructed with a SART algorithm[8] with 1 mm slice thickness and 148 μm in-plane pixel size.

3   Results and Discussion

Pre-sampled MTF was calculated from the center (0°) projection view for both step and shoot mode and continuous motion mode. From Figure 2, the degradation of MTF from the continuous tube motion scheme was clearly demonstrated.

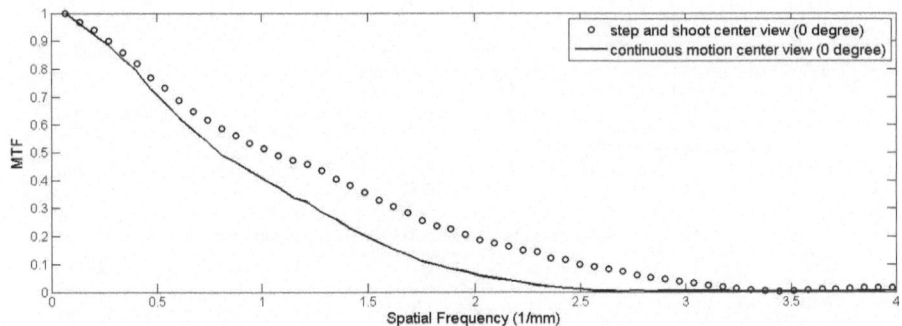

Fig. 2. Pre-sampled MTFs for step-and-shoot mode and continuous motion mode

Reconstructed data sets were analyzed using methods similar to some of the methods described by Zhang et al[3]. In order to investigate the impact on in-plane image quality of different tube motion modes, we analyzed the blur of the top microcalcification from the smallest speck group that could be clearly visualized (0.32 mm) in the phantom with all those different imaging geometries.

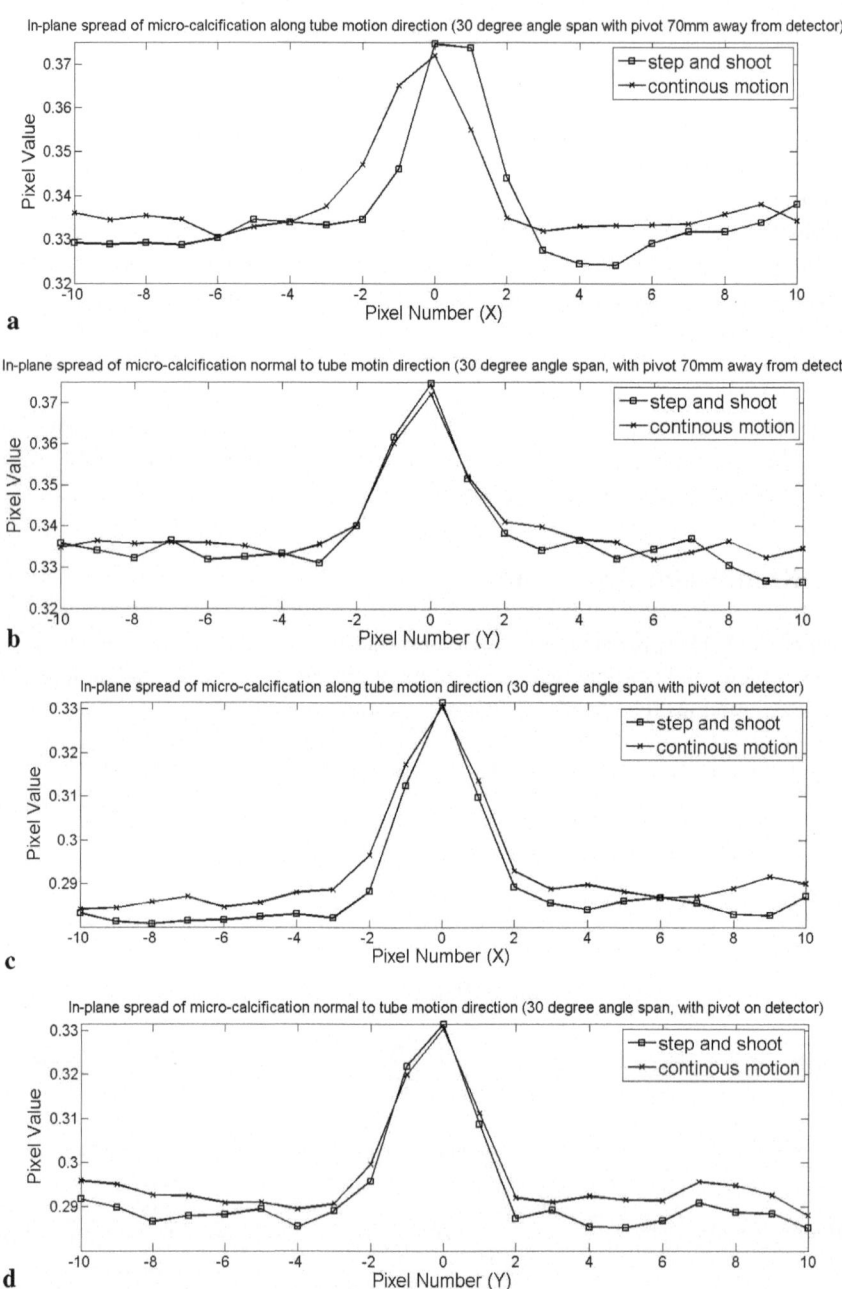

Fig. 3. Pivot-to-detector distance is 70mm: (a) The in-plane spread for the micro-calcification along the tube-motion direction. (b) The in-plane spread for the micro-calcification normal to the tube-motion direction. (c) and (d) is for the pivot on detector case.

Figures 3a and 3b show the line profiles for this specific speck parallel to (3a) and normal to (3b) the tube-motion direction, respectively, for the 30° angle span case, while 3c and 3d show the same. The difference in the full-width-at-half-max (FWHM) values for the line profiles shown is 0.4 pixel along (X) and 0.1 pixel normal to(Y) the tube-motion direction, respectively. Similar results were observed for the 15° and 60° data sets.

In order to compare our results with the simulation study of Shaheen et al. [6] that compared continuous motion with step-and-shoot, we calculated the peak contrast for the set of six 0.32mm micro-calcification specks in the focal plane, for each acquisition mode, using the relation Peak contrast $= \frac{\mu_{smax} - \mu_b}{\mu_b}$, where μ_{smax} is the maximum pixel value for the micro-calcification, and μ_b is the mean pixel value for a 36×36 ROI that was chosen as the background.

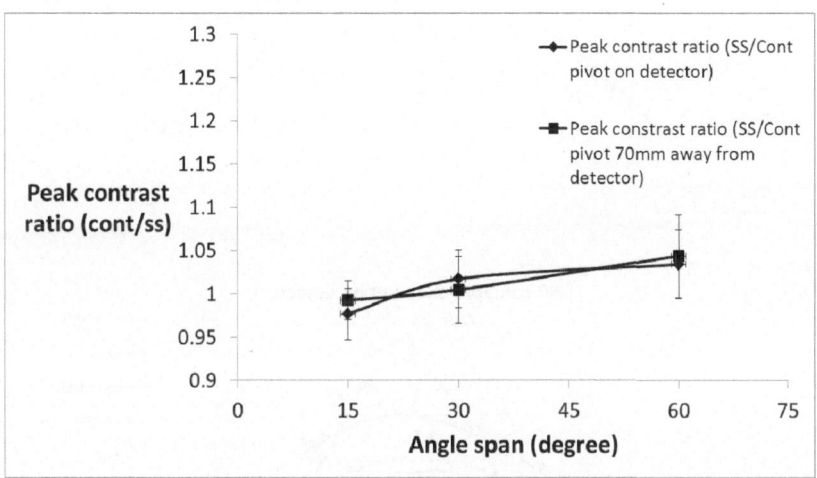

Fig. 4. Average ratio of peak contrast for the same speck group (averaged over all six micro-calcification in the group) with different angle span. Peak contrast ss is the peak contrast in Step-and-shoot mode, while peak contrast cont is that in the continuous motion mode.

Figure 4 is a plot of the average ratios of peak contrast in continuous-motion mode to peak contrast in the step-and-shoot mode. The averages are over the six specks in the nominal 0.32 mm group. Average values were used because the ratios for individual specks showed considerable variation. The simulation study found higher peak contrast for the step-and-shoot mode, with differences of 8% to 9% for 3, 5, and 7 cm breast sizes. Our results show about slightly higher peak contrast for the 15° angular span in step and shoot mode and slightly higher peak contrast for the 30° and 60° angular spans in continuous-motion mode for both geometries. We are looking into possible causes for the differences, and for the variability from speck to speck that we observed.

To study the propagation of artifacts, the contrast-to-noise ratio for the largest mass in the ACR phantom insert was analyzed. A 36×36 ROI was chosen within the mass to calculate the mean signal intensity μ_s. Another 36×36 ROI was chosen in a surrounding area away from features and boundaries. The mean value μ_b and the standard deviation σ_b of this ROI were calculated as the background mean intensity and noise respectively. The equation $CNR = \frac{\mu_s - \mu_b}{\sigma_b}$ was used to calculate the contrast-to-noise ratio.

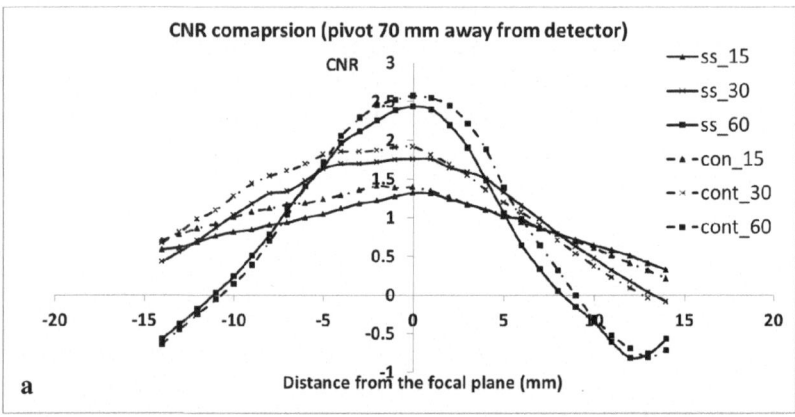

a

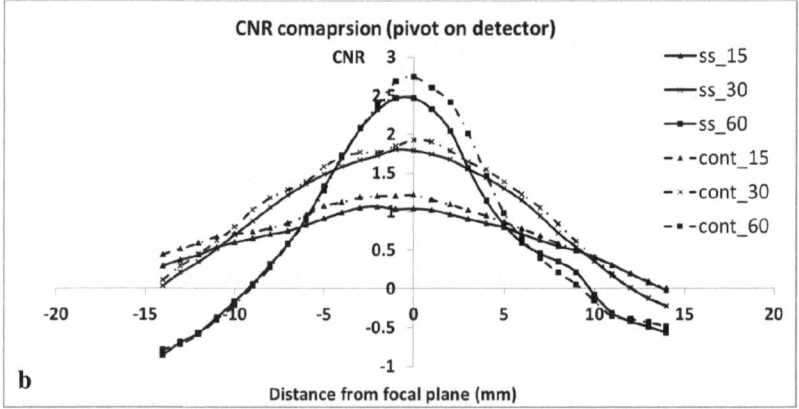

b

Fig. 5. CNR of the mass at different reconstructed planes from six different acquisition protocols in (a) pivot to detector distance=70mm and (b) pivot is on the detector surface

The variation of CNR of the chosen ROIs under six different acquisition modes is plotted in Figure 5 to show the artifact spread away from the focal plane. We found that in-plane CNR, the value at distance zero from the focal plane, and artifact CNR increase with angular span while the spread of the artifact CNR decreases. We are currently investigating whether the differences in CNR between continuous and step-and-shoot modes, for all three of the angular spans, are statistically significant.

4   Conclusion

We have described a bench-top 3D breast imaging system that is capable of acquiring tomosynthesis data in both step-and-shoot and continuous motion mode. A preliminary experimental study using this system to compare in-plane blur and artifact propagation for the two acquisition modes has been presented. From the pre-sampled MTF measurements, a degradation of spatial resolution from continuous tube motion was clearly shown, however results from reconstructed slices show little difference between the two modes for both in-plane blurring and artifact spread, for the conditions studied, which might be attributed to the inaccuracies in geometry calibration and the induced reconstruction blur.

References

1. Wu, T., et al.: A comparison of reconstruction algorithms for breast tomosynthesis. Medical Physics 31(9), 2636–2647 (2004)
2. Sechopoulos, I., Ghetti, C.: Optimization of the acquisition geometry in digital tomosynthesis of the breast. Medical Physics 36(4), 1199–1207 (2009)
3. Zhang, Y., et al.: A comparative study of limited-angle cone-beam reconstruction methods for breast tomosynthesis. Medical Physics 33(10), 3781–3795 (2006)
4. Zhao, B., Zhao, W.: Imaging performance of an amorphous selenium digital mammography detector in a breast tomosynthesis system. Medical Physics 35(5), 1978–1987 (2008)
5. Li, B., et al.: The impact of acquisition angular range on the z-resolution of radiographic tomosynthesis. International Congress Series, vol. 1268, pp. 13–18 (2004)
6. Shaheen, E., Marshall, N., Bosmans, H.: Investigation of the effect of tube motion in breast tomosynthesis: continuous or step and shoot? SPIE (2011)
7. de las Heras Gala, H., et al. A versatile laboratory platform for studying x-ray 3D breast imaging. In: IEEE Medical Imaging Conference (2011)
8. Zeng, R., Myers, K.J.: Task-based comparative study of iterative image reconstruction methods for limited-angle x-ray tomography. SPIE (2011)

Application of a Dynamic 4D Anthropomorphic Breast Phantom in Contrast-Based Imaging System Optimization: Dual-Energy or Temporal Subtraction?

Nooshin Kiarashi[1,2,3], Sujata V. Ghate[3], Joseph Y. Lo[1,2,3,4,5], Loren W. Nolte[2], and Ehsan Samei[1,2,3,4,5,6]

[1] Carl E. Ravin Advanced Imaging Laboratories, Duke University Medical Center, Durham, NC
{nooshin.kiarashi,joseph.lo,samei}@duke.edu
[2] Department of Electrical and Computer Engineering, Duke University, Durham, NC
[3] Department of Radiology, Duke University Medical Center, Durham, NC
[4] Medical Physics Graduate Program, Duke University, Durham, NC
[5] Department of Biomedical Engineering, Duke University, Durham, NC
[6] Department of Physics, Duke University, Durham, NC

Abstract. We previously developed a dynamic 4D anthropomorphic breast phantom, which can be used to optimize contrast-based breast imaging systems, accounting for patient variability and contrast kinetics [1]. In this study we aim to compare the performance of contrast-enhanced mammographic and tomosynthesis imaging protocols followed by temporal subtraction and dual-energy subtraction, qualitatively and quantitatively across a couple of patient models. Signal-difference-to-noise ratio (SDNR) is measured for the six paradigms of contrast enhanced, temporally subtracted, and dual-energy subtracted mammography and tomosynthesis and compared. The results show how the performance is more dependent on the breast model in mammography than in tomosynthesis. Also, it is observed that dual-energy subtraction can be beneficial in mammography, whereas it is not advantageous in tomosynthesis. Lastly, the results suggest that temporal subtraction in general outperforms dual-energy subtraction.

Keywords: Virtual Breast Model, Anthropomorphic Breast Model, Tomosynthesis, Mammography, Dual-energy Subtraction, Temporal Subtraction.

1 Introduction

The increased blood supply requirements of malignancies and hence the process of angiogenesis have motivated the application of contrast agents to increase lesion conspicuity. To further augment the lesion visibility, post-processing contrast enhancement techniques have been introduced that involve multiple acquisitions before and/or after administration of the contrast agent at one or more energies. In the particular case of x-ray imaging, contrast agents are usually iodine-based solutions that are injected to the patient at a rate of 1 ml/kg of patient's weight.

A.D.A. Maidment, P.R. Bakic, and S. Gavenonis (Eds.): IWDM 2012, LNCS 7361, pp. 658–665, 2012.

One contrast enhancement technique is temporal subtraction, which involves acquiring images before and after the administration of the contrast agent and then subtracting them. The principal behind this technique is the fact that after administration of the contrast agent, the areas with most blood infusion show the highest contrast. Hence, when the two images are subtracted most of the anatomy is subtracted out and the malignant lesions that have blood pooling around them will be what remain.

Another contrast enhancement technique, dual-energy subtraction, involves acquiring images after the administration of the contrast agent at energies below and above the k-edge of iodine, which happens at 33.2 keV. At the higher energy acquisition, areas with most blood infusion will result in highest attenuation and hence highest contrast. Therefore, if the two images are subtracted, most of the anatomy could cancel out and malignancies could remain visible.

In order to design and optimize breast imaging systems that involve contrast enhancement there are many questions that need to be answered. First, the optimal enhancement technique needs to be selected. Next, beam parameters such as the energies and filters to be used need to be optimized. Also, system timing should be studied and optimized. Furthermore, issues such as patient motion, contrast kinetics, and angulation mismatch, which can affect the performance should also be considered.

In a previous study we presented a suite of 4D dynamic anthropomorphic breast phantoms for contrast-based breast imaging, which are capable of modeling patient variability and kinetics of contrast agent uptake in the breast [1]. In the present study we incorporate these phantoms in order to compare temporal and dual-energy subtractions in contrast-enhanced breast imaging, specifically mammography and tomosynthesis. The present study is specifically different from [1] in a few ways. The focus of the current work is on the application of the phantoms in imaging system optimization rather than the development of the phantoms themselves. The present work targets six more clinically relevant imaging paradigms and carefully compares them numerically. Furthermore, two patient-based models are used for inferring the conclusions rather than just one patient-based model to represent a wider range of patients. As a result, very interesting conclusions have been possible.

2   Methods

There have been studies on the performance of contrast-enhanced breast imaging techniques incorporating physical phantoms or real patients. However, these studies were mainly limited to one patient model and rarely incorporated the kinetics of contrast agent uptake in the breast tissues, which are essential in extension of the results of such studies.

In this study, we adopt our 4D dynamic anthropomorphic breast phantoms to evaluate the contrast enhancement techniques. The phantoms are based on denoised, scatter-corrected, and segmented real-patient dedicated breast CT data [3-4]. The phantoms were further equipped by modeling contrast uptake kinetics in normal tissue, benign and malignant lesions to accommodate studies involving contrast agents over a wide range of patients. We essentially aim to compare temporal subtraction and dual-energy subtraction in both mammography and tomosynthesis. We assume typical low-energy (W/Rh 28 kVp) and high-energy (W/Cu 49 kVp) acquisitions. Contrast-enhanced low-energy mammography and tomosynthesis, temporally subtracted low-energy mammography and tomosynthesis, and dual-energy subtracted mammography and tomosynthesis amount to a total of six imaging paradigms to be compared.

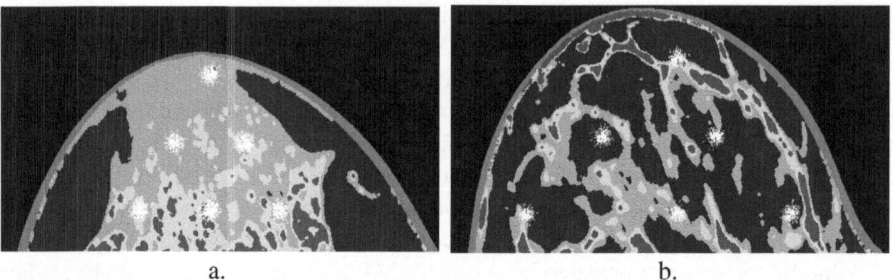

a.   b.

Fig. 1. A slice through the mid-depth of the 44% dense (a) and 28% dense (b) breast models. The grey levels are representative of tissue density

A 28% dense and a 44% dense breast model were picked from the family of breast models for this study to present a wide majority of patients with denser breasts (Fig. 1). Each breast model was compressed to 50% of its thickness. Six lesions were then added to these models at the mid-depth of the compressed volumes. The same lesion model as in [2] was used.

A ray-tracing algorithm simulates projection images, where we include x-ray source spectrum and the geometry of a prototype MAMMOMAT Inspiration tomosynthesis unit (Siemens, Erlangen, Germany). When operating in tomosynthesis mode, 25 images are acquired over a 50° arc centered at the normal position of the x-ray tube to the detector. A filtered back-projection algorithm is then used to reconstruct these images into the compressed breast volume.

The 4D breast phantom enables the simulation of temporal subtraction at arbitrary time points. The breast model at T_0 is considered as the pre-contrast instance (Fig. 2). For the purpose of this study we consider T_1 as the post-contrast instance. Temporal subtraction is performed by subtracting the images at T_0 from images at T_1. Dual-energy subtraction on the other hand is performed by subtracting the weighted normalized low-energy image at T_1 from the normalized high-energy image at T_1. The weighting factor is empirically optimized to result in best anatomical noise cancellation according to measured signal-difference-to-noise ratio (SDNR) values.

Numerical comparison of the six paradigms was done by calculating SDNR as a first-order figure of merit. A circular region of interest (ROI) was selected inside each lesion. Signal was measured by taking the average of the mean values of ROI's in all the lesions. A number of circular ROI's were selected in the background (internal areas of the breast farther from the edges and excluding the lesions). Noise was measured by taking the average of the mean values of the ROI's in the background.

The difference between the signal and noise was divided by the standard deviation of the mean values of the ROI's in the background. We did not include quantum noise or scattering in this first trial of our phantoms.

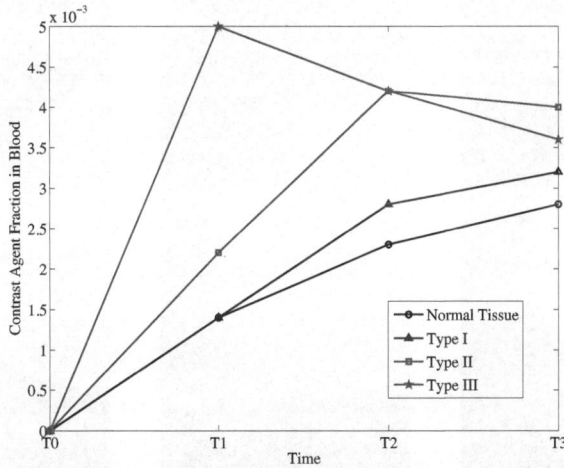

Fig. 2. Contrast agent concentration over time for each type of enhancement pattern: Type II and III patterns are suggestive of malignancy, while lesions following a Type I pattern are mostly benign

3   Results and Discussion

Here we present the results of temporal subtraction and dual-energy subtraction simulations applied to a 28% dense and a 44% dense breast model with six lesions inserted in the mid-plane. Fig. 3 shows contrast-enhanced low-energy mammography, temporally subtracted mammography, and dual-energy subtracted mammography on the 28% dense and 44% dense models respectively. Fig. 4 shows the slice through mid-depth of the reconstructed breast volume acquired by contrast-enhanced low-energy tomosynthesis, temporally subtracted tomosynthesis, and dual-energy subtracted tomosynthesis on the 28% dense and 44% dense models respectively. Lastly, the measured SDNR values for all examined acquisition paradigms are shown in Fig. 5 for comparison.

It is observed in Fig. 3 and 4 that the performance is more dependent on the breast model in mammography compared to tomosynthesis in general, which is expected due to the 3D nature of tomosynthesis. As presented in Fig. 5, in mammography, as a result of temporal subtraction, we evaluated about 10-fold increase in SDNR in a denser breast, compared to about 4-fold increase in a less dense breast. In tomosynthesis on the other hand, the same 4-fold increase is observed in the two breast models.

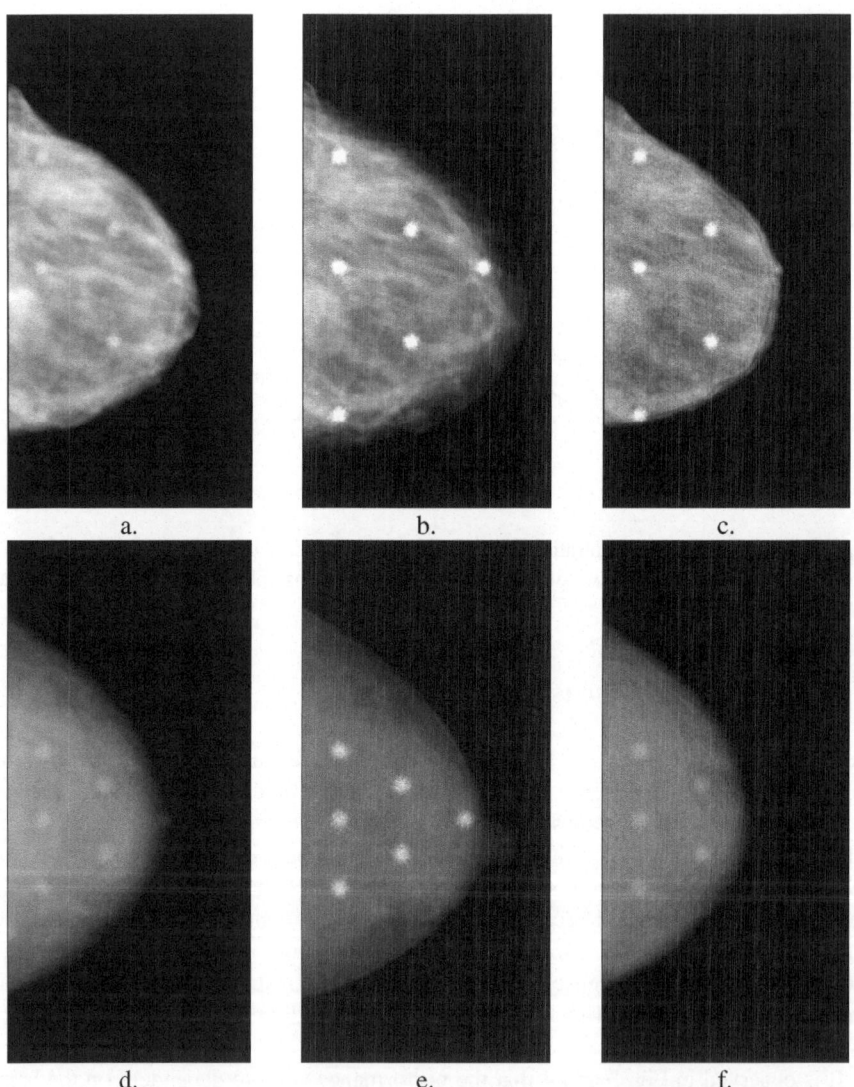

Fig. 3. Contrast-enhanced low-energy mammography (a,d), temporally-subtracted low-energy mammography (b,e), and dual-energy subtracted mammography (c,f) on the 28% dense (top) and the 44% dense (bottom) breast models with lesions following a washout pattern

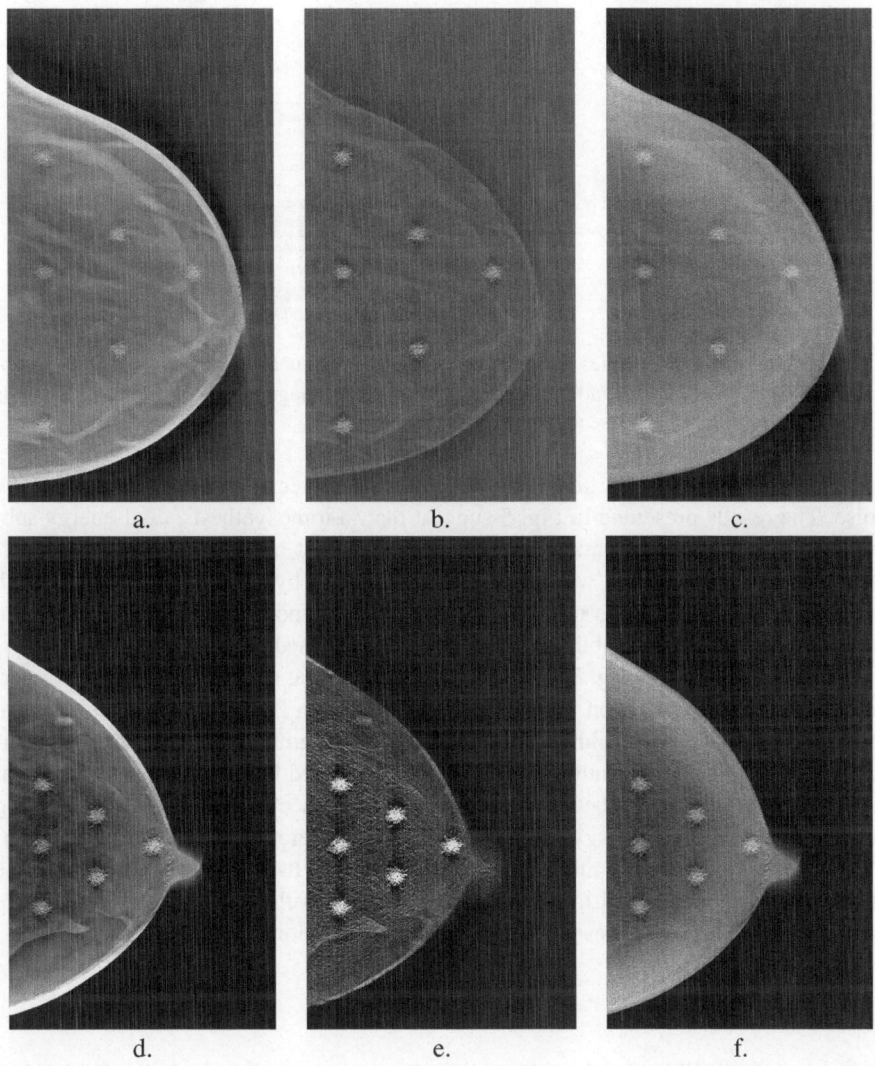

Fig. 4. Slice through the mid-depth of the reconstructed breast volume acquired by contrast-enhanced low-energy tomosynthesis (a,d), temporally-subtracted low-energy tomosynthesis (b,e), and dual-energy subtracted tomosynthesis (c,f) on the 28% dense (top) and the 44% dense (bottom) breast models with lesions following a washout pattern

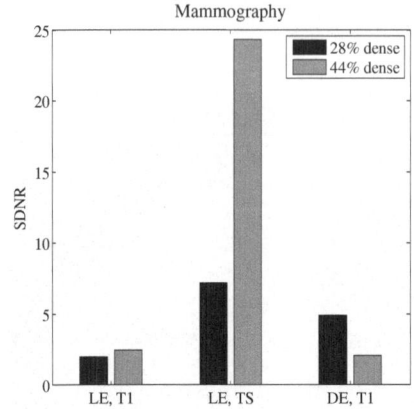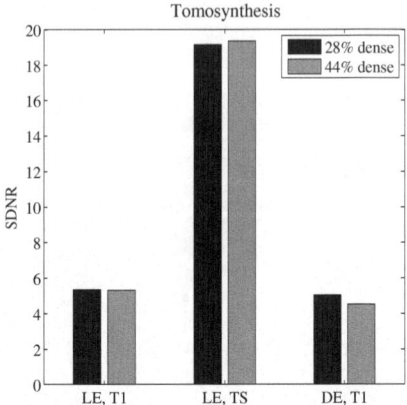

Fig. 5. Measured SDNR values for contrast-enhanced low-energy (LE, T_1), temporally subtracted low-energy (LE, TS), and dual-energy (DE, T_1) mammography (left) and tomosynthesis
(right) applied to the 28% dense and 44% dense breast models

Both dual-energy subtraction and tomosynthesis are techniques to reduce anatomic
noise. The results presented in Fig. 5 suggest that in tomosynthesis, dual-energy subtraction is in fact not advantageous due to the inherent noise enhancement in dual-
energy subtraction; SDNR was decreased on average by 10%. On the other hand,
mammography, which does not have the luxury of tomosynthesis's 3D nature, can
benefit from dual-energy subtraction; SDNR was increased on average by 56%.

Finally, the results in Fig. 3 and 4. show that temporal subtraction tends to outperform dual-energy subtraction in general. As presented in Fig. 5, on average, temporal
subtraction provided a 7-fold increase in SDNR in mammography and a 4-fold increase in SDNR in tomosynthesis. This can be explained by the fact that in temporal
subtraction the difference between absence and presence of contrast agent is being
captured, while in dual-energy subtraction only the differential absorption of the contrast-agent at two different energies is being captured. It is observed that due to the
absorption of contrast agent in normal breast tissue as well as the malignancies, there
is more anatomical noise present in dual-energy subtraction.

4   Conclusion

In this paper we attempted to answer the question of whether to perform temporal
subtraction or dual-energy subtraction in contrast-based breast imaging. Our approach
to this problem was to employ the newly developed 4D dynamic anthropomorphic
breast phantoms and simulate six imaging paradigms: contrast-enhanced low-energy
mammography and tomosynthesis, temporally subtracted low-energy mammography
and tomosynthesis, and dual-energy subtracted mammography and tomosynthesis.
The results suggested that temporal subtraction in general outperforms dual-energy
subtraction. In future, we aim to increase the number of breast models used to
represent a wider population. Furthermore, we can investigate the effects of timing,
patient motion, and weighting factor optimization into the final results.

References

1. Kiarashi, N., Lin, Y., Segars, W.P., Ghate, S.V., Ikejimba, L., Chen, B., Lo, J.Y., Dobbins III, J.T., Nolte, L.W., Samei, E.: Development of a Dynamic 4D Anthropomorphic Breast Phantom for Contrast-based Breast Imaging. In: Proc. SPIE, vol. 8313, pp. 0C1–0C7 (2012)
2. Chen, B., Shorey, J., Saunders, R.S., Richard, S., Thompson, J., Nolte, L.W., Samei, E.: An anthropomorphic breast model for breast imaging simulation and optimization. Acad. Radiol. 18(5), 536–546 (2011)
3. Li, C.M., Segars, W.P., Lo, J.Y., Dobbins III, J.T., Veress, A.I., Boone, J.M.: Three-dimensional computer generated breast phantom based on empirical data. In: Proc. SPIE, vol. 6913, pp. 14.1–14.8 (2008)
4. Li, C.M., Segars, W.P., Dobbins III, J.T., Tourassi, G.D., Boone, J.M.: Methodology for generating a 3D computerized breast phantom from empirical data. Med. Phys. 36(7), 3122–3131 (2009)

Image Processing and Registration of Opposed View 3D Breast Ultrasound

Sumedha Sinha[1,2], Fong-Ming Hooi[1,2], Renee Pinsky[1],
Oliver Kripfgans[1], and Paul Carson[1,2]

[1] Department of Radiology, University of Michigan, Ann Arbor
[2] Department of Biomedical Engineering, University of Michigan, Ann Arbor
pcarson@umich.edu

Abstract. We are studying opposed view ultrasonic imaging (OVI) of the breast in the mammographic geometry, with probable future automation and alignment with X-ray tomosynthesis. OVI through a filament mesh paddle results in improved spatial resolution, contrast, and signal-to-noise ratio. We expect these images will be of a quality that justifies their use for screening purposes, especially for subjects with dense breasts. A previous study assessed machine learning for isolating image artifacts, which included posterior acoustic shadowing from cancers and enhancement arising from cysts. The image volumes were acquired on a custom breast-mimicking phantom containing multiple cysts and solid masses. This paper reports that 3D non-linear registration of opposed view image volumes was robust for the segmented image volumes with noisy areas excluded.

Keywords: breast cancer screening, automated breast ultrasound, ABUS, ultrasonic imaging, shadow segmentation, image registration.

1   Introduction

Hand held ultrasound is commonly used in conjunction with mammography as a diagnostic aid to distinguish benign breast masses from malign lesions [1]. Berg et al.

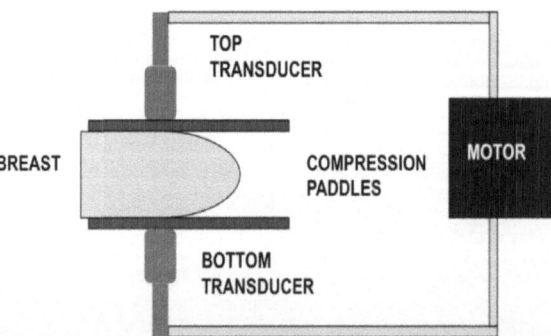

Fig. 1. Schematic of setup for automated dual sided imaging of the breast in mammographic compression. The software-driven motorized transducer carriage moves over each compression paddle.

A.D.A. Maidment, P.R. Bakic, and S. Gavenonis (Eds.): IWDM 2012, LNCS 7361, pp. 666–672, 2012.

[2] observed a diagnostic accuracy for mammography in high-risk women of 0.78 (95% CI, 0.67-0.87) that increased to 0.91 (95% CI, 0.84-0.96) for mammography with expert hand held ultrasound. We propose that automated 3D ultrasound imaging [3, 4, 5] can contribute to breast cancer screening [6], particularly for younger women and women with dense breasts for whom mammography is less sensitive [7].

We have developed a technique to image the breast from both sides in the mammographic geometry to retain the resolution of high frequency ultrasound. This technique is known as dual sided or opposed view imaging, OVI (see Fig. 1, and [8]). OVI is a viable technique for better quality images formed by registering and fusing opposite views since less depth penetration is needed. This allows for the use of higher frequencies that provide finer resolution, an aid to observation of tumor margins, micro-calcifications and improved characterization of internal contents.

2   Materials and Methods

To eventually achieve successful registration of dual-sided in vivo images, we conducted early experiments with the simpler, reproducible case of a breast-mimicking phantom containing 39 lesions in all, 21 of which simulate cancers and 18 of which simulate cysts. These lesions produce realistic artifacts and provide contrast detectability. Our first goal was the automated detection and removal of artifacts such as shadows that would impede registration. Shadow detection on breast ultrasound was attempted before by Drukker et al. [9] using a nonlinear filtering technique. Machine learning was our choice since it has been used with considerable success for identifying suspicious masses on ultrasound images [10, 11].

2.1   Machine Learning for Image ROI Classification

Machine learning classifiers were used to classify image regions in the bottom half of the ultrasound images, which is the region of overlap between opposed views, into useful and less useful information for image fusion and registration purposes. The classifiers we selected were support vector machines (SVMs) and Artificial Neural Networks (ANNs). See [12, 13]. In order to train our classifiers, the phantom image regions of interest (ROIs) were manually labeled. Data was decompressed prior to feature extraction and ROIs were proportionately distributed amongst training, testing and validation sets. First order image statistics of overlying image pixel columns were sufficient features for the SVM and ANN. Six features were extracted: mean and standard deviation of the ROI itself and two ROIs above it. The SVM used a linear kernel, and the ANN used 20 neurons in a feed-forward network with one hidden layer. The procedure is described in full in [8].

2.2   Non-linear Registration of Opposed View Phantom Images

After segmenting the image with our classifiers, registration was performed with mutual information for automatic multimodality image fusion (MIAMI FuseTM, University of Michigan) non-rigid 3D registration [14] on the AVS platform (Advanced Visual Systems, Waltham, MA) [15]. This technique is based on the mutual information objective function (see Equation 1) and thin plate spline interpolation [16].

$$I = \sum_{}^{a} \sum_{}^{b} p(a,b) \log_2\left(\frac{p(a,b)}{p(a)p(b)}\right)$$

$$(1)$$

where 'a' and 'b' are the two data sets to be registered.

Thin-plate spline interpolation is analogous to the warping or bending of a thin sheet of metal. The radial basis function for its kernel is written as below in Equation 2:

$$\varphi(r) = r^2 \log r$$

$$(2)$$

One image set was selected as the reference (usually the top image volume; either can be selected). The other image set (called the target or homologous image) was spatially transformed to align with the reference frame. We registered the two 3D image sets by selecting 9 or more corresponding control points placed at key features, e.g. edges of lesions or echogenic knots. These points were employed as control points by the software and were moved to optimize the so-called mutual information (MI) of the two image volumes.

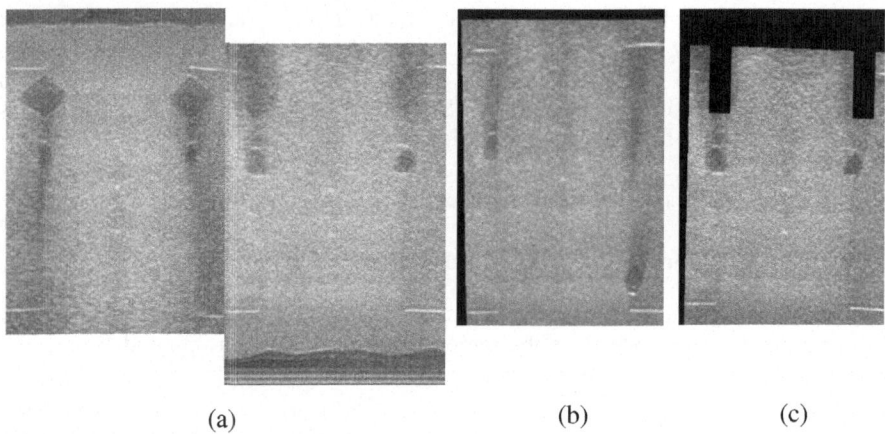

(a)   (b)   (c)

Fig. 2. (a) Reference image and homologous image taken from opposite sides of different phantom region. (b) Misregistered homologous image slice, using a warp transform on the original image. (c) Same registered homologous image slice, using a warp transform on the segmented image.

3   Results and Discussion

3.1   Machine Learning for Image ROI Classification

For guided classification of ROIs chosen from areas below lesions and in the central background of the breast phantom we obtained near-perfect accuracy of 98%, using an SVM with a linear kernel. The SVM and ANN both achieved excellent accuracy of about 97% for the automated classification of true and corrupt image regions in ultrasound data obtained from the breast phantom. For both classifiers, using the first two features alone (mean and standard deviation) gave us an accuracy of 90%. Using different kernels and median filtering images prior to feature selection did not significantly impact accuracy. The computation time was negligible for both classifiers.

3.2   Non-linear Registration of Opposed View Phantom Images

A full affine transform did not succeed in aligning the two opposed views during early trial run. Fig 3 shows an example of 3D misalignment where the two registered image slices do not belong to the same vertical cross-section of the phantom.

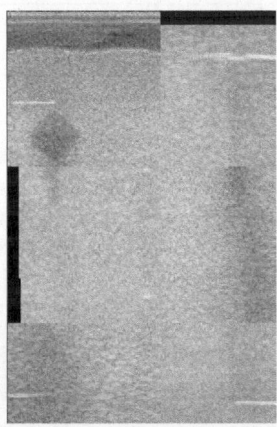

Fig. 3. Checkerboard image of misregistered homologous image, using a full affine transform

Non-linear registrations were carried out for 6 cases with good results. Tables 1 and 2 show the registration error values over multiple runs for the original phantom images and the segmented phantom images, respectively. Mutual information values were actually slightly lower for segmented images, and not indicative of registration accuracy. Errors were calculated by averaging the distances between lesion centers in the reference images and the registered homologous images. The centers were marked by hand and then shifted slightly to a more optimal position by correlating the surrounding region with a lesion-sized mask. The mean error was significantly large for cases 2, 3 and 5, because the original phantom images were grossly misregistered.

Table 1. Registration error in x and y for the unsegmented original images; note that cases 2, 3 and 4 did not register at all

Case	Mean error and standard deviation in x (mm)	Mean error and standard deviation in y (mm)
Original 1	0.49 +/- 1.06	0.27 +/- 1.01
Original 2	9.54 +/- 14.22	8.61 +/- 15.69
Original 3	13.92 +/ -6.89	11.94 +/- 13.09
Original 4	0.5 +/- 0.46	0.85 +/- 0.69
Original 5	12.57 +/- 7.85	9.26 +/- 7.77
Original 6	0.69 +/- 0.43	1.08 +/- 0.85

Table 2. Registration error in x and y for the segmented images

Case	Mean error and standard deviation in x (mm)	Mean error and standard deviation in y (mm)
Segmented 1	0.71 +/-0.74	1.39 +/- 1.91
Segmented 2	0.57 +/-1.28	0.53 +/- 1.84
Segmented 3	0.78 +/- 0.8	1.34 +/- 2.31
Segmented 4	0.83 +/-0.97	1.72 +/-2.83
Segmented 5	0.83 +/-0.88	1.74 +/-2.76
Segmented 6	0.77 +/-0.81	1.58 +/-2.06

Since the natural structure of the phantom is such that lesions are divided into four zones depth-wise (1.25 cm each), CNR (contrast-to-noise ratios) for these zones show where the signal begins to degrade substantially. There is only a slight reduction in average lesion CNR while moving from the surface down to the zone directly below it (4.5% and 2.1% respectively for each view), and average CNR dropped by 25% one zone further down. Decisions must be made regarding the selection of image regions in the central two zones, where quality is highly variable and overlap from the two views is usual.

The proposed technique for constructing the combined image set retains the original image information in the top and bottom, while fusing the central zone post-registration as follows: if certain image regions have been masked as corrupt on both sides, then fill in those pixels with a pixel by pixel average of the original image information. If an image region is masked only on one side, retain pixels from the un-masked side. Finally, if the machine learning algorithm has not eliminated a particular image region on either side, replace those pixels with the maximum of the two sides.

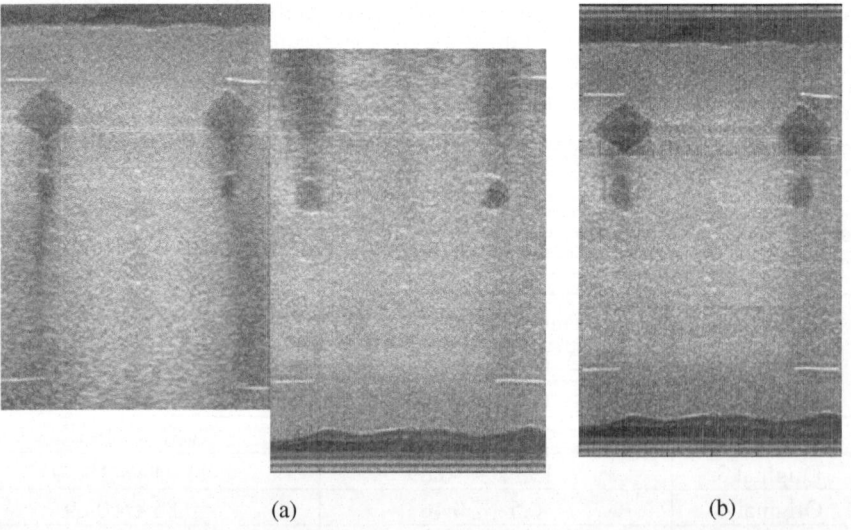

(a)   (b)

Fig. 4. (a) Reference image and homologous image taken from opposite sides of different phantom region (b) Fused image after registration

An example of fused images from the phantom is in Fig. 4. Note the improvement in visibility of underlying lesions in Fig. 4(b). However, resolution is lost on the filaments seen in cross section on a line down the center. The averaging of data from both views causes blurred or even duplicate target points due to registration error or imperfect focusing in either image.

4   Conclusions

Machine learning classifiers accurately identified regions of corrupted data on a breast-mimicking phantom. Registration of opposed view image volumes after segmentation was less vulnerable to error when using the non-linear thin-plate spline warping alignment technique.

Acknowledgements. We are grateful to E.L. Madsen, Z.H. Syed, J.A. Fessler, G.L. Frank, M.M. Goodsitt and J. B. Fowlkes for their contributions. This work was supported in part by NIH Grants CA115267 and CA91713.

References

1. Kolb, T.M., Lichy, J., Newhouse, J.H.: Occult cancer in women with dense breasts: detection with screening US–diagnostic yield and tumor characteristics. Radiology 207(1), 191–199 (1998)
2. Berg, W.A., Blume, J.D., Cormack, J.B., Mendelson, E.B., Lehrer, D., Böhm-Vélez, M., et al.: Combined Screening With Ultrasound and Mammography vs Mammography Alone in Women at Elevated Risk of Breast Cancer. JAMA 299(19), 2151–2163 (2008)
3. Carson, P.L., LeCarpentier, G.L., Roubidoux, M.A., Erkamp, R.Q., Fowlkes, J.B., Goodsitt, M.M.: Physics and Technology of Ultrasound Breast Imaging Including Automated 3D. In: Karellas, A., Giger, M.L. (eds.) Syllabus, Advances in Breast Imaging: Physics, Technology, and Clinical Applications, RSNA Categorical Course in Diagnostic Radiology Physics, pp. 223–232. RSNA (2004)
4. Kapur, A., Carson, P.L., Eberhard, J., Goodsitt, M.M., Thomenius, K., Lokhandwalla, M., Buckley, D., Roubidoux, M.A., Helvie, M.A., Booi, R.C., LeCarpentier, G.L., Erkamp, R.Q., Chan, H.P., Fowlkes, J.B., Thomas, J.A., Landberg, C.E.: Combination of digital mammography with semi-automated 3d breast ultrasound. Technol. Cancer Res. Treat 3(4), 325–334 (2004)
5. Sinha, S.P., Goodsit, M.M., Roubidoux, M.A., Booi, R.C., LeCarpentier, G.L., Lashbrook, C.R., Thomenius, K.E., Chalek, C.L., Carson, P.L.: Automated Ultrasound Scanning on a Dual Modality Breast Imaging System. Journal of Ultrasound in Medicine 26, 645–655 (2007)
6. Kelly, K., Dean, J., Comulada, W.S., Lee, S.J.: Breast cancer detection using automated whole breast ultrasound and mammography in radiographically dense breasts. Eur. Radiol. 20(3), 734–742 (2010)
7. Stacey-Clear, A., McCarthy, K.A., Hall, D.A., Pile-Spellman, E., White, G., Hulka, C.A., Whitman, G.J., Halpern, E.F., Kopans, D.B.: Mammographically detected breast cancer: location in women under 50 years old. Radiology 186, 677–680 (1993)

8. Sinha, S.P., Hooi, F.M., Syed, Z., Pinsky, R., Thomenius, K., Carson, P.L.: Machine learning for noise removal on breast ultrasound images. In: 2010 IEEE Int. Ultrasonics Symp., Inst. Elect. Electr. Engrs., San Diego, October 10-13 (2010)
9. Drukker, K., Giger, M.L., Mendelson, E.B.: Computerized analysis of shadowing on breast ultrasound for improved lesion detection. Med. Phys. 30(7), 1833–1842 (2003)
10. Kotropoulos, C., Pitas, I.: Segmentation of ultrasonic images using Support Vector Machines. Pattern Recognition Letters 24, 715–727 (2003)
11. Piliourasa, N., Kalatzisa, I., Dimitropoulos, Cavouras, D.: Development of the cubic least squares mapping linear-kernel support vector machine classifier for improving the characterization of breast lesions on ultrasound. Computerized Medical Imaging and Graphics 28, 247–255 (2004)
12. Vapnik, V.: Statistical learning theory. Wiley (1998)
13. Widrow, B., Lehr, M.: 30 Years of Adaptive Neural Networks: Perceptron, Madaline, and Backpropagation. Proceedings of IEEE 78, 1415–1444 (1990)
14. Meyer, C.R., Boes, J.L., Kim, B., Bland, P.H., Lecarpentier, G.L., Fowlkes, J.B., Roubidoux, N.A., Carson, P.L.: Semiautomatic registration of volumetric ultrasound scans. Ultrasound Med. Biol. 25, 339–347 (1999)
15. Krucker, J.F., Meyer, C.R., LeCarpentier, G.L., Fowlkes, J.B., Carson, P.L.: 3-D spatial compounding of ultrasound images using image-based nonrigid registration. Ultrasound Med. Biol. 26(9), 1475–1488 (2000)
16. Bookstein, F.: Morphometric tools for landmark data: geometry and biology. Cambridge University Press (1997)

Detecting Low-Conspicuity Mammographic Findings – The Real Added Value of CAD

Isaac Leichter[1,2], Richard Lederman[3], and Alexandra Manevitch[2]

[1] Department of Medical Engineering, Jerusalem College of Technology, Jerusalem, Israel
[2] Siemens Israel, CAD division, Jerusalem, Israel
[3] Department of Radiology, Hadassah University Hospital, Jerusalem, Israel
leichter@jct.ac.il

Abstract. This study investigates the effectiveness of CAD for low-conspicuity malignant lesions that are subtle and sometimes missed in conventional analysis. 280 malignant cases were retrospectively reviewed by a non-blinded radiologist, who identified 676 findings. A conspicuity score was assigned to each finding on each view, and 171 findings were of low conspicuity. CAD sensitivity of a prototype CAD algorithm (Siemens), for the high-conspicuity findings was 91.5%. The sensitivity for the 67 cases with low-conspicuity findings in both views (65.7%) was considerably higher than that reported for similar cases in conventional interpretation (40.2%). For the 2688 normal cases, CAD generated 1.24 false marks per case. CAD sensitivity for low-conspicuity findings did not significantly depend on breast density, and was significantly better for non-invasive lesions and for masses in younger women. Thus, CAD should be most beneficial for avoiding oversight of low-conspicuity breast cancers, particularly non-invasive lesions and masses in younger women.

Keywords: CAD, screening mammography, FFDM, low-conspicuity findings.

1 Introduction

Computer Aided Detection (CAD) has been described as useful for avoiding oversights in mammography due to distraction or fatigue. It is expected that CAD should also assist the novice to detect more subtle lesions and even allow experts to detect lesions in earlier stages. Studies have provided conflicting results regarding the usefulness of CAD, some showing improved cancer detection [1, 2] while others reporting decreased specificity [3].

While CAD is impressive technology, its current intended use in mammography is as a "second reader", after a conventional interpretation of the mammogram without CAD assistance, has been completed. Thus, it is irrelevant whether CAD is able to detect a lesion which has been detected in the initial, conventional interpretation. However, it is essential that CAD should detect a cancer missed in the conventional evaluation. It is also important that, ultimately, in the final phase of the CAD-assisted interpretation, the reader accepts the true CAD prompt. The lower the false mark (FM) rate, the higher the likelihood of the reader to accept the CAD marks for the less

A.D.A. Maidment, P.R. Bakic, and S. Gavenonis (Eds.): IWDM 2012, LNCS 7361, pp. 673–681, 2012.

conspicuous malignant lesions which are more subtle, and often do not have the typical malignant characteristics. Therefore, the sensitivity of the CAD algorithm for low-conspicuity findings, as well as the FM rate of the CAD algorithm should be investigated. To our knowledge, no published study has described the usefulness of CAD in detecting subtle, low-conspicuity findings that are occasionally missed in conventional interpretation.

Since no added value of CAD is expected for highly conspicuous lesions, CAD performance could be most beneficial for lesions with low conspicuity. The current study was designed to evaluate the prevalence of low-conspicuity malignant findings and the CAD performance on these findings by lesion type, breast density, histopathology and patient age.

2   Material and Methods

2.1   Case Acquisition and Review

Two thousand nine hundred and eighty-six Full Field Digital Mammography (FFDM) cases were culled retrospectively from 6 screening facilities. Two hundred and eighty of the cases were pathology proven cancers, including 186 cases with mass lesions and 94 cases with clusters and the remaining 2706 cases were normal. Both the malignant cases and the normal cases were collected in a consecutive manner,

All the malignant cases were retrospectively reviewed by a non-blinded expert radiologist with more than 30 years of experience in mammography. The radiologist examined the 4 standard views of each case and identified, on a per-view basis, a total of 676 findings which correlated with the pathology reports (477 masses and 199 clusters). The pathology codes, the patient age and the breast density for the pathology proven malignant cases were also recorded. BI-RADS breast density categories 1 and 2 were considered "non-dense" breast composition, while categories 3 and 4 were considered "dense" breast composition.

2.2   Analysis of Conspicuity

This study evaluates the CAD performance on low-conspicuity findings which are challenging for conventional interpretation. In order to identify the low-conspicuity findings, the conspicuity of each finding in each view was assessed. The conspicuity of mass findings depends on the density of the lesion, its contrast compared to the surrounding tissue, its shape, its margins and the presence of architectural distortion or asymmetry. Although it would seem that smaller masses should be less conspicuous, lesion size was not included among the factors affecting the conspicuity of a mass lesion. However, the conspicuity of the mass lesions was evaluated as a function of lesion size. The conspicuity of a cluster depends on the brightness of the calcifications, the contrast of the calcifications compared to the background, the size of the calcifications, and their individual shape. Based on these parameters, each finding was assigned a conspicuity score, using a five-point scale. This score was assigned separately to each finding for each view, since the conspicuity of a finding may differ from one view to the other. The distribution of the 477 mass findings and the 199 clusters was evaluated by the conspicuity score. Findings with a score of 1-3 were considered to be of low conspicuity, while those with a score of 4-5 were considered to be of high conspicuity.

Of the 676 malignant findings analyzed per view, 171 were found to be of low conspicuity, including 118 masses and 53 clusters. Of the 171 findings with low conspicuity per view, 126 were invasive ductal carcinoma, 16 were invasive lobular carcinoma, 12 were ductal carcinomas in-situ and for 17 findings only cytology results were available. In 67 of the 280 malignant cases, the findings were of low conspicuity in both views (45 masses, 22 clusters).

2.3   CAD Methodology

All the cases were run with a prototype CAD algorithm (Siemens)[1].The CAD algorithm was designed to detect and mark suspicious findings on standard FFDM views. The algorithm is intended to diminish oversights by bringing the CAD marks to the attention of the radiologist after the initial reading has been completed. As described elsewhere [4], the system consists of two separate algorithms, one for detecting masses and the other for detecting micro-calcifications. A large library of digital mammograms was used to train and optimize the performance of the algorithms in order to detect the suspicious findings while minimizing the generation of false marks. The 2986 cases analyzed in the present study were "unseen cases" and none of them, had been used for the training of the algorithms.

The CAD algorithm initially performs a very sensitive detection process in order to generate candidates for any potentially malignant finding. Then, for each candidate, the algorithm extracts quantitative features, which characterize the potential finding and its surrounding tissue. Based on this characterization, the algorithm automatically assigns each candidate a level of suspicion. Then, a threshold is applied to the levels of suspicion [5] and each candidate with a level below the threshold is filtered out. The filtering process decreases the number of CAD false marks, which distract the radiologist and decrease the likelihood of accepting the true CAD marks. After filtering, only the most suspicious findings are marked by CAD and displayed on the mammogram.

2.4   Statistical Analysis

A lesion was considered detected by CAD, if it was correctly marked by the algorithm on at least one of the views. The overall sensitivity of the CAD algorithm was calculated as the ratio of the cases with detected lesions to the total number of malignant cases. Each CAD mark on a normal case was considered false. The FM rate for the normal cases was calculated as the ratio of the number of marks to the total number of normal cases.

---

[1] Not for sale in the US.

The performance of the CAD algorithm for the 67 cases with findings of low-conspicuity in both views was evaluated by lesion type and breast density. The CAD performance by age and by histopathology, for the 171 low-conspicuity findings, was evaluated per finding per view, rather than per case, due to the limited sample size in each of these subgroups. Statistical significance was determined by Student's t-test, assuming unequal variances, with one-tailed p-values.

3   Results

3.1   The Relationship between the Conspicuity and Size of Findings

Figure 1 displays the distribution of the mass lesions by size for the low and the high-conspicuity masses. The figure shows that the distribution of cases by lesion size is similar, regardless of conspicuity and that small masses are not more prevalent amongst the low-conspicuity findings.

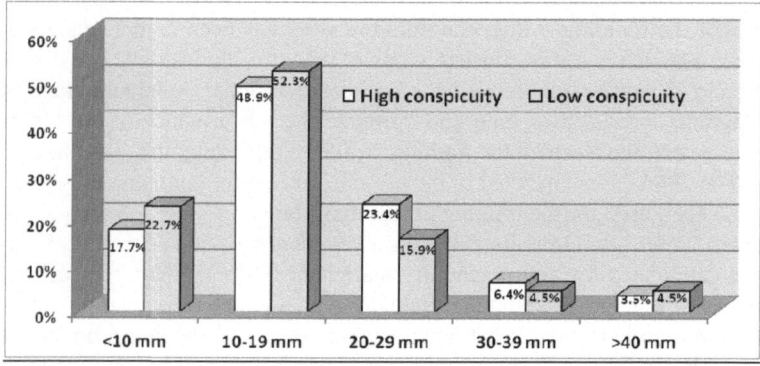

Fig. 1. The distribution of mass lesions by size for the low and the high-conspicuity masses

3.2   CAD Sensitivity for Low-Conspicuity Findings by Lesion Type

The CAD sensitivity for the 213 cases with high-conspicuity findings in at least one view was 91.5%. The sensitivity for the 67 subtle cases with findings of low conspicuity in both views (65.7%) was considerably higher than reported for similar cases [6] in conventional interpretation (40.2%). Figure 2 displays the CAD sensitivity per case, by the type of finding, for the 67 cases with findings of low conspicuity in both views and for the 213 cases with findings of high conspicuity in at least one view. The FM rate per case for the 2706 normal cases was 1.24. The FM rate for masses was higher in dense breasts, while the FM rate for clusters was higher in older women mainly due to CAD marking vascular calcifications.

Figure 2, which displays the CAD sensitivity per case by the type of finding, shows that the sensitivity was lower both for cases with low-conspicuity mass lesions and low-conspicuity clusters. The prevalence of cases with low-conspicuity findings can be derived from the number of cases in each subgroup shown in Figure 2. Forty-five cases had low-conspicuity masses in both views and 22 cases had low-conspicuity clusters in both views. Thus, 24.2% of the cases with masses (45/186) were of low-conspicuity and 23.4% of the cases with clusters (22/94) were of low-conspicuity. Radiologists are most likely to require CAD assistance specifically for these cases, which represents nearly one fourth of the population.

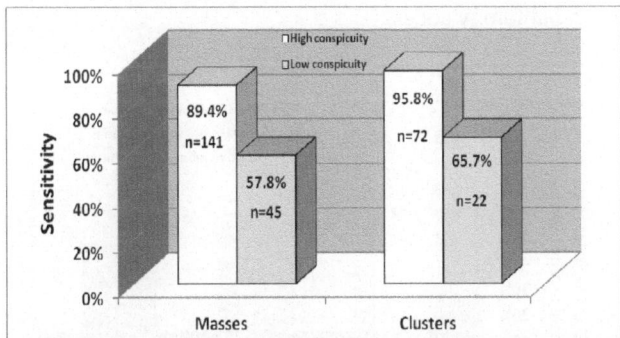

Fig. 2. The CAD sensitivity for cases with findings of high and low conspicuity, by the type of finding. The numerical values in the bars refer to the actual number of cases in each subgroup.

3.3   CAD Sensitivity for Low-Conspicuity Findings by Breast Density

Figure 3 displays the CAD sensitivity for cases with low-conspicuity findings by breast density.

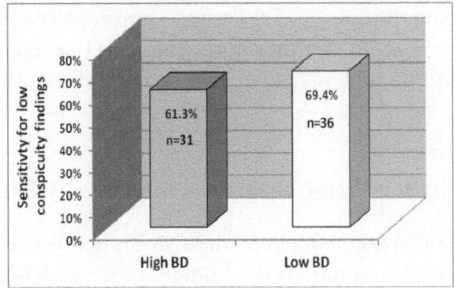

Fig. 3. The CAD sensitivity for the 67 cases with low conspicuity findings by breast density. The numerical values in the bars refer to the actual number of cases in each subgroup.

The figure shows that although the CAD sensitivity for cases with low-conspicuity findings in both views was slightly lower in women with high density breast composition, the difference was not statisticaly significant (p=0.25).

3.4   CAD Sensitivity for Low-Conspicuity Findings by Histopathology

The analysis of the CAD sensitivity for the low-conspicuity findings by histopatholo-gy was performed per finding, per view, and not per case due to the small number of cases with non-invasive findings of low-conspicuity in both views (5 cases). It should be noted that the CAD analysis per finding per view yields, by definition, lower sensi-tivity than that calculated per case, since in the latter, detection in only one view is considered sufficient, while per finding the sensitivity would be only 50%. Figure 4 displays the CAD sensitivity, by pathology code, for the 154 low-conspicuity find-ings, with known pathology codes.

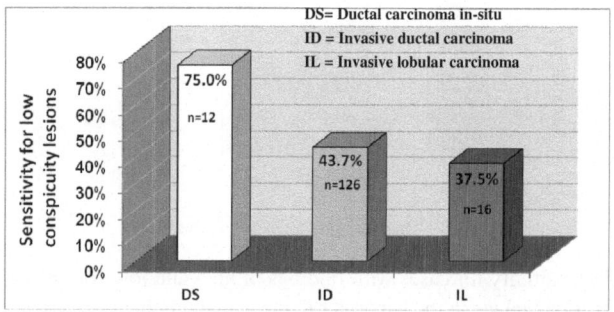

Fig. 4. The CAD sensitivity by histopathology, for the 154 low-conspicuity findings per view, with known pathology codes. The numerical values in the bars refer to the actual number of findings in each subgroup.

Figure 4 shows that for the low-conspicuity findings, CAD performed better on non-invasive lesions compared to invasive lesions. The sensitivity for the low-conspicuity non-invasive findings (75.0%) was significantly higher (p<0.02) than for the invasive findings (43.0%). Furthermore, the CAD sensitivity for findings with invasive ductal carcinoma and invasive lobular carcinoma was similar (43.7% and 37.5%).

3.5   CAD Sensitivity for Low-Conspicuity Findings by Patient Age

The CAD sensitivity of low-conspicuity findings by age was also analyzed per find-ing per view and not per case, due to the limited number of women below the age of 50 with low conspicuity findings in both views (10 cases). The CAD sensitivity of low-conspicuity findings analyzed per view, in women under the age of 50 (56.5%) was not significantly different (p = 0.16) from that in women of age 50 and above (45.3%). However, as shown in figure 5, when the analysis by age was performed only for the 118 low-conspicuity mass lesions, the CAD sensitivity per view was much higher for younger women.

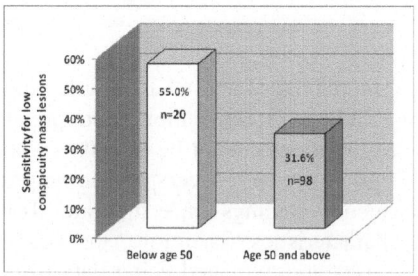

Fig. 5. The CAD sensitivity , by age, for the 118 low-conspicuity mass findings per view. The numerical values in the bars refer to the actual number of findings in each subgroup.

Figure 5 shows that of the 20 low conspicuity mass lesions in women under the age of 50, the CAD algorithm detected 11 findings (55.0%)   while of the 98 low-conspicuity masses in women of age 50 or above, only 31 findings were detected (31.6%).   Thus, CAD performed significantly better (p<0.04) for low conspicuity masses in women under 50, compared to older women.

In order to determine the prevalence of low-conspicuity masses in women under 50, the data shown in figure 6 were used. Figure 6 displays the distribution of mass lesions by conspicuity score for women younger than 50 and women of age 50 and above.

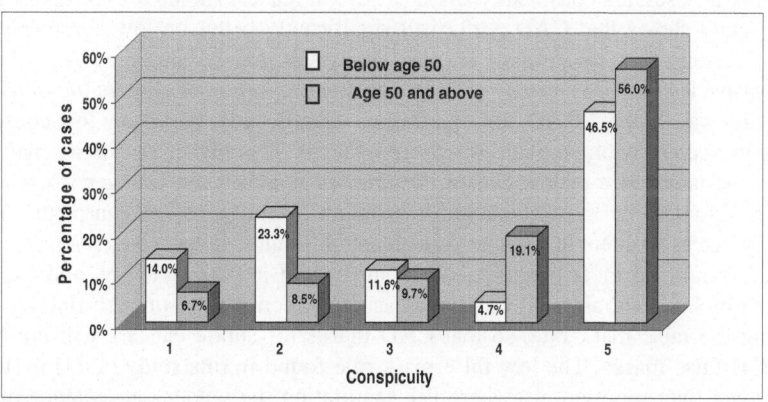

Fig. 6. The distribution of mass lesions by conspicuity for women younger than 50 and women of age 50 and above

This figure shows that the prevalence of low-conspicuity mass lesions (conspicuity scores 1-3) in younger women is 48.8%, while in older women it is only 24.9%. Thus, while low conspicuity mass lesions are twice as frequent in younger women, the CAD sensitivity for those masses in younger women is significantly higher.

4   Discussion

Since to our knowledge, no published study has reported the performance of radiologists on low-conspicuity findings in conventional interpretation, the CAD sensitivity for subtle, low-conspicuity findings cannot be directly compared to the conventional sensitivity on such findings. However, cancers missed on prior mammograms may be comparable to low-conspicuity findings since they are also subtle, possibly lacking the typical malignant characteristics. Therefore, the conventional performance on low-conspicuity findings was approximated using data from a study which reported the detection sensitivity for blinded radiologists who analyzed, in retrospect, visible findings that were missed on prior mammograms [6]. In that study, of 286 cases with visible findings on prior examinations, only 115 cases were considered actionable by the combined weighted assessments of 5 experienced radiologists, yielding a sensitivity of 40.2% (115/286). The CAD algorithm in the current study performed much better (65.7%) on cases with low-conspicuity in both views.

The overall sensitivity of the CAD algorithm, used in the above study [6], for visible findings missed on prior mammograms was reported to be 60%, which is similar to the sensitivity of the CAD algorithm in the current study for the low-conspicuity lesions (65.7%). Therefore, cases with low-conspicuity malignant findings may serve for the evaluation of CAD performance, rather than visible cancers that were overlooked on prior mammograms, since prior mammograms are not always available.

One of the limitations of the study was that only one reading was used to determine conspicuity, hence intra and inter-variability could not be evaluated. In future studies the variability in assessing conspicuity amongst several readers should also be investigated.

Our study shows that CAD performed significantly better on low conspicuity non-invasive lesions, than on invasive lesions. This result may be attributed to the fact that non-invasive lesions (DS) usually include a greater proportion of clusters for which CAD sensitivity was higher. CAD also performed significantly better on low-conspicuity masses in younger women, than in women over 50. This higher sensitivity may be related to the larger size of low-conspicuity masses found in the younger women in the study. CAD could be most valuable for avoiding oversight of low-conspicuity masses that are twice as frequent in younger women and difficult to detect conventionally.

CAD should be most beneficial for lesions with low conspicuity, and future refinement of CAD should emphasize increasing the sensitivity for such findings while lowering the false mark rate, so that CAD marks for subtle cancers will not be dismissed as false marks. The low false mark rate found in this study (1.24) is substantially lower than reported elsewhere [7], facilitating the reader's acceptance of CAD prompts for these subtle findings.

References

1. Birdwell, R.L., Bandodkar, P., Ikeda, D.M.: Computer-aided detection with screening mammography in a university hospital setting. Radiology 236, 451–457 (2005)
2. Romero, C., Almenar, A., Pinto, J.M., Varela, C., Muñoz, E., Botella, M.: Impact on breast cancer diagnosis in a multidisciplinary unit after the incorporation of mammography digitalization and computer-aided detection systems. Am. J. Roentgenol. 197(6), 1492–1497 (2011)

3. Fenton, J.J., Abraham, L., Taplin, S.H., Geller, B.M., Carney, P.A., D'Orsi, C., Elmore, J.G., Barlow, W.E.: Breast Cancer Surveillance Consortium. Effectiveness of computer-aided detection in community mammography practice. J. Natl. Cancer Inst. 103(15), 1152–1161 (2011)
4. Bamberger, P., Leichter, I., Merlet, N., Ratner, E., Fung, G., Lederman, R.: Optimizing the CAD Process for Detecting Mammographic Lesions by a New Generation Algorithm Using Linear Classifiers and a Gradient Based Approach. In: Krupinski, E.A. (ed.) IWDM 2008. LNCS, vol. 5116, pp. 358–365. Springer, Heidelberg (2008)
5. Leichter, I., Lederman, R., Ratner, E., Merlet, N., Fung, G., Krishnapuram, B., Bamberger, P.: Does a Mammography CAD Algorithm with Varying Filtering Levels of Detection Marks, Used to Reduce the False Mark Rate, Adversely Affect the Detection of Small Masses? In: Krupinski, E.A. (ed.) IWDM 2008. LNCS, vol. 5116, pp. 504–509. Springer, Heidelberg (2008)
6. Warren Burhenne, L.J., Wood, S.A., D'Orsi, C.J., Feig, S.A., Kopans, D.B., O'Shaughnessy, K.F., Sickles, E.A., Tabar, L., Vyborny, C.J., Castellino, R.A.: Potential contribution of computer-aided detection to the sensitivity of screening mammography. Radiology 215(2), 554–562 (2000)
7. Skaane, P., Kshirsagar, A., Stapleton, S., Young, K., Castellino, R.A.: Effect of computer-aided detection on independent double reading of paired screen-film and full-field digital screening mammograms. Am. J. Roentgenol. 188(2), 377–384 (2007)

Potential of a Standalone Computer-Aided Detection System for Breast Cancer Detection in Screening Mammography

Jaime Melendez, Clara I. Sánchez, Rianne Hupse,
Bram van Ginneken, and Nico Karssemeijer

Radboud University Nijmegen Medical Centre, Department of Radiology,
Geert Grooteplein Zuid 18, 6525 GA Nijmegen, The Netherlands
j.melendezrodriguez@rad.umcn.nl

Abstract. Current computer-aided detection (CAD) systems for mammography screening work as prompting devices that aim at drawing radiologists' attention to suspicious regions. In this paper, we investigate utilizing a CAD system based on a support vector machine classifier as a standalone tool for recalling additional abnormal cases missed at screening, while keeping the associated recall rate at low levels. We tested the system on a large database of 5800 cases containing abnormal instances (1%) corresponding to prior examinations missed at screening. The results showed that 26% of the missed cases could be detected with a low additional recall rate of 2%. Moreover, after extrapolating this result to a screening program, we determined that, with our system, 0.73 additional cancers per 20 additional recalls could be potentially detected. We also compared the proposed system with a regular CAD system intended for non-standalone operation. The performance of the proposed system was significantly better.

Keywords: Screening mammography, breast cancer, computer-aided detection, support vector machine.

1 Introduction

Breast cancer is one of the leading causes of death among women. Therefore, it is essential to detect the presence of any sign of this disease as early as possible. To accomplish this objective, screening programs have been deployed in several countries, being mammography the preferred examination method. However, it is known that screening mammography tends to be difficult for radiologists and screening errors cannot be avoided. For instance, previous work (e.g., [1,2,3]) has shown in a retrospective study that between 57% and 67% of the cancers detected at screening examination are already visible on a prior mammogram.

Taking into account these findings, the importance of developing tools that aid radiologists in their work, such as computer-aided detection (CAD) systems, becomes evident. In the last decades, CAD systems for screening mammography have been introduced in clinical practice and, for instance, in the United States,

A.D.A. Maidment, P.R. Bakic, and S. Gavenonis (Eds.): IWDM 2012, LNCS 7361, pp. 682–689, 2012.

they are nowadays applied on about three of four screening mammograms [4]. The aim of these systems is to prompt radiologists to any suspicious region on a mammogram, thus they are designed to achieve high sensitivity, at the expense of obtaining low specificity. In fact, they operate at a false positive rate that is at least an order of magnitude higher than that of radiologists.

In this paper, we investigate a rather different application of CAD that, instead of prompting suspicious regions, aims at detecting malignant cases potentially missed by screening radiologists. The idea is to run the CAD system on the set of not recalled cases in order to generate an additional set with the most suspicious exemplars and then send these exemplars back to radiologists for reconsideration. To operate at a low recall rate, the system is trained using data following the distribution encountered in screening setting, i.e., high prevalence of normal cases. Additionally, the CAD parameters are optimized to operate at a recall rate of 2%, which closely matches the numbers observed in some screening programs [5].

2 Materials and Methods

2.1 Image Database

A total of 18242 scanned film mammography images from Preventicon screening center (Utrecht, the Netherlands) have been used in our experiments. They correspond to 5800 patients and comprise 188 images from 58 prior exams with visible masses and architectural distortions that were not detected until a later screening round. The remaining 18054 images (5742 exams) correspond to normal cases with no sign of pathology. For both normal and abnormal exams, either two or four views have been included depending on their availability.

2.2 Overview of the CAD System

The developed CAD system consists of a pre-processing stage, an initial detection stage and an interpretation stage that aims at reducing the number of false positive detections.

During the pre-processing stage, mammograms are segmented into three regions: breast tissue, pectoral muscle and background. The image background is labeled by marking pixels with high exposure and low gradient values. This operation is followed by morphological transformations to remove labels and to fill small gaps. Subsequently, the pectoral muscle in the mediolateral oblique (MLO) views is segmented as a straight line using a method based on the Hough transform [6].

After pre-processing, locations in the tissue area are sampled on a regular grid and, at each location, five features based on gradient and spiculation measures are computed to determine the presence of a potentially suspicious pattern [7,8]. These features are fed into an ensemble of five neural networks that are randomly initialized and trained on a small data set. In this way, a more powerful classifier than with a single network is obtained. For each location at the grid, a likelihood score is computed by averaging the five network outputs. Together, these likelihood scores form a likelihood map. After smoothing this map, each local maximum that exceeds a threshold is selected as a candidate region and is segmented using the dynamic programming method described in [9].

In the interpretation stage, the segmented regions are classified into normal or malignant tissue by means of a soft margin support vector machine (SVM) configured with a radial basis function (RBF) kernel. For this stage, a new set of features measuring region contrast, location, linear texture, density, region size, compactness and contextual information is computed. In addition, the five gradient and spiculation features and the likelihood score computed in the initial detection stage are also used. Therefore, a total of 73 features is processed. Each of these features is normalized to have zero mean and unit standard deviation before classification.

2.3   CAD System Training

Training of a CAD system to operate at low recall rates involves a large number of normal cases (more than 4000 per fold considering the four-fold cross-validation evaluation scheme explained in Section 2.4). This is necessary for two reasons: first, to achieve the high specificity required for standalone operation and, second, to be able to accurately measure the performance of the system at that high-specificity operation point. In this work, this set of normal cases corresponds to a random sample of the whole population available in the complete Preventicon database and thus aims at modeling the actual distribution of the data.

Another key point during training is the optimization of the SVM classifier used in the interpretation stage. In this work, two of its parameters: the penalization parameter for the abnormal instances, C^+, and a coefficient related to the width of the RBF kernel, γ, have been determined using a grid search procedure.

The first parameter, C^+, derives from the formulation of the soft margin SVM, which aims at dealing with non-separable classification problems [10]. Since a hyperplane that perfectly separates the two analyzed classes may not always exist, the soft margin method determines a hyperplane that splits the classes as cleanly as possible, while allowing some of their instances to lie inside the margin or even be misclassified. These elements are penalized during optimization by a penalty parameter C by following the formulation shown below:

$$\min_{\mathbf{w},\xi,b} \quad \left\{ \frac{1}{2}\|\mathbf{w}\|^2 + C\sum_i \xi_i \right\}$$
$$\text{subject to} \quad y_i(\mathbf{w} \cdot \mathbf{x}_i - b) \geq 1 - \xi_i,$$
$$\xi_i > 0 \,, \tag{1}$$

where $\mathbf{w}$ denotes the separating hyperplane. The larger the value of C, the larger the impact of those elements on the resulting model. Essentially, C can be regarded as a tuning parameter and, in problems with highly imbalanced data, such as the one dealt with in this paper, separate parameters, C^+ and C^-, are used for abnormal and normal instances, respectively. Furthermore, in order to keep the tuning process tractable, one of them is usually kept constant and the other one is varied [11]. In this work, C^- has been set to one and C^+ has been searched over $C^+ \in \{1, 5, 10, 50\}$.

The second parameter, γ, derives from the fact that the sets to be discriminated are usually not linearly separable in the original space, thus an SVM often maps the input data into a higher (maybe infinite) dimensional space in which separation is expected to be easier. This mapping is achieved by means of a kernel function $K(\mathbf{x}, \mathbf{x}')$, which in our case corresponds to the RBF:

$$K(\mathbf{x}, \mathbf{x}') = \exp(-\frac{\|\mathbf{x} - \mathbf{x}'\|^2}{\gamma}) , \tag{2}$$

where γ is related to the kernel width and must also be tuned appropriately. In this work, the search grid for γ has been constructed by randomly sampling 1000 data points, computing their pairwise distances, deriving the 30-, 50- 70- and 90- percentile and averaging the results after ten trials.

The selected values for both C^+ and γ correspond to those yielding the highest sensitivity at 2% recall rate after classifying the training set using a three-fold cross-validation.

2.4 Evaluation Method

A four-fold cross validation scheme was used for the evaluation of the proposed CAD system. Image sets corresponding to individual cases have not been distributed among the cross-validation subsets. Moreover, the ratio of abnormal to normal cases has been roughly the same in each subset. Afterwards, a curve with case sensitivity values for different, increasing recall rates has been computed for each classifier. The partial area under this curve (PAUC) from 0 to 2% recall rate has been used as a performance measure. The statistical analysis has been carried out using the bootstrap method [12]. Cases were sampled with replacement from the compete cross-validation set 5000 times.

3 Results

The performance curve obtained for the developed system is shown in Fig. 1 (solid line). The mean PAUC from 0 to 2% recall rate is 3.39×10^{-3} (95% CI $= 1.75 \times 10^{-3}$ to 5.25×10^{-3}), while the mean case sensitivity at 2% recall rate is 0.264 (95% CI $= 0.150$ to 0.389), which indicates that 15 of the missed cases could be detected. Furthermore, at a lower recall rate of 1%, the mean case sensitivity is 0.202 (95% CI $= 0.086$ to 0.317) and thus 11 cases could still be detected. Some examples of detected cases are shown in Fig. 2.

We have extrapolated our results to the Dutch screening program carried out at Preventicon screening center. In a previous study, a detection rate of 0.49%

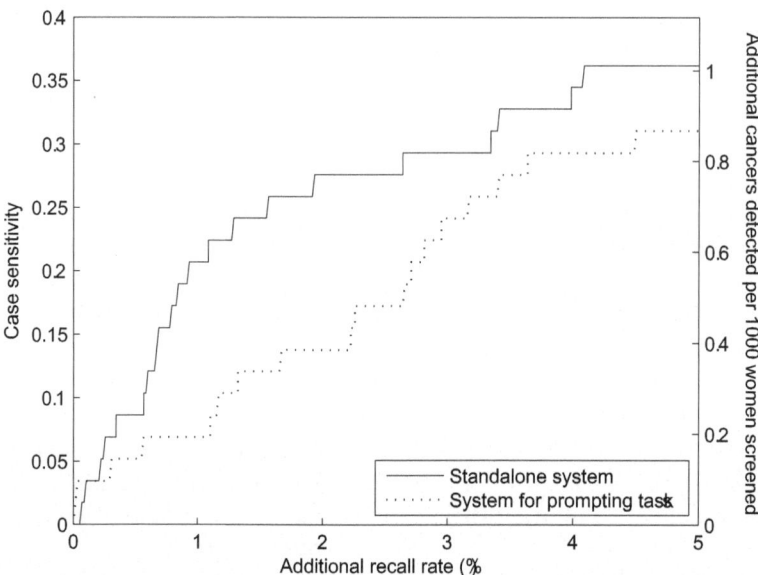

Fig. 1. Case-based performance curve for the standalone system proposed in this paper and the system intended for prompting tasks previously developed by our group [13]

for film-based mammography was obtained [5]. Assuming that 57% of these detected cancers should be visible on a prior mammogram as stated before [1,3], the additional number of detected cancers expected by applying our CAD system can be computed. They are associated with the right vertical axis in Fig. 1. Therefore, considering an additional recall rate of 2%, 0.73 additional detected cancers per 20 additional recalls are expected.

For the sake of comparison, a CAD system previously developed by our group and designed for prompting tasks has been evaluated [13]. This system comprises the same pre-processing and detection stages as the standalone system and processes the same features, but utilizes an ensemble of five neural networks in the interpretation stage. Training of these networks involves a stopping criterion based on a validation learning curve generated using an independent set of images (additional to the training set). In our experiments, these networks have been configured with 12 nodes in the hidden layer, a learning rate of 0.005 and a sampling ratio of 9:1 negative to positive instances presented during training. These settings correspond to the ones used in normal operation.

The performance curve for this system is also shown in Fig. 1 (dotted line). The mean PAUC from 0 to 2% recall rate is 1.61×10^{-3} (95% CI = 0.46×10^{-3} to 2.99×10^{-3}), while the mean case sensitivity at 2% recall rate is 0.147 (95% CI = 0.051 to 0.258). Comparing this performance with the one achieved by the standalone system, there is a clear and statistically significant advantage in favor of the latter ($p < 0.05$).

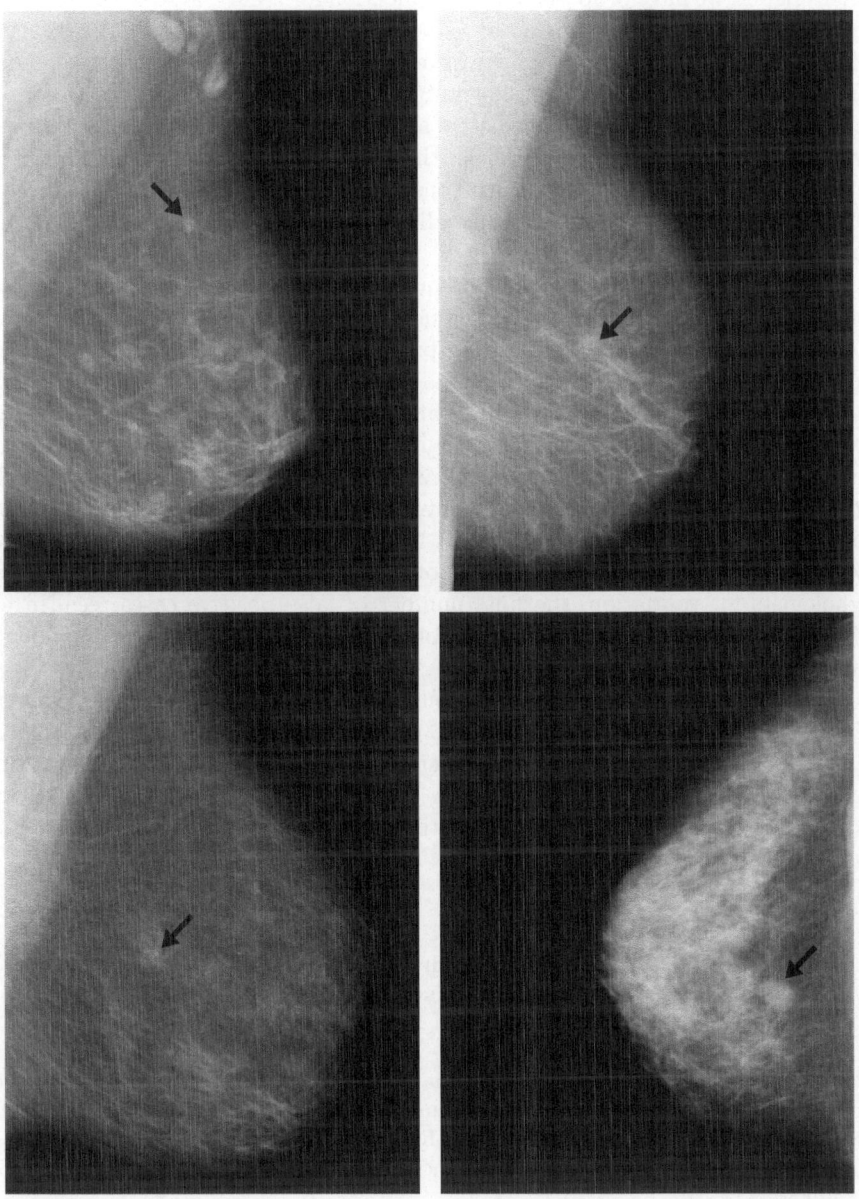

Fig. 2. Examples of malignant cases missed during screening that were detected by the proposed standalone system. The detected lesions are indicated with an arrow.

4 Discussion and Conclusion

In this paper, we have proposed a new application for a CAD system consisting of detecting suspicious cases missed by radiologists during screening, while keeping a low additional recall rate. We have developed a highly specific system intended for standalone operation by training an SVM classifier with a large set of normal cases and by optimizing its parameters at 2% recall rate. This system has been evaluated on a large image database that aims at approximating the typical setting observed in screening, which consists of a large number of normal cases (99% in our database) and a very small number of abnormal ones (1% in our database).

Moreover, to demonstrate the potential of the developed system, we have selected the set of abnormal cases in such a way that it corresponds to examinations missed by radiologists during prior screening rounds. The preliminary experimental results showed that, operating at a similar recall rate as screening radiologists, the developed system was able to detect 26% of these missed cases. Extrapolating this result to a mammography screening program, the obtained detection sensitivity corresponds to 0.73 additional detected cancers per 1000 women screened. As a consequence, several late screen-detected cancers could be detected earlier at the expense of a 2% additional recall rate. However, we hypothesize that, by referring the set of cases selected by the system back to radiologists for validation, the final number of false positive cases recalled for further examination could be considerably lowered. We are currently planning a study to assess this hypothesis.

As part of this work, we have also compared the proposed standalone system with a CAD system for prompting. The results showed that the performance of the standalone system is significantly better, which is mainly due to the specific optimization procedure followed during training, as well as the generalization capabilities of the SVM and its ability to deal with high-dimensional spaces.

References

1. van Dijck, J.A., Verbeek, A.L., Hendriks, J.H., Holland, R.: The Current Detectability of Breast Cancer in a Mammographic Screening Programme: A Review of the Prior Mammograms of Interval and Screen-Detected Cancers. Cancer 72, 1933–1938 (1993)
2. Warren Burhenne, L.J., et al.: Potential Contribution of Computer-Aided Detection to the Sensitivity of Screening Mammography. Radiology 215, 554–562 (2000)
3. Otten, J.D.M., et al.: Effect of Recall Rate on Earlier Screen Detection of Breast Cancers Based on the Dutch Performance Indicators. J. Natl. Cancer I. 97, 748–754 (2005)
4. Rao, V.M., Levin, D.C., Parker, L., Cavanaugh, B., Frangos, A.J., Sunshine, J.H.: How Widely is Computer-Aided Detection Used in Screening and Diagnostic Mammography? J. Am. Coll. Radiol. 7, 802–805 (2010)
5. Karssemeijer, N., et al.: Breast Cancer Screening Results 5 Years after Introduction of Digital Mammography in a Population-Based Screening Program. Radiology 253, 353–358 (2009)

6. Karssemeijer, N.: Automated Classification of Parenchymal Patterns in Mammograms. Phys. Med. Biol. 43, 365–378 (1998)
7. Karssemeijer, N., te Brake, G.M.: Detection of Stellate Distortions in Mammograms. IEEE T. Med. Imaging 15, 611–619 (1996)
8. te Brake, G.M., Karssemeijer, N.: Single and Multiscale Detection of Masses in Digital Mammograms. IEEE T. Med. Imaging 18, 628–639 (1999)
9. Timp, S., Karssemeijer, N.: A New 2D Segmentation Method Based on Dynamic Programming Applied to Computer Aided Detection in Mammography. Med. Phys. 31, 958–971 (2004)
10. Cortes, C., Vapnik, V.: Support-Vector Networks. Mach. Learn. 20, 273–297 (1995)
11. Lesniak, J., et al.: Computer Aided Detection of Breast Masses in Mammography using Support Vector Machine Classification. In: Proc. SPIE, vol. 7963 (2011)
12. Samuelson, F.W., Petrick, N., Paquerault, S.: Advantages and Examples of Resampling for CAD Evaluation. In: Proc. IEEE Int. Symp. Biomed. Imag., pp. 492–495 (2007)
13. Hupse, R., Karssemeijer, N.: Use of Normal Tissue Context in Computer-Aided Detection of Masses in Mammograms. IEEE T. Med. Imaging 28, 2033–2041 (2009)

Estimating Sensitivity and Specificity
in an ROC Experiment

Robert M. Nishikawa

Carl J. Vyborny Translational Laboratory for Breast Imaging Research
Department of Radiology
and the Committee on Medical Physics
The University of Chicago
5841 S Maryland Ave. MC-2026
Chicago, IL 60636 USA
r-nishikawa@uchicago.edu

Abstract. Observer studies and clinical studies are used to evaluate imaging technologies and to compare two different technologies. The area under the receiver operating characteristic (ROC) curve is often used as the endpoint. However, in clinical practice, radiologists will operate at a single point on the ROC curve and this will define the sensitivity and specificity of the radiologist using the technology. In an ROC study, sensitivity and specificity are often estimated based on the ratings that the radiologist gave each case, which are needed to generate the ROC curve. Unfortunately, because of intra-reader and inter-reader variability, estimates of sensitivity and specificity based on these ratings can lack accuracy and precision. We demonstrate using an observer study of computer-aided diagnosis in diagnostic mammography that estimates of sensitivity of a given radiologist can be either over or under estimated by as much as 100%. Further, the statistical power of the experiment is substantially reduced because of increased variability between readers. By simply asking the observer explicitly their recommendation (e.g., biopsy on no biopsy), sensitivity and specificity can be measured directly and the power of the study can be maximized.

1   Introduction

Receiver operating characteristic (ROC) analysis is a popular method for evaluating the effectiveness of different medical imaging technologies both in reader studies [1] and in clinical studies [2, 3]. The area under of the ROC curve (AUC) is often used as a figure of merit to summarize the ROC curve. This allows the evaluation of a technology or the comparison of two technologies that is independent of whether the radiologist is a conservative or an aggressive reader. Conservative readers tend to read with lower sensitivity, but higher specificity than aggressive readers who can have very high sensitivity, but much lower specificity. The assumption is that a radiologist can choose to read aggressively or conservatively, but they will maintain the same AUC. That is, they will slide on their ROC curve to the right when they read aggressively and to the left if they read conservatively.

A.D.A. Maidment, P.R. Bakic, and S. Gavenonis (Eds.): IWDM 2012, LNCS 7361, pp. 690–696, 2012.

In clinical practice, a radiologist usually operates at one fixed point on the ROC curve and that point will determine their sensitivity and specificity. While the AUC is an overall measure of performance, the fixed operating point has important clinical implications, for example on positive predictive value, recall or biopsy rates, and efficacy estimations, such as clinical utility and cost effectiveness. Therefore, it is important to estimate sensitivity and specificity as accurately as possible.

In an ROC study, the radiologist uses a rating scale to indicate their confidence that the case is positive or negative. The rating scale can be a 5-point scale, a 100-point scale or something else. In this paper, the number of points in the scale is unimportant. The scale is an indirect reflection of the actual clinical recommendation that the radiologist would make clinically. For example, in screening mammography, the scale can be used to determine whether the radiologist would recall the woman or not. Therefore, applying a threshold value to the rating scale would allow sensitivity and specificity to be estimated. The alternative would be to directly ask the radiologist what their recommendation would be. While this easy and straightforward and as we will show the most accurate method, it is often not done or not used to estimate sensitivity and specificity.

Accurate estimates of the sensitivity and specificity could be obtained using the rating scale, if the radiologists used the scale consistently. That is, there is a threshold point on the scale above which the radiologist would always recall the woman and below which they would never recall the woman. If the radiologist could consistently use that threshold for recalling women, then sensitivity can be estimated accurately. If the radiologist is inconsistent and uses a different threshold for different women, then there can be an error in estimating sensitivity. Further, if multiple radiologists participate in the study, then all radiologists would have to use the same threshold value in order to get accurate estimates of sensitivity and specificity. Unfortunately, inter-reader variability is known to be large [4] and so it is unlikely that all radiologists would use the rating scale in a similar manner.

In this study, we will demonstrate that estimating sensitivity and specificity based on ROC rating data can either overestimate or underestimate the actual sensitivity and specificity of a radiologist. The majority of ROC studies have in the literature asked only for rating data or rating data and recommendation, and in either design used only the rating data to estimate sensitivity and specificity.

2   Method

Previously, we conducted an observer study to demonstrate that computer-aided diagnosis (CADx) of clustered calcifications on mammograms can improve radiologist's ability to recommend breast biopsies [5]. In that study 10 radiologists each read the same 104 cases, containing 46 malignant lesions and 58 benign lesions. All cases contained at least one cluster of calcifications that was biopsy proven. All cases consisted of standard screening views, craniocaudal and mediolateral oblique, along with any magnification views of the breast containing the calcifications.

Each reader read the case once without any knowledge of the CADx analysis and once with the CADx output that was the computer's estimate that the cluster in question was associated with a malignancy. The two reads were done independently (i.e., in different reading sessions). Under each reading condition, the readers were asked:

1. their degree of suspicion that a lesion was malignant; and
2. their recommendation for the patient from four choices:

   a. surgical biopsy;
   b. alternative tissue sampling;
   c. short-term follow-up; and
   d. routine follow-up.

The first question was answered using a visual analog scale in which the left side of the scale was marked benign and the right side malignant. Using a pen, the radiologists were instructed to mark near the benign end if they had a low level of suspicion for malignancy and near the malignant end if they had a high level of suspicion. The marks were converted to a distance using a ruler. The distances were used as the rating for the case. The answer to question 2 was dichotomized into either "biopsy" for choices (a) and (b) or "no biopsy" for the choices (c) and (d). The rating data were used to estimate AUC using MRMC ROC analysis and the biopsy/no biopsy data were used to determine sensitivity, specificity, and positive predictive value. It is also possible to estimate sensitivity and specificity by applying a threshold to the rating data.

For this study, we examined the relationship between the rating data and the recommendation data. We computed the sensitivity and specificity for each observer using the two different scales. This was straightforward for the recommendation since those data were binary. For the rating scale, we applied different thresholds and computed sensitivity and specificity as a function threshold. We also computed the p-value for the differences in these metrics from the aided and unaided reading conditions. While we looked at each individual observer's data, we applied the same threshold to all readers as would be done in actual practice. The goal was to determine whether sensitivity and specificity can be estimated accurately and with the same statistical power from the rating scale compared to the direct measurement from the simply asking the observer their recommendation.

3   Results

Table 1 gives the ratings for a subset of the 58 benign cases in ascending order for each reader. The numbers in red are cases for which the radiologist recommended biopsy, whereas the ones in black are for cases in which a biopsy was not recommended. Table 2 gives the comparable data for the 46 malignant cases. For the malignant cases, 70% of the readers were consistent in their use of the rating scale, that is, all cases recommended for biopsy had higher scores than all the cases that were not recommended for biopsy. However, readers R3, R7 and R9 were inconsistent. For the benign cases, only readers R1, R5, and R6 were consistent in their use of the rating scale. These inconsistencies resulted in inaccuracies in estimating sensitivity.

Table 1. Readers' rating data near the division between biopsy and no-biopsy cases for benign cases. The cases in black italics were not recommended for biopsy, while the cases in red were. For each reader the cases were sorted by biopsy recommendation and then within each group the cases were sorted in numerical order. The visual analog scale marking was converted to a value between 0 and 50, in 0.5 increments.

R1	R2	R3	R4	R5	R6	R7	R8	R9	R10
			4.5						
			5.5						
			5.5						
			6.5						
			7						
			7						
			7.5						
			8						
			8.5						
			9						
			9						
			9						
			9.5						
			12.5						
			13						
			13				10.5		
			13.5				10.5		
			14.5				10.5		
		22	15.5				11		
		22	16.5				11	5	14.5
		22.5	18.5	10.5		4.5	11.5	7	14.5
		25	24	11		9	12	9	15
16	10.5	25.5	26.5	11	8	13.5	13.5	9.5	15
17.5	11.5	25.5	26.5	11	8.5	17	17.5	10.5	15
21	14	26.5	32.5	13	8.5	19.5	18	11.5	18
22	14	22.5	5.5	15	11	8	12	6	15.5
22	15	24	30	15.5	11.5	8	17	8.5	16
22.5	15	24.5	30	16.5	12.5	8	17.5	10	17.5
		26	30.5	17		8.5	30.5	10	21
		26.5	31.5	17		9		10.5	
		26.5	31.5			9.5		11	
		27	32			10		12	
		27.5	32			10		12	
		28	32.5			12.5		13	
		28	33			12.5		13	
		28	34			13.5			
		28				14			
						18.5			
						20			

Table 2. Readers' rating data near the division between biopsy and no-biopsy cases for malignant cases. The cases in black italics were not recommended for biopsy, while the cases in red were. For each reader the cases were sorted by biopsy recommendation and then within each group the cases were sorted in numerical order. The visual analog scale marking was converted to a value between 0 and 50, in 0.5 increments.

R1	R2	R3	R4	R5	R6	R7	R8	R9	R10
						9			
						10		*7*	
		21.5				*14.5*		*7.5*	
13.5	*12.5*	*22.5*	*14.5*	*12.5*	*8*	*15*	*12*	*8.5*	*12*
15.5	*12.5*	*23.5*	*16.5*	*12.5*	*8*	*22.5*	*12.5*	*10*	*12.5*
15.5	*13*	*25*	*18*	*14*	*8*	*23.5*	*12.5*	*15.5*	*13*
20	20	22	18.5	16.5	15.5	9.5	32.5	7	16
23.5	20	24	25.5	17	16	11	32.5	7	17
24.5	21	25.5	31	18	16	11.5	33.5	7	18
		26.5				12		8	
						13.5		12.5	
						14.5		13.5	
						20.5		16	
						21			
						21			
						25.5			

Shown in Table 3 are the estimated sensitivities and specificities for the 10 readers for a threshold of 14. While the estimated sensitivity for some readers is correct, other estimates are either too high or too low. Estimates can be as much as 20% in error. The situation for specificity is much more variable – the estimated value was up to 100% in error. Thus, estimating sensitivity and specificity from rating data can be inaccurate.

Shown in Table 4 are the estimated sensitivities averaged over the 10 readers when applying different threshold values to the readers' rating data. A threshold of 14 produced the closest estimates to the actual sensitivity. Note that in an experiment where the readers are not directly asked for their recommendation, there is no method for determining what the best threshold should be, and from Table 2, the estimated sensitivities are very sensitive to the threshold value. Even though the estimates from a threshold of 14 are close to the actual values, the statistical power for determining the difference in sensitivity reading without and with CADx is much lower when the rating scale is used to estimate sensitivity, as can be seen by the higher p-values. The lower power is caused by inter-reader variability. That is, a single threshold is not optimal for all readers.

Table 3. Comparison of the actual and estimated sensitivities and specificities for the 10 readers. The estimates are for a threshold of 14 on the unaided reading condition.

Reader	Actual Sensitivity	Estimated Sensitivity	% error	Actual Specificity	Estimated Specificity	% error
R1	0.761	0.804	6%	0.310	0.241	-22%
R2	0.761	0.761	0%	0.155	0.172	11%
R3	0.826	1.000	21%	0.362	0.069	-81%
R4	0.522	0.587	13%	0.534	0.414	-23%
R5	0.870	0.870	0%	0.086	0.086	0%
R6	0.761	0.761	0%	0.276	0.345	25%
R7	0.717	0.696	-3%	0.259	0.431	67%
R8	0.609	0.609	0%	0.466	0.448	-4%
R9	0.870	0.761	-13%	0.190	0.379	100%
R10	0.652	0.652	0%	0.517	0.414	-20%
Ave	0.735	0.750		0.316	0.300	
Stdev	0.113	0.124		0.154	0.146	

Table 4. Estimated sensitivities averaged over the 10 readers for different thresholds applied to the rating data

Threshold	Unaided			Aided			p-value
	mean	stdev	%diff	mean	stdev	%diff	
10	0.83	0.10	13%	0.93	0.06	6%	0.0065
11	0.81	0.11	10%	0.91	0.07	4%	0.0039
12	0.79	0.13	7%	0.89	0.07	2%	0.0055
13	0.76	0.12	4%	0.88	0.07	1%	0.0017
14	0.75	0.12	2%	0.87	0.07	0%	0.0029
15	0.74	0.13	1%	0.86	0.07	-2%	0.0047
16	0.72	0.13	-2%	0.84	0.08	-3%	0.0029
17	0.71	0.13	-4%	0.83	0.08	-4%	0.0029
18	0.69	0.13	-6%	0.83	0.09	-5%	0.0020
19	0.68	0.14	-7%	0.82	0.09	-6%	0.0034
20	0.67	0.14	-9%	0.81	0.09	-8%	0.0037
actual	0.73	0.11		0.87	0.09		0.0006

4   Discussion

Accurate estimates of sensitivity and specificity are important because they directly reflect the clinical use of technologies. These metrics are often used compare different medical imaging technologies. More importantly, analyses of utility and cost-effectiveness rely on sensitivity and specificity (or derivatives of these, such as positive predictive value).

The Breast Cancer Screening Consortium (BCSC) and the American College of Radiology Imaging Network (ACRIN) DMIST threshold rating scale when in many situations sensitivity and specificity can be directly and unambiguously by simply asking and recording the radiologists for their recommendation (e.g., recall or no recall; biopsy or no biopsy). In fact, in the assessment of efficacy of a medical technology, the Food and Drug Administration (FDA) requires the manufacturer to submit data on sensitivity and specificity estimated from thresholding the rating scale, using multiple thresholds. That is, obtaining more than one set of estimates of sensitivity and specificity. It is not clear how the FDA evaluates the multiple estimates.

One limitation of the study is that we used the likelihood of malignancy as a rating scale. In clinical practice, radiologists use the BI-RADS assessment scale, which for diagnostic breast imaging is a-5 point scale (1-5) or a 7-point scale, where 4 is subdivided into 4a, 4b, and 4c. It is possible that a given radiologist can use the BI-RADS scale more consistently. Unfortunately, this study was conducted before BI-RADS was the clinical standard. A study examining BI-RADS, a 100-point rating scale, and directly asking radiologists their clinical recommendation would address this issue.

5   Conclusions

Using the rating scale data to estimate sensitivity and specificity reduces the statistical power of the study and can produce inaccurate estimates. We strongly recommend that reader studies should directly ask the readers their recommendation for each case. This permits a direct estimate of sensitivity and specificity, at little or no cost to conducting the study. While there may be other approaches to obtaining accurate and precise estimates of sensitivity and specificity, this is a simple solution.

Acknowledgements. RM Nishikawa is a shareholder in and receives royalties from Hologic, Inc. He is a consultant to USystems, Inc.

References

1. Shiraishi, J., Pesce, L.L., Metz, C.E., Doi, K.: Experimental Design and Data Analysis in Receiver Operating Characteristic Studies: Lessons Learned from Reports in Radiology from 1997 to 20061. Radiology 253, 822–830 (2009)
2. Berg, W.A., Blume, J.D., Cormack, J.B., Mendelson, E.B., Lehrer, D., Bohm-Velez, M., Pisano, E.D., Jong, R.A., Evans, W.P., Morton, M.J., Mahoney, M.C., Larsen, L.H., Barr, R.G., Farria, D.M., Marques, H.S., Boparai, K.: Combined screening with ultrasound and mammography vs mammography alone in women at elevated risk of breast cancer. Jama 299, 2151–2163 (2008)
3. Pisano, E.D., Gatsonis, C., Hendrick, E., Yaffe, M., Baum, J.K., Acharyya, S., Conant, E.F., Fajardo, L.L., Bassett, L., D'Orsi, C., Jong, R., Rebner, M.: Diagnostic performance of digital versus film mammography for breast-cancer screening. N. Engl. J. Med. 353, 1773–1783 (2005)
4. Beam, C., Sullivan, D.: Variability in mammogram interpretation. Adm. Radiol. J. 15, 47, 49–50, 52 (1996)
5. Jiang, Y., Nishikawa, R.M., Schmidt, R.A., Metz, C.E., Giger, M.L., Doi, K.: Improving breast cancer diagnosis with computer-aided diagnosis. Acad. Radiol. 6, 22–33 (1999)

Level Set Breast Mass Segmentation in Contrast-Enhanced and Non-Contrast-Enhanced Breast CT

Hsien-Chi Kuo[1], Maryellen L. Giger[2], Ingrid Reiser[2] John M. Boone[3], Karen K. Lindfors[3], Kai Yang[3], and Alexandra Edwards[2]

[1] Dept. of Bioengineering, University of Illinois at Chicago, Chicago, IL 60607, USA
hkuo6@uic.edu
[2] Dept. of Radiology, The University of Chicago, Chicago, IL 60637, USA
[3] Dept. of Radiology, University of California at Davis, Sacramento, CA 95817, USA

Abstract. Dedicated breast CT (bCT) is an emerging technology that produces 3D reconstructed images of the breast, thus allowing radiologists to detect and evaluate breast lesions in 3D. In previous work, we have developed an algorithm that combines radial gradient index (RGI) segmentation and a modified level set model for segmentation of lesions in contrast-enhanced bCT images; yielding an average overlap ratio (OR) of 0.69, which is higher than 0.4, the overlap ratio that is generally deemed "acceptable". In this study, this segmentation algorithm, with the same parameter settings, was applied to the corresponding non-contrast-enhanced bCT images. The results show that the OR obtained on non-contrast images was 0.62, with the segmented lesion volumes tending to be slightly smaller as compared with those obtained on the corresponding contrast-enhanced images. These results imply that while use of contrast improves segmentation performance, the increase may not be significant, and thus, the role of non-contrast-enhanced breast CT should be further investigated.

1 Introduction

Over the past three decades, mammography has been widely accepted as a screening tool for breast cancer. Although the mortality was significantly reduced by 30% to 40% in screened population [1], the very poor positive predictive value of 10% to 30% [2] demonstrates a big room to improve the accuracy. The high rate of misdiagnoses is in part due to tissue superimposition, which occurs when 3D tissue structures with similar x-ray attenuation, such as fibroglandular and tumor tissues, are projected onto a plane [1]. This results in substantial anatomical noise in the background, which can make visualization of suspected lesions difficult [2].

Recently developed dedicated breast bCT provides 3D visualization that mitigates superimposition effects in mammography [1,2]. The excellent morphologic detail makes this emerging modality likely to play an important role in future breast cancer screening and diagnosis.

With the large amount of image data that is generated by bCT [2], computer-aided-diagnosis (CAD) methods are expected to support the radiologist and help alleviate the burden due to the large number of images to be reviewed. In our previous study

A.D.A. Maidment, P.R. Bakic, and S. Gavenonis (Eds.): IWDM 2012, LNCS 7361, pp. 697–704, 2012.
© Springer-Verlag Berlin Heidelberg 2012

[3], we have shown that a level-set-based segmentation method can be applied on contrast-enhanced bCT images and yielded an average overlap ratio of greater than 0.65. In this study, the level-set based segmentation algorithm was applied to non-contrast enhanced bCT images.

2   Method

2.1   Database

The dataset included 23 contrast/non-contrast breast CT image pairs (13 malignant masses and 10 benign masses) acquired at the University of California at Davis under an IRB approved protocol. All 46 CT images were manually outlined in the coronal, sagittal and axial planes by a research technologist with more than 10 years experience in mammography.

2.2   Segmentation

Lesion segmentation is performed in two steps. First, RGI segmentation [5,6] is performed to generate an initial lesion outline, which then serves as the starting contour for the active contour segmentation.

RGI segmentation is a seeded lesion segmentation technique performed on a volume of interest (VOI) centered on the lesion center. For a given contour $d\Omega$, the 3D RGI is given by [5]

$$RGI_{3D} = \frac{\sum_{d\Omega} \vec{G}(x,y,z) \cdot \hat{r}(x,y,z)}{\sum_{d\Omega} |\vec{G}(x,y,z)|} \quad (1)$$

where $\vec{G}$ is the image gradient, and $\hat{r}$ is a unit vector in the radial direction.

To segment the RGI contour, the VOI is first multiplied with a 3D Gaussian constraint function. Next, a series of contours $d\Omega_i$ is generated by applying multiple gray-level thresholds to the constraint VOI. The resulting RGI contour is the contour with the greatest RGI value defined as [5,6]:

$$d\Omega_{RGI} = \arg\max_{d\Omega_i} RGI\{d\Omega_i\} \quad i = 1,..,n \quad (2)$$

To ensure that the RGI contour, which served as the input to the subsequent active contour segmentation, was completely contained within the lesion, we applied morphological erosion to shrink RGI contour. The side length of the cubic structural element for erosion is 3rd root proportional to the RGI segmented lesion volume. This eroded RGI contour served as the starting contour for the level set model segmentation.

Second, modified level-set segmentation is performed, which was previously developed for segmentation of contrast-enhanced lesions in bCT [3]:

$$\frac{\partial \phi}{\partial t} = \mu g_s \left[\Delta \phi - \text{div} \left(\frac{\nabla \phi}{|\nabla \phi|} \right) \right] + \lambda \delta(\phi) \text{div} \left(g \frac{\nabla \phi}{|\nabla \phi|} \right) + \nu g \delta(\phi) \qquad (3)$$

where $\phi(\mathbf{x}, t)$ is the level-set function. The contour $d\Omega$ is the zero level set of ϕ, i.e., $d\Omega = \{(\mathbf{x}, t) : \phi(\mathbf{x}, t) = 0\}$, $\mathbf{x}$ is position vector $\in \mathbf{R}^3$ and t parameterizes the curve evolution. $\mu > 0$ is a parameter of penalizing term, $\lambda > 0$ and ν are constants. δ, g, and g_s denote the Dirac function

$$(x) = \begin{cases} 0, & |x| > \varepsilon \\ \frac{1}{2\epsilon} \left[1 + \cos \left(\frac{\pi x}{\varepsilon} \right) \right], & |x| \leq \varepsilon \end{cases} \qquad (4)$$

indicator function

$$g = \frac{1}{1 + |\nabla G_\sigma * I|^2} \qquad (5)$$

and "softened" indicator function [4]

$$g_s = \frac{1}{1 + |\nabla G_\sigma * I|} \qquad (6)$$

2.3   Termination of Contour Evolution

Due to the ambiguous margin of lesion in medical images, it is necessary to provide a stopping criterion for the evolving contour. Here we employ the stopping criterion based on the difference of mean value changing rate of the foreground and background (Δv_w) proposed by Yuan et al [7]:

$$\Delta v_w = \frac{1}{L - s} \cdot (c_1 - c_2) \cdot \left[2 \cdot \overline{I(d\Omega)} - 0.7(c_1 + c_2) \right]^2 \cdot \hat{v} \qquad (7)$$

L denotes the volume of the effective VOI, s denotes the lesion volume, c_1 denotes the mean value within the lesion, c_2 denotes the mean gray value within the background, $\overline{I(d\Omega)}$ denotes the mean value of contour, $\hat{v}$ is outward unit vector, and w denotes the weighted factor $1/(L - s)$. Starting curve evolution from inside the lesion, the changing rate of the mean in the foreground decreases less than the background. This is due to that the foreground is more homogeneous than the background. However, when the evolving contour crosses lesion margin, the changing rate of the foreground becomes faster. Therefore we used $\Delta v_w = 0$ as the sign to terminate the curve evolution.

2.4   Evaluation

Manual lesion outlines on 3 orthogonal planes were obtained to evaluate the segmentation results. The performance of segmentation was evaluated by the overlap ratio (OR), computed as

$$OR = \frac{1}{3}\left(\left(\frac{\Omega \cap \omega_{man}}{\Omega \cup \omega_{man}}\right)_{xy} + \left(\frac{\Omega \cap \omega_{man}}{\Omega \cup \omega_{man}}\right)_{xz} + \left(\frac{\Omega \cap \omega_{man}}{\Omega \cup \omega_{man}}\right)_{yz}\right) \tag{8}$$

where Ω is the computer-segmentation in a plane through the lesion centers, with the indices (x,y), (x,z), (y,z) denote the orientation of the plane. ω_{man} is the human-outlined region in the same slice.

3   Results

Shown below are examples of segmentation results on contrast images and non-contrast images. Note that once the center of the lesion on the bCT is indicated, the 3D segmentation is fully automated.

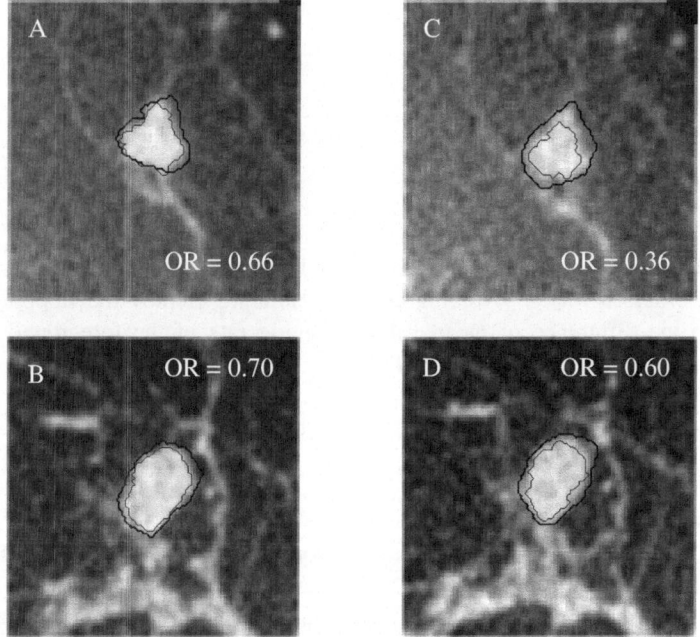

Fig. 1. Examples of lesion segmentation in contrast-enhanced bCT images (A, B), and non-contrast-enhanced bCT images (C, D). Bold: human outline. Thin: computer-segmented outlines.

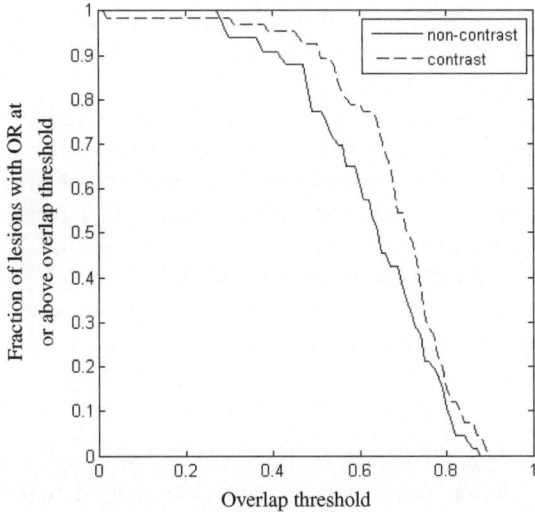

Fig. 2. Comparison of segmentation performance between contrast and non-contrast images with radiologist's outlines

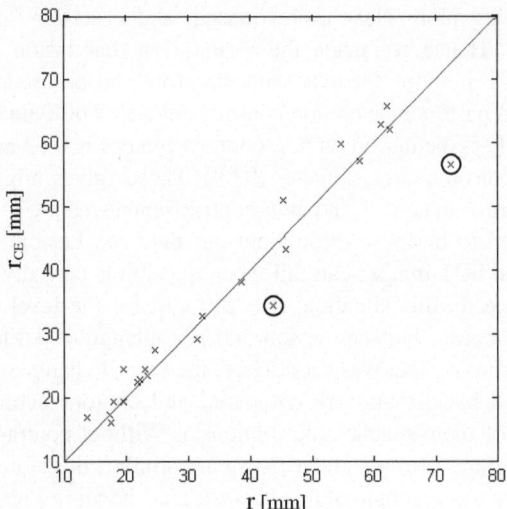

Fig. 3. Comparison of lesion volume obtained from lesion segmentation in non-contrast or contrast-enhanced breast CT images. Plotted here is the radius of the equivalent sphere. The 2 circled data points represent failed segmentation cases on non-contrast images. $r_{CE} = \sqrt[3]{\frac{3V_{CE}}{4\pi}}$ and $r = \sqrt[3]{\frac{3V_{NCE}}{4\pi}}$. ($V_{CE}$: contrast-enhanced volume; V_{NCE}: non-contrast-enhanced volume)

The average OR in contrast-enhanced bCT images was 0.69 while the average OR in non-contrast-enhanced bCT images was 0.62. Figure 2 shows the cumulative overlap ratios for all lesions. Segmentation performance on contrast images is better than on non-contrast images in terms of their respective OR.

Figure 3 shows the relationship between segmented lesion volumes in the non-contrast and contrast-enhanced bCT images. Each data point represents one lesion. Overall, lesion volume for both segmentations is similar, except for two outliners which corresponded to failed segmentations on non-contrast bCT images. Examining segmentation results for the two outliners, which are circled in Fig. 3, revealed that segmentation in the non-contrast bCT images had failed.

To assess the differences in lesion volume, a paired t-test was performed. Excluding these two failed segmentations, a p-value of 0.09 was found.

4   Discussion

In a study comparing lesion conspicuity in contrast-enhanced bCT with that in unenhanced bCT images, Prionas *et al.* [4] found that lesion conspicuity was greater in contrast-enhanced bCT images than in non-contrast-enhanced bCT images, evaluated by mean conspicuity scores. This is intuitive because lesions are enhanced by 55.9 HU and 17.6 HU in average for malignant and benign lesions, respectively [4]. Therefore, the lesion margin tends to be better visualized in contrast-enhanced bCT images, displaying more clear lesion margin and is easier for active contour algorithm to capture. Hence we made the assumption that lesion segmentation in contrast-enhanced bCT is more accurate, and therefore can be used as a baseline to evaluate segmentation perfomance on non contrast-enhanced bCT images.

The average OR of segmentation on non-contrast images is 0.62 and is not significantly smaller than that on contrast images (0.69). These values might be lower than reality for both contrast-enhanced and non-contrast-enhanced bCT images because human outlines tended to be loose throughout our data set. Lesion segmentation on non-contrast-enhanced bCT images can fail when a lesion is partially or fully embedded in glandular tissue. In this situation, it is difficult for the level set algorithm to correctly identify the border between lesion and fibrograndular tissues. This may be due to the stopping criterion that was used. Here, the rate of change of mean intensity in the foreground and background are compared and contour evolution is stopped when the difference of them reaches the minimum. Without contrast agent, the CT values of lesion tissue and fibrograndular tissue are similar; therefore the lesion contour tends to overgrow. An example of this occurring is shown in Fig. 4.

While non-contrast and contrast bCT images were acquired without changes in patient positioning for most cases, there was a time lapse between the two acquisitions, during which the contrast agent was injected. This resulted in patient motion, causing the lesion locations in the two images to be different. Therefore human outlining had to be performed separately on contrast images and non-contrast images. However, human outlines are very similar in the contrast and non-contrast image pairs: in the example shown in Fig. 1B and 1D, the overlap ratio of the human outlined regions is

0.99. When comparing with the computer segmentation, the OR still differs: 0.7 for contrast and 0.6 for non-contrast. This helps demonstrate that the active contour might tend to stop evolving earlier without contrast agent because the lesion is less emphasized. Although the p-value of 0.09, yielded by t-test for contrast and non-contrast segmented volumes, might not be strongly significant, this still indicates the trend that segmentation in non-contrast bCT images tends to produce smaller lesion volumes than when segmenting the lesion in contrast-enhanced images.

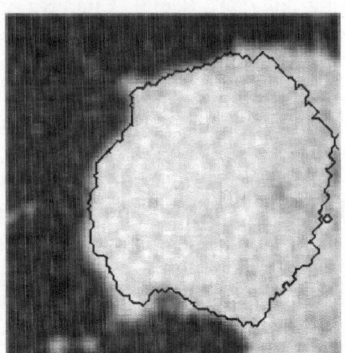 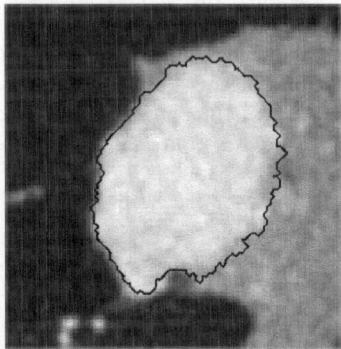

Fig. 4. An example showing failed segmentation when lesion is surrounded by glandular tissue. Left: non-contrast. Right: contrast.

5   Conclusion

A level set algorithm that was developed and optimized for contrast-enhanced breast CT, has been applied to non-contrast breast CT without any modification of algorithm parameters. The average OR value of 0.62 is slightly below the average OR of 0.69 for contrast-enhanced breast CT, but still well above 0.4, which is generally deemed "acceptable". This indicates that the segmentation procedure is robust and does not depend strongly on whether contrast agent was used.

The p-value suggests a trend that our level-set-based active contour algorithm might tend to segment smaller lesion volumes on non-contrast images compared to contrast ones. While more data and analysis is required to investigate whether active contour tends to stop evolving earlier in non-contrast images, this similarity does demonstrate that our segmentation method can be applied on non-contrast images. Potentially, this modified level set segmentation method could be improved by optimizing the parameters and increasing sensitivity to the difference of glandular and tumor tissues in non-contrast breast CT images.

Acknowledgement. This work is partially supported by NIH grants R01-EB002138 and S10-RR021039.   M.L.G. is a stockholder in R2 Technology/Hologic and receives royalties from Hologic, GE 740 Medical Systems, MEDIAN Technologies, Riverain Medical, Mitsubishi and Toshiba. It is the University of Chicago Conflict of

Interest Policy that investigators disclose publicly actual or potential significant financial interest that would reasonably appear to be directly and significantly affected by the research activities.

References

[1] Lindfors, K.K., Boone, J.M., Newell, M.S., D'Orsi, C.J.: Dedicated Breast computed tomography: The optimal cross-sectional imaging solution? Radiol. Clin. N. Am. 48, 1043–1054 (2010)
[2] Glick, S.J.: Breast CT. Annu. Rev. Biomed. Eng. 9, 501–526 (2007)
[3] Kuo, H., Giger, M.L., Reiser, I., Boone, J.M., Lindfors, K.K., Yang, K., Edwards, A.: Evaluation of stopping criteria for level set segmentation of breast masses in contrast-enhanced dedicated breast CT. In: Proc. SPIE (in press)
[4] Prionas, N.D., Lindfors, K.K., Ray, S., Huang, S., Beckett, L.A., Monsky, W.L., Boone, J.M.: Contrast-enhanced dedicated breast CT: Initial clinical experience. Radiology 256(3), 714–723 (2010)
[5] Reiser, I., Joseph, S.P., Nishikawa, R.M., Giger, M.L., Boone, J.M., Lindfors, K.K., Edwards, A., Packard, N., Moore, R.H., Kopans, D.B.: Evaluation of a 3D lesion segmentation algorithm on DBT and breast CT images. In: Proc. SPIE, vol. 7624, pp. 119–129 (2010)
[6] Kupinski, M.A., Giger, M.L.: Automated seeded lesion segmentation on digital mammograms. IEEE Trans. Med. Img. 17(8), 510–517 (1998)
[7] Yuan, Y., Giger, M.L., Li, H., Suzuki, K., Sennett, C.: A dual-stage method for lesion segmentation on digital mammograms. Med. Phys. 34(11), 4180–4193 (2007)

Methods for Evaluating the Effectiveness of Screening Mammography Are Not Necessarily Valid for Evaluating the Effectiveness of Computer-Aided Detection in Screening Mammography

Robert M. Nishikawa

Carl J. Vyborny Translational Laboratory for Breast Imaging Research
Department of Radiology
and The Committee on Medical Physics
The University of Chicago
5841 S Maryland Ave. MC-2026
Chicago, IL 60636 USA
r-nishikawa@uchicago.edu

Abstract. It is important that the clinical effectiveness of computer-aided detection (CADe) systems be evaluated. Since CADe is used to improve the effectiveness of screening mammography, it might be expected that the same methods and endpoints that are used to evaluate screening mammography can be used to evaluated screening mammography when CADe is used. Unfortunately, this is not always true and when the assumption fails, erroneous conclusions are often made. In clinical studies the choice of endpoints, estimation of sensitivity, and the significance of DCIS are potential problem areas. Further, the use of ROC versus FROC can affect the measured performance.

1 Introduction

Clinical studies [1-15] and observer studies [16-19] have been used to measure the effectiveness of computer-aided detection systems (CADe) for screening mammography. The methodology used in these studies often follows those used to evaluate the effectiveness of screening mammography by itself. This is not unreasonable since CADe is an adjunct to screening mammography. That is, if CADe is effective, it should enhance the outcome produced by screening mammography alone. Unfortunately, this approach is not always suitable. In this paper, we describe several subtleties in methodology, data analysis and interpretation when CADe is being evaluated. In many studies, these differences can make the difference of whether or not CADe is beneficial when interpreting screening mammograms.

A.D.A. Maidment, P.R. Bakic, and S. Gavenonis (Eds.): IWDM 2012, LNCS 7361, pp. 705–712, 2012.

2   Clinical Studies

2.1   Cancer Detection Rate in Case Control Studies

In a case control study of CADe, two populations of women are used: the control group, which does not undergo CADe, and the study group in which CADe is used by radiologists. In these studies, cancer detection rate is often used as the endpoint. That is, the number of cancers detected per 1000 women screened are compared between the two groups. Cancer detection rate is used instead of sensitivity, because the cancer detection rate is easier to compute. To calculate sensitivity, one needs to know the number of false negative cases, which can be problematic. There have been four clinical studies published to date that use cancer detection rate in a case control study design [2, 5, 10, 14].

For the case control study to be valid, the two patient groups need to be identical or at least made to be identical statistically. This can be done approximately when studying screening mammography alone. However, when CADe is used this is very difficult if not impossible. CADe will change the cancer prevalence in the population being screened by an unknown amount. When the cancer prevalence decreases, the cancer detection rate will decrease. Therefore, even if CADe were effective, no appreciable difference in the cancer detection rate between the control and study group will be seen. Determining the effectiveness of CADe using cancer detection rate in a case-control study is biased against CADe. This was demonstrated in Ref. [20].

A good example of this is from the clinical study by Gromet [14]. His study used a case control design, but in addition he performed follow-up on the 231,211 mammographic exams used in the study using the cancer registries from the major hospital systems in the Charlotte, NC, area. The study and control groups had 118,808 and 112,413 examinations respectively. As expected, based on the argument above, the cancer detection rate per 1000 women screened was relatively unchanged: 4.12 in the control group and 4.20 in the study group, a 2% relative change. The sensitivity in the control group was 81.4% and 90.4% in the study group, an 11.1% relative change. Although, no corrections were made to make the study and control groups comparable statistically, this study does show that there can be an increase in sensitivity even though the cancer detection rate does not change (appreciably). That is, using cancer detection rate as the endpoint in a case-control study design will underestimate the effectiveness of CADe. In fact one would conclude from this type of study design – case control with cancer detection rate as the endpoint – that CADe is not effective [2, 10] when in fact it may be.

This point is important when performing meta-analyses or systematic reviews of CADe. Inclusion of case-control studies can bias the results and they should be omitted from the analyses, although in the past they have not been [21-23].

2.2   Estimation of Sensitivity

Sensitivity can be estimated using the equation:

$$\text{Sensitivity=Se} = Ns/(Ns+Ni) \ , \tag{1}$$

where Ns is the number of cancers detected by screening (without using CADe) and Ni is the number of interval cancers (i.e., cancers found outside of screening, for example by palpation). When CADe is used, the sensitivity is given by:

$$\text{Sensitivity (with CADe)} = Se(CADe) = (Ns+Nc)/(Ns+Ni+Nc) \tag{2}$$

where Nc is the number of cancers detected because CADe is used. The denominator of the two equations is the known number of cancers in the population being screened. In principle, they should be the same, assuming comparable populations are being screened. However, because CADe is used, more cancers will be detected and therefore the denominator in Eq. 2 will be greater than the denominator in Eq. 1. For a fair comparison of sensitivity, the denominator in Eq. 1 needs an additional term:

$$\text{Sensitivity} = Se(\text{no CADe}) = Ns/(Ns+Ni+Na) \tag{3}$$

where Na is an estimate of the number of cancers present in the screening population that would have been detected by the radiologist if CADe were used. Without such a term, determining the effectiveness of CADe based on sensitivity is biased against CADe.

Using data from Fenton et al. [10], sensitivity without CADe using Eq. 1 was 80.4 and using Eq. 2, 84.0. This results in a percentage increase of 4.5%. If we assume that Na=Nc (corrected for the differences in population size of the with CADe and without CADe cohorts) then the sensitivity when CADe is not used is 77.6%. This would give a percentage increase in sensitivity of 8.2%, which is more consistent with the data published from other clinical CADe studies.

To examine this effect in more detail, we used data from an observer study that we previously performed to measure the effect of CADe on radiologists reading screening mammograms [18]. In that study there were 69 cancers in mammograms from 66 women and 234 mammograms from women who did not have breast cancer. All the cancer cases were collected from clinically missed cancers. Eight MQSA-qualified radiologists read the case in a sequential reading method (i.e., first without CADe and after scoring the cases, reading with CADe and rescoring the case). When available, a previous exam was provided. For this study, we randomly assigned a fraction of the cases to be potential interval cancers. That is, if the cancer was not detected and the cases was selected as a potential interval cancer, then we assumed that it would be detected in the interval between screens and the case was scored a false negative. If the cancer was not detected and it was not assigned to be a potential interval cancer, then the case was scored as a true negative. We repeated the randomization 1000 times and computed the three different sensitivities given in Eqs. 1-3. We randomly assigned 30% of the cancers cases as potential interval cancers and we bootstrapped over cases.

The three sensitivities, as given by Eqs. 1-3 were: 80.3% (unaided sensitivity), 83.6% (aided sensitivity), and 76.1 (unaided sensitivity corrected as in Eq. 3). These are in close agreement with the values estimated by Fenton at al. (see Table 1). Further, after applying a Bonferoni correction for multiple testing – the critical p-value became p=0.16 – the difference between the aided and unaided (uncorrected) sensitivities was not statistically significant (p=0.21), the relative differences in sensitivity between the aided and unaided (with correction) and the sensitivity between the corrected and uncorrected unaided sensitivities were statistically significant $p<0.001$ and $p=0.004$, respectively.

Thus estimating sensitivity between reading with and without CADe needs to be done by properly estimating the number of false negative mammograms. For reading without CADe, the number of cancers that would have been detected if CADe were used needs to be estimated and added to the number of interval cancers to estimate the number of false negative cases.

Table 1. The effect of correcting for the number of false negative cases on the measured benefit on sensitivity of using CADe

	Clinical Study Fenton (15)	Simulation using Observer Study (18)		
		Average	95% CI	p-value
Sensitivity Unaided (Eq. 1)	80.4	80.3	[70,90]	n/a
Sensitivity Aided (Eq. 2)	84.0	83.6	[74,92]	n/a
Sensitivity Unaided corrected (Eq. 3)	77.6	76.1	[67,85]	n/a
Relative increase Aided vs. Unaided	4.5%	4.1%	[2.5%,8.5%]	<0.001
Relative increase Aided vs. Unaided corrected	8.2%	9.9%	[6.1%,14.5%]	0.004
Relative difference Unaided vs. Unaided corrected	3.6%	5.3%	[1.4%,6.1%]	0.021

2.3 Significance of Detecting DCIS

One of the drawbacks of screening mammography is overdiagnosis: the detection of cancers that would not cause death if left untreated. Not all ductal carcinoma in situ (DCIS) will become an invasive cancer and potentially life threatening. Therefore, many screening opponents argue that it is detrimental to detect DCIS.

Fenton et al. [15] have shown that the use of CADe is associated with a higher rate of detection of DCIS. This could lead one to argue that CADe exacerbates the problem with DCIS. However, this is not true. All cancers (including DCIS) that are detected using CADe are visible mammographically. Therefore, if CADe was not used and the cancer was missed, it would be detected on a subsequent screening mammogram. That is, all cancers detected because CADe was used would eventually be detected if CADe were not used. Therefore, the detection of DCIS by CADe will not amplify overdiagnosis, but in fact will lead to earlier detection, which is the goal of screening mammography.

2.4 ROC versus FROC

In an ROC experiment, which can be either a clinical study or an observer study, the reader either calls a case negative or positive. The reader does not have to specify where the lesion is located. This can lead to the reader correctly calling a cancer case positive, but by identifying a false lesion and missing the actual location of the cancer. The solution to this is to use an analysis that requires the reader to localize the lesion correctly. Two examples are localization ROC (LROC) and free-response ROC (FROC). In both of these paradigms, the reader needs to specify the location of a suspicious lesion and if it is close to the location of the true lesion, it is considered a true-positive detection, otherwise it is scored as a false-negative case (for LROC), and a false positive (for FROC) with the true lesion being missed.

When comparing two different imaging systems, this "error" in location may not be important because it may be that the location error is equally likely on either imaging system. However, when comparing CADe to no CADe, this is not the case. CADe identifies the exact location of a lesion in the image. Therefore, a reader could call a case positive, but not recognize the correct location of the cancer. If CADe correctly identified the cancer, then when using CADe the reader may recognize the true location and correct their response. Thus in a ROC experiment CADe will not be beneficial, but in LROC or FROC experiment, the reader will increase their sensitivity.

We analyzed the data from the observer study [18]described in Section 2.2 to compare the performance of radiologists reading mammograms without and with CADe, without considering location in scoring. We applied bootstrapping over readers and cases and computed the sensitivities of reading with and without CADe when scoring by location (i.e., the radiologist needed to mark the location of the cancer in the image within 2 cm of the center of the actual cancer) and when not considering location (i.e., the radiologists is given credit for detecting the cancer as long as he or she recalls the patient, regardless of where he or she indicates where the cancer was). In Table 2, the percentage increase in sensitivity when using CADe was 10.0% when the radiologist was required to localize the cancer and only 4.7% when localization was not required. Further, the increase in sensitivity was statistically significant when location was considered in scoring and not significant (after correcting for multiple testing) when location was not considered in scoring. (See Table 2).

We note that in clinical studies this problem of not requiring localization also exists, since a patient is recalled or not recalled whether the cancer has been correctly identified or not. However, once a patient is recalled and undergoes diagnostic workup, it is possible that even if the screening mammogram identified the wrong location of the actual cancer, it may be correctly located on ultrasound or with the use of specialized mammographic views.

Table 2. Computed sensitivities and relative % increase in sensitivities for reading with and without CADe when considering correct localization of the cancer for scoring a case. After correcting for multiple testing, critical p-value is 0.025 (not 0.05).

Reading Condition	Sensitivity	Relative % increase in Sensitivity from unaided to aided	95% CI for increase in Sensivitity	p-value
Unaided Location	53.6	10.0%	[3.3%,20%]	0.017
Aided Location	58.8			
Unaided No Location	72.9	4.70%	[0.8%,10%]	0.048
Aided No location	76.4			

3   Conclusions

The evaluation of the clinical effectiveness of CADe requires careful attention to the planning and interpretation of study results. Applying methods of and interpretation to evaluating screening mammography for comparing screening with and without CADe are not necessarily valid. Specifically, we showed that:

1. Using cancer detection rate as the endpoint in a case-control study, will underestimate the benefits of using CADe.
2. When comparing sensitivity with and without CADe measured in a clinical study, one needs to estimate the number of cancers that would have been detected if CADe were used in the without CADe reading condition. If this is not estimated and used to correct the number of false negatives, then the relative gain in sensitivity when CADe is used will be underestimated.
3. If correct localization of the cancer is not required when scoring cancer detection, then the gain in sensitivity from using CADe will be underestimated.
4. CADe will not contribute to overdiagnosis by detecting more CADe then if CADe were not used.

These four aspects have not always been considered in clinical and observer studies published. As a result the benefits of CADe have been underestimated [2, 10, 15, 24], and some of the negative effects overestimated [10, 24].

Acknowledgements. RM Nishikawa is a shareholder in and receives royalties from Hologic, Inc. He is a consultant to USystems, Inc.

References

1. Freer, T.W., Ulissey, M.J.: Screening mammography with computer-aided detection: prospective study of 12,860 patients in a community breast center. Radiology 220, 781–786 (2001)
2. Gur, D., Sumkin, J.H., Rockette, H.E., Ganott, M., Hakim, C., Hardesty, L., Poller, W.R., Shah, R., Wallace, L.: Changes in breast cancer detection and mammography recall rates after the introduction of a computer-Aided detection system. Journal of the National Cancer Institute 96, 185–190 (2004)
3. Helvie, M.A., Hadjiiski, L., Makariou, E., Chan, H.-P., Petrick, N., Sahiner, B., Lo, S.-C.B., Freedman, M., Adler, D., Bailey, J., Blane, C., Hoff, D., Hunt, K., Joynt, L., Klein, K., Paramagul, C., Patterson, S.K., Roubidoux, M.A.: Sensitivity of noncommercial computer-aided detection system for mammographic breast cancer detection. Radiology 231, 208–214 (2004)
4. Birdwell, R.L., Bandodkar, P., Ikeda, D.M.: Computer-aided detection with screening mammography in a university hospital setting. Radiology 236, 451–457 (2005)
5. Cupples, T.E., Cunningham, J.E., Reynolds, J.C.: Impact of computer-aided detection in a regional screening mammography program. AJR Am. J. Roentgenol. 185, 944–950 (2005)

6. Khoo, L.A., Taylor, P., Given-Wilson, R.M.: Computer-aided detection in the United Kingdom National Breast Screening Programme: prospective study. Radiology 237, 444–449 (2005)
7. Dean, J.C., Ilvento, C.C.: Improved cancer detection using computer-aided detection with diagnostic and screening mammography: prospective study of 104 cancers. AJR Am. J. Roentgenol. 187, 20–28 (2006)
8. Ko, J.M., Nicholas, M.J., Mendel, J.B., Slanetz, P.J.: Prospective Assessment of Computer-Aided Detection in Interpretation of Screening Mammography. Am. J. Roentgenol. 187, 1483–1491 (2006)
9. Morton, M.J., Whaley, D.H., Brandt, K.R., Amrami, K.K.: Screening mammograms: interpretation with computer-aided detection–prospective evaluation. Radiology 239, 375–383 (2006)
10. Fenton, J.J., Taplin, S.H., Carney, P.A., Abraham, L., Sickles, E.A., D'Orsi, C., Berns, E.A., Cutter, G., Hendrick, R.E., Barlow, W.E., Elmore, J.G.: Influence of computer-aided detection on performance of screening mammography. The New England Journal of Medicine 356, 1399–1409 (2007)
11. Georgian-Smith, D., Moore, R.H., Halpern, E., Yeh, E.D., Rafferty, E.A., D'Alessandro, H.A., Staffa, M., Hall, D.A., McCarthy, K.A., Kopans, D.B.: Blinded comparison of computer-aided detection with human second reading in screening mammography. AJR Am. J. Roentgenol. 189, 1135–1141 (2007)
12. Gilbert, F.J., Astley, S.M., Gillan, M.G., Agbaje, O.F., Wallis, M.G., James, J., Boggis, C.R., Duffy, S.W.: Single reading with computer-aided detection for screening mammography. The New England Journal of Medicine 359, 1675–1684 (2008)
13. Gilbert, F.J., Astley, S.M., Gillan, M.G., Agbaje, O.F., Wallis, M.G., James, J., Boggis, C.R., Duffy, S.W.: Single reading with computer-aided detection for screening mammography. The New England Journal of Medicine 359, 1675–1684 (2008)
14. Gromet, M.: Comparison of computer-aided detection to double reading of screening mammograms: review of 231,221 mammograms. American Journal of Radiology 190, 854–859 (2008)
15. Fenton, J.J., Abraham, L., Taplin, S.H., Geller, B.M., Carney, P.A., D'Orsi, C., Elmore, J.G., Barlow, W.E.: For the Breast Cancer Screening Consortium: Effectiveness of Computer-Aided Detection in Community Mammography Practice. JNCI 103, 1152–1161 (2011)
16. Ciatto, S., Rosselli Del Turco, M., Burke, P., Visioli, C., Paci, E., Zappa, M.: Comparison of standard and double reading and computer-aided detection (CAD) of interval cancers at prior negative screening mammograms: blind review. British Journal of Cancer 89, 1645–1649 (2003)
17. Gilbert, F.J., Astley, S.M., McGee, M.A., Gillan, M.G., Boggis, C.R., Griffiths, P.M., Duffy, S.W.: Single reading with computer-aided detection and double reading of screening mammograms in the United Kingdom National Breast Screening Program. Radiology 241, 47–53 (2006)
18. Nishikawa, R., Schmidt, R., Linvers, M., Edwards, A., Papaioannou, J., Stull, M.: Clinically Missed Cancers: How Effectively Can Radiologists Use Computer-Aided Detection (CADe). American Journal of Roentgenology (2011) (in press)
19. Taylor, P., Champness, J., Given-Wilson, R., Johnston, K., Potts, H.: Impact of computer-aided detection prompts on the sensitivity and specificity of screening mammography. Health Technol. Assess. 9, 1–70 (2005)

20. Nishikawa, R.M., Pesce, L.L.: Computer-aided detection evaluation methods are not created equal. Radiology 251, 634–636 (2009)
21. Taylor, P., Potts, H.W.: Computer aids and human second reading as interventions in screening mammography: two systematic reviews to compare effects on cancer detection and recall rate. Eur. J. Cancer 44, 798–807 (2008)
22. Noble, M., Bruening, W., Uhl, S., Schoelles, K.: Computer-aided detection mammography for breast cancer screening: systematic review and meta-analysis. Arch. Gynecol. Obstet. 279, 881–890 (2009)
23. Eadie, L.H., Taylor, P., Gibson, A.P.: A systematic review of computer-assisted diagnosis in diagnostic cancer imaging. European Journal of Radiology 81, e70–e76 (2012)
24. Hall, F.M.: Breast imaging and computer-aided detection. The New England Journal of Medicine 356, 1464–1466 (2007)

Joint Registration and Limited-Angle Reconstruction of Digital Breast Tomosynthesis*

Guang Yang[1],**John H. Hipwell[1], Christine Tanner[2],
David J. Hawkes[1], and Simon R. Arridge[1]

[1] Centre for Medical Image Computing, Department of Computer Science and
Medical Physics, University College London (UCL), London, WC1E 6BT, UK
[2] Computer Vision Lab, Eidgenössische Technische Hochschule, Zürich, 8092, CH
G.Yang@cs.ucl.ac.uk

Abstract. Digital breast tomosynthesis (DBT), an emerging imaging modality, provides a pseudo-3D image of the breast. Algorithms to aid the human observer process these large datasets involve two key tasks: reconstruction and registration. Previous studies separated these steps, solving each task independently. This can be effective if reconstructing using a complete set of data, *e.g.*, in cone beam CT, assuming that only simple deformations exist. However, for ill-posed limited-angle problems such as DBT, estimating the deformation is complicated by the significant artefacts associated with DBT reconstructions, leading to severe inaccuracies in the registration. In this paper, we present an innovative algorithm, which combines reconstruction of a pair of temporal DBT acquisitions with their simultaneous registration. Using various computational phantoms and in vivo DBT simulations, we show that, compared to the conventional sequential method, jointly estimating image intensities and transformation parameters gives superior results with respect to reconstruction fidelity and registration accuracy.

1 Introduction

Digital breast tomosynthesis (DBT) involves acquiring a small number of low dose X-ray images, over a limited angle, and reconstructing this data into a pseudo-3D image of the breast [1]. It is of considerable interest to the research community [2], as a potential replacement for conventional mammography, but has been slow to be adopted into routine clinical practice.

In a breast cancer screening or diagnostic setting, radiologists routinely compare conventional current and prior mammograms to detect suspicious changes that might be indicative of malignancy. DBT has the potential to improve the sensitivity and/or specificity of this task by reducing the confounding influence

---

* This work has been funded by DTI Project *Digital Breast Tomosynthesis* TP/7/SEN/6/1/M1577G. The authors would like to thank the UK MR Breast Screening Study (MARIBS) [6] for providing the data for this study.
** Corresponding author.

A.D.A. Maidment, P.R. Bakic, and S. Gavenonis (Eds.): IWDM 2012, LNCS 7361, pp. 713–720, 2012.
© Springer-Verlag Berlin Heidelberg 2012

of overlaying tissue, but only if the large quantity of data acquired can be efficiently incorporated into the clinical workflow [3] [4] [5]. To enable the data to be viewed as a pseudo-3D volume, it must first be reconstructed. Although not currently a component of routine clinical practice, image registration algorithms could be used to aid the clinician in comparing temporal data sets. This would enable image features to be transformed into a common coordinate system where abnormal differences due to disease progression can be distinguished from differences due to patient position and breast deformation.

In other modalities, such as MRI or CT, registration has generally been performed after the images have been reconstructed. In DBT however, the presence of reconstruction artefacts due to the not insignificant null space, complicates the registration process. Rather than separate these two tasks and perform them sequentially therefore, we investigate an algorithm which performs them simultaneously, and test the hypothesis that the performance of the joint estimation will benefit both processes.

In the following sections we describe this algorithm and present a comparison of its performance with the sequential alternative. We test and validate the methods using phantom data and DBT simulations generated from breast MRI. Breast MRI is a fully 3D imaging modality which provides good visibility of internal breast anatomy. It is therefore a good surrogate source of breast data with which to test the performance of our algorithms.

2   Method

Two sets of limited angle X-ray acquisitions, $y_1 \in \mathbb{R}^{N_2}$ and $y_2 \in \mathbb{R}^{N_2}$, obtained at different times, can be expressed in terms of a 3D volume, $x \in \mathbb{R}^{N_3}$, in two positions related by the transformation, R, with parameters, $\zeta_p \in \mathbb{R}^n$, and the system matrix $A : \mathbb{R}^{N_3} \mapsto \mathbb{R}^{N_2}$ (where N_2 is the projection dimension and N_3 is the volume dimension) via

$$y_1 = Ax, \tag{1}$$

and

$$y_2 = Ax^\dagger = AR_{\zeta_p}x. \tag{2}$$

Rather than perform the two tasks sequentially or iteratively [7, 8], we propose a fully coupled algorithm using a *simultaneous* reconstruction and registration framework summarised in Algorithm 1.

The objective function is given by

$$\min_{x,\zeta_p \in \mathbb{R}^n} \Phi_{\mathrm{RR}} = \frac{1}{2}\left(\left\| Ax - y_1 \right\|_2^2 + \left\| AR_{\zeta_p}x - y_2 \right\|_2^2 \right). \tag{3}$$

We combine optimisation of the two temporal reconstructions with the 12 degrees of freedom ζ_p, $(p = 1, 2, \ldots, 12)$, of an affine transformation, which globally describes the translation, scaling, rotation and shearing between the two time points. We can also substitute other non-rigid deformations for the affine transformation in this framework, but considered an affine transformation in the first instance due to its simplicity.

In addition, we can also derive the gradient with respect to the image intensities x and transformation parameters ζ_p as follows:

$$\Psi_x = A^T (Ax - y_1) + R_{\zeta_p}^T A^T (AR_{\zeta_p} x - y_2), \tag{4}$$

$$\Psi_{\zeta_p} = (AR'_{\zeta_p} x)^T (AR_{\zeta_p} x - y_2). \tag{5}$$

To minimise issues of memory usage associated with processing these large datasets, we opt for a Quasi-Newton (L-BFGS) solver.

Algorithm 1. Simultaneous Reconstruction and Registration

Input: y_1, y_2.
Output: $x^\star$, $\zeta_p^\star$.

begin

    % Initialise x^0 to a vector with all zero entries
    % Initialise $\zeta_p{}^0$ to a vector of the reshaped identity matrix I
    $x^0 := 0$;
    $\zeta_p := \text{RESHAPE}(I)$;

    % Calculate matrix A for the forward projection
    % Matrix A^T represents the backward projection
    $A := \text{RAYCASTING}(\text{SIZE}(x))$;

    % Simultaneous reconstruction and registration
    for $(i = 0;\ i < m;\ i{+}{+})$ **do**

        % Ψ_x and Ψ_{ζ_p} are the analytical gradients
        % of the x and ζ_p for the L-BFGS solver

        $\Psi_{x^i} := A^T (Ax^i - y_1) + R_{\zeta_p}^T A^T (AR_{\zeta_p} x^i - y_2)$;

        $\Psi_{\zeta_p{}^i} := (AR'_{\zeta_p} x^i)^T (AR_{\zeta_p} x^i - y_2)$;

        $x^{i+1} := x^i + (A^T A)^{-1} \Psi_{x^i 1} + (A^T R_{\zeta_p}^T R_{\zeta_p} A)^{-1} \Psi_{x^i 2}$;
        $\zeta_p{}^{i+1} := \zeta_p{}^i + (x^T A^T Ax)^{-1} \Psi_{\zeta_p{}^i}$;

    % Output the $x^\star$ and $\zeta_p^\star$
    $x^\star := x^{i+1}$; $\zeta_p^\star := \zeta_p{}^{i+1}$.

end

---

3   Results

In the following three experiments we compare the performance of (a) a *sequential* reconstruction and registration, in which $n = 1000$ iterations of the reconstruction of projection images, y_1 and y_2, is followed by a single registration of the reconstructed volumes x_1 and x_2 ($m = 1$) and (b) our *simultaneous* approach in which $n = 50$ iterations of the reconstruction are followed by a registration and the process repeated $m = 20$ times. In both cases the total number of iterations is the same ($m \times n = 1000$). Our test data is created from a 3D data set, x, which is transformed by a known transformation to produce a second volume $x^\dagger$. From each of these, 11 projections covering ±25 degrees are created to simulate the pair of temporal DBT acquisitions y_1 and y_2. In all experiments the affine transformation parameters were selected from random uniform distributions with the following limits: ±20 degrees for rotation, ±5 pixels for translation, 0.9 to 1.1 for the scale factor and a small amount of shearing.

In the first experiment, a 3D toroidal phantom image was created, and subjected to 20 affine transformations to test the robustness of our simultaneous method. The *simultaneous* results are much more compact and accurate than the *sequential results*, and the out of plane blurring is reduced (Fig. 1 (d)-(f) vs. Fig. 1 (m)-(o)). In the second experiment, 15 randomly generated affine transformations were applied to a 3D breast MR image and similar performance was observed (Fig. 2 (d)-(f) vs. Fig. 2 (m)-(o)). The specific parameters recovered are shown in Figs. 3 and 4. In a third experiment, we tested the methods using two MRI acquisitions obtained before and after application of a lateral-to-medial plate compression of the breast. There is no ground truth for the deformation of this dataset, however from both the image appearance (Fig. 5 (d)-(f) vs. Fig. 5 (m)-(o)) and the mean squared error (MSE in Table 1), we can conclude that our simultaneous method outperformed the sequential method.

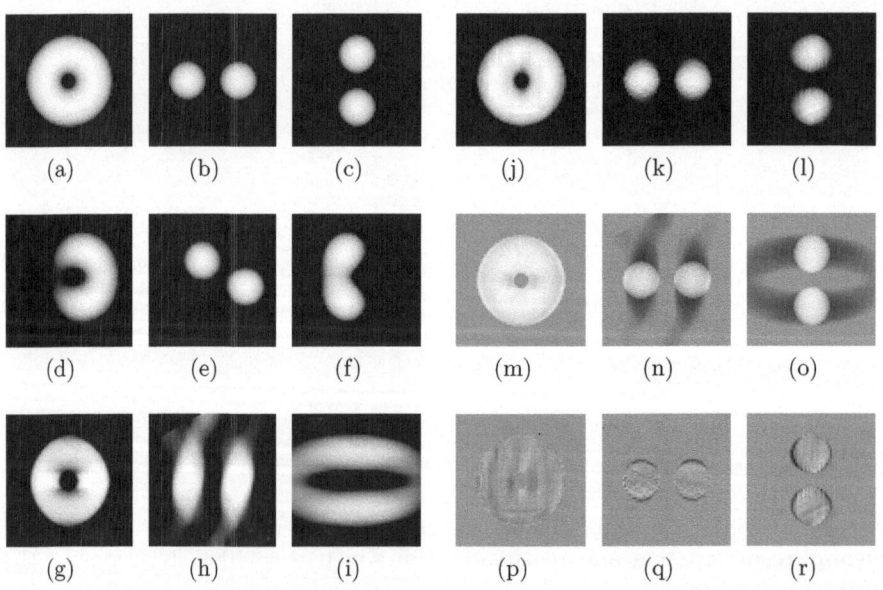

Fig. 1. Test case 1: Toroid phantom image. (a)-(c): Fixed image; (d)-(f): Moving image; (g)-(i): Sequential result, i.e., transformed moving image reconstruction; (j)-(l): Simultaneous result; (m)-(o): Difference between the sequential result and the fixed image; (p)-(r): Difference between the simultaneous result and the fixed image. (For each set of three sub-figures: Left: Coronal view; Middle: Transverse view; Right: Sagittal view.)

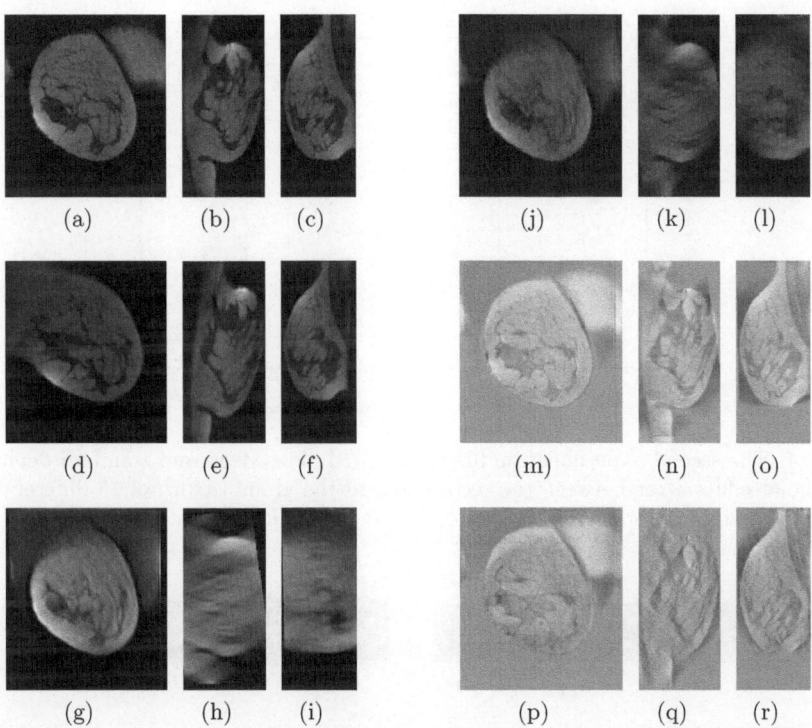

Fig. 2. Test case 2: 3D breast MR image. (a)-(c): Fixed image; (d)-(f): Moving image; (g)-(i): Sequential result, i.e., transformed moving image reconstruction; (j)-(l): Simultaneous result; (m)-(o): Difference between the sequential result and the fixed image; (p)-(r): Difference between the simultaneous result and the fixed image. (For each set of three sub-figures: Left: Coronal view; Middle: Transverse view; Right: Sagittal view.)

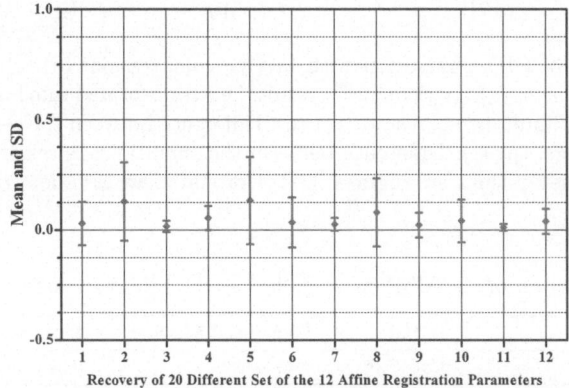

Fig. 3. The first experiment on a 3D toroidal phantom image. The Mean and standard deviation of the absolute error between the recovered and the ground truth of 20 different sets of affine transformations. Parameters 4, 8, and 12 are the translations along each axis.

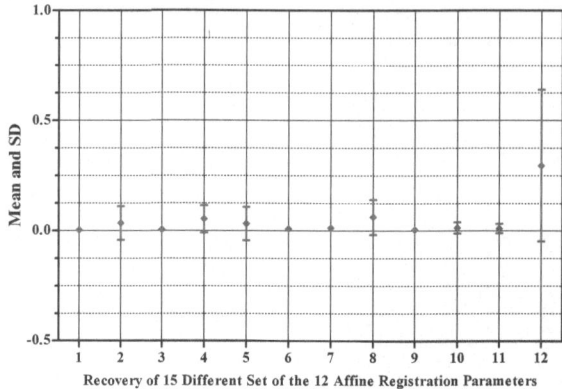

Fig. 4. The second experiment on 3D breast MRI. The Mean and standard deviation of the absolute error between the recovered and the ground truth of 15 different sets of affine transformations. Parameters 4, 8, and 12 are the translations along each axis.

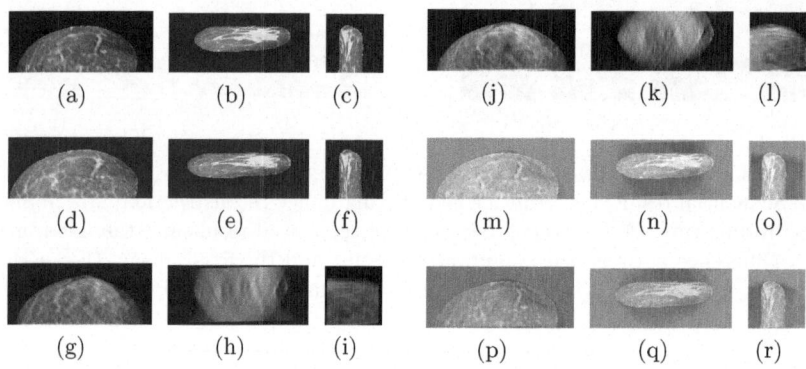

Fig. 5. Test case 3: DBT simulation with in vivo compression. (a)-(c): Fixed image; (d)-(f): Moving image; (g)-(i): Sequential result, i.e., transformed moving image reconstruction; (j)-(l): Simultaneous result; (m)-(o): Difference between the sequential result and the fixed image; (p)-(r): Difference between the simultaneous result and the fixed image. (For each set of three sub-figures: Left: Coronal view; Middle: Transverse view; Right: Sagittal view.)

Table 1. Comparison of the MSE error $\frac{1}{N_3}\left\|x^\star - x\right\|_2^2$ (N_3 is the number of voxels).

	Initial	Sequential Method	Simultaneous Method
Toroid Phantom	1.31×10^6	7.46×10^3	0.24×10^3
Uncompressed Breast MRI	1.18×10^6	6.04×10^3	3.01×10^3
In vivo DBT simulation	5.32×10^6	3.68×10^4	3.22×10^4

4 Discussion

As far as we aware this is the first time that the simultaneous reconstruction and registration of DBT data sets using a unified optimisation framework has been demonstrated to be superior to the conventional sequential method. This approach jointly considers reconstruction and registration components of DBT, and it is capable of recovering both the deformation parameters, and an enhanced, reconstructed image. By integrating the registration directly into the framework of the reconstruction problem, we are able to fully explore the interdependence between the transformation parameters and the 3D volume to be reconstructed.

Significantly, compared to previous research on combining reconstruction and registration (or motion correction), our combined limited angle DBT problem has a much larger null space and is severely ill-posed, which makes the inverse problem more intriguing and more challenging. From Table 2, we can see that for a typical 2D super-resolution problem previous studies used 5 low resolution images to restore a high resolution image recovering only rotations and translations, and 32 low resolution images for the affine registration. In general 3D problems, the authors used at least 60 and up to 799 forward projections covering a full-range of views, *i.e.*, 180 degrees or 360 degrees, to perform the joint estimations. However, for our DBT application, we have two sets of data which are observed at two time-points. Each of the data is acquired using only 11 forward projections covering just 50 degrees (± 25 degrees), and the two data sets overlap to a certain degree according to the original unknown deformations.

Table 2. Comparison of different applications of simultaneous inverse problem. (SR: super-resolution; LR: low resolution; fwdProjs: forward projections; Recon.+Regn.: reconstruction and registration; "–": not mentioned; Data collected according to [9]).

Publications	Application	Dimension	Optimiser	Data
Chung et al. 2006	SR	2D Affine	Gauss-Newton	32 LR images
He et al. 2007	SR	2D Rigid	Conjugate Gradient	5 LR images
Yap et al. 2009	SR	2D Rigid	Linear Interior Point	5 LR images
Jacobson and Fessler 2003	PET	3D Affine	Gradient Descent	64 fwdProjs 180°
Fessler 2010	PET	3D –	Conjugate Gradient	–
Odille et al. 2008	MRI	3D Affine	GMRES	–
Schumacher et al. 2009	SPECT	3D Rigid	Gauss-Newton	60 to 64 fwdProjs 360°
Yang et al. 2005	Cryo-EM	3D Rotation	Quasi-Newton (L-BFGS)	84 fwdProjs
Chung et al. 2010	Cryo-EM	3D Rigid	Quasi-Newton (L-BFGS)	799 fwdProjs
Our Recon.+Regn. Model	DBT	3D Affine	Conjugate Gradient or L-BFGS	22 fwdProjs 50° ($\pm 25°$)

We analysed our simultaneous method with various data sets using an affine transformation model, and the simultaneous method has clearly achieved superior results compared to the conventional sequential method. First, the experiment on the 3D toroid image demonstrates the potential of this approach over the conventional method to increase the depth resolution of the reconstructed image. Second, the results of the breast MR image have further strengthened our confidence in the hypothesis that the reconstruction and registration have a reciprocal relationship. In addition, the recovery of the transformation parameters was consistently accurate for both the 3D toroid and the breast MR data sets. Next, we attempted to reconstruct and register simulated DBT data sets created from real medio-lateral compressions of a breast imaged using MRI. As anticipated, the simultaneous approach still outperformed the conventional sequential method as demonstrated by the image appearance and MSE comparison (Figure 5 and Table 1). Although the improvements were modest in this experiment, this can be attributed, at least in part, to the fact that the affine transformation, which is a global parametric model, is insufficient to capture such a non-rigid breast deformation.

5   Conclusion

We have presented a method to simultaneously reconstruct and register temporal DBT datasets and compared it with performing the two tasks sequentially. Our simultaneous method produced superior results in both registration accuracy and reconstructed image appearance. In future work we will incorporate B-spline transformations and address the application to combine reconstruction and registration of two view (cranial-caudal/mediolateral-oblique) DBT data sets, to overcome the null-space limitation.

References

[1] Niklason, L.T., et al.: Digital Tomosynthesis in Breast Imaging. Radiology 205(2), 399–406 (1997)
[2] Dobbins III, J.T., et al.: Digital X-ray Tomosynthesis: Current State of the Art and Clinical Potential. Physics in Medicine and Biology 48(19), R65 (2003)
[3] Poplack, S.P., et al.: Digital Breast Tomosynthesis: Initial Experience in 98 Women with Abnormal Digital Screening Mammography. American Journal of Roentgenology 189(3), 616–623 (2007)
[4] Gur, D., et al.: Digital Breast Tomosynthesis: Observer Performance Study. American Journal of Roentgenology 193(2), 586–591 (2009)
[5] Spangler, M.L., et al.: Detection and Classification of Calcifications on Digital Breast Tomosynthesis and 2D Digital Mammography: A Comparison. American Journal of Roentgenology 196, 320–324 (2011)
[6] Leach, M.O., et al.: Screening with MRI and Mammography of a UK Population at High Familial Risk of Breast Cancer. The Lancet 365, 1769–1778 (2005)
[7] Yang, G., Hipwell, J.H., Clarkson, M.J., Tanner, C., Mertzanidou, T., Gunn, S., Ourselin, S., Hawkes, D.J., Arridge, S.R.: Combined Reconstruction and Registration of Digital Breast Tomosynthesis. In: Martí, J., Oliver, A., Freixenet, J., Martí, R. (eds.) IWDM 2010. LNCS, vol. 6136, pp. 760–768. Springer, Heidelberg (2010)
[8] Yang, G., et al.: Combined Reconstruction and Registration of Digital Breast Tomosynthesis: Sequential Method versus Iterative Method. In: Medical Image Understanding and Analysis (MIUA 2010), University of Warwick, Coventry, pp. 1–5 (2010)
[9] Yang, G.: Numerical Approaches for Solving the Combined Reconstruction and Registration of Digital Breast Tomosynthesis, Ph.D. Thesis, University College London (2012)

Dose Reduction for Digital Breast Tomosynthesis by Patch-Based Denoising in Reconstruction

Gang Wu[1,2], James G. Mainprize[2], and Martin J. Yaffe[1,2]

[1] Department of Medical Biophysics, University of Toronto
[2] Sunnybrook Research Institute, 2075 Bayview Avenue, Toronto, ON. Canada M4N 3M5
{Gang.wu,james.mainprize,martin.yaffe}@sri.utoronto.ca

Abstract. In digital breast tomosynthesis (DBT), it is desirable to achieve an appropriate level of image quality while keeping the radiation dose as low as reasonably achievable. The purpose of this study is to examine the effectiveness of a patch-based denoising algorithm in reducing noise while preserving details in DBT reconstruction. Low-dose DBT projection images were simulated with various levels of entrance exposure, based on the stochastic property of incident photons from the x-ray source. The patch-based algorithm estimates the true value of a pixel as a weighted average of all pixels in the projection image, where the weights depend on the similarity between the patches. Compared with local smoothing or filtering methods, patch-based techniques can reduce noise while preserving details. The preliminary results have demonstrated that the image quality of DBT can be potentially improved by the proposed technique by incorporating appropriate denoising into the iterative reconstruction algorithm. The suppressed noise was found to resemble the desired white noise except at sharp edges. The contrast is enhanced by more than 10% and the mean lesion signal-difference-to-noise ratio (SDNR) in homogeneous regions was increased by 131.8% and 76.4% for the entrance exposure of 0.1 R and 1 R per projection respectively. The proposed algorithm can further reduce the total imaging dose in DBT by allowing a reduced exposure for each projection view.

Keywords: Tomosynthesis, Reconstruction, Denoising, Non-local means.

1 Introduction

Digital breast tomosynthesis (DBT) is an x-ray acquisition and processing technique which is based on a set of projection images acquired over a range of angles. From the reconstruction of the projection images a series of cross-sectional images or slices is obtained. The advantage of DBT over conventional mammography is that much of the effect of superposition of the anatomic structures that occurs over the thickness of the breast is mitigated from the slice images. Resolving the depth in the image to a selected slice eliminates some of the image complexity caused by structures at other depths and can, therefore, enhance the conspicuity of a tumour as well as facilitate spatial localization within the breast. Moreover, the systems are designed to operate such that the patient does not incur additional radiation dose compared to mammo-

A.D.A. Maidment, P.R. Bakic, and S. Gavenonis (Eds.): IWDM 2012, LNCS 7361, pp. 721–728, 2012.

graphy. In current DBT imaging, one acquires data with a small number of projection views with approximately the equivalent radiation dose of a standard two-view mammography exam.

However the reconstruction of a three-dimensional (3D) breast volume is challenging in DBT because the dataset is sparse and/or noisy; only a limited number of low-dose projections are acquired over an arc. Consequently spatial resolution through the thickness of the breast (z-direction) is typically inferior to the resolution within the plane of the detector (x-y). Iterative methods for calculating the reconstruction are preferred when projections are sparse, noisy, or when sampling is non-uniform. Progress has recently been made on image reconstruction from sparse-view data, which can potentially allow reduction of the radiation dose [1]. For cases where data are highly sparse, such as when only a few (e.g. <10) projections are available, accurate image reconstruction becomes more difficult.

2   Methods

The acquisition of the digital breast tomosynthesis was simulated for a partial-isocentric geometry. The detector was stationary while the x-ray tube rotated around a pivot point. Nine (9) projections were taken over an angular range of -20° to 20°, at 5° increments, using monoenergetic (20 keV) x-rays. A series of mathematical phantoms representing the compressed breast were created with a uniform distribution of 50% fibroglandular and 50% adipose tissue as background. They are rectangular prisms in shape and each contains a simulated small tumour with various diameters (from 0.6 mm to 8 mm) at the centre. The attenuation coefficients of the simulated tumours are equivalent to those measured for infiltrating ductal carcinoma (IDC) [2]. Three levels of entrance exposure per projection (0.1 R, 1 R and noise-free, implying infinite dose) were evenly distributed over the projections in the DBT simulation.

A patch-based algorithm was used to suppress the random variations of pixel intensity in the projection views before reconstruction. Patches of an image are simple objects defined as local square neighborhood regions of image pixels. Compared to pixel-based algorithms, patch-based methods are more powerful because image patches contain more relatively large-scale structures and textures present in natural images than single pixels. The patch $P^I_{(x,y)}$ located at pixel $p(x, y)$ on the grey image I is defined as the set of image intensities belong to a spatially discretized local $m \times m$ neighborhood region of I centered at pixel (x, y). The size m is usually chosen to be an odd number, $i.e.$ $m = 2n + 1$ (n is a natural number). Therefore, a patch $P^I_{(x,y)}$ can be ordered in an m^2-dimensional vector as:

$$P^I_{(x,y)} = (I_{(x-n,y-n)}, ..., I_{(x+n,y+n)})^T \qquad (1)$$

Similar to the Non-Local Means scheme [3], our denoising algorithm estimates the true intensity value of a pixel p as a weighted average of all patches in the projection image, where the weights depend on the similarity (both structural and intensity-based) between the patches. A mathematical form of the weighting factor is given as following,

$$\omega_{(p,q)} = \frac{1}{W_p} \sum_{q \in S} \exp\left(-\frac{\|p-q\|^2}{2\sigma_s^2}\right) \exp\left(-\frac{\left\|P_p^{I_{noisy}} - P_q^{I_{noisy}}\right\|^2}{2\sigma_r^2}\right) \tag{2}$$

where p and q are the coordinates of any pixel located within the noisy image S and ‖.‖ indicates the L2 norm. Compared with the local smoothing or filtering methods, patch-based techniques can reduce noise while preserving details.

An iterative reconstruction method, maximum likelihood convex (ML) has been implemented in C++ for image reconstruction. The contrast and lesion signal-difference-to-noise ratio (SDNR) were used as figures of merit (FOM) to evaluate the image quality in the reconstructed slices.

Images were taken from a digital mammography unit Senographe DS (GE Healthcare, Chalfont St. Giles, UK) system for testing the denoising algorithm in projection views. In addition, a 5-cm-thick biopsy phantom was imaged with anode/filter combination of Rh/Rh, at 29 kV and 4 mAs to produce a noisy image. The proposed method has been also tested on the projection images for a clinical DBT exam.

3   Results

3.1   Biopsy Phantom

Those digital images of the biopsy phantom acquired at a very low exposure (4 mAs) were first converted and normalized to a log-compressed image, in which the intensity of each pixel is the sum of x-ray attenuation coefficients along the x-ray path, shown in Fig. 1a. The denoised version of the projection image by the patch-based algorithm

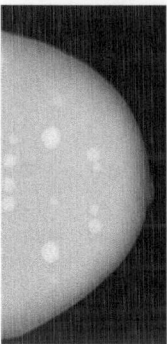 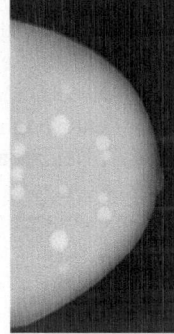 

Fig. 1a. Original projection image of a biopsy phantom

Fig. 1b. Projection image of the phantom denoised by the patch-based technique

Fig. 1c. Difference image displayed in the gray scale window of [-0.1, 0.1]

is shown in Fig. 1b and the difference between the original and the denoised projection is shown in Fig. 1c. The suppressed noise appears like white noise with different intensities in the phantom area and the background, consistent with the quantum noise in mammography being content dependent.

A profile of the biopsy phantom along one column is plotted in Fig. 2a. As expected, the fine details in the image were preserved while random noise was removed. The noise power spectrum (NPS) measured by the multitaper method [4] for the difference image (Fig. 1c) between the original and the denoised projection view of the biopsy phantom is shown in Fig. 2b. The NPS of the difference image approaches that of the noisy projection above 2 mm^{-1}, suggesting that the original projection of the phantom was dominated by quantum noise for higher frequencies. The suppressed noise resembled white noise for a wide range of frequencies while, as desired, the lower frequencies (< 2 mm^{-1}), which contain more information about the main structures of the phantom are removed to a much lesser extent.

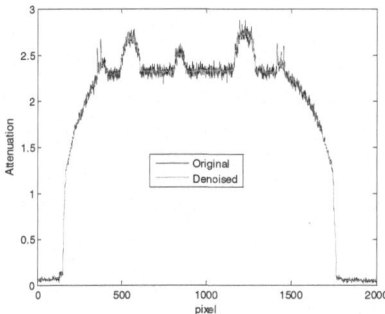
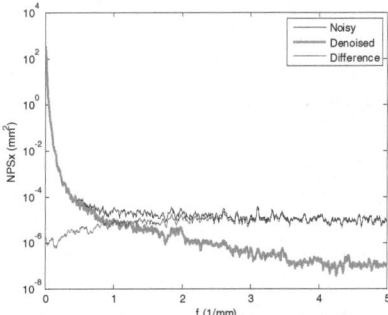

Fig. 2a. Profiles of the original and denoised projection image of a biopsy phantom

Fig. 2b. Power spectra of the projection, the denoised image and the difference

3.2   Clinical Mammograms

The proposed method was also applied to de-identified screening mammograms (courtesy Dr. Roberta Jong, Sunnybrook Health Sciences Centre), as in Fig. 3a. The denoised projection image by the patch-based algorithm is shown in Fig. 3b and the difference between the original and the denoised projection is shown in Fig. 3c. The suppressed noise appears like white noise. Neither anatomic details nor any microcalcifications were observed in the difference image.

A profile of the mammogram along one column through several microcalcifications is plotted in Fig. 4a. As expected, the fine details in the image were preserved while random noise was removed. The power spectra of the difference image (Fig. 3c) between the original and the denoised projection view of the breast are shown in Fig. 4b. The NPS of the difference image approaches that of the noisy projection above 3 mm^{-1}, indicating that the original mammogram was dominated by quantum noise for higher frequencies. The suppressed noise is essentially white for a wide range of frequencies and, the lower frequencies (< 3 mm^{-1}), which contain most of the information about the anatomic structures of the breast are removed to a much less extent. The cause of the peak near the frequency of 3.5 mm^{-1} in the NPS of the original mammogram is believed to be the improper cancellation of the anti-scatter grid during flat-fielding [4], which can be completely eliminated by our denoising algorithm as demonstrated in the noise component of the difference image shown in Fig. 4b (arrow). The removal of the anti-scatter grid effect is also obvious in Fig. 3c. This implies that our proposed patch-based denoising method could also be a powerful candidate for flat-fielding and pre-processing for projection images.

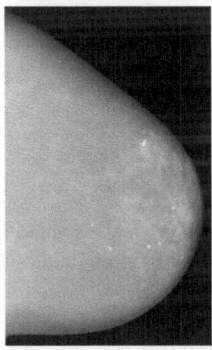
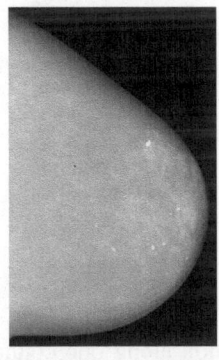

Fig. 3a. Original screening mammogram   **Fig. 3b.** Mammogram denoised   **Fig. 3c.** Difference image displayed in [-0.02, 0.02]

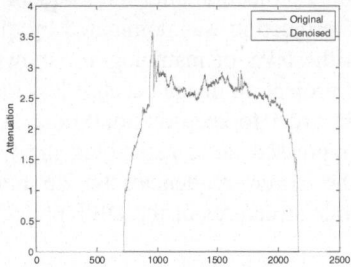
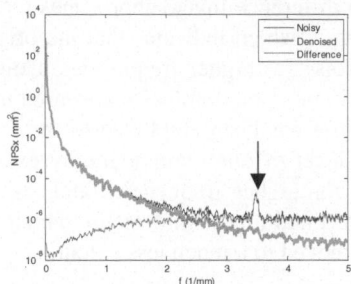

Fig. 4a. Profiles of the original and denoised mammogram   **Fig. 4b.** Power spectra of the mammogram, the denoised image and the difference

3.3   Clinical DBT Exam, Projection Image

The proposed method was also applied to the projection views of a clinical DBT exam, one of which was shown in Fig. 5a. The denoised version of the projection image by the patch-based algorithm was shown in Fig. 5b and the difference between the original and the denoised projection was shown in Fig. 5c. The suppressed noise appears like white noise with different intensities in the breast area and the air region in background, which agrees with the fact that the quantum noise in mammography is content dependent. Virtually no anatomic detail was observed in the difference image.

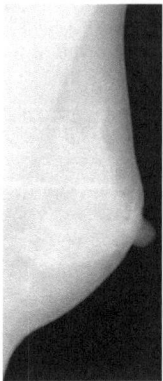 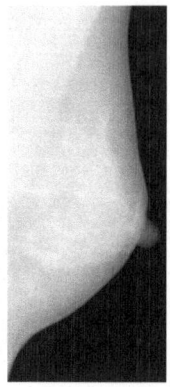 

Fig. 5a. Original projection view of a clinical DBT exam

Fig. 5b. Projection view of the DBT exam denoised by the patch-based technique

Fig. 5c. Noise component, displayed in the gray scale window of [-0.05, 0.05]

A profile of the DBT projection along one column is plotted in Fig. 6a. As expected, the fine details in the image were preserved while random noise was removed. The power spectra of the noisy projection, the denoised version and the difference image (Fig. 5c) between the two of the DBT projection is shown in Fig. 6b. The NPS of the difference image approaches that of the noisy projection after the frequency of 2.5 mm^{-1}, which indicates that the original DBT projection was dominated by quantum noise for higher frequencies. Comparing to the NPS of mammogram shown in Fig. 4b, more random noise appeared in the DBT projection image because less radiation dose has been employed to the each view in order to keep the total dose at the same level of one mammography exam. The suppressed noise resembled the white noise for higher frequencies and, as desired, the lower frequencies (< 2.5 mm^{-1}), which contain most information about the anatomic structures of the DBT projection are removed to a much less extent.

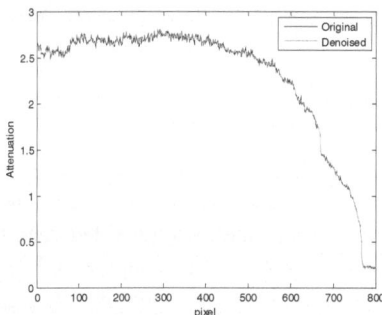 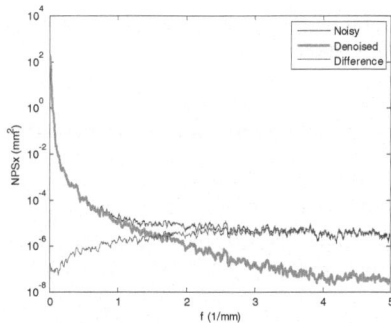

Fig. 6a. Profiles of the original and denoised projection image of a DBT exam

Fig. 6b. Power spectra of the DBT projection, the denoised view and the difference

3.4   Simulation of Uniform Phantoms

The image quality was evaluated in terms of the contrast and the lesion SDNR in the reconstructed central slices in the simulated phantoms with uniform background. For example, results for a 2 mm diameter lesion are shown as a function of reconstruction iteration numbers in Fig. 7 and Fig. 8. Both the contrast and lesion SDNR were enhanced by the denoising technique for the two levels of the entrance exposure simulated in the DBT projections. On average, the contrast is increased by 16.6% and 12.2% for 0.1 R and 1 R per projection respectively. The lesion SDNR is increased by 131.8% and 76.4% on average for 0.1 R and 1R respectively. More importantly, the contrast of the 0.1 R exposure was boosted by denoising to almost the same performance as obtained at 1 R without denoising. This shows a great potential of the integration of patch-based denoising in low-dose DBT reconstructions for low contrast objects, such as mass tumours.

4   Discussion

Results from the biopsy phantom, the screening mammogram and the clinical DBT projection data demonstrated that the proposed technique effectively reduces noise while preserving most fine details in DBT. The suppressed noise appears like white noise and virtually no anatomic details or microcalcifications were observed in the difference image. It also implies that our proposed patch-based denoising method could be a powerful candidate tool for flat-fielding and pre-processing projection images. The preliminary results from the simulated phantom study have demonstrated that the image quality of DBT can potentially be improved by the proposed technique by incorporating appropriate denoising into the iterative reconstruction algorithm. Further investigation will be carried on images with heterogeneous background such as anatomic clusters in both simulation phantoms and patient data in clinical DBT exams.

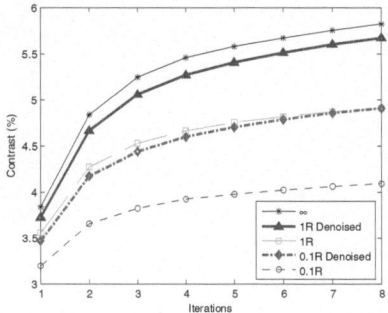   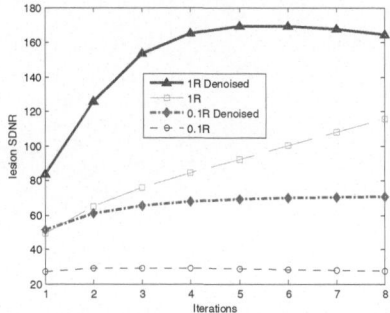

Fig. 7. Contrast enhanced in the reconstructed slices by the patch-based denoising technique for both levels of exposure

Fig. 8. The lesion SDNRs in the reconstructed slices were increased by the denoising technique for both levels of exposure

References

[1] Sidky, E.Y., Pan, X., Reiser, I.S., Nishikawa, R.M., Moore, R.H., Kopans, D.B.: Enhanced imaging of microcalcifications in digital breast tomosynthesis through improved image-reconstruction algorithms. Medical Physics 36, 4920 (2009)

[2] Johns, P.C., Yaffe, M.J.: X-ray characterisation of normal and neoplastic breast tissues. Physics in Medicine and Biology 32, 675–695 (1987)

[3] Buades, A., Coll, B., Morel, J.M.: A Non-Local Algorithm for Image Denoising. In: 2005 IEEE Computer Society Conference on Computer Vision and Pattern Recognition, CVPR 2005, vol. 2, pp. 60–65 (2005)

[4] Wu, G., Mainprize, J.G., Yaffe, M.J.: Spectral analysis of mammographic images using a multitaper method. Med. Phys. 39, 801–810 (2012)

Out-of-Plane Artifact Reduction
in Tomosynthesis Based on Regression Modeling
and Outlier Detection

Shiras Abdurahman[1,2], Anna Jerebko[1], Thomas Mertelmeier[1],
Tobias Lasser[2,3], and Nassir Navab[2]

[1] Siemens AG, Healthcare Sector, Erlangen, Germany
[2] Chair for Computer Aided Medical Procedures (CAMP),
Technische Universität München, Garching, Germany
[3] Institute for Biomathematics and Biometry,
Helmholtz Zentrum München, Munich, Germany
anna.jerebko@siemens.com

Abstract. We propose a method for out-of-plane artifact reduction in digital breast tomosynthesis reconstruction. Because of the limited angular range acquisition in DBT, the reconstructed slices have reduced resolution in z-direction and are affected by artifacts. The out-of-plane blur caused by dense tissue and large masses complicates reconstruction of thick slices volumes. The streak-like out-of-plane artifacts caused by calcifications and metal clips distort the shape of calcifications which is regarded by many radiologists as an important malignancy predictor. Small clinical features such as micro-calcifications could be obscured by bright artifacts. The proposed technique involves reconstructing a set of super-resolution slices and predicting the artifact-free voxel intensity based on the corresponding set of projection pixels using a statistical model learned from a set of training data. Our experiments show that the resulting reconstructed images are de-blurred and streak-like artifacts are reduced, visibility of clinical features, contrast and sharpness are improved and thick-slice reconstruction is possible without the loss of contrast and sharpness.

Keywords: Tomosynthesis, filtered back projection, out-of-plane artifacts, outlier detection, regression modeling.

1 Introduction

In Digital Breast Tomosynthesis (DBT), the 3D representation of the breast is reconstructed from projections acquired only within a limited angular range. There are many algorithms designed to reduce the out-of-plane artifacts, inevitable in reconstructed DBT images [1]. While iterative reconstruction approaches reduce artifacts better than Filtered Back Projection (FBP) methods, they do not completely remove streak-like artifacts from metal clips and calcifications and require much longer computation time. The metal artifact reduction methods coming

A.D.A. Maidment, P.R. Bakic, and S. Gavenonis (Eds.): IWDM 2012, LNCS 7361, pp. 729–736, 2012.

from CT are often based on segmenting the metal objects in sinograms or projection images, removing them before the reconstruction by interpolation and then restoring them again in the resulting volume [2]. Such methods are of very limited use in DBT, where artifacts are often caused by dense tissue or masses with amorphous shape or by calcifications, detection and removal of which in low dose projections is not feasible. One of the state of art artifact reduction methods specific to tomosynthesis is the slice thickness filter which is used in FBP reconstructions [3]. The slice thickness filter is a low pass filter which reduces the frequency response in z direction. It allows maintaining constant slice thickness and limits the out-of-plane artifacts but reduces the sharpness of high frequency features in the projections with high angle of incidence. Other methods suggest using statistical outlier detection tests during back projection to further reduce artifacts [4]. The goal of such methods is to separate projection pixels contributing to each reconstructed voxel into two categories: normal pixels and outliers which introduce artifacts to that voxel. The popular statistical tests based on mean and standard deviation (including Grubb's, Chauvenet's, Peirce's test, etc.) assume unimodal data distribution and are not well suited to deal with limited data samples from few projection views with considerable fraction of them containing the artifact. In this paper we suggest designing a smoothed statistical model that reflects distribution parameters of the normal artifact free voxels and using the predicted parameters instead of explicitly computing them during the reconstruction.

2   Method

2.1   Baseline Reconstruction Method

We used FBP with filters designed specifically for mammography images as a baseline reconstruction method. The polynomial filter kernel in Fourier domain was designed so that reconstructed volume resembles iterative reconstruction results [5] with mammogram-like image impression and well differentiated tissue densities. The filter parameters were derived from Simultaneous Iterative Reconstruction Technique (SIRT) applied to a wire phantom.

2.2   Super-Resolution Reconstruction

The reconstructed voxels in DBT are highly anisotropic. For example, the data sets acquired with MAMMOMAT Inspiration system[1], Siemens, Erlangen are typically reconstructed into 1 mm thick slices with high in-plane resolution of 0.085×0.085 mm^2. Such voxels project into several projection pixels for high incidence angles (see Fig. 1) resulting in non-uniform sampling for different projection angles. This problem is usually solved by slice thickness filter.

---

[1] Breast tomosynthesis with Siemens MAMMOMAT Inspiration is an investigational practice and is limited by U.S. law to investigational use. It is not commercially available in the U.S. and its future availability cannot be ensured.

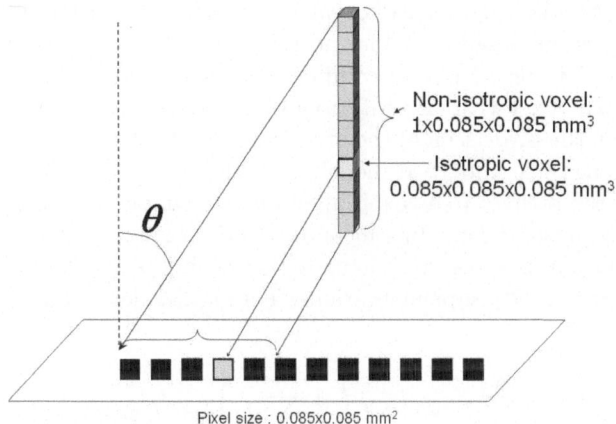

Fig. 1. Projection of a voxel on the detector plane

However, to eliminate the blurring of micro-calcifications in the projections with high angle of incidence θ, slice thickness filter is not used in our approach. Instead, we suggest reconstructing slabs consisting of 'super resolution' thin slices with the total thickness S (eg. 1 mm) acceptable for clinical reading routine. Each slab should consist of several slices ($n = S/p$), thin enough so that each voxel's projected footprint area for all incidence angles is approximately equal to the pixel size p of acquired projections. Bilinear interpolation on the detector plane could be used to account for overlap of voxel's projection with more than one pixel on the detector plane. After the artifact reduction step the stack of thin slices could be collapsed into a slab with thickness S with average or maximum intensity projection (MIP) of thin slices in the direction orthogonal to the slice plane or with an angle of one of the acquired projections.

2.3 Artifact Reduction Based on Outlier Detection and Regression Modeling

While the method suggested in this paper could be used with different outlier detection tests, the following mean and standard deviation test was chosen here for artifact reduction as an example because of it's simplicity and ease of implementation:

$$if \; I_t > \frac{1}{N} \sum_{j=1}^{N} I_j + k\sigma \Rightarrow I_t \; is \; an \; outlier \tag{1}$$

where I_t, I_j are intensities of pixels contributing to the same voxel, $j = 1, .., N$, σ - standard deviation of pixels I_j, k - constant parameter determining the strength of outlier detection, N - number of projections, and pixels contributing to the same voxel.

The idea is the following: instead of calculating the standard deviation, predict it with the regression based model for normal, outlier-free data for a given mean intensity of pixel values. Directly computed standard deviation of pixel values contributing to a voxel with an artifact can be too high when a large fraction of samples contain the projection of the artifact (which is often the case with a limited angular range). A smoothed model that reflects the statistical distribution parameters of the artifact free voxels allows more reliable outlier-pixel rejection during image reconstruction. Only mean intensities of pixel values are computed and the distribution parameter is predicted according to the smoothed model f (sigmoid function in our implementation). The outlier detection rule now looks as follows:

$$if \ I_t \ > \ \frac{1}{N} \sum_{j=1}^{N} I_j + k \times f \left(\frac{1}{N} \sum_{j=1}^{N} I_j \right) \ \Rightarrow \ I_t \ is \ an \ outlier \qquad (2)$$

Since the distribution parameter is predicted based on the average value of both normal and outlier pixels, the tests based on mean are not always optimal. While more robust statistical tests (e.g. based on median) could give better results, in practice the mean based test gives reasonably good results in wide angle DBT images.

2.4   Regression Modeling

The training data for the regression modeling of statistical distribution parameters was collected from 58 patient cases generated with Siemens MAMMOMAT Inspiration at four different clinical sites. The reconstructed volumes were randomly sampled and the mean and standard deviation of the pixel values which contribute to the sampled voxel were used as a training set to fit the regression model (see Fig. 2). It is highly unlikely that any of the micro-calcifications later used to test the model were present in the training set.

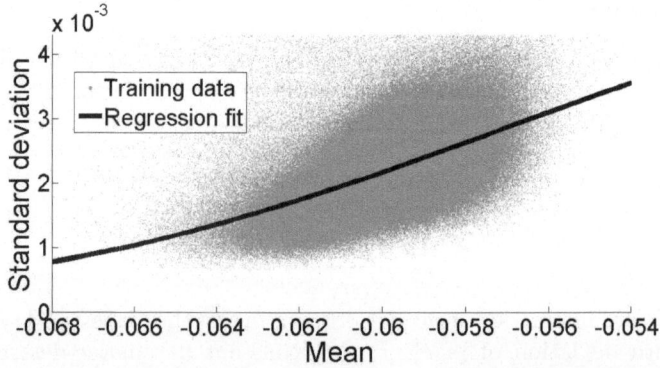

Fig. 2. Regression modeling with sigmoid function

3   Results

3.1   Reduction of Out-of-Plane Artifacts

Out-of-plane artifacts caused by the high attenuation structures like large calcifications and metals are very visible in tomosynthesis images. Fig. 3 shows that artifacts from calcifications (A and B) were reduced considerably with the method based on modeled statistical distribution parameters (as in Eq. 2) compared with standard statistical test with computed standard deviation (as in Eq. 1) and with the baseline reconstruction. Artifact reduction strength is the same in both statistical artifact reduction methods. Fig. 4 provides similar visualization of the effectiveness of artifact reduction method for an ROI containing a metal clip. Although the noise was slightly higher in reconstructions with 1 mm thick slices in the new method compared to the baseline, it was considered acceptable by the radiographer. MIP of the reconstructed volume can be used as one of the quality measures for artifact reduction. The volume without artifact reduction yield MIP images where artifacts obscure some of the calcifications. Fig. 5 shows the improvement of MIP image quality with statistical artifact reduction.

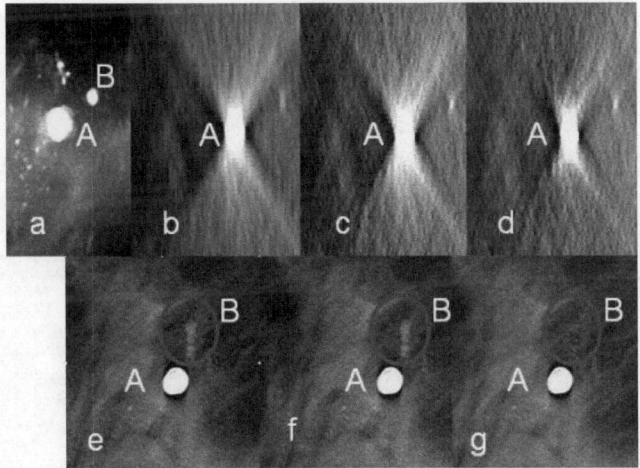

Fig. 3. ROI containing calcifications, top: (a) MIP image. Coronal slices through calcification A, visualizing the artifacts; (b) Baseline reconstruction with slice thickness filter; (c) Artifact reduction with computed standard deviation; (d) Artifact reduction with regression-modeled standard deviation. Bottom, axial slices showing calcification A in focus and artifacts from calcification B: (e) Baseline reconstruction with slice thickness filter; (f) Artifact reduction with computed standard deviation; (g) Artifact reduction with regression-modeled standard deviation. Images courtesy of Malmo University Hospital, Sweden.

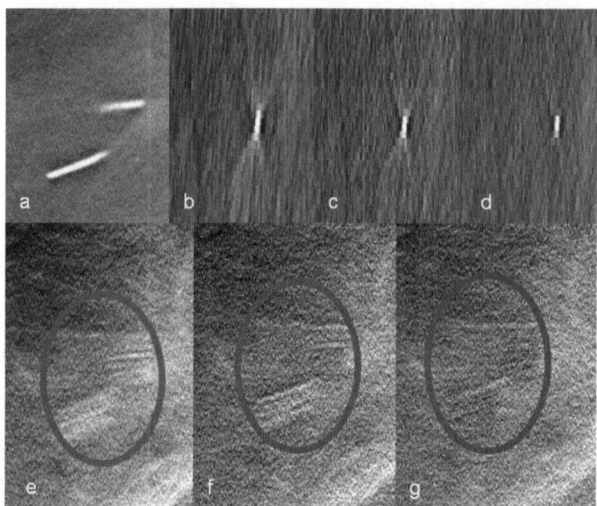

Fig. 4. ROI containing metal clip of 0.5 mm diameter, top: (a) Axial slice, in-focus plane. Coronal slices: (b) Baseline reconstruction with slice thickness filter; (c) Artifact reduction with computed standard deviation; (d) Artifact reduction with regression-modeled standard deviation. Bottom, axial slices, 5 mm distance from in-focus plane: (e) Baseline reconstruction with slice thickness filter; (f) Artifact reduction with computed standard deviation; (g) Artifact reduction with regression-modeled standard deviation. Images courtesy of Leuven University Hospital, Belgium.

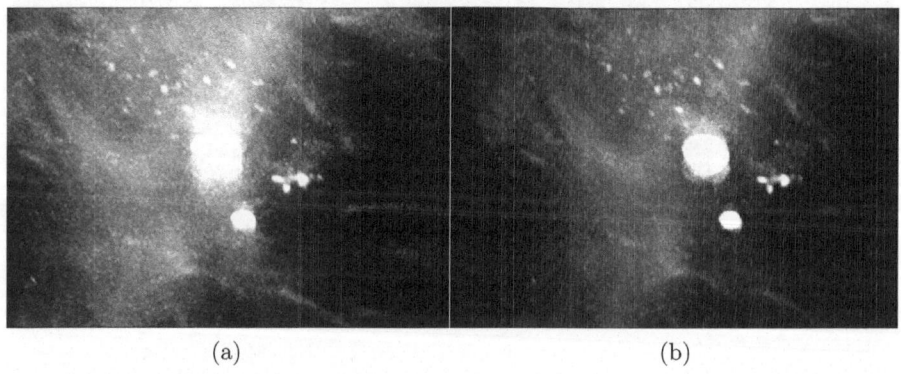

(a)   (b)

Fig. 5. Maximum intensity projection: (a) Baseline reconstruction with slice thickness filter; (b) Artifact reduction with regression-modeled standard deviation

3.2   Quantitative Evaluation

The experiments were designed to test the possible limitation of this method that for certain values of the strength of artifact reduction (k), the contrast of micro-calcifications could be reduced, leading to potential loss of faint micro-calcification clusters. To test this hypothesis we have segmented 212 faint micro-calcifications in baseline reconstructions (FBP with slice thickness filter) of 58 patient images. The same segmentations were used in the images reconstructed with our statistical artifact reduction approach to compare the contrast of the micro-calcifications for varying levels of artifact reduction strength k with the baseline method. We analyzed the relative contrast of calcification computed as the ratio of contrast of calcification in images reconstructed with statistical artifact reduction to their contrast in base line reconstruction. As it could be seen from Fig. 6a, the mean relative contrast of micro-calcifications is higher than 1 for $k > 1$. The strength of the outlier detection in the next experiment was set such that the mean contrast of the calcification set is maximal. Fig. 6b shows the histogram of the contrast of all micro-calcifications relative to the baseline approach for the fixed value of $k = 2.3$. As it could be seen from the figure, the relative contrast has improved for majority of calcifications (92%) with the average improvement of 27%, a statistically significant improvement with the p value of 0.00005 and [24:29%] confidence interval for the mean. The contrast-to-noise ratio (CNR) was reduced by 17% on average, partially because the segmentations were done on the baseline FBP reconstructions and did not fully overlap with sharper reconstructions with artifact reduction.

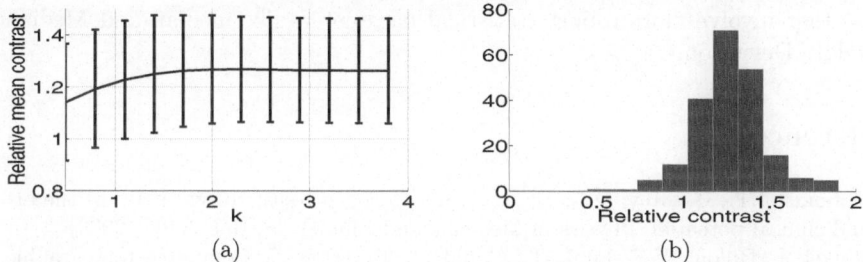

(a)   (b)

Fig. 6. Relative contrast of calcifications: (a) Selection of artifact reduction strength; (b) Histogram for $k = 2.3$

Both contrast and CNR are not the most appropriate measures to characterize image quality. While we use relative contrast analysis to make sure that no micro-calcifications were lost with the proposed method, we rely on the qualitative feedback of a human observer to make a conclusion about the quality of the reconstruction.

3.3   Visual Qualitative Assessment

An experienced radiographer inspected 58 patient images reconstructed with statistical artifact reduction with 1 mm and 2 mm slice thickness side by side with the images with 1 mm slice thickness reconstructed with the baseline approach. It was observed that the contrast of calcifications has improved in 1 mm reconstructions with slightly higher noise level compared to the baseline

approach while 2 mm thick slices appeared less noisy than the 1 mm reconstructions. No calcifications visible in the baseline images have been missed. The
contrast and appearance of masses was improved and the out-of-plane artifacts
were noticeably diminished in both 1 and 2 mm reconstructions (see Fig. 3).

4   Conclusion

Our preliminary experiments have shown that statistical artifact reduction based
on regression modeling and outlier detection visibly reduces the out-of-plane
artifacts, especially those caused by calcifications and metals. Although the main
assumption was that this method should help to reduce streak-like out-of-plane
artifacts, we observed that it also removes some of the out-of-plane blur caused
by dense tissue, noticeably improving the visualization of mass's morphology.
The proposed approach allows to increase the sharpness and contrast of microcalcifications. That, in turn, makes the reconstruction of thicker slices possible
without the loss of sharpness and contrast. In addition to improved artifact
reduction, using the distribution parameters predicted with a regression model
is computationally less expensive than of computing them on-line. The statistical
artifact reduction approach with modeled distribution parameters suggested in
this paper is applicable to other statistical outlier detection tests, for example
those that involve more robust statistical parameters like median and Median
Absolute Deviation.

References

1. Dobbins, J.T., Godfrey, D.J.: Digital x-ray tomosynthesis: current state of the art
   and clinical potential. Physics in Medicine and Biology 48, R65–R106 (2003)
2. Rinkel, J., Dillon, W.P., Funk, T., Gould, R., Prevrhal, S.: Computed tomographic
   metal artifact reduction for the detection and quantitation of small features near
   large metallic implants: a comparison of published methods. Journal of Computer
   Assisted Tomography 32, 621–629 (2008)
3. Mertelmeier, T., Orman, J., Haerer, W., Dudam, M.K.: Optimizing filtered backprojection reconstruction for a breast tomosynthesis prototype device. In: Proc. SPIE,
   vol. 6142, p. 61420F (2006)
4. Wu, T., Moore, R.H., Kopans, D.B.: Voting strategy for artifact reduction in digital
   breast tomosynthesis. Medical Physics 33, 2461–2471 (2006)
5. Kunze, H., Härer, W., Orman, J., Mertelmeier, T., Stierstorfer, K.: Filter determination for Tomosynthesis aided by iterative reconstruction techniques. In: 9th
   International Meeting on Fully Three-Dimensional Image Reconstruction in Radiology and Nuclear Medicine, Lindau, Germany, pp. 309–312 (2007)

Investigating Oblique Reconstructions
with Super-Resolution in Digital Breast Tomosynthesis

Raymond J. Acciavatti, Stewart B. Mein, and Andrew D.A. Maidment

University of Pennsylvania, Department of Radiology, Physics Section, 1 Silverstein Building,
3400 Spruce St., Philadelphia PA 19104-4206
racci@seas.upenn.edu, Andrew.Maidment@uphs.upenn.edu

Abstract. In digital breast tomosynthesis (DBT), the image of an object is shifted in sub-pixel detector element increments with each increasing projection angle. As a consequence of this property, we have previously demonstrated that DBT is capable of super-resolution in reconstruction planes parallel to the breast support. This study demonstrates that super-resolution is also achievable in obliquely pitched reconstruction planes. To this end, a theoretical framework is developed in which the reconstruction of a sinusoidal input is calculated. It is demonstrated that frequencies exceeding the detector alias frequency can be resolved over many pitches. For experimental validation of this finding, a bar pattern phantom was imaged on a goniometry stand using a commercial DBT system. With a commercial prototype reconstruction solution, high frequency patterns were resolved in oblique reconstructions, and modulation contrast was determined at various pitches and frequencies. This work demonstrates the existence of super-resolution in oblique DBT reconstructions.

Keywords: Digital breast tomosynthesis (DBT), aliasing, super-resolution, image reconstruction, filtered backprojection (FBP), Fourier transform, spectral leakage, oblique reconstruction.

1   Introduction

Digital breast tomosynthesis (DBT) is a 3D imaging modality in which tomographic sections of the breast are generated from a limited range of x-ray projections. Because the image of an object is translated along the detector in sub-pixel detector element increments with each increasing projection angle, our prior work [1] has demonstrated that DBT is capable of super-resolution (*i.e.*, sub-pixel resolution).

By convention, DBT reconstructions are created in planes parallel to the breast support. The feasibility of reconstructions in planes with oblique pitches relative to the breast support has not yet been explored based on the conventional interpretation of the Central Slice Theorem [2]. According to that theorem, Fourier space is sampled only within double-napped cones (DNCs) whose opening angle matches the angular range of the scan. This paper demonstrates that super-resolution is achievable in reconstruction planes whose pitch is well outside the scanning range.

A.D.A. Maidment, P.R. Bakic, and S. Gavenonis (Eds.): IWDM 2012, LNCS 7361, pp. 737–744, 2012.
© Springer-Verlag Berlin Heidelberg 2012

2   Methods

An analytical framework for investigating super-resolution in obliquely pitched DBT reconstructions is now proposed. Accordingly, we calculate the reconstruction profile along the long axis of a thin input object whose linear attenuation coefficient varies as $C \cdot \cos(2\pi f_0' x')$. In this formulation, f_0' denotes the input spatial frequency, which may be chosen to be higher than the detector alias frequency. In addition, C denotes the amplitude of the input waveform, and x' measures position along the oblique angular pitch ζ relative to point A (Figure 1). The midpoint of the waveform at A is taken to be positioned at the height z_0 above the detector. Under these assumptions, DBT acquisition with a stationary detector and a parallel x-ray beam geometry is modeled for each projection. Although a more general formulation would consider the possibility of a rotating detector and a divergent x-ray beam geometry, the proposed formulation is approximately applicable to measurements made near the midpoint of the chest wall side of a clinical DBT detector.

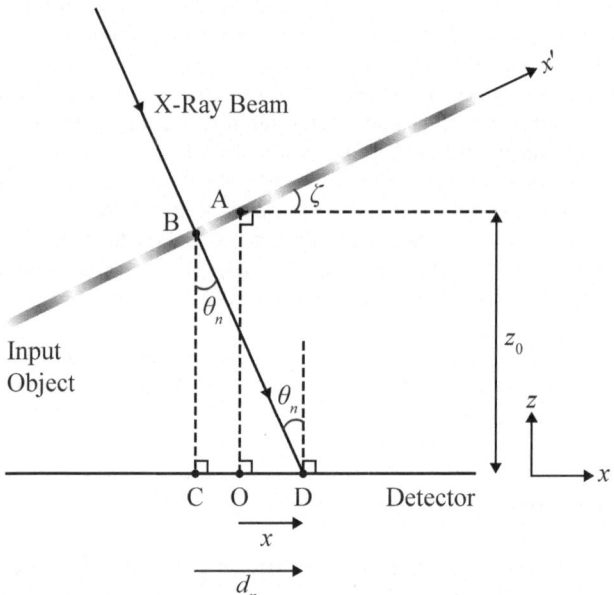

Fig. 1. A schematic diagram of the DBT acquisition geometry is shown (figure not to scale). The thin input object has an attenuation coefficient which varies sinusoidally along the angular pitch ζ. A stationary detector and a parallel beam geometry are modeled for each projection.

As diagrammed in Figure 1, each point along the input object is translated across the detector by the increment d_n in the nth projection. Applying trigonometry to triangle BCD, one can derive an expression for the translational shift d_n as

$$\tan\theta_n = \frac{\overline{CD}}{\overline{BC}} = \frac{d_n}{z_0 + (x - d_n)\tan\zeta} \quad , \quad d_n = \frac{(z_0 + x\tan\zeta)\tan\theta_n}{1 + \tan\zeta\tan\theta_n} \quad , \tag{1}$$

where θ_n is the angle of x-ray incidence on the detector for each projection and x is the position along the detector relative to the origin O. In terms of these parameters, the signal recorded by the mth detector element for the nth projection is thus

$$\mathcal{D}\mu(m,n) = \int_{\left[a(m-1/2)-d_{mn}^-\right]\sec\zeta}^{\left[a(m+1/2)-d_{mn}^+\right]\sec\zeta} C \cdot \cos(2\pi f_0' x)\frac{dx}{a} \; , \tag{2}$$

where a denotes the length of the detector elements, which are taken to be centered on $x = ma$, and where $d_{mn}^{\pm} \equiv d_n\big|_{x=a(m\pm1/2)}$. This integral can be evaluated as

$$\mathcal{D}\mu(m,n) = C\sec(\zeta)\text{sinc}(af_0'\sec\zeta)\cos\left(\frac{2\pi f_0'\left[ma - z_0\tan\theta_n\right]\sec\zeta}{1+\tan\zeta\tan\theta_n}\right) , \tag{3}$$

where $\text{sinc}(u) \equiv \sin(\pi u)/(\pi u)$. Using Eq. (3), the reconstructed attenuation coefficient (μ_{FBP}) can now be determined at any point (x, z). The filtered backprojection (FBP) reconstruction is given by the expression

$$\mu_{\text{FBP}} = \frac{1}{N}\sum_m\sum_n \mathcal{D}\mu(m,n)\cdot\left[\phi(t)*\text{rect}\left(\frac{t\sec\theta_n - ma}{a}\right)\right]\Bigg|_{t=x\cos\theta_n+z\sin\theta_n} , \tag{4}$$

where ϕ is the filter and $*$ is the convolution operator [1]. Assuming N projections, the index n ranges from $+(N-1)/2$ to $-(N-1)/2$; the special case $n = 0$ defines the central projection. Following linear systems theory for DBT, the reconstruction filter should be written as the product of a ramp (RA) filter and a spectrum apodization (SA) filter in the Fourier domain, where the SA filter is typically given by a Hanning window function [2]. Both filters are truncated at the frequencies $f = \pm\xi$. The net filter can be calculated in the spatial domain using the inverse Fourier transform [1].

To determine μ_{FBP} along the pitch of the input object, one must evaluate Eq. (4) with the constraints $x = x'\cos\zeta$ and $z = z_0 + x'\sin\zeta$. Finally, to investigate the frequency dependence of the reconstruction, its Fourier transform may also be calculated.

3   Results

3.1   Analytical Modeling

Reconstruction is now simulated for the Selenia Dimensions x-ray unit with 15 projections taken at a uniform angular spacing ($\Delta\theta$) of 1.07°, assuming $C = 1.0$ mm^{-1}, $a = 140$ μm, $f_0' = 0.7a^{-1}$ (5.0 lp/mm), $z_0 = 50.0$ mm, and $\zeta = 20°$. To illustrate the potential for super-resolution, the input frequency has been specified to be higher than the detector alias frequency, $0.5a^{-1}$ (3.6 lp/mm). Also, the pitch of 20° has been chosen since it is well outside the DNCs with an opening angle spanning $-7.5°$ to $+7.5°$ in frequency space.

Figure 2 demonstrates that simple backprojection (SBP) reconstruction is capable of resolving the input frequency, while the central projection alone is not. In acquiring the central projection, the input waveform projects onto the detector as if it were the frequency $f_0' \sec \zeta$ (5.3 lp/mm). Due to aliasing, this frequency is represented as if it were $(1 - 0.7 \sec \zeta) a^{-1}$, or 1.8 lp/mm. Consequently, the Fourier transform of the central projection possesses a major peak at 1.8 lp/mm, and has minor alias peaks at $0.7 a^{-1} \sec \zeta$ (5.3 lp/mm), $(2 - 0.7 \sec \zeta) a^{-1}$ (9.0 lp/mm), and $(1 + 0.7 \sec \zeta) a^{-1}$ (12.5 lp/mm). By contrast, the SBP Fourier transform correctly possesses a major peak at the input frequency, 5.0 lp/mm.

FBP reconstructions and their Fourier transforms are also shown using either the RA filter alone or the RA and SA filters together, assuming a filter truncation frequency (ξ) of 10.0 lp/mm. Although ξ is often specified to be the detector alias frequency $0.5 a^{-1}$ (3.6 lp/mm), it is necessary to choose a higher value in order to achieve super-resolution. Like SBP, the FBP Fourier transforms possess their major peak at the input frequency, 5.0 lp/mm. Filtering provides an improvement over SBP by smoothing pixilation artifacts in the spatial domain and increasing modulation. The two FBP reconstructions differ in that reconstruction with the RA filter alone has greater modulation than reconstruction with the RA and SA filters together. This finding is expected, since the SA filter places more relative weight on low frequencies to reduce high frequency noise. The drawback of reconstruction with the RA filter alone is increased high frequency spectral leakage in the Fourier domain.

3.2   Experimental Validation

The feasibility of super-resolution in an oblique reconstruction has been verified experimentally using a lead bar pattern phantom. The phantom was placed on a goniometry stand at a height of 7.6 cm above the breast support of a Selenia Dimensions DBT system. The goniometry stand was adjusted to vary the pitch of the bar patterns. At 30 kV and 14 mAs, 15 projections were acquired with a W/Al target-filter combination and a 0.3 mm focal spot. Reconstruction was then performed along the pitch of the bar patterns using a commercial prototype backprojection filtering algorithm (Briona™, Real Time Tomography, Villanova, PA). The pixel size of the reconstruction grid (14.0 µm) was much smaller than that of the detector elements (140 µm), so that the alias frequency of the reconstruction grid (35.7 lp/mm) was significantly higher than the alias frequency of the detector (3.6 lp/mm).

In Figure 3, the central projection is shown at a 0° pitch. As expected, frequencies up to 3 lp/mm can be resolved, since 3 lp/mm is less than the alias frequency of the detector (3.6 lp/mm). Classical signs of aliasing at higher frequencies include Moiré patterns [3] at 4 lp/mm and the misrepresentation of 5 lp/mm as a lower frequency (~3 lp/mm). At the same magnification, the central projection is also shown at a 20° pitch. Its aliasing artifacts are similar to the image at the 0° pitch; the main difference relative to the 0° pitch is compression of the alternating bright and dark bands over a smaller length, increasing the effective frequency projected onto the detector.

Unlike an individual projection, reconstructions along both 0° and 20° pitches clearly show frequencies up to 5 lp/mm (Figure 4). The existence of super-resolution along the 20° pitch is significant because the input frequency is well outside the DNCs in frequency space having an opening angle between −7.5° to +7.5°.

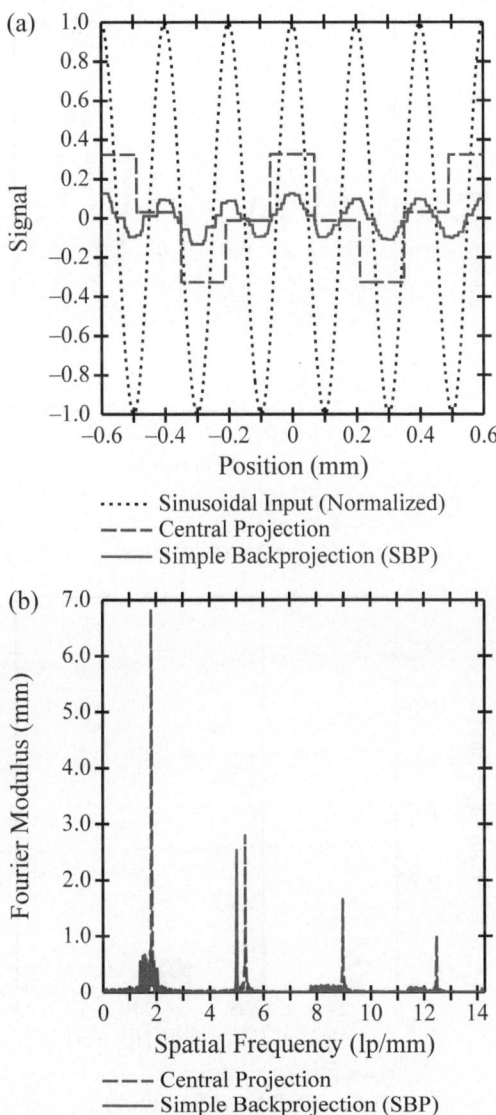

Fig. 2. Assuming $N = 15$, $\Delta\theta = 1.07°$, $C = 1.0$ mm^{-1}, $a = 140$ μm, $f_0' = 5.0$ lp/mm, $\zeta = 20°$, and $z_0 = 50.0$ mm, the central projection and SBP reconstruction are plotted in both the spatial and Fourier domains. The central projection represents the input frequency as 1.8 lp/mm. By contrast, SBP reconstruction performed along the pitch of the input correctly resolves the object. Adding filters to the reconstruction smoothens pixilation artifacts in the spatial domain and increases the modulation relative to SBP. Although the reconstruction with the RA filter alone has the benefit of the highest modulation, it presents the trade-off of increased high frequency spectral leakage. The SA filter suppresses such high frequency Fourier content. The existence of super-resolution along a 20° pitch would not initially be expected from the conventional interpretation of the Central Slice Theorem.

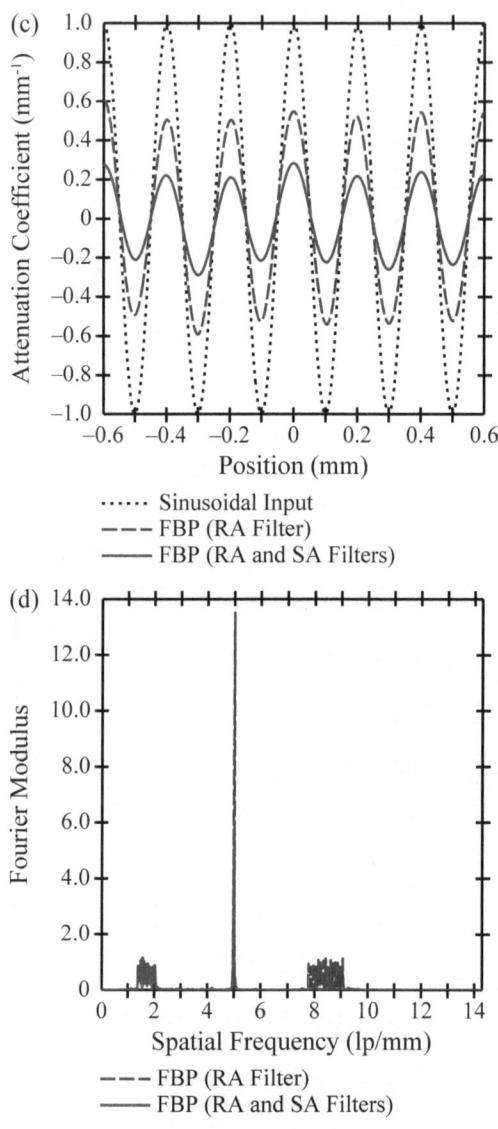

Fig. 2. (*continued*)

Although high frequencies are resolved along a 20° pitch, there is a slight reduction in image quality relative to the 0° pitch. To investigate distortions in visibility, modulation contrast [4] may be calculated as $(I_1 - I_2)/(I_1 + I_2)$, where I_1 and I_2 are the mean signal intensities in the bright and dark bands at a fixed frequency. At 5 lp/mm, modulation contrast is 0.0034 and 0.0020 for 0° and 20° pitches, respectively (41% decrease). The analogous values at 4 lp/mm are 0.0074 and 0.0059 (20% decrease).

Central Projection (0° Pitch)   Central Projection (20° Pitch)

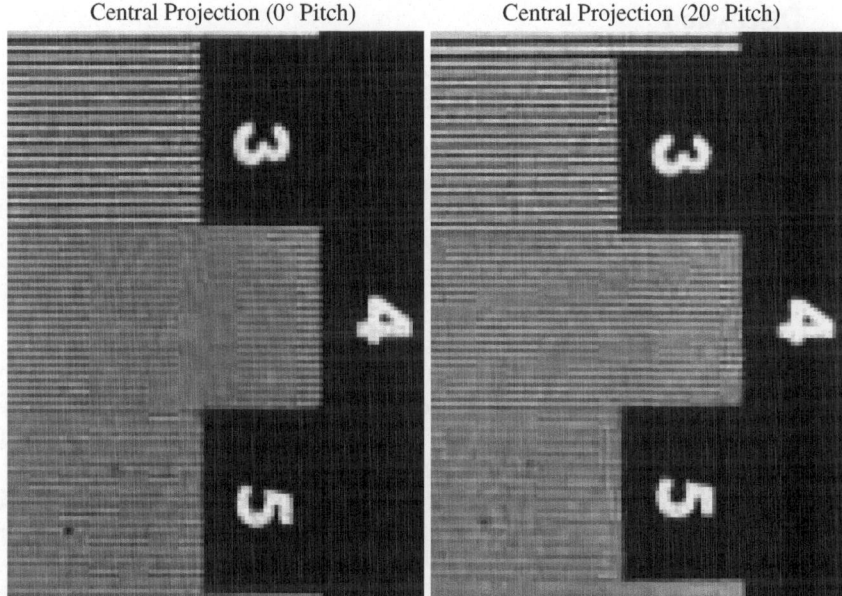

Fig. 3. With a goniometry stand, a lead bar pattern phantom was imaged at various pitches using the Selenia Dimensions DBT system. A single projection can only resolve frequencies less than the alias frequency of the detector, 3.6 lp/mm for 140 μm detector elements. Evidence of aliasing at higher frequencies includes Moiré patterns at 4 lp/mm and the misrepresentation of 5 lp/mm as a lower frequency (~3 lp/mm).

Reconstruction (0° Pitch)   Reconstruction (20° Pitch)

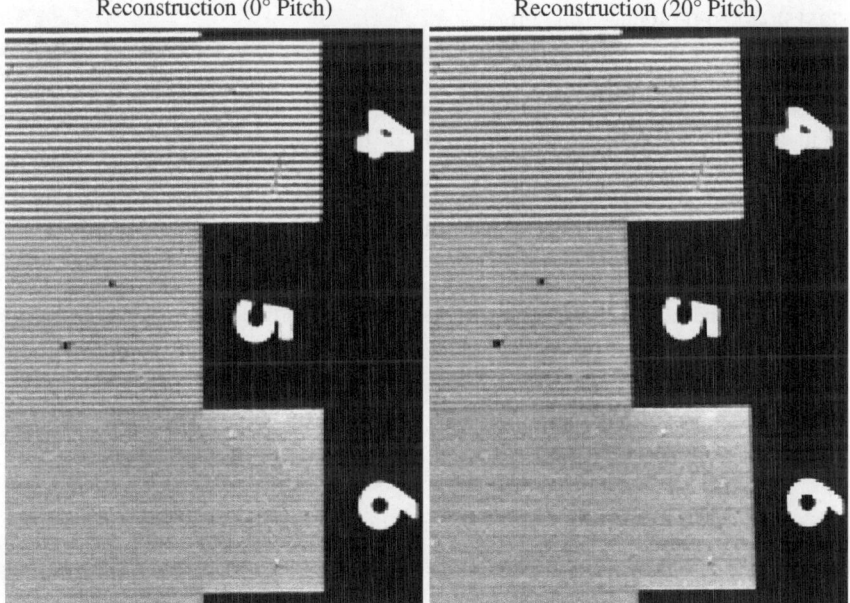

Fig. 4. Reconstructions performed within planes along 0° and 20° pitches can resolve higher frequencies than a single projection (Figure 3), providing experimental evidence of super-resolution.

4   Discussion

This paper demonstrates that high frequency objects can be resolved in obliquely pitched reconstruction planes for DBT. The range of pitches for which super-resolution is feasible is much broader than one would initially expect from the Central Slice Theorem. These analytical predictions were verified experimentally. In future work, the analytical model can be refined by simulating additional subtleties of the imaging system, such as focal spot blur [2] and noise [5, 6]. Also, filters with more parameters can be modeled, and the parameters can be optimized for different pitches.

Acknowledgments. We thank Roshan Karunamuni (UPenn) for his help assembling the goniometry stand, as well as Johnny Kuo, Susan Ng, and Peter Ringer (Real Time Tomography) for their assistance reconstructing the bar pattern images. The project described was supported by predoctoral training Grant No. W81XWH-11-1-0100 through the Department of Defense Breast Cancer Research Program. The content is solely the responsibility of the authors and does not necessarily represent the official views of the funding agency. Andrew D. A. Maidment is the chair of the Scientific Advisory Board of Real Time Tomography.

References

1. Acciavatti, R.J., Maidment, A.D.A.: Investigating the potential for super-resolution in digital breast tomosynthesis. In: Pelc, N.J., Samei, E., Nishikawa, R.M. (eds.) Proc. of SPIE, Medical Imaging 2011: Physics of Medical Imaging, vol. 7961, pp. 79615K-1–79615K-12. SPIE, Bellingham (2011)
2. Zhao, B., Zhao, W.: Three-dimensional linear system analysis for breast tomosynthesis. Med. Phys. 35(12), 5219–5232 (2008)
3. Albert, M., Beideck, D.J., Bakic, P.R., Maidment, A.D.A.: Aliasing effects in digital images of line-pair phantoms. Med. Phys. 29(8), 1716–1718 (2002)
4. Barrett, H.H., Swindell, W.: Radiological Imaging: The Theory of Image Formation, Detection, and Processing, New York (1981)
5. Barrett, H.H., Myers, K.J.: Foundations of Image Science. Bahaa E.A. Saleh, Hoboken (2004)
6. Hu, Y.-H., Masiar, M., Zhao, W.: Breast Structural Noise in Digital Breast Tomosynthesis and Its Dependence on Reconstruction Methods. In: Martí, J., Oliver, A., Freixenet, J., Martí, R. (eds.) IWDM 2010. LNCS, vol. 6136, pp. 598–605. Springer, Heidelberg (2010)

Improving Image Quality of Digital Breast Tomosynthesis by Artifact Reduction

Yao Lu, Heang-Ping Chan, Jun Wei, Lubomir Hadjiiski, and Chuan Zhou

Department of Radiology, University of Michigan, Ann Abor, MI
{yaol,chanhp,jvwei,lhadjisk,chuan}@med.umich.edu

Abstract. Digital breast tomosynthesis (DBT) is a new breast imaging modality for which the factors that affect image quality and methods for improvement are still under investigation. Various reconstruction artifacts arise from factors including the limited scan angular range, the limited detector field-of-view, the collimator shadows near the detector boundary, and the inaccurate estimation of path-length for x-rays near the breast periphery and the detector boundary. In this work, we studied the causes of some major reconstruction artifacts and developed correction methods for the artifacts by compensation for the tissue attenuation coefficient utilizing accurate geometric information of the DBT system and breast boundary. We will discuss the different artifacts and the correction methods in DBT reconstruction. The effectiveness of the methods will be demonstrated by comparison of reconstructed DBT images with and without artifact reduction.

Keywords: digital breast tomosynthesis, artifact reduction, ray-tracing, 3D breast surface, iterative reconstruction.

1 Introduction

Digital breast tomosynthesis (DBT) is an emerging breast imaging modality that provides quasi-three-dimensional (3D) volumetric information for the breast [1-3]. In DBT, a small number of low-dose x-ray projection view (PV) mammograms are acquired when the x-ray source is moved over a limited angular range. A stack of DBT slices are then reconstructed from the limited-angle PVs. The reconstructed DBT volume provides high-resolution 2D slices parallel to the detector plane and limited resolution in the depth direction, which depends on the tomographic angle. DBT has superior structural information of the breast compared to conventional mammography but inferior depth information compared to breast computed tomography.

A number of factors in DBT imaging may cause artifacts in the reconstructed images. The effects of these factors on lesion detection and the correction methods for the artifacts are still under investigation. These factors include the limited scan angular range, the limited detector field-of-view (FOV), the collimator shadows near the boundary of the detector, and the inaccurate estimation of path-length for x-rays near the breast periphery and the detector boundary. They may create artificial edges, discontinuities in the tissue voxel values, and overestimation or underestimation of linear

A.D.A. Maidment, P.R. Bakic, and S. Gavenonis (Eds.): IWDM 2012, LNCS 7361, pp. 745–752, 2012.
© Springer-Verlag Berlin Heidelberg 2012

attenuation coefficients around the boundary regions of the reconstructed DBT images. The artifacts affect the image quality and may impact the accuracy of detection and diagnosis of breast cancer in DBT.

In this work, we studied the causes of some major reconstruction artifacts and developed correction methods for these artifacts in DBT reconstruction to improve the image quality. The effectiveness of the methods will be demonstrated by comparison of reconstructed DBT images with and without artifact reduction.

2   Methods

2.1   DBT Systems

A General Electric (GE) GEN2 prototype DBT system at the University of Michigan was used to acquire DBT scans in this study. The distance from x-ray focal spot to the fulcrum of the rotation is 64 cm and the x-ray source rotation plane is parallel to the chest wall and perpendicular to the detector plane. The system has a CsI phosphor/a:Si active matrix flat panel digital detector with a matrix size of 1920 x 2304 pixels and a pixel pitch of 0.1 mm x 0.1 mm. The system uses a step-and-shoot design and acquires PV images from a total of 21 angles in 3° increments over a ±30° range in less than 8 seconds. The detector is stationary during the DBT scan. DBT images were reconstructed by the simultaneous algebraic reconstruction technique (SART). DBT imaging of human subjects was performed with IRB approval and written informed consent.

2.2   Artifact Correction

X-ray attenuation artifacts

In DBT reconstruction, estimation of the x-ray path-length through the breast tissue is an important step during backward and forward projections. Underestimation (or overestimation) of the x-ray path-length within the breast tissue will cause overestimation (or underestimation) of the tissue attenuation coefficients and thus artifacts appearing as bright (or dark) shadows in the reconstructed DBT slices. Underestimation of the path-length can occur near the top and bottom boundaries (perpendicular to the x-ray source motion direction) of the DBT reconstruction volume if the breast tissue that may extend beyond the reconstruction volume is not taken into consideration. This can occur for the pectoral muscle in the oblique views or in cases that the breast is larger than the FOV of the PVs.

Figure 1(a) shows the top view of the imaged volume intersected by a radial plane of the cone beam perpendicular to the X-Y (detector) plane and Figure 1(b) shows the side view of the radial plane in which the ray $\overline{SD}$ intersects the imaged volume at B and D. Consider that the breast tissue extends beyond the left boundary, the segment $\overline{AB}$ of the selected x-ray path is outside the imaged volume, while the x-ray intensity detected by the PV has actually been attenuated by the tissue along the entire path including $\overline{AB}$. If the x-ray attenuation outside the reconstruction volume is not properly estimated, the error will cause over- or underestimation of the tissue attenuation coefficients in voxels within the reconstructed volume along the ray, depending on the approximation used.

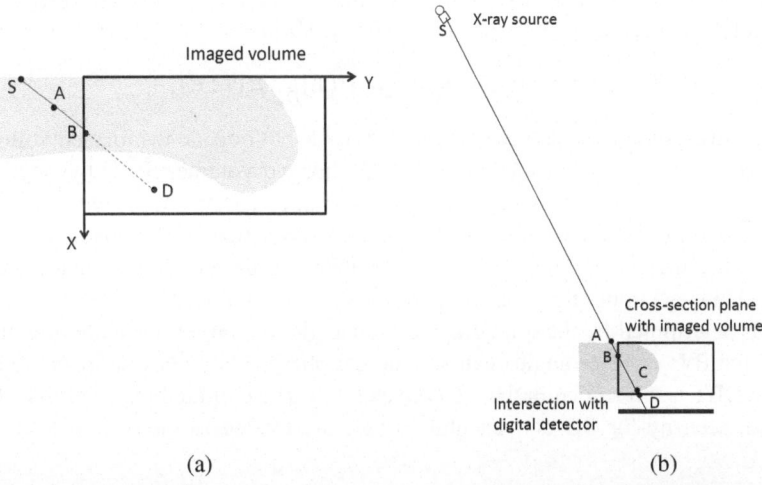

(a)   (b)

Fig. 1. Underestimation of path-length across pectoral muscles because of limited imaged volume (a) top view, for a PV where S is the x-ray source location, showing a radial plane of the cone beam perpendicular to the X-Y plane intersecting the breast volume, $\overline{SA}$ is the ray path in air above the breast volume, (b) side view showing the radial plane of the cone beam containing the ray $\overline{SD}$. The ray $\overline{SD}$ intersects the imaged volume at B and D, The segment $\overline{AB}$ and $\overline{CD}$ have to be correctly treated as tissue and air, respectively.

To calculate the x-ray attenuation, both the path-length and the tissue attenuation coefficient have to be estimated. The length of the segment $\overline{AB}$ can be estimated from from the imaging geometry. Since the tissue attenuation outside the imaged volume is not calculated in the reconstruction process, its attenuation value has to be estimated from the values of the adjacent voxels inside the imaged volume. Previously we used a fixed threshold method to determine whether a ray path is partially outside the boundary and estimated the tissue attenuation outside the imaged volume by averaging all voxel values along the path-length within the imaged volume, $\overline{BD}$, which caused underestimation of the voxel values within the reconstructed volume and created dark shadows in some cases [4]. In this study, a binary two-dimensional (2D) mask is first generated to identify the breast region on each PV by automated breast boundary detection. Using the imaging geometry of the DBT system, the 2D breast masks are back-projected to estimate the three-dimensional (3D) shape of the breast periphery[5]. Combining the breast periphery with the compressed breast thickness, the breast volume can then be defined by a 3D convex hull breast surface. At the anterior breast periphery, the intersection of the x-ray path with the 3D convex hull, the path segment $\overline{BC}$ in Figure 1(b), determines the path-length in the breast tissue.

At the left and right boundaries in Figure 1(b) of the imaged volume, the x-ray path outside the volume is treated as passing through tissue if the breast volume extends beyond the 3D convex hull at that intersection, or air if otherwise. If it is treated as tissue, the voxel value of the x-ray path outside the imaged volume will be estimated as the average of the current voxel values within the volume along the same x-ray path. The total attenuation calculation along the ray $\overline{AD}$ in Figure 1 is formulated as

$$\text{Total attenuation} = \int_{\overline{AB}} \bar{\mu}_{\overline{BC}} \, dl + \int_{\overline{BD}} \mu(l) \, dl,$$

where $\overline{AB}$ is the segment of the ray in the breast tissue but outside the imaged volume, volume, $\overline{BD}$ is the segment of the ray within the imaged volume, $\overline{BC}$ is the segment within the breast tissue, $\bar{\mu}_{\overline{BC}}$ is the average linear attenuation coefficient along the segment $\overline{BC}$ and $\mu(l)$ is the current linear attenuation coefficient of a voxel along the path $\overline{BD}$ in the imaged volume. $\overline{CD}$ is the segment in air due to the round breast periphery. How accurate the bottom part of the round breast periphery can be estimated is determined by the tomographic scan angle; the larger the angle, the more accurately the PVs at large angles can see the periphery. The breast periphery shape seen by the DBT is embedded in the 3D convex hull surface of the breast volume. The air gaps not seen by the 3D convex hull surface are treated as breast tissue so that $\overline{BC}=\overline{BD}$.

Collimator artifacts
Due to the changing angle of the incident x-ray beam, the collimator blades perpendicular to the x-ray source motion direction have to be adjusted to collimate the beam to the detector area at each angle. Small inaccuracy in the collimator position may leave a shadow at the top and/or bottom boundaries of the PV images. Each of the shadows will create a band of white voxels on each DBT slice along the edge of the steps due to the truncated FOV of the PVs, aggravating the truncated projection artifacts (discussed below). We developed an automated algorithm to detect the collimator shadows using edge detection methods. The collimator shadows, on each PV, are trimmed before the reconstruction.

Truncated projection artifacts
For each PV, the collimated x-ray beam only exposes the breast volume within the detector FOV. Due to the cone-beam geometry, the changing angular position of the x-ray source during PV acquisition, and the limited detector size, the breast tissue volume projected within the FOV of the detector varies from one PV to another and varies at different depths of the breast. If uncorrected, the reconstructed DBT slices will contain truncated projection artifacts (TPA) because, for a given PV updating, the voxel values beyond the FOV boundary cannot be updated, causing a discontinuity in voxel values at the FOV boundary, as illustrated in Figure 2. The TPAs appear as staircase strips at the FOV boundaries of the PVs perpendicular to the motion direction of the x-ray source. Previously we designed a diffusion-based TPA reduction method [6]. The method can reduce the TPAs well for cases that do not have large, dense tissue or object in the TPA region. However, in cases where the steps intersect a high density object, it may not approximate the structured background closely, thus

creating shadows around these objects that can propagate to other steps via diffusion. In this study, the diffusion-based correction method was refined, in which the difference between the updated voxel values inside the FOV and the un-updated voxel values is calculated along the edge of the FOV after updating with each PV. A compensating image is generated by smoothly diffusing the differences from the edge of the FOV over the entire step. The compensated image is then updated by the next PV. This method preserves the structured details of the DBT image over any number of iterations while reducing the TPAs.

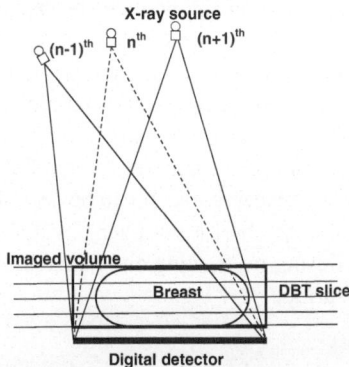

Fig. 2. The change of the field of view (FOV) causes the discontinuity of X-ray exposure across the boundary of the FOV, which results in discontinuity of linear attenuation coefficient updating

3   Results

Figures 3(a)-(c) show an example of a reconstructed DBT slice with artifact due to underestimation of path-lengths, the corrected image using the method in [4] and the corrected image using our current correction method, respectively. Figure 3(a) demonstrated that underestimation of path-lengths in the tissue due to truncation of x-ray path beyond the imaged volume created bright artifacts in the boundary region where the pectoral muscle extended beyond the reconstruction volume. Figure 3(b) shows that previous correction method could eliminate the bright region [4], but it might have overestimated the attenuation through breast tissue near the breast periphery and outside the top boundary of the imaged volume, thereby causing underestimation of the attenuation coefficients (dark shadow) at the top region within the imaged volume. The new method more closely estimated the attenuation of the breast tissue outside the top boundary thereby removing the dark shadow, and improving the visibility of the area, as seen in Figure 3(c).

Figures 4(a)-(c) show an example of a reconstructed DBT slice with TPAs, TPA-corrected image using the method in [6] (correction 1) and TPA-corrected image using the new correction method (correction 2), respectively. Figure 4(a) shows that without TPA correction, the step artifacts appear at both the top and bottom parts of the reconstructed image, which correspond to the discontinuity of voxel values across the FOV boundaries in the forward and backward PV updating directions. Figure 4(b) demonstrates that, with the method developed in [6], the step artifacts are largely eliminated, but the high density tissue at the top region creates a bright shadow. With the new correction method, both the TPA and the bright shadow are removed as shown in Figure 4(c). Note that the voxel values along the boundary of the pectoral muscle at the top and the dense tissue at the bottom of the slice are more continuous after TPA reduction. Figure 5(a)-(b) show selected line profiles along the yellow lines (a) at the top part and (b) at the bottom part in Figure 4. As evident from the line profiles, both the method in [6] and the new correction method reduced the step artifacts. However, the new corrected method maintained the background intensity while the previous method increased the background intensity (see Figure 5(a)) when TPA intersected a structure that had very different intensity than the background. Table 1 shows that both correction methods reduced the average step height by above 90% at the top part and by above 95% at the bottom part.

Figures 6(a)-(b) show an example of a reconstructed DBT slice with attenuation artifact and the corrected image, respectively. It can be seen that overestimation of path-lengths caused a darker rim at the breast periphery, which was reduced by improving the path-length estimation during ray-tracing and hence the tissue attenuation by using the 3D convex hull breast surface.

Table 1. Average step height along the selected line profiles (the yellow lines) at the top part and the bottom part in Figure 5

Average Step height	No correction	Correction 1	Correction 2
Top	93.8	7.8	6.7
Bottom	187	7.3	9.7

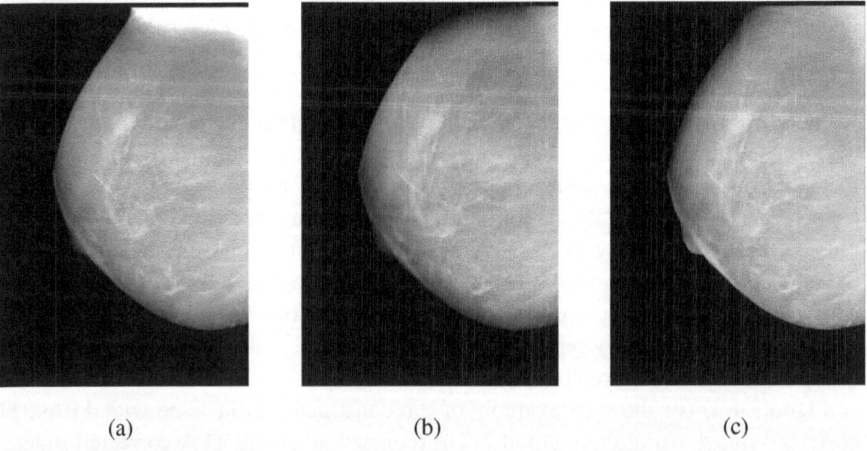

(a)   (b)   (c)

Fig. 3. Reconstructed DBT slice with one SART iteration (a) with underestimation of the path-length at the top reconstruction volume boundary, (b) with correction method developed in [4], and (c) with correction method developed in this study

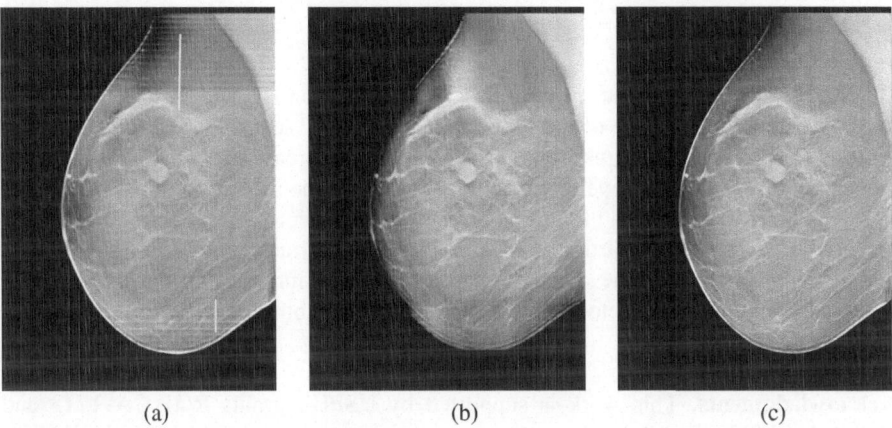

(a)   (b)   (c)

Fig. 4. Reconstructed DBT slice with five SART iterations (a) with no truncated projection artifact correction, (b) with correction method developed in [6] (correction 1), and (c) with correction method developed in this study (correction 2)

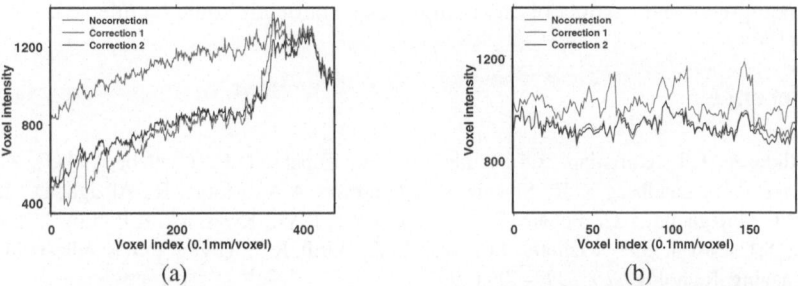

(a)   (b)

Fig. 5. Line profiles along the yellow lines (a) at the top part and (b) at the bottom part in Figure 4

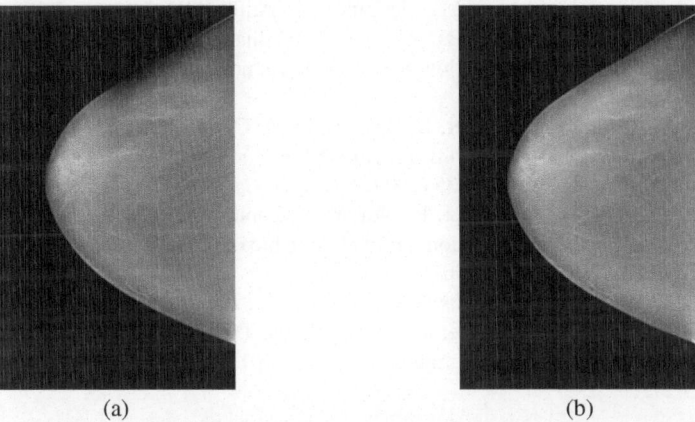

(a)   (b)

Fig. 6. Reconstructed DBT slice with five SART iterations (a) with overestimation of the path-length and (b) with 3D convex hull breast surface information for ray-tracing

4   Discussion

Our study demonstrated that many artifacts can appear on DBT reconstructed images due to the limited coverage of the breast volume in DBT scans and other factors. The artifacts can affect image quality and the visibility of breast structures and potential lesions. In this study, we developed methods to correct the reconstruction artifacts due to the imaging geometry and breast shape. The results demonstrated that our methods can effectively reduce the artifacts. Reduction of the artifacts can improve the image quality of DBT, reduce the distraction to radiologists interpreting the images, and potentially may improve detection and assessment of subtle breast lesions that are in the areas with artifacts.

Acknowledgments. This work is supported by USPHS grants RO1 CA91713 and RO1 CA151443. The digital breast tomosynthesis system was developed by the GE Global Research Group, with input and some revisions from the University of Michigan investigators, through the Biomedical Research Partnership (USPHS grant CA91713, PI: Paul Carson, Ph.D.) collaboration. The content of this paper does not necessarily reflect the position of the funding agencies and no official endorsement of any equipment and product of any companies mentioned should be inferred.

Reference

1. Niklason, L.T., Christian, B.T., Niklason, L.E., Kopans, D.B., Castleberry, D.E., Opsahl-Ong, B.H., Landberg, C.E., Slanetz, P.J., Giardino, A.A., Moore, R., Albagli, D., DeJule, M.C., Fitzgerald, F.C., Fobare, D.F., Giambattista, B.W., Kwasnick, R.F., Liu, J., Lubowski, S.J., Possin, G.E., Richotte, J.F., Wei, C.Y., Wirth, R.F.: Digital tomosynthesis in breast imaging. Radiology 205, 399–406 (1997)
2. Kopans, D.B.: Novel approaches and newer imaging modalities. Course 815: Problem-solving Breast Imaging. RSNA Program 2001, 97 (2001)
3. Wu, T., Stewart, A., Stanton, M., McCauley, T., Phillips, W., Kopans, D.B., Moore, R.H., Eberhard, J.W., Opsahl-Ong, B., Niklason, L., Williams, M.B.: Tomographic mammography using a limited number of low-dose cone-beam projection images. Medical Physics 30, 365–380 (2003)
4. Zhang, Y., Chan, H.P., Sahiner, B., Wei, J., Zhou, C., Hadjiiski, L.M.: Artifact reduction methods for truncated projections in iterative breast tomosynthesis reconstruction. J. Comput. Assist. Tomogr. 33, 426–435 (2009)
5. Zhang, Y., Chan, H.-P., Sahiner, B., Wu, Y.-T., Zhou, C., Ge, J., Wei, J., Hadjiiski, L.M.: Application of boundary detection information in breast tomosynthesis reconstruction. Medical Physics 34, 3603–3613 (2007)
6. Lu, Y., Chan, H.P., Wei, J., Hadjiiski, L., Zhou, C.: Improving Image Quality of Iterative Reconstruction for Digital Breast Tomosynthesis: Diffusion-Based Truncated Projection Artifact Reduction. RSNA Program Book SSE23 (2011)

Automatic Volumetric Glandularity Assessment from Full Field Digital Mammograms

André Gooßen, Harald S. Heese, and Klaus Erhard

Philips Research, Röntgenstr. 24-26, 22335 Hamburg, Germany
{andre.goossen,harald.heese,klaus.erhard}@philips.com

Abstract. Estimation of breast density suffers from high inter-observer variability. A fully automated solution for objective and consistent assessment of breast density from full field digital mammography (FFDM) data is presented. For the computation of glandularity a region of interest (ROI) with a corresponding height model is automatically extracted from the mammograms. Assessment of adipose and glandular tissue volumes is performed by means of calibration data. Volumetric breast density is finally computed as the fraction of glandular tissue volume to overall breast volume with respect to the ROI. The fully automated approach provides volumetric breast density estimates that show strong non-linear correlation with the manual reference ($R^2 = 0.80$) and high intra-patient consistency ($R \in [0.92, 0.97]$) among mammograms of different orientation or laterality.

Keywords: volumetric breast density, glandularity, breast cancer risk assessment, digital mammography.

1 Introduction

Breast density is associated with an increased risk of developing breast cancer [16,12,1]. Moreover, detecting early stages of breast cancer in women with dense breasts is more difficult than in women with mainly adipose breast tissue. In [11], for example, it has been shown that breast density is a major risk factor for interval breast cancer, i.e. women with dense breast tissue have an increased risk that a developing breast cancer is missed during routine screening. Recently, regulation authorities have acted by requiring the enlisting of breast density in the mammographic report with a recommendation for subsequent ultra-sound or MRI examinations for women with dense breasts [15].

In contrast to *mammographic percent density* as a pure area measure, *volumetric breast density* or more precise breast composition [7] estimates the volume fraction of glandular tissue within the complete breast tissue either expressed in a percentage or an actual volume. Thus, *mammographic percent density* and *volumetric breast density* are not interchangeable [8]. Nevertheless, Kontos et al. found a quadratic relation between *mammographic percent density* estimated via Cumulus [2] and *volumetric breast density* estimated via Quantra [9].

A.D.A. Maidment, P.R. Bakic, and S. Gavenonis (Eds.): IWDM 2012, LNCS 7361, pp. 753–760, 2012.
© Springer-Verlag Berlin Heidelberg 2012

The assessment of volumetric breast density is based on a physical model of the mammographic image formation process. Several methods for estimating volumetric breast density have been proposed that either require the simultaneous acquisition of the breast with a calibration phantom [3] or try to estimate the attenuation of an adipose pixel value directly from the image [5,14].

In the following, we present a method for the fully-automatic assessment of volumetric breast density and breast composition that is reference free and is based on a 3D breast model and a calibration of linear attenuation coefficients for the two major tissue types found within the breast. The proposed method has been validated on clinical data of 334 patients.

2   Methods and Materials

The suggested approach for volumetric breast density assessment has been developed using pre-processed data ($0.085 \times 0.085 \, \text{mm}^2$ resolution, 2084×2800 pixel matrix) from Philips MammoDiagnost DR 1.0 X-ray mammography systems (Philips Medical Systems DMC GmbH, Hamburg, Germany) as input data.

The applied pre-processing comprises interpolation over defect pixels, offset and gain correction. The images have been collected in a proprietary image file format using anonymized headers, thus removing the patient information but preserving all image acquisition related parameters.

2.1   Image and Ground Truth Data

Image data of 100 patients (age: 29 - 84 years, median age: 50 years) have been collected from 4 different diagnostic institutions between July 2007 and August 2009. For each patient, bilateral standard views, i.e. cranio-caudal (CC) and medio-lateral oblique (MLO), were acquired. Only patients that had unsuspicious findings and no implants were included in the collection. Distribution of clinical density classification was chosen to adequately represent all categories (ACR I: 24; ACR II: 26; ACR III: 38; ACR IV: 12). Each image was rated by 5 readers on a 10 percent scale between $0 - 100\%$.

Additional image data in terms of the bilateral views of 245 patients (age: 34-89, median age: 60 years) have been collected from 2 different diagnostic institutions and were used for intra-patient consistency checking.

2.2   System Calibration

In order to derive physical measurements from a digital mammography system we calibrate the system using material with known attenuation extending on prior work [6]. Phantom studies on different mammography systems show that the measurements are stable. We thus calibrate the algorithm once for each type of system and do not need to perform a dedicated calibration on each installed clinical system.

The observed intensity $\mathcal{I}$, measured by the detector, depends on the linear attenuation coefficients μ_{adp} and μ_{gland} of adipose and glandular tissue, respectively, and on the initial non-attenuated intensity $\mathcal{I}_0$ according to Beer's law

$$\mathcal{I} = \mathcal{I}_0 \cdot e^{-\mu_{\mathrm{adp}} \cdot (1-g)h - \mu_{\mathrm{gland}} \cdot g \cdot h} \quad \rightarrow \quad \mu = \frac{\ln(\mathcal{I}_0/\mathcal{I})}{h} \; , \tag{1}$$

where h denotes the total thickness of the radiated object and $g \in [0, 1]$ denotes the glandularity, i.e. the fraction of glandular tissue along the beam path. In practice, we observe a total attenuation μ that results from the attenuation of the composite tissue along the beam path.

For calibration of the attenuation coefficients a set of dedicated step wedge phantoms (cf. Figure 1a) composed of two materials with attenuations equivalent to adipose and glandular breast tissue was used (CIRS Inc., Norfolk, VA).

By help of these phantoms effective linear attenuation coefficients have been derived for all combinations of specified tube voltages $U \in 23, 24, \ldots, 35\,\mathrm{kV}$ and tissue heights $h \in 10, 20, \ldots, 120\,\mathrm{mm}$. Using biquadratic regression allows to represent $\mu_{\mathrm{adp}}(U, h)$ and $\mu_{\mathrm{gland}}(U, h)$ as polynomials,

$$\mu(U, h) = a_0 + a_1 U + a_2 U^2 + a_3 h + a_4 h^2 + a_5 U h \; . \tag{2}$$

With an average deviation of 1.5 % for adipose and 2.0 % for glandular tissue from the measured attenuation, a precise and compact model for the attenuation of breast tissue within the specified system boundaries has been derived. Figure 1b depicts the models for μ_{adp} and μ_{gland} in a combined plot.

2.3   Tissue Segmentation

Typical mammograms contain four different major regions (background, uncompressed breast tissue, compressed breast tissue, pectoral muscle – cf. Figure 2a) that need to be identified in preprocessing steps in order to extract a region of interest (ROI) for volumetric density estimation. According to the BI-RADS atlas for mammography [4], the pectoral muscle should not be included in the evaluation of breast density.

We detect the skinline using a Gauss-Deriche filter followed by a connected component analysis [6], and classify the regions with high intensities as background. Subsequently, we extract the pectoral muscle outline by directional gradient filtering [17] and a Hough transform through local feature points of plausible orientation [6].

2.4   Breast Height Modelling

Volumetric breast density assessment relies on the exact height of the breast, i.e. the thickness of irradiated tissue. Hence, it has to be modelled using prior knowledge and assumptions about the tissue thickness. Observations indicate that the thickness of the peripheral tissue (cf. Figure 2a) follows a semi-circular behavior. Hence, similar to [13], the breast height $h(x, y)$ is modelled as a block

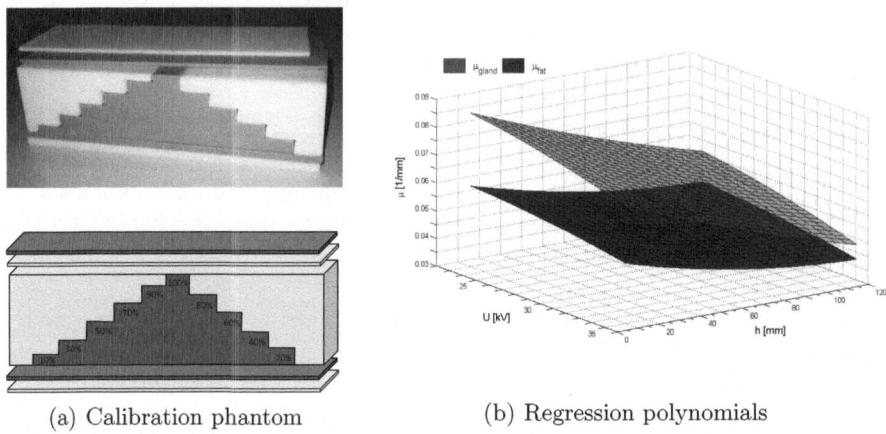

(a) Calibration phantom   (b) Regression polynomials

Fig. 1. System calibration. (a) A calibration phantom consisting of adipose and glandular tissue equivalent material, assembled in a step wedge. With a constant height, the phantom contains steps with 0, 10, ..., 100 % of either tissue type. In order to cover the full range of possible tissue heights the step wedges exist in different sizes, and additional thin plates can be used to measure intermediate heights. (b) Results of a biquadratic regression through the measured effective linear attenuation coefficients for adipose and glandular tissue equivalent material plotted against tube voltage U and tissue height h. The polynomials serve as model for adipose and glandular breast tissue attenuation at a given voltage and tissue height.

of compressed tissue with constant height h_0 in the interior, and by semi-circles of matching diameter perpendicular to the skinline in the periphery, i.e.

$$h(x,y) = \begin{cases} 2\sqrt{d_s(x,y)(h_0 - d_s(x,y))}, & d_s(x,y) < 0.5h_0 \\ h_0, & d_s(x,y) \geq 0.5h_0 \end{cases}, \qquad (3)$$

where h_0 is the compression height (i.e. distance between compression paddle and detector cover), and $d_s(x,y)$ is the distance to the extracted skinline.

2.5   Breast Composition Estimation

Using the calibration polynomials for μ_{adp} and μ_{gland} (cp. Eq. (2)), it is possible to directly derive the volumetric fraction of glandular tissue, also called glandularity or volumetric breast density. We avoid estimating attenuation references from the image [5,14], since there are many cases where such an approach is deteriorated. Such comprise positioning artifacts (skin folds or dips – cf. Figure 2b) or very dense breasts, where any ray through the breast necessarily passes through glandular tissue (cf. Figure 2c). In our approach we neglect uncompressed peripheral breast tissue with a height $h(x,y) < 0.5h_0$ of less than half of the compressed breast height according to our height model. This is due to the fact that the influence of the skin tissue (with constant height) as well as errors

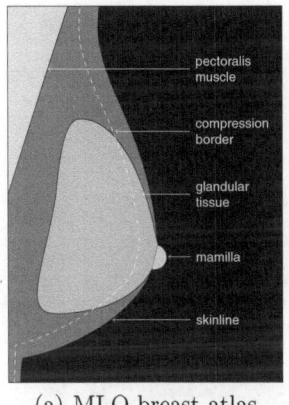 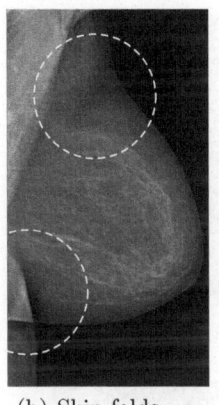 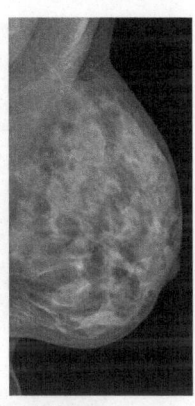

(a) MLO breast atlas   (b) Skin folds   (c) Dense breast

Fig. 2. Modelling the breast. (a) Atlas of an MLO view of the breast with the relevant regions. The peripheral regions are separated by a dashed line. Frequently occuring examples of failure for estimating an adipose reference value comprise (b) skin folds and (c) very dense breasts resulting in an under- and overestimation of μ_{adp}, respectively.

in the height model have stronger influence on the estimation for small overall tissue heights.

For each position we compute the actual tissue attenuation $\mu(h(x,y))$ as well as the calibrated attenuation values $\mu_{\mathrm{adp}}(U, h(x,y))$ and $\mu_{\mathrm{gland}}(U, h(x,y))$. In order to deal with outlier values in the attenuation map, we clamp the glandularity for each position to the interval $[0\%, 100\%]$, i.e. by defining the attenuation

$$
\hat{\mu}(h(x,y)) = \begin{cases} \mu_{\mathrm{adp}}(U, h(x,y)), & \text{if } \mu(U, h(x,y)) < \mu_{\mathrm{adp}}(U, h(x,y)) \\ \mu_{\mathrm{gland}}(U, h(x,y)), & \text{if } \mu(U, h(x,y)) > \mu_{\mathrm{gland}}(U, h(x,y)) \\ \mu(h(x,y)), & \text{else} \end{cases} \tag{4}
$$

The local glandularity $g(x,y)$ is given by

$$
g(x,y) = \frac{\hat{\mu}(U, h(x,y)) - \mu_{\mathrm{adp}}(U, h(x,y))}{\mu_{\mathrm{gland}}(U, h(x,y)) - \mu_{\mathrm{adp}}(U, h(x,y))} \; , \tag{5}
$$

and the corresponding glandular tissue volume, $V_{\mathrm{gland}}(x,y)$, is given by

$$
V_{\mathrm{gland}}(x,y) = g(x,y) \cdot h(x,y) \cdot p_x \cdot p_y \; , \tag{6}
$$

with p_x and p_y denoting the pixel spacing in horizontal and vertical direction, respectively. We derive the fraction of glandular tissue by summation over all individual contributions and by relating it to the total breast volume, i.e.

$$
g = \frac{\sum_{\Omega} g(x,y) \cdot h(x,y)}{\sum_{\Omega} h(x,y)} \; , \text{ where } \Omega = \left\{ (x,y)^{\mathsf{T}} \;\middle|\; h(x,y) \ge \frac{h_0}{2} \right\} \; . \tag{7}
$$

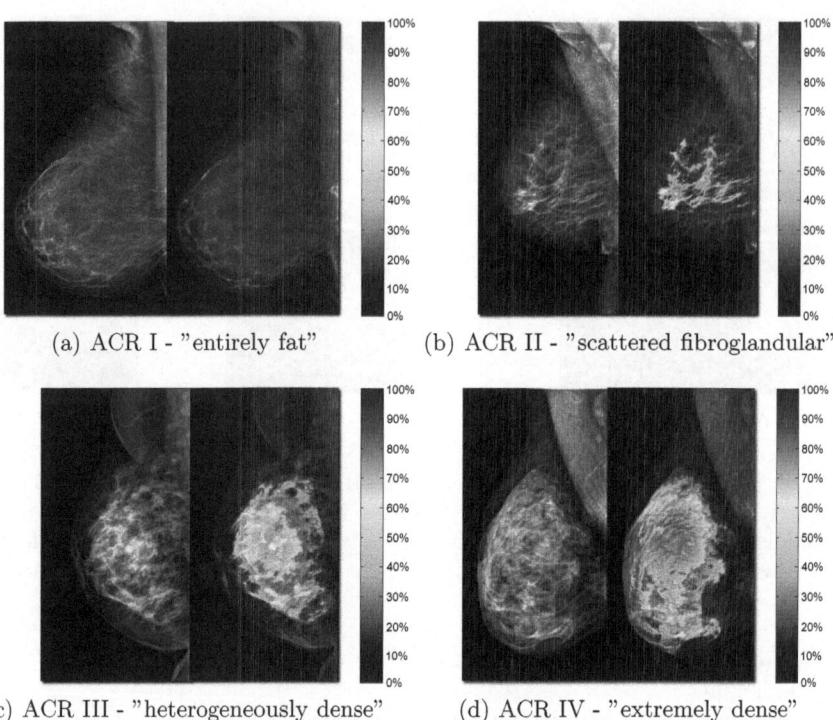

(a) ACR I - "entirely fat"   (b) ACR II - "scattered fibroglandular"

(c) ACR III - "heterogeneously dense"   (d) ACR IV - "extremely dense"

Fig. 3. Mammograms of the four ACR classes [4] overlaid with their corresponding colour-coded volumetric density maps (shown for $h > 0.2h_0$)

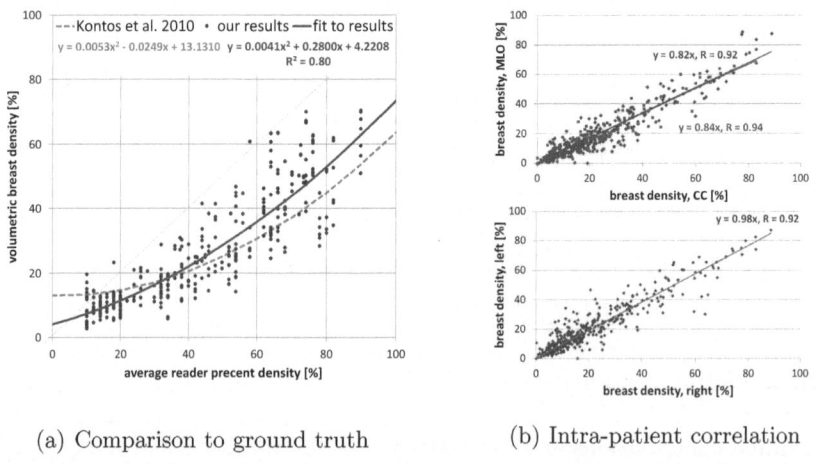

(a) Comparison to ground truth   (b) Intra-patient correlation

Fig. 4. *Volumetric breast density* compared against (a) *percent density* scores for 82 patients determined by human readers via visual inspection only and (b) Intra-patient comparison of 245 patients for MLO and CC view as well as left and right laterality

3   Results and Discussion

Figure 3 depicts four example mammograms together with an overlay of the glandularity map. The map is colour-coded between blue and red, reflecting 0 % to 100 %, respectively. Note the different spread and density of the tissue for the four categories ranging from "entirely fat" to "extremely dense".

In addition to qualitative visual assessment, we compare the results of automatic *volumetric breast density* assessment against averaged percent density ratings of 5 readers (cf. Figure 4a). Following the assumption of Kontos et al. [9], the dependency has been modelled by a second order polynomial. It is evident that, with a maximum of 70.4%, *volumetric breast density* does not reach highest *percent density* values. Generally *percent density* is overestimated by the reader [10], especially for high *percent density* values. With a regression of $R^2 = 0.80$ the agreement is significant, but still deviations of up to 25% occur between human readers and the automatically computed glandularity. Comparing the results to Kontos et al. [9], it is evident that the regression derived similar coefficients, however, with a slightly steeper regression curve.

Figure 4b evaluates the robustness of the proposed method by comparing computed glandularity values for the two mammographic views (MLO and CC) as well as for the two lateralities (left and right breast). All correlations range between $R = 0.92$ and $R = 0.97$. The mean volumetric breast density in the patient population was computed as 22.3%, which is in accordance with the previously reported mean density value 21.9% of Kontos et al. [9] using $Quantra^{TM}$.

Regarding the excellent intra-patient correlation of results among different lateralities or views, we conclude that the method yields very reproducible *volumetric breast density* values, which are in accordance with comparable methods [3,9]. The results show a strong non-linear relationship with estimated *percent density* scores of human readers. Since the clinical data originated from a diagnostic rather than from a screening setting the distribution of densities might significantly differ for an actual screening population.

4   Conclusion and Outlook

We presented a method for volumetric breast density assessment that shows excellent stability in terms of correlation for left and right breasts as well as MLO and CC views. These results fit very well with the results of manual assessment by experienced clinical readers. With the ability to compute the real volume of glandular tissue, the method is well suited for a screening workflow, assisting the selection of the appropriate screening interval and additional modalities.

Computation of volumetric breast density assessment requires the estimation of the breast composition into adipose and glandular tissue compartments. This information can only be estimated from one single mammogram by introducing additional information, such as a model for the breast thickness. Therefore, future work will address the accurate measurement of breast thickness with spectral mammography, where two mammograms are available for a decomposition into the adipose and glandular tissue volumes.

References

1. Boyd, N.F., Martin, L.J., Rommens, J.M., et al.: Mammographic density: a heritable risk factor for breast cancer. Methods Mol. Biol. 472, 343–360 (2009)
2. Byng, J.W., Boyd, N.F., Fishell, E., et al.: The quantitative analysis of mammographic densities. Phys. Med. Biol. 39(10), 1629–1638 (1994)
3. Diffey, J., Hufton, A., Astley, S., Mercer, C., Maxwell, A.: Estimating Individual Cancer Risks in the UK National Breast Screening Programme: A Feasibility Study. In: Krupinski, E.A. (ed.) IWDM 2008. LNCS, vol. 5116, pp. 469–476. Springer, Heidelberg (2008)
4. D'Orsi, C.J., Bassett, L.W., Berg, W.A., et al.: BI-RADS: Mammography. In: D'Orsi, C.J., Mendelson, E.B., Ikeda, D.M., et al. (eds.) Breast Imaging Reporting and Data System: ACR BI-RADS - Breast Imaging Atlas, 4th edn. American College of Radiology, Reston (2003)
5. van Engeland, S., Snoeren, P.R., Huisman, H., et al.: Volumetric breast density estimation from full-field digital mammograms. IEEE Trans. Med. Imaging 25(3), 273–282 (2006)
6. Heese, H., Erhard, K., Gooßen, A.: Fully-automatic breast density assessment from full field digital mammograms. In: Proc Workshop on Breast Image Analysis, pp. 113–120 (2011)
7. Highnam, R., Brady, S.M., Yaffe, M.J., Karssemeijer, N., Harvey, J.: Robust Breast Composition Measurement - Volpara^{TM}. In: Martí, J., Oliver, A., Freixenet, J., Martí, R. (eds.) IWDM 2010. LNCS, vol. 6136, pp. 342–349. Springer, Heidelberg (2010)
8. Jeffreys, M., Harvey, J., Highnam, R.: Comparing a New Volumetric Breast Density Method (Volpara^{TM}) to Cumulus. In: Martí, J., Oliver, A., Freixenet, J., Martí, R. (eds.) IWDM 2010. LNCS, vol. 6136, pp. 408–413. Springer, Heidelberg (2010)
9. Kontos, D., Bakic, P.R., Acciavatti, R.J., Conant, E.F., Maidment, A.D.A.: A Comparative Study of Volumetric and Area-Based Breast Density Estimation in Digital Mammography: Results from a Screening Population. In: Martí, J., Oliver, A., Freixenet, J., Martí, R. (eds.) IWDM 2010. LNCS, vol. 6136, pp. 378–385. Springer, Heidelberg (2010)
10. Makaronidis, J., Berks, M., Sergeant, J., et al.: Assessment of breast density: reader performance using synthetic mammographic images. In: Proc. SPIE Med Imaging 2011, vol. 7966, p. 796603. SPIE (2011)
11. Mandelson, M.T., Oestreicher, N., Porter, P.L., et al.: Breast density as a predictor of mammographic detection: comparison of interval- and screen-detected cancers. J. Natl. Cancer Inst. 92(13), 1081–1087 (2000)
12. Saftlas, A.F., Hoover, R.N., Brinton, L.A., et al.: Mammographic densities and risk of breast cancer. Cancer 67(11), 2833–2838 (1991)
13. Snoeren, P.R., Karssemeijer, N.: Thickness correction of mammographic images by means of a global parameter model of the compressed breast. IEEE Trans. Med. Imaging 23(7), 799–806 (2004)
14. Tromans, C., Brady, M.: An Alternative Approach to Measuring Volumetric Mammographic Breast Density. In: Astley, S.M., Brady, M., Rose, C., Zwiggelaar, R. (eds.) IWDM 2006. LNCS, vol. 4046, pp. 26–33. Springer, Heidelberg (2006)
15. U.S. Connecticut Senate (ed.): Bill No. 458. Public Act No. 09-41 (2009)
16. Wolfe, J.N.: Breast patterns as an index of risk for developing breast cancer. AJR Am. J. Roentgenol. 126(6), 1130–1137 (1976)
17. Zhou, C.A., Wei, J., Chan, H.P., et al.: Computerized image analysis: Texture-field orientation method for pectoral muscle identification on MLO-view mammograms. Med. Phys. 37(5), 2289–2299 (2010)

A Breast Density-Dependent Power-Law Model for Digital Mammography

James G. Mainprize[1] and Martin J. Yaffe[1,2]

[1] Sunnybrook Research Institute, Sunnybrook Health Sciences Centre, Toronto, Canada
james.mainprize@sri.utoronto.ca
[2] Department of Medical Biophysics, University of Toronto, Canada

Abstract. In mammograms, the parenchymal patterns have been described by a Wiener power spectrum that has an inverse power-law shape at low spatial frequencies. Its frequency content can then be described by the parameter, β. Previously, we have shown that there is some dependence of β on the relative amount of fibroglandular tissue or volumetric breast density (VBD). Here, we develop a mathematical model that simulates the distributions of β as a function of VBD. This model will be useful for clinically-relevant task-based image analyses that incorporate realistic tissue backgrounds.

Keywords: parenchymal texture, anatomic noise, power spectra, cascaded systems model.

1 Introduction

The detectability of lesions in a mammogram is generally reduced by the "background" image signal arising from the complex parenchymal and stromal structures in the breast. Others [1] have shown that this "anatomic noise" reduces the lesion detection accuracy compared to a uniform noise background. Anatomic noise textures typically display a power spectral content that decreases on a log-log graph with a slope, $-\beta$. It has been shown that $\beta \sim 3$ for mammographic backgrounds [2].

Several techniques exist to simulate mammographic backgrounds (e.g. [3–5]). For example, we have a developed a simple model that has a nearly analytic form for a cascaded systems model of mammographic backgrounds that can be incorporated into task-based model observer studies [6].

Any of these models have the capability of varying the texture by means of changing β along with all of the other parameters describing the compressed breast (e.g tissue composition). The selection of the value for β in these models will affect image quality [7]. The question that is raised is, how should β be modeled to represent conditions in a real mammogram?

In a recent retrospective clinical study [8] of 2762 de-identified screening mammograms, the volumetric breast density (VBD) and β were measured. Volumetric breast density was measured using an in-house software package (Cumulus V) [9]. The power spectral parameter β was measured using techniques similar to those

A.D.A. Maidment, P.R. Bakic, and S. Gavenonis (Eds.): IWDM 2012, LNCS 7361, pp. 761–768, 2012.
© Springer-Verlag Berlin Heidelberg 2012

published by other authors [10, 11]. It was found that there was a trend between β and volumetric breast density as shown in Fig. 1. It was estimated that approximately 25% of the variation seen in β could be explained by differences in breast density. It appeared that β increases as VBD increases until a plateau is reached at roughly 40% VBD.

We have previously developed an analytic cascaded systems model for predicting the Wiener spectra for simulated power-law backgrounds [6]. Here, we extend the model to include β dependence on VBD and to compare image statistics of the prediction with those of clinical mammograms. Such a clinically-relevant model will be useful in the evaluation of image quality for task-based observer analysis.

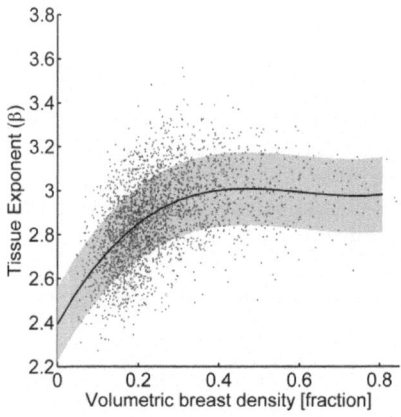

Fig. 1. A scatter plot of tissue power exponent β versus measured volumetric breast density measured in screening mammograms. The solid curve is the polynomial fit (Eq. (5)) and the gray region is the approximate 50% confidence interval.

2   Model

The model used here follows the approach given in Mainprize *et al.* [6] This model assumes the breast is a rectangular tissue block. The transmission through a uniformly compressed heterogeneous breast reaching any given point (x,y) on the detector is modeled by the Beer's law expression for monoenergetic x-rays

$$m(x,y) = \exp\left(-\left(\mu_{\text{fat}} + \Delta\mu\tilde{\theta}(x,y)\right)t\right) \tag{1}$$

where μ_{fat} is the linear attenuation of breast adipose tissue, $\Delta\mu = \mu_{\text{fib}} - \mu_{\text{fat}}$ is the difference in linear attenuation between fibroglandular and fat tissue, t is the compressed breast thickness, and $\tilde{\theta}(x,y)$ represents a random variable that is a map of the texture of the mammographic background. To simulate mammographic texture, $\theta_0(x,y)$ is generated from a uniform distribution and filtered by

$$F(f) = \frac{1}{\left(1 + \dfrac{f}{f_0}\right)^{\beta(v)/2}},$$ (2)

where $\beta(v)$ is the power-law parameter as a function of breast density, $v \in [0,1]$, and $f_0=0.05$ mm^{-1}. This yields a random structured background, $\theta_F(x,y)$. To control the range of attenuation values, the image is rescaled such that $\theta(x,y) = (\theta_F(x,y) - \bar{\theta}_F)/b + \bar{\theta}_F$, where b is a normalization constant. The selection of b is somewhat arbitrary but it will dictate the scale of the tissue variation seen in an image. A convenient form was selected where $b = 2w\sigma_{\theta_F}$, and

$$\sigma_{\theta_F}^2 = 2\pi\sigma_{\theta_0}^2 p^2 \int_0^{f_{max}} \frac{1}{\left(1 + \dfrac{f}{f_0}\right)^{\beta}} df,$$ (3)

giving a b that spans $\pm w$ standard deviations of $\theta_F(x,y)$.

If $\theta_0(x,y)$ is generated from a uniform distribution, this yields a filtered image with a mean value $\bar{\theta}_F = 0.5$. To generate a different tissue fraction, the following empirical transformation is used

$$\tilde{\theta}(x,y,v) = \theta(x,y)^a,$$ (4)

where $a = \ln(v)/\ln(0.5)$. Note that here we have assumed that linear attenuation (Eq. (1)) is linear with breast density, v. A more appropriate model would include the mass density changes of the tissue with, $\mu = (\mu_{fat} + v\Delta\mu)/\left(\dfrac{v}{\rho_{flb}} + \dfrac{1-v}{\rho_{fat}}\right)$, but the model equations would become much more complicated.

From our clinical study [8], the relationship for $\beta(v)$ can be partly described by a third-order polynomial fit of the form,

$$\beta(v) = p_3 v^3 + p_2 v^2 + p_1 v + p_0,$$ (5)

with $p_3=3.19$, $p_2=-5.8$, $p_1=3.33$ and $p_0=2.39$, which fit over a range of $0<v<0.82$. This yields the mean β as a function of breast density. If a clinically relevant distribution is required, β can be selected as a random variable from a distribution model that encompasses the variation seen in Fig. 1.

Following an approach similar to Mainprize et al. [6], an analytic form of the cascaded signal and noise equations can be generated for task-based analysis as a function of breast density. Briefly, the latent total noise power spectrum $S(f)$ exiting the breast can be described by

$$S(f) = \langle\bar{m}\rangle\Phi_0 + \Phi_0 var_\theta\{\bar{m}\} + \Phi_0^2 T_m(f),$$ (6)

where $\langle\bar{m}\rangle$ is the mean transmission (Eq. (1)) through the breast based on VBD averaged over all possible values of θ and breast thickness, and Φ_0 is the incident photon fluence, $var_\theta\{\bar{m}\}$ is the variance of the transmission through the tissue over all possible values of the random variable θ, and $T_m(f)$ is the Fourier transform of the spatial covariance of m. Following Mainprize et al.,

$$T_m(f) = \left|\frac{\partial m}{\partial \theta}\right|^2 \frac{\sigma_{\theta_0}^2 p^2}{\left(1 + \frac{f}{f_0}\right)^\beta}, \tag{7}$$

and assuming $\mathrm{var}_\theta\{\overline{m}\}$ is small, then

$$S(f) \approx \langle \overline{m} \rangle \Phi_0 + \frac{\langle \overline{m} \theta^{a-1} \rangle^2 \Phi_0 \Delta \mu^2 t^2 \sigma_{\theta_0}^2 p^2}{b^2} \frac{\Phi_0^2}{\left(1 + \frac{f}{f_0}\right)^\beta}, \tag{8}$$

where $\sigma_{\theta_0}^2$ is the expected variance in original random map $\theta_0(x, y)$, and p is the detector element pitch. For simplicity we assume that the expectations reduce to

$$\langle \overline{m} \rangle \approx \exp(-(\mu_{\mathrm{fat}} + \Delta \mu \overline{\theta_F})t), \text{ and} \tag{9}$$

$$\langle \overline{m} \theta^{a-1} \rangle \approx \langle \overline{m} \rangle \overline{\theta_F}^{a-1}. \tag{10}$$

This provides a predictive model that can be applied to image quality analysis such as evaluating detection tasks through model observers. Combined with the clinically relevant relationship between VBD and β, the performance of an imaging system can be evaluated both analytically and through simulation over a broad range of breast types.

To help validate the model, a simulation of mammograms was also created as follows:

1. A random uniform deviate map in the range [0,1] of size $2N \times 2N$ was generated and subsequently filtered by a radial filter of the form in Eq. (2). The mean value is 0.5 and the variance is equal to $\sigma_{\theta_0}^2 = 1/12$. Here, $N=512$.
2. To avoid edge effects and aliasing, only the central $N \times N$ region was extracted, called $\theta_{F_{ij}}$. Here, ij denote the pixel coordinates for a discretized image.
3. A normalized tissue map was created $\theta_{ij} = \left(\theta_{F_{ij}} - \frac{1}{2}\right)/b + \frac{1}{2}$, where $b = 8\sigma_{\theta_F}$. Unphysical values of $\theta_{ij} < 0$ or $\theta_{ij} > 1$ were truncated. Careful selection of b is required to minimize effects due to this truncation.
4. A tissue map with an appropriate density is created: $\tilde{\theta}_{ij} = \left(\theta_{ij}\right)^a$.
5. A transmission image is created using the attenuation equation, $M_{ij} = \exp(-(\mu_{\mathrm{fat}} + \Delta \mu \tilde{\theta}_{ij})t)$.
6. An $N \times N$ Poisson quantum noise image (I_{ij}) is generated with pixel averages equal to $M_{ij}\Phi_0 p^2$.

Wiener spectra were extracted from $n=20$ images for each $\beta(v)$ using the multi-taper method of Wu et al. [12] As another useful parameter to compare model images and mammograms, the average variance of $\{I\}$ was also measured and compared to that measured in Mainprize et al. [8]

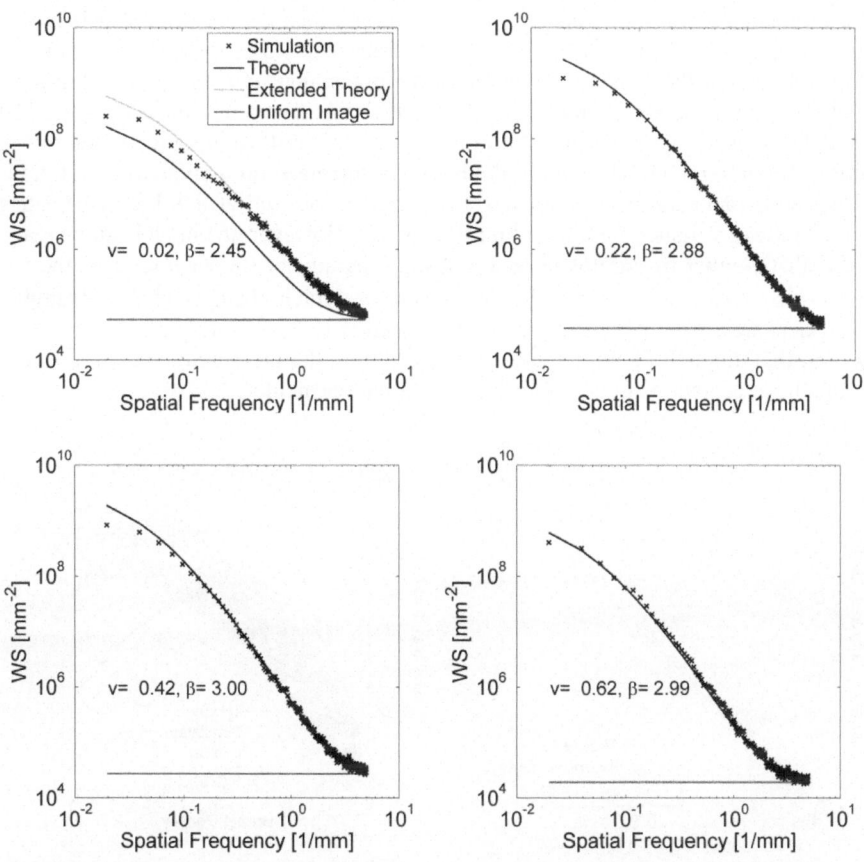

Fig. 2. Examples of simulated and predicted Wiener spectra (Eq. (8)) for anatomic tissue simulated images for clinically relevant breast density and values of β. The heavy dashed curve corresponds to the noise power spectrum of a uniform Poisson noise image through a block with transmission equal to $\langle \bar{m} \rangle$. Gray dashed curves correspond to the model when the expectations for $\langle \bar{m} \rangle$ and $\langle \bar{m}\theta^{a-1} \rangle$ are calculated assuming Gaussian statistics for θ.

3   Results

Wiener spectra predicted via Eq. (8) and simulated as described above are shown for four breast density values, v, in Fig. 2. In all cases, a mean energy of 20 keV, a breast thickness of 5 cm and an incident exposure of 10 mR was used. It was noted that for very small densities $v<0.1$, the simulations deviated from the analytic curve. This is believed to be due to limitations from the approximations of the expectations of Eqs. (9) and (10). If instead, the expectations are calculated numerically by assuming Gaussian probability density functions for θ_F ("extended theory"), the predicted curve yields a much closer match as shown by the dashed curves in Fig. 2. At higher densities, there is little difference between the theoretical curves suggest that the Eqs.

(9) and (10) are reasonable. One important caveat is that the measured breast densities in the simulated images are generally 0.0-0.02 larger than expected for densities less than v=0.5 and 0.0-0.015 smaller for densities larger than 0.5 as shown in Fig. 3(a).

Fig. 3(b) shows the standard deviation of the breast density calculated within individual images for the simulations and compared to that found in clinical images. The shaded region is the approximate 50% confidence interval illustrating the variations in anatomic texture, *i.e.* in the standard deviation, occurring from individual to individual. The model appears to yield greater variance than desired at low breast densities and much lower variance for higher breast densities. However, the model can be made more realistic either by careful selection of the b parameter (larger b reduces the variance) or by changing the input random generator, which changes σ_θ^2. For example, for low densities, the b parameter can be increased to reduce the tissue variance. Note however, that this will likely increase the distortion in the measured mean breast density and the expectations in Eq. (8) must be accurately calculated.

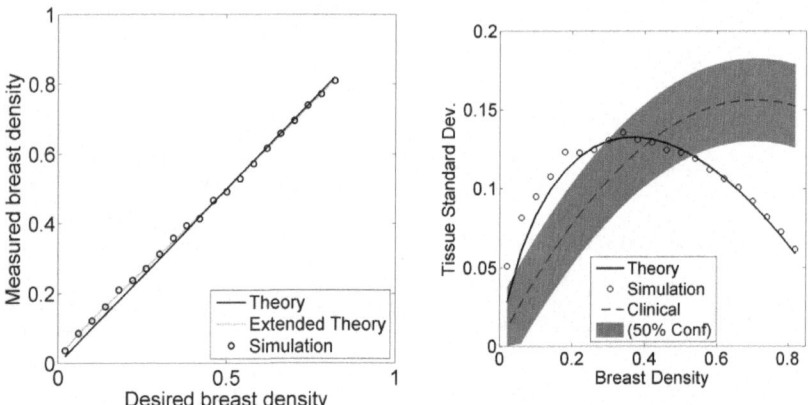

Fig. 3. (a) The measured breast density as a function of the input density for the simulations and model. The extended theory includes the Gaussian approximation for determining the expectation terms in Eq. (8) and shows much better agreement with the simulation results (open circles). (b) The tissue standard deviation from the model and simulation shown in comparsion to the range of breast densities seen in clinical images.

Fig. 4 shows examples of three simulated tissue backgrounds and three mammograms with the corresponding VBD and β. The parameter b was rescaled based on the ratio between the theoretical curve and the clinical data presented in Fig. 3(b). Although a simple inverse power-law model does not capture linear structures in the mammographic images, simulated images do appear to have the granularity or roughness seen in the mammographic textures. Fig. 5 shows the histograms of pixel-by-pixel breast density for both the mammograms and simulated textures for four measurements of breast density and β. Note that v and β are quoted for the whole breast for the mammogram, not just the regions used in Fig. 4 and Fig. 5, causing some discrepancies between the histograms for the mammogram and the simulation.

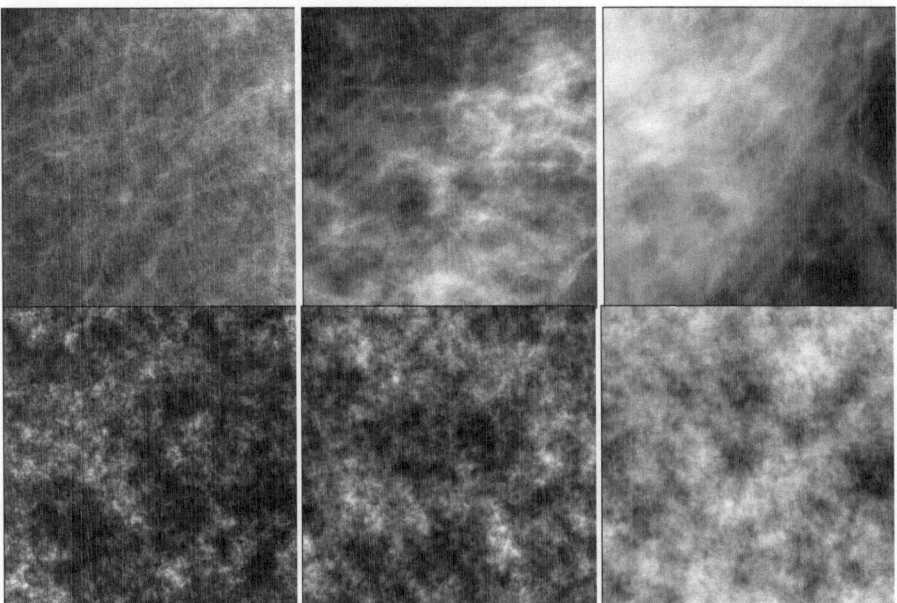

Fig. 4. Examples of real mammographic backgrounds (upper) and corresponding simulated mammographic backgrounds (lower). From left to right, $\beta=\{2.6, 2.96, 3.24\}$ and $\nu=\{0.053, 0.20, 0.53\}$. The grey scale display is set to extend between the maximum and minimum pixel values in each image.

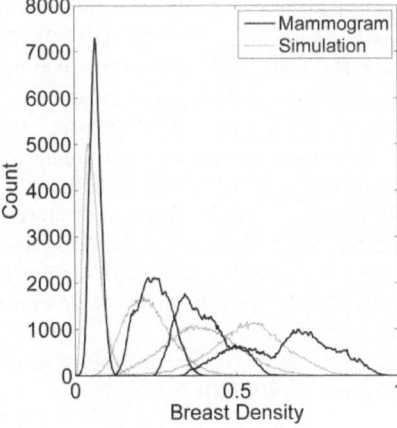

Fig. 5. Histograms of the pixel-by-pixel tissue density estimated from mammograms by Cumulus V and from simulation. From left to right, $\beta=\{2.6, 2.96, 3.2, 3.24\}$ and $\nu=\{0.053, 0.20, 0.35, 0.53\}$.

4   Summary

Using clinically relevant inverse power-law parameters and volumetric breast densities, a mathematical model is used to create simulated mammographic images. Both an analytic form and a simulation algorithm can be used from the model. These models can be adjusted to match image parameters from a clinical population. The approached described here will be extended to task-based observer models for digital mammography and potentially to breast tomosynthesis and CT.

Acknowledgements. This project is funded in part by the Canadian Cancer Society Research Institute. We thank Olivier Alonzo-Proulx and Mei Ge for their expertise in volumetric breast density evaluation.

References

1. Burgess, A.E.: Statistically defined backgrounds: performance of a modified nonprewhitening observer model. J. Opt. Soc. Am. A. 11, 1237–1242 (1994)
2. Burgess, A.E.: On the detection of lesions in mammographic structure. In: Proc. SPIE, vol. 3663, pp. 419–437 (1999)
3. Reiser, I., Nishikawa, R.M.: Task-based assessment of breast tomosynthesis: Effect of acquisition parameters and quantum noise. Med. Phys. 37, 1591–1600 (2010)
4. Park, S., Jennings, R., Liu, H., Badano, A., Myers, K.: A statistical, task-based evaluation method for three-dimensional x-ray breast imaging systems using variable-background phantoms. Med. Phys. 37, 6253 (2010)
5. Bakic, P.R., Albert, M., Brzakovic, D., Maidment, A.D.A.: Mammogram synthesis using a 3D simulation. I. Breast tissue model and image acquisition simulation. Med. Phys. 29, 2131 (2002)
6. Mainprize, J.G., Yaffe, M.J.: Cascaded analysis of signal and noise propagation through a heterogeneous breast model. Med. Phys. 37, 5243–5250 (2010)
7. Burgess, A.E., Jacobson, F.L., Judy, P.F.: Human observer detection experiments with mammograms and power-law noise. Med. Phys. 28, 419–437 (2001)
8. Mainprize, J.G., Tyson, A.H., Yaffe, M.J.: The relationship between anatomic noise and volumetric breast density for digital mammography. Med. Phys. (accepted April 2012)
9. Alonzo-Proulx, O., Packard, N., Boone, J.M., Al-Mayah, A., Brock, K.K., Shen, S.Z., Yaffe, M.J.: Validation of a method for measuring the volumetric breast density from digital mammograms. Phys. Med. Biol. 55, 3027–3044 (2010)
10. Engstrom, E., Reiser, I., Nishikawa, R.: Comparison of power spectra for tomosynthesis projections and reconstructed images. Med. Phys. 36, 1753 (2009)
11. Burgess, A.E.: Mammographic structure: data preparation and spatial statistics analysis. In: Hanson, K.M. (ed.) Medical Imaging 1999: Image Processing. Proc. SPIE, vol. 3661, pp. 642–653. SPIE, San Diego (1999)
12. Wu, G., Mainprize, J.G., Yaffe, M.J.: Spectral analysis of mammographic images using a multitaper method. Med. Phys. 39, 801 (2012)

A Calibration Approach for Single-Energy X-ray Absorptiometry Method to Provide Absolute Breast Tissue Composition Accuracy for the Long Term

Serghei Malkov, Jeff Wang, Fred Duewer, and John A. Shepherd

University of California, San Francisco, Department of Radiology
1Irving Street, AC-109, San Francisco, CA 94141
{Serghei.Malkov,Jeff.Wang2,
Frederick.Duewer,john.shepherd}@ucsf.edu

Abstract. We report on development of a new calibration approach for the Single-Energy X-ray Absorptiometry method (SXA) to provide absolute breast tissue composition accuracy in clinical conditions for the long term and realize cross-calibration between machines, sites and manufacturers.

The proposed method takes into account both geometric and image related factors that impact the calibration of grayscale image into absolute tissue composition. A specially designed phantom (GEN III) is imaged in place of the breast and analyzed as if it were a breast. An automatic algorithm was developed to extract all necessary parameters for recalibration. Subsequently, the thickness correction factors and recalibration procedures were applied during calculations of density.

A breakpoint stepwise approach was used to correct the thickness variations. It provides the thickness measurement variations over time with a typical standard deviation of 0.2-0.3 mm. After recalibration, the recalculated %FGV of the GEN III region of interests are consistent over time, with a typical standard deviation around 1%.

Keywords: full-field digital mammography, volumetric breast density, single x-ray absorptiometry, breast cancer.

1 Introduction

The relationship between high breast tissue density and breast cancer has shown that breast density is one of the strongest predictors of breast cancer risk in women. Current mammography methods, such as scoring methods and mammographic density, estimate areal breast density and are semi-quantitative as well as subjective. Recently, research has focused on automated calibrated volumetric density measures that are both quantitative and accurate. Methods that use an image reference phantom, calibration and model based approaches have been reported. A full review of methodologies was recently published by Yaffe et al [1]. More recently, another calibration approach was developed by Heine et al [2]. MRI and CT can create accurate 3D images of

A.D.A. Maidment, P.R. Bakic, and S. Gavenonis (Eds.): IWDM 2012, LNCS 7361, pp. 769–774, 2012.
© Springer-Verlag Berlin Heidelberg 2012

dense breast volume and have been used to accurately quantify breast density. However, these modalities are generally used for diagnostic imaging because the exams are more expensive and, in the case of CT, expose the patient to higher dose than screening mammography. Thus, there are advantages to measuring breast density in a mammography environment and there is a demand for method with absolute accuracy to serve as a "gold" standard for different approaches. The Single-Energy X-ray Absorptiometry method (SXA) quantifying percentage of fibroglandular tissue volume (%FGV) and absolute fibroglandular dense tissue volume (FGV) has been developed earlier by our group and demonstrated strong breast cancer risk prediction [3, 4]. The method estimates breast density by combining thickness and density measures determined from a calibration phantom present in each image. In contrast to other volumetric calibrated and modeling methods, the accuracy of our approach can be verified using simple phantoms of known compositions, which also allow for cross-calibration between machines, and phantom quality control procedures. These procedures allow us to monitor and recalibrate the SXA outputs when necessary and take into account both geometric and imaging parameter variations of mammography systems in their clinical application. The paper reports recent develops of a new calibration approach for the SXA method in order to provide absolute breast tissue composition accuracy in clinical conditions for the long term and realize cross-calibration between machines, sites and manufactures.

2   Method

Although SXA is stable and reproducible in clinical conditions in a short term of a few months, the accuracy of this method is sensitive to mammography system geometrical changes, service procedures and detector degradation over longer periods of time such as several years. In order to take into account these variations, we modified our calibration method. A specially designed phantom (GEN III) is imaged in place of the breast and analyzed as a breast. It incorporates numerous innovative features to test and monitor mammographic system performance for accurate breast volume and density measures. Features of this approach include the ability to monitor reference grayscale values at several thicknesses and densities, paddle compression height and tilt angle accuracy, as well as to detect major hardware changes such as detector array replacement in order to recalibrate. The GEN III phantom is composed of 9 regions of interest (ROI) covering 0 to 100 %FGV at 2, 4 and 6 cm thicknesses. 14 lead markers embedded in the phantom at specific locations allow for registering the detector array coordinate system to reveal whether a detector array replacement has occurred. Two "bookends" on each side of the density steps offer angled/tapered surfaces to which the mammographic compression paddle conforms to when imaging. This feature allows for the compression paddle height and tilt angle to be explicitly known. 6 metal wires were embedded on the surface and used as markers at known thicknesses. Images of the GEN III phantom were weekly acquired on 22 Hologic Selenia machines at 5 different sites (California Pacific Medical Center, University of California San Francisco, Marin General Hospital, Novato Community Hospital, and University of Vermont) over 2.5 years. The top view of the GEN III and SXA phantom, side view of the GEN III phantom with the paddle compressed to its top surface as during the imaging procedure is presented in Fig. 1, left and right, respectively. An automatic algorithm was developed to extract all necessary parameters for recalibration - converting grayscale into density and correcting thickness map estimation. Subsequently, the thickness correction factors and recalibration procedures were applied during calculations of density. Fig. 2 demonstrates the GEN III x-ray image after processing. The algorithm identifies 6 metal wires at locations with known thicknesses, extracts the thicknesses at their locations and calculates the thicknessses of 9 ROIs. It also locates 8 lead markers, projects lines to find the source point at their intersection and save the values to a database. Next, the calculated and known thicknesses under wires are compared and correction factors are updated relative to the image's acquisition date, if necessary. Then, a standard recalibration procedure using the 9 GEN III ROI attenuation values and the SXA phantom 9 thickness attenuation values is applied to update the database table which captures two calibration parameters (k_{lean} and k_m) described in [3]. Multiple consecutive images of the GEN III phantom were also obtained and analyzed to estimate the paddle compression error.

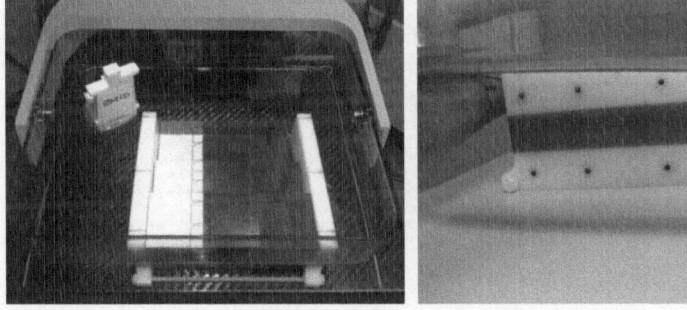

Fig. 1. The top view of the GEN III and the SXA phantom (left), side of the GEN III phantom with the paddle compressed to its top surface

3   Results

To test the paddle compression-decompression variations, 8 consecutive scans of the GEN III phantom were obtained during one day. They demonstrated the %FGV error around 1% due to accumulative deviations of the paddle angles, compression thicknesses, and imaging attenuation. Using the weekly GEN III phantom measurements under the same conditions we validated the thicknesses at 6 locations, paddle angles,

ROI attenuations and %FGV of 9 steps on the phantom. We found significant deviations of thicknesses and ROI attenuation pixel values from the values obtained during initial calibration over the monitored period of time. Time dependence of thickness differences between actual and calculated thicknesses at wire 1 (thickness = 6.26 cm) is shown in Fig. 3 before correction and in Fig. 4 after correction. A break point stepwise approach was used to correct the thickness variations. After correction the thickness errors are characterized by typical standard deviations between 0.2-0.3 mm.

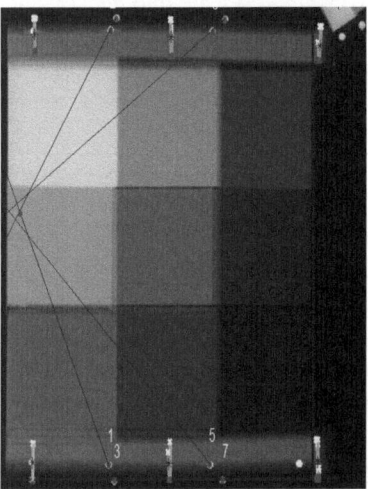

Fig. 2. The GEN III x-ray image after processing. The algorithm identifed 6 metal wires at locations with known thicknesses, 8 lead markers are connected with projected lines to find the source point at their intersection.

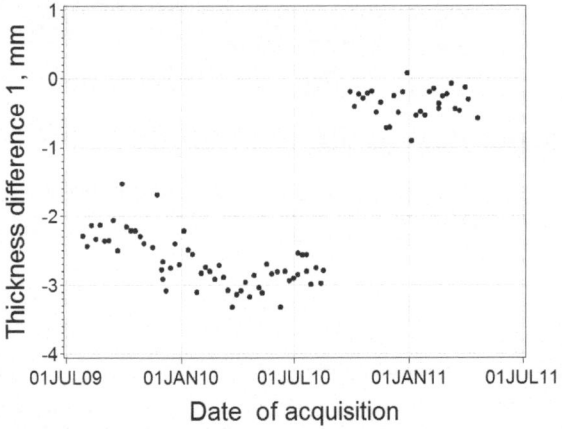

Fig. 3. Time dependence of thickness differences between actual and calculated thicknesses at wire 1 (thickness = 6.26 cm) before correction

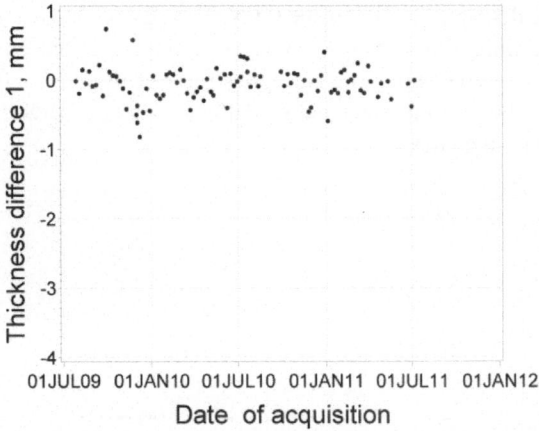

Fig. 4. Time dependence of thickness differences between actual and calculated thicknesses at wire 1 (thickness = 6.26 cm) after correction.

Fig. 5 shows time dependence of ROI attenuation at thickness 6cm. In the case of ROI attenuations, we can observe the periods of continuous changes alongside relatively flat periods. This is apparently due to either continuous degradation of the mammography imaging system performance over time variation or after service procedure changes. Although the SXA phantom looks after small attenuation changes, it is not able to follow significant changes. Thus, mammography imaging system performance and thickness measurement variations give rise to %FGV errors up to 15% To solve this problem weekly recalibration was applied and a new look up table of calibration coefficients generated. Fig. 6 demonstrates calculated %FGV after weekly recalibration of data presented in Fig. 5. It clearly shows efficiency of the chosen

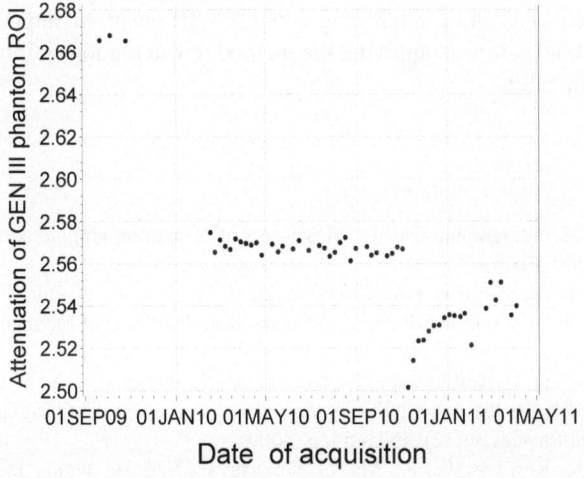

Fig. 5. Time dependence of ROI attenuations at thickness 6cm

approach. The recalculated %FGV of the GEN III ROIs are consistent over time. This recalibration procedure allows us to achieve standard deviations around 1% over the period of 2.5 years. The initial clinical application of the new calibration approach demonstrated significant improvements of data consistency between different mammography machines and sites.

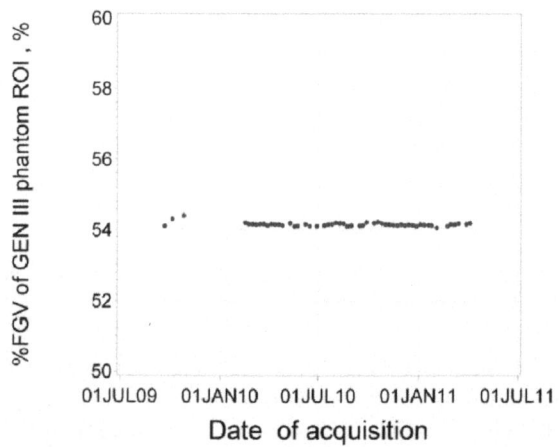

Fig. 6. Time dependence of calculated %FGV after weekly recalibration

4   Conclusions

A new calibration approach for the SXA method has been developed. It provides stable thickness measurements and grayscale to density pixel conversion and different machine cross-calibration. The cross-calibration between sites and machines could be achieved by Quality Control monitoring with GEN III phantom outputs. An extension of this approach is underway applying the method to calculations of breast %FGV and validating it clinically.

References

1. Yaffe, M.J.: Mammographic density. Measurement of mammographic density. Breast Cancer Res. 10, 209 (2008)
2. Heine, J.J., Cao, K., Thomas, J.A.: Effective radiation attenuation calibration for breast density: compression thickness influences and correction. BioMedical Engineering Online 9, 73 (2010)
3. Malkov, S., Wang, J., Kerlikowske, K., Cummings, S., Shepherd, J.A.: Single x-ray absorptiometry method for the quantitative mammographic measure of fibroglandular tissue volume. Medical Physics 36(12), 5525–5536 (2009)
4. Shepherd, J.A., Kerlikowske, K., Ma, L., Duewer, F., Fan, B., Wang, J., Malkov, S., Vittinghoff, E., Cummings, S.R.: Volume of mammographic density and risk of breast cancer. Cancer Epidemiol. Biomarkers Prev. 20(7), 1473–1482 (2011)

Local versus Whole Breast Volumetric Breast Density Assessments and Implications

Baorui Ren, Andrew P. Smith, and Zhenxue Jing

Hologic Inc., 35 Crosby Drive, Bedford, MA 01730 USA
bren@hologic.com

Abstract. Mammographic breast density is very important in the area of cancer risk evaluation, dosimetry and image quality optimization. Many studies have shown that a breast consisting of 50% glandular and 50% adipose tissues is not a representative model of typical breast composition, as the mean volumetric breast density has been found to be less than 20%, much lower than the commonly assumed value of 50/50. In this paper we investigate the characteristics of local breast density distribution of a breast in a large population. We find that the maximum local breast density, calculated from a densest region of a breast, is about 2.3X as high as the mean whole breast density. Therefore the maximum local breast density seems to match the 50/50 model better. Since modern mammography systems employ automatic exposure control (AEC) to ensure acceptable image quality for dense regions of a breast, and since the local breast density over AEC sensor regions often fall into the range of 40% and higher, the 50/50 breast model and physical phantoms should continue to be used in development of x-ray technique and clinical evaluation of mammography systems.

Keywords: volumetric breast density, local breast density, 50/50 model, automatic exposure control, AEC.

1 Background

Mammography density is a reflection of the amount of glandular tissue as opposed to adipose tissue in the breast. It is measured using either area based or volume based methods, with result expressed as percentage breast density. Breast is a highly heterogeneous human organ, often showing significant local density variation in a mammogram. It is commonly expected to have higher breast density values when we perform local breast density analysis with a mammogram. There are papers discussing characteristics of local breast density distributions and their relations to clinical cancer risk [1, 2], but we have not seen studies on technical aspects of local density distributions, e.g., mammography instrument development, dosimetry, and x-ray techniques optimizations. Actually mammographic breast density is an important topic both clinically and technically. Studies [3] have shown that a breast model consisting of 50% glandular and 50% adipose tissues may not be a good representative model of breast composition, as the mean volumetric breast density over large patient population is found to be less than 20%. Therefore there have been

A.D.A. Maidment, P.R. Bakic, and S. Gavenonis (Eds.): IWDM 2012, LNCS 7361, pp. 775–782, 2012.
© Springer-Verlag Berlin Heidelberg 2012

suggestions to reduce the density of mammography model and phantom to better match the density of clinical breast. However in certain applications, the local breast density is a more important consideration than the averaged density over the entire breast. For example, modern mammography systems employ automatic exposure control (AEC), which pre-images the breast with a low dose exposure to identify dense regions in a breast and then determines an x-ray technique accordingly to achieve satisfactory image quality for these dense regions. In practice a very fatty breast could have a very dense region inside and result in a high x-ray exposure by AEC control. To evaluate the clinical performance of a mammography system, the density of phantom should better match the highest local density of a clinical breast instead of the breast density averaged over the entire breast volume.

In this paper, we apply the volumetric breast density (Vbd) method to study the characteristics of local breast density distributes in a breast, and the result will provide guidance in phantom design, x-ray technique development, and clinical evaluation of mammography systems.

2   Methods

We carried out volumetric breast density calculation with 17623 mammograms in this study with a FDA-approved breast density calculation software package – Quantra^{TM}. The software was developed based on physical modeling of mammography system, and can perform volumetric assessment of breast tissue compositions [4]. Quantra can produce a map of glandular tissue thickness at each pixel location, and we then perform regional breast density analysis based on this map with an offline program, in which the computation time is about 10 seconds per image. The pixel size is 70 microns in the original mammogram, and we select a local ROI size of 8.75 x 8.75 mm^2 (125 x 125 pixels, referred as super pixel) and then divide the mammogram into a matrix of super pixels (Fig. 1). The super pixel is selected to be of a square shape for convenience, and mammograms taken with large or small paddles will result to different super pixel matrix sizes. These super pixels are similar to the ROI sizes that an AEC algorithm uses in Selenia and Selenia Dimensions systems. If the AEC's sensor region is too small the exposure technique can be dictated by small dense objects such as calcifications, and if it is too large the exposure is insensitive to local density variations.   In each ROI region, we integrate the total glandular tissue volume and the total breast tissue volume, and the ratio of the two becomes the local Vbd of the region. The software package has a configurable option of either including the skin or excluding the skin in Vbd calculation. In this study the skin content is included in breast density result. This is because we are interested in the impact of local breast density to AEC. The skin contributes to the local density measurement during the AEC process, so the skin effect needs to be considered from the AEC point of view. In general the presence of skin in volumetric breast density calculation only adds an offset to the final breast density result but does not change the underlining physics and clinical cancer risk. Among all super pixels, the one with maximum local Vbd (ML-Vbd) is marked in Fig. 1. We refer the whole breast Vbd as WB-Vbd as against the term of ML-Vbd in discussions. Each mammogram is processed to obtain its WB-Vbd and ML-Vbd, and then the results are analyzed all together or in each category like thickness, age and so on.

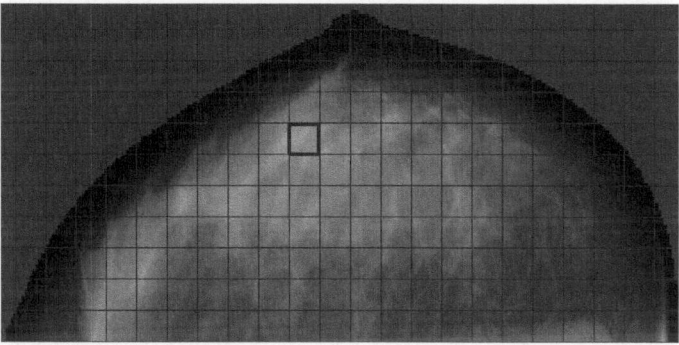

Fig. 1. A mammogram is sub-divided into matrix of super pixels with each element containing 125 x 125 pixels (8.8x8.8 mm^2). Local volumetric breast density (L-Vbd) is calculated within the volume of each super pixel, and the one with maximum local Vbd is marked. The breast has a WB-Vbd of 29% and a ML-Vbd of 67%. The histogram of L-Vbd is given in Fig.2.

3   Results

3.1   Characteristics of the Database

The database consists of 17623 mammograms, with both CC and MLO views. The mean patient age is 53.6 year old (σ=11), with a range from 21 to 96 year old. The mean breast thickness is 5.8 cm (σ=1.4). The mean volumetric breast density Vbd is 17.3% (σ=8.1%).

3.2   Local Breast Density Distribution

The histogram of local Vbd of the case in Fig 1 is given in Fig. 2. The histogram is dominated by large numbers for Vbd less than 5%, which are from these fatty regions. For local Vbd greater than 5%, the height of the Vbd histogram is limited within 10 counts and is scattered approximately uniformly versus the Vbd. The shape of this histogram distribution seems to agree well with the visual appearance of that mammogram, as the glandular tissues are scattered around uniformly inside the breast.

We also change the size of super pixel from 125x125 pixels to other choices like 50x50, 75x75, 150x150 and 200x200, and investigate how the size of super pixel affects the result. The histograms of these choices are shown in Fig.3a-3d. Compared with all five super pixel sizes, the ML-Vbd decreases slightly as the super pixel size is increased, which is straightforward to understand. The larger the size or volume of a super pixel, the more chance the local Vbd is averaged to become smaller in that super pixel. However, the shape of histogram seems to hold consistent, as for Vbd larger than 5%, the histogram tends to be more flat and uniformly spreading out against the horizontal Vbd axis, with the maximum Vbd decreases as pixel size becomes larger. For the rest of analysis in this paper, we fix our choice of super pixel size to be 8.8 x 8.8 mm^2 (125 x 125 pixels) as this size matches to the size of AEC sensor in many clinical mammography systems.

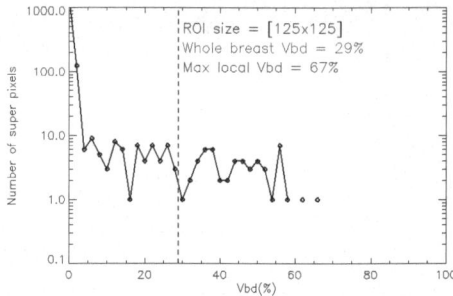

Fig. 2. Histogram of local Vbd of the case in Fig.1. The WB-Vbd is 29%, labeled by the dash line in the plot. The ML-Vbd is 67%. The super pixel size is 125 x125 pixels (8.8 x 8.8 mm).

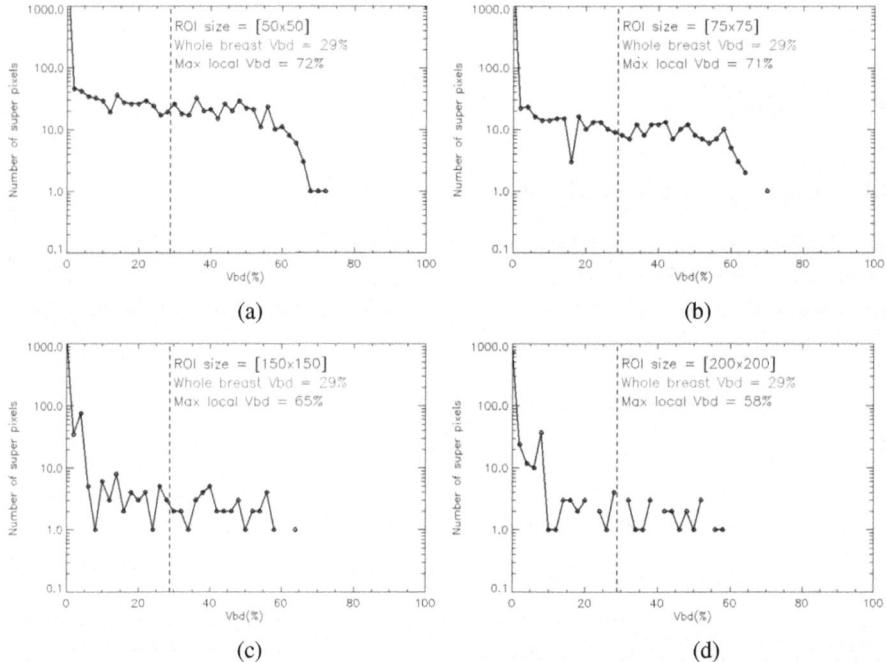

Fig. 3a-3d. Histograms of Vbd versus the size of super pixel, for a) 3.5 x 3.5 mm^2; b) 5.3 x 5.3 mm^2; c) 10.5 x 10.5 mm^2; and d) 14 x 14 mm^2, respectively

3.3   The Distribution of Whole Breast Vbd vs. Maximum Local Vbd

In Fig. 4, histograms of WB-Vbd and ML-Vbd of the entire database are co-plotted. The shape of WB-Vbd is skewed and has a mean Vbd value of 17.3%, and with few breasts exceeding 40% Vbd. However, the maximum local Vbd follows a very different distribution. The ML-Vbd extends all the way up to 100% Vbd, and has a mean Vbd value of 41.3%.

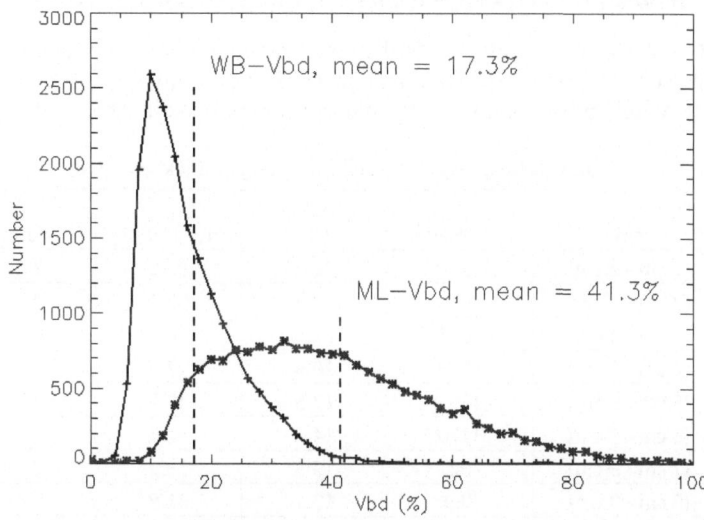

Fig. 4. Histogram of WB-Vbd vs. ML-Vbd from all 17623 mammograms in the study

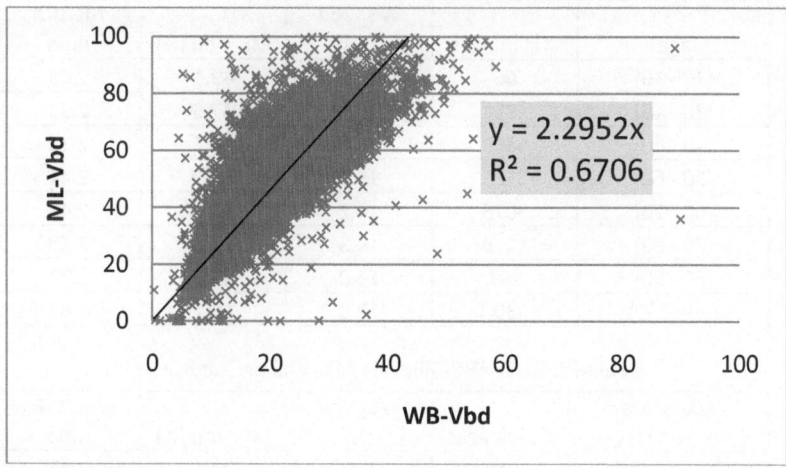

Fig. 5. The scatter plot of WB-Vbd vs. ML-Vbd, and the linear regression with a slope of 2.30

In Fig.5, we show the ML-Vbd versust Wb-Vbd of each mammogram with a scatter plot. The linear regression of the data (passing through the origin of zero) has a slope of 2.30. The ratio of mean WB-Vbd and mean ML-Vbd is 2.39 (=41.3%/17.3%) in the study. In average, ML-Vbd is about 2.3X times as high as WB_Vbd for a breast.

3.4   WB- and ML-Vbd Per Thickness, Age and Abd-Score, View Groups

The WB- and ML-Vbd results are further analyzed in each category against thickness, age, Abd-score (a BIRADS-equivaalent score derived from WB-Vbd, renamed from the "ACR-score" in [5]), and view. Results are summarized in tables 1-4.

Table 1. Mean WB-Vbd and ML-Vbd per thickness group

cm	# of images	WB_Vbd (%)	ML_Vbd (%)	ML/WB ratio
(1 cm - 2 cm]	34	39.6	82.0	2.07
(2 cm - 3 cm]	530	23.7	51.1	2.15
(3 cm - 4 cm]	1676	22.8	50.2	2.20
(4 cm - 5 cm]	3123	20.4	47.6	2.33
(5 cm - 6 cm]	4272	17.5	42.7	2.45
(6 cm - 7 cm]	4470	14.8	37.1	2.50
(7 cm - 8 cm]	2621	13.3	33.2	2.50
(8 cm - 9 cm]	759	13.1	31.8	2.43
(9 cm - 10 cm]	115	14.9	35.1	2.36

Table 2. Mean WB-Vbd and ML-Vbd per age group

age	# of images	WB_Vbd (%)	ML_Vbd (%)	ML/WB ratio
(20 - 30]	66	24.2	49.1	2.03
(30 - 40]	1754	20.5	47.3	2.30
(40 - 50]	5830	19.8	45.8	2.31
(50 - 60]	5485	15.9	38.7	2.44
(60 - 70]	3078	14.2	35.1	2.48
(70 - 80]	1128	14.3	37.1	2.59
(80 - 90]	247	16.0	43.7	2.73
(90 - 100]	30	18.0	48.1	2.67

Table 3. Mean WB-Vbd and ML-Vbd per Abd-score

Abd-score (WB_Vbd range)	# of images	WB_Vbd (%)	ML_Vbd (%)	ML/WB ratio
1: (0% - 11.9%)	5070	9.8	24.1	2.45
2: (11.9% - 20.2%)	7553	15.6	39.9	2.56
3: (20.2% - 35%)	4478	25.6	58.3	2.28
4: (35% - 100%)	519	42.0	82.2	1.96

Table 4. Mean WB-Vbd and ML-Vbd per view

View	# of images	WB_Vbd (%)	ML_Vbd (%)	ML/WB ratio
R_MLO	4377	17.3	41.5	2.40
R_CC	4407	17.2	41.1	2.38
L_MLO	4339	17.3	41.5	2.40
L_CC	4500	17.2	41.0	2.39

4   Discussion

The analysis of local Vbd in our study confirms a common expectation that the maximum local Vbd is much higher than the whole breast Vbd. The exact value of the ratio depends on the size of ROI used in the analysis. A smaller ROI will have a slightly higher ratio while a large ROI will lead to a slightly lower ratio. Based on the patient population in this study, the ML-Vbd is likely to be about a factor of two or higher than the WB-Vbd in general.

From histograms in Fig.4, while it is rare to see a clinical breast with a WB-Vbd larger than 40%, it is quite common to find the ML-Vbd of a breast larger than 50%. This finding could have important practical implication. Modern mammography systems all employ some kinds of automatic exposure control to optimize x-ray exposure for different breasts. In particular, the AEC ensures that the densest portion of breast achieves satisfactory image quality in the mammogram. A breast may appear very low in whole breast density but the x-ray technique and the patient dose can be still high as they are actually set by densest portion of the breast. Therefore local breast density is more important than the whole breast density in AEC control.

Recent developments in breast density study have brought in consent that the average breast density is generally below 20%, much lower than the 50/50 reference that were widely adopted in x-ray dosimetry and phantom study in the past. There have been proposals that breast imaging dose should be lowered accordingly to match that well-agreed low value of Vbd; some suggestions also propose that image quality evaluation should be done with a fattier phantom instead of the 50/50 ACR phantom. So there are two questions related to breast density here: what density should be used to do dose calculation and what density phantom should be used to evaluate a mammography system? In mammography the mean glandular dose (MGD) is calculated by the product of entrance surface exposure (ESE) and the dose conversion DgN factor as $MGD = ESE \times DgN$. Breast density affects both terms here. For uniform phantom, both DgN and ESE are set by the mean density (WB-Vbd). For heterogeneous breast, DgN is set by WB-Vbd, and the ESE is set the densest part of the breast (ML-Vbd) through AEC. In table 5, we give typical ratios to do a quantitative comparison for 4.2 cm thickness phantoms and breast. AEC maintains constant detector count under AEC sensor so ESE is lower for the 20% density phantom. From table 5, if one uses a fatty 20% density phantom to evaluate the AEC of a system, the x-ray exposure could be off by 25% in comparison with the clinical scenario that a breast with the same WB-Vbd is imaged.

Table 5. AEC dose comparison of 20% and 50% density 4.2 cm thick phantom

	phantom 20%	phantom 50%	breast with WB-Vbd=20%, ML-Vbd=50%
DgN	1.12x	1	1.12X
ESE	0.75X	1	1
AEC dose	0.84X	1	1.12X

According to the finding in this study, when we consider breast as a heterogeneous organ with large local density variation, the x-ray imaging dose will be dictated by the maximum local density that is at least 2X as high as its WB-Vbd. Since the mean ML-Vbd is usually around 40% or higher, the 50/50 based mammography phantom should continue to be used to evaluate AEC dose and clinical image quality.

In Tables 1-4, WB- and ML-Vbd results are evaluated against thickness, age, Abd-score and view. We find that breast density drops as thickness, age and Abd-score go up. Abd-score serves as the BIRADS-equivalent score for a patient, which is derived from the Wb-Vbd result of the patient. The result also does not depend on whether it is the CC or MLO view, and the left or right breast. In particular, our results of ML-Vbd of thickness group can be used as breast density reference for each thickness in dose calculation and system evaluation.

5   Conclusion

In this paper, we describe our study on the assessment of local breast density distribution in a mammogram. First, we confirm the general expectation that local breast density can be much higher than the whole breast density; and we further quantify our result that the ML-Vbd is about a factor of two or higher than the WB-Vbd. Second, we find the distribution of ML-Vbd spreads out nicely toward the upper limit of 100% breast density, unlike the distribution of WB-Vbd that is highly skewed towards a low value. While mean value of WB-Vbd in the study is only17.3%, the mean value of ML-Vbd is found to be as high as 41.3%. Therefore there are significant numbers of breast with ML-Vbd beyond the 50% reference clinically. Our results suggest that while in certain dosimetry applications, the reference value of breast composition needs to be set low to match the WB-Vbd value, in AEC related dose and image quality applications, the 50% reference and the 50/50 based physical phantom should continue to be used as they match the ML-Vbd of a breast well, which can better simulate the dense region of a breast to generate relevant x-ray technique and image quality during testing.

References

[1] Malkov, S., Ma, L., Kerlikowske, K., Wang, J., Cummings, S., Shepherd, J.: Comparison of Subregional Breast Density with Whole Breast Density. In: Martí, J., Oliver, A., Freixenet, J., Martí, R. (eds.) IWDM 2010. LNCS, vol. 6136, pp. 402–407. Springer, Heidelberg (2010)

[2] Pinto Pereira, S.M., et al.: The spatial distribution of radiodense breast tissue: a longitudinal study. Breast Cancer Res. 11(3), R33 (2009)

[3] Yaffe, M.J., et al.: The Myth of the 50-50 breast. Med. Phys. 36, 5437–5443 (2009)

[4] Hartman, K., Highnam, R.P., Warren, R., Jackson, V.: Volumetric Assessment of Breast Tissue Composition from FFDM Images. In: Krupinski, E.A. (ed.) IWDM 2008. LNCS, vol. 5116, pp. 33–39. Springer, Heidelberg (2008)

[5] Ren, B., Smith, A.P., Marshall, J.: Investigation of Practical Scoring Methods for Breast Density. In: Martí, J., Oliver, A., Freixenet, J., Martí, R. (eds.) IWDM 2010. LNCS, vol. 6136, pp. 651–658. Springer, Heidelberg (2010)

Author Index